# Nutrition and Health

**Series Editors**

Adrianne Bendich
Wellington, FL, USA

Connie W. Bales
Durham VA Medical Center
Duke University School of Medicine
Durham, NC, USA

The Nutrition and Health series has an overriding mission in providing health professionals with texts that are considered essential since each is edited by the leading researchers in their respective fields. Each volume includes: 1) a synthesis of the state of the science, 2) timely, in-depth reviews, 3) extensive, up-to-date fully annotated reference lists, 4) a detailed index, 5) relevant tables and figures, 6) identification of paradigm shifts and consequences, 7) virtually no overlap of information between chapters, but targeted, inter-chapter referrals, 8) suggestions of areas for future research and 9) balanced, data driven answers to patient/health professionals questions which are based upon the totality of evidence rather than the findings of a single study.

Nutrition and Health is a major resource of relevant, clinically based nutrition volumes for the professional that serve as a reliable source of data-driven reviews and practice guidelines.

More information about this series at http://www.springer.com/series/7659

Debbie L. Humphries
Marilyn E. Scott • Sten H. Vermund
Editors

# Nutrition and Infectious Diseases

## Shifting the Clinical Paradigm

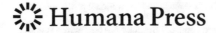 Humana Press

*Editors*
Debbie L. Humphries
Yale School of Public Health
Yale University
New Haven, CT
USA

Marilyn E. Scott
Institute of Parasitology
McGill University
Ste-Anne de Bellevue, QC
Canada

Sten H. Vermund
Yale School of Public Health
Yale University
New Haven, CT
USA

Nutrition and Health
ISBN 978-3-030-56915-0        ISBN 978-3-030-56913-6   (eBook)
https://doi.org/10.1007/978-3-030-56913-6

This Humana imprint is published by the registered company Springer Nature Switzerland AG
The registered company address is: Gewerbestrasse 11, 6330 Cham, Switzerland

# Foreword

The year 2019 marks the 50th anniversary of the World Health Organization monograph titled *Interactions of Nutrition and Infection* by the late Nevin Scrimshaw, Carl Taylor, and John Gordon. This groundbreaking work by three pioneers of public health was the first scientific compilation to describe the synergistic relationship between an individual's nutritional state and risk of infectious diseases in the context of the high burden of under-five child mortality prevalent in those days. This relationship became widely known and described as the "vicious cycle of malnutrition and infection" that underpinned the high mortality rates among children, especially in low-resource settings. These concepts and research done in this area are as salient today as they were 50 years ago; nearly half of all global child deaths attributed to infectious syndromes such as pneumonia and diarrhea have underlying undernutrition. Additionally, undernourished children also experience increased severity and frequency of infections and slow recovery, causing irrevocable long-term impact. At the Bill & Melinda Gates Foundation, dedicated to the maxim that all individuals have an equal opportunity to lead a healthy and productive life, our mission and work in maternal, newborn, and child health (MNCH) embodies understanding and addressing the close synergistic link between undernutrition and infection. Our approach is evidence-based in the recognition that the vulnerability that marks being undernourished and micronutrient deficient can exponentially increase the risk of death due to an infection in populations living in low-income settings. For example, data from a study we supported found undernutrition to be one of the most powerful risk factors, increasing the risk of pneumonia mortality by more than fivefold.

Improvements in maternal, newborn, and child survival are among the most significant achievements in global health during the twenty-first century. Under-five child deaths have declined from 12.5 million in 1990 to 5.4 million per year in 2017. Yet, 149 million children under 5 are estimated to be stunted, 58 million experience wasting annually, 20.5 million are born low-birth weight, and 240 million women of reproductive age are undernourished (low BMI). Additionally, micronutrient deficiencies are common and multiple ones coexist in over a billion if not up to 2 billion people. Understanding the epidemiologic, biologic, molecular, and cellular mechanisms by which undernutrition can exacerbate both the occurrence of and survival from infectious disease is key, as is the role of infectious morbidity in preventing optimal growth and development.

As public health researchers who hail from two high-disease burden countries in South Asia, having spent years studying and clinically observing undernutrition and infection coexist to exacerbate risk of mortality, we are excited that these conditions are again being comprehensively reviewed. Over the past few decades, numerous advances have been made in our understanding of the field of nutrition and infection, spanning from unravelling the important linkages between infections and specific micronutrients to recognizing the emerging role of inflammation in linear growth failure (pre- and postnatal) and poor neurodevelopment. This book covers a vast array of topics with deep expositions into links between nutrition and a range of bacterial, viral, protozoan, and helminth infections and their health implications. Also, appropriately, it addresses these issues taking into account the current context of a world experiencing a nutrition and demographic transition leading to more noncommunicable diseases and obesity, even while climate change challenges our global food systems and causes an emergence or resurgence of infectious diseases and epidemics.

Undernutrition and infectious diseases disproportionately impact the under-resourced populations of the world, and the imperative for accelerated progress toward achieving the sustainable development goals will only be fulfilled with a combined focus on the areas of health and nutrition. This well-written book and its state-of-the art compilation of a breadth of topics contributed by global experts provides its readership a closer and deeper understanding of the connection between nutrition and infectious diseases and the significant implications of that connection for addressing important challenges facing clinical and public health practice in the twenty-first century.

Parul Christian
Department of International Health, Program in Human Nutrition
The Johns Hopkins Bloomberg School of Public Health
Baltimore, MD, USA

Anita Zaidi
Department of Global Health
Bill and Melinda Gates Foundation,
Seattle, WA, USA

# Preface

Undernutrition is estimated to affect over 800 million individuals, or more than one in ten persons on Earth [1]. This number includes those who are undernourished based on anthropometric measurements and those for whom at least one nutrient deficiency has been diagnosed. Though less well documented, many of these individuals likely have been diagnosed with multiple macronutrient and/or micronutrient deficiencies, and many others may have suboptimal health attributable to nutritional deficiencies that have not been diagnosed. The combined prevalence of overweight and obesity, currently estimated to affect over half of adults worldwide [2], was recognized as a global crisis in 2000 with the publication of the World Health Organization (WHO) Technical Report on preventing and managing obesity [3]. Key to the recognition of the crisis was a growing awareness of the contribution of obesity and overweight to a variety of noninfectious diseases including heart disease and type-2 diabetes [4, 5]. While estimates of excess nutrition are most commonly based on overweight and obesity, the importance of considering micronutrient status as a U-shaped curve, with negative health impacts at both low and high levels of intake, is increasingly recognized [6, 7]. The magnitude of both undernutrition and overnutrition is emphasized by data indicating that, among 5–19-year-old children and adolescents in 2016, 192 million (range 114–295) were moderately or severely underweight while 124 million (range 53–214) were obese [8]. Yet nutrition is often neglected within medical schools and clinics as a critical variable influencing human health [9–11] including outcomes of infectious diseases.

Statistics for infectious diseases are even more dramatic than those for malnutrition. For example, it is estimated that, in 2016, diarrhea was the eighth leading cause of death overall, and the fifth leading cause of death in children under five [12], that 3–5 million are infected with influenza annually, that there were 219 million cases of malaria and 435,000 deaths in 2017 [13], and that 1.5–2 billion people are infected with helminth parasites [14]. Despite high rates of infectious diseases, such infections are often overlooked as contributors to, or consequences of, malnutrition. This is most recently and dramatically evident in the vast impacts of the COVID-19 pandemic on food production, distribution, and affordability [15–22].

A 1968 World Health Organization (WHO) monograph by Scrimshaw, Gordon and Taylor highlighted the intersections between nutrition and infectious disease [23]. Built on a much shorter review published 9 years earlier [24], the 1968 monograph described the conceptual pathways of influence between nutrition and infectious disease and provided an in-depth analysis of associations between diarrhea and nutrition in India and Guatemala [23]. Through this monograph, Scrimshaw and colleagues were among the first to comprehensively describe both synergistic and antagonistic relationships between malnutrition and infection, noting that malnutrition was sometimes associated with increased infection severity and other times with decreased severity of infection [23]. Their monograph represented a critical synthesis the state of knowledge at that time derived from some 900+ references. This key conceptual document addressed interactions between nutrition and infection, highlighted the impacts of malnutrition on immune responses to pathogens, emphasized the reliance of pathogens on the host for their nutrients, and cited the energetic costs imposed on the host by infections.

Now, over 50 years later, our knowledge base has expanded dramatically. Many concepts described by Scrimshaw and colleagues have been further substantiated, underlying mechanisms have been clarified, breadth of examples have expanded, and range of possible points of interface between nutrition and infection have emerged. Our book thus provides a follow-up to the 1968 WHO monograph [23] by exploring what is currently known, and not known, about how malnutrition influences infectious diseases. To this end, we have brought together a diverse group of specialists who are intrigued by broader concepts. We have challenged authors to think "outside the box," to consider questions that may not have previously occurred to them, and to dig into the literature to see what insights might exist. We have also asked authors to frame their remarks in a way that can be understood by nonspecialists. In this way, we hope that the chapters will be accessible to the nonexpert and provocative for the specialist.

The book is structured into four parts. Part I lays out a conceptual framework for the book and introduces nonspecialists to key concepts in nutrition and immunology. Part II provides primers on the four traditional types of pathogens, viruses, bacteria, protozoans, and helminths. Part III addresses nutrition issues in several major diseases and conditions. Part IV addresses cross-cutting topics.

## Part I: The Foundations of the Nutrition-Infection Nexus

This section begins with a conceptual model linking nutritional status and infectious diseases, followed by primers on nutrition and immune function that can serve as resources for students, researchers, and practitioners.

Chapter 1 presents the linkage framework for nutritional status and infectious disease and explores the theory of causation in the context of nutrition-infection interactions [25]. Authors Humphries, Scott, and Vermund highlight the biological, physiological, and social determinants of both malnutrition and infection such that they represent a clinical and public health syndemic. More vulnerable populations (age, sex, immunosuppression, food insecure, unhygienic environment) are both more likely to have compromised nutritional status and increased exposure to infectious agents. The conceptual framework considers the effect of host nutrition on pathogen exposure, on the pathogen's ability to break through natural host barriers and reach its target tissues, and on its ability to replicate and be transmitted to others. Whether infection can be self-cured via immune responses will depend upon how severe and immunogenic the infection is and whether the immune response is effective in limiting the infection or leads to immunopathology. When treated with antibiotics, antivirals, antifungals, or anthelmintics, the effectiveness of drug interventions can be altered by intake of specific foods and/or underlying nutritional status (Chap. 1) [25]. Authors of all subsequent chapters were encouraged to allow this conceptual framework to shape how they approached their individual chapters.

In Chap. 2, Barffour and Humphries examine human nutritional needs in the context of metabolism and physiology, as well as their influences on infections [26]. The chapter highlights evidence that immune responses relevant to infectious disease outcomes are altered by macro- and micronutrient deficiencies and supplementation, while noting the gaps in our current grasp of the origin and underpinning of these interactions. As a background to clinical needs and complexities, the authors review the specific macronutrients (carbohydrates, proteins, fats) and micronutrients (vitamins and minerals) that have metabolic relevance to infection-mediated disease states and attendant immune responses. The chapter serves as a pithy nutritional primer to give context to the rest of the book.

Chapter 3 provides an invaluable "short course" on how the immune response to infection combines with various states of malnutrition to alter clinical outcomes [27]. Stephensen highlights how mammalian immune systems have evolved to respond to specific infectious challenges with innate effector mechanisms that can clear such infections without harming those microbes in the oral and digestive tract microbiome that are essential for health. When innate responses do not clear infections, the adaptive immune system generates pathogen-specific immunity to clear the initial infection and prevent further infections. A vigorous immune system depends on energy supplied by diet, thus the immune response of nutritionally marginal persons may not be optimum. With severe, chronic, or repeated infections, the nutritional status of even a previously normal host can be compromised through damage of host tissues, suboptimal food intake or tolerance, malabsorption and nutrient loss, higher metabolic demands for nutrients, and perturbed nutrient transport or storage. That malnutrition compromises host immune defenses is a fundamental underpinning of risk of increased virulence of organisms and pathogenicity of infections [28].

## Part II: Types of Infectious Diseases and Influences of Nutrition

This section provides accessible overviews of major categories of pathogens and is intended to be used as antecedents of pathogen-focused subsequent chapters, as well as to serve as discrete educational resources for students, researchers, and practitioners.

In Chap. 4, Berkley examines the specific elements of bacterial infections vis-à-vis nutritional status [29]. The human microbiome is dominated by bacteria that can be beneficial or neutral or harmful, depending upon the mutual adaptation and coevolution of the human host and its diverse array of bacteria. How host nutritional status and selected specific nutrients affect bacterial colonization, invasion, severity, chronicity, as well as recovery or mortality from bacterial infections is placed into context of undernutrition is a principal chapter focus. Of further clinical relevance are the impact of undernutrition on vaccine responses and the efficacy of antimicrobial drugs. Malnutrition in children is highlighted since they experience the greatest burden and mortality risk, in large part due to their metabolic needs for growth, immaturity of the early immune system, and lack of memory immune responses when prior bacterial challenge has not yet been experienced. Perturbations of the commensal bacteria in the gastrointestinal tract are highlighted, particularly their effect on child growth and development.

Chapter 5 is of special interest now as the COVID-19 pandemic rages across the world. This chapter, containing over 250 relevant references, reviews basic virology, several well known viruses including measles, herpes, Ebola, HIV and provides a number of up-to-date references with regard to the data concerning COVID-19 and obesity available in September, 2020. The chapter concentrates on the complex interactions between influenza virus infection, nutritional status and specific nutrient deficiencies. The chapter reviews the cycle of viral replication and causes of infectivity as well as the annual development of flu vaccines. The data clearly indicate that poor nutritional status is a strong risk factor for viral infections and that infection severity as well as robust response to vaccination are dependent upon nutritional adequacy especially in young children. There is an in-depth discussion of the "triple burden of malnutrition" in resource poor nations where undernutrition, essential micronutrient deficiencies and obesity are seen in the population. There is a bidirectional interaction between viral infection and nutritional status; of interest, undernutrition of key micronutrients can foster virus mutation that then reduces the efficacy of vaccines. Also, obesity has been shown to independently and significantly increase morbidity and mortality from H1N1 infection. There is a detailed review of the roles of vitamins A and D in the maintenance of epithelial tissue integrity and thus the essentiality in reducing the risk of lung epithelial viral infections including influenza. Vitamin E and C's unique roles in enhancing immune responses and affecting the flu virus directly are reviewed. Minerals associated with enhancing the immune system and/or affecting the virulence of viruses are reviewed. Additionally, there is a discussion of the different life stages, immune function and nutritional status.

In Chap. 6, Wiser presents both a primer on protozoan parasites and background on how nutrition and protozoan parasites interact [35]. These eukaryotic microbes may infect the gastrointestinal track via ingestion and cause diarrheal disease, as seen for *Entamoeba histolytica*, *Giardia* spp., and *Cryptosporidium* spp. These can decrease nutritional absorption when they are found in high numbers, exacerbating the problem of childhood undernutrition in resource-limited settings with food insecure families. A second transmission route of protozoans is via an insect vector, such as transmission of malaria by mosquitoes. Malaria is the most common and lethal protozoan infection, particularly in children in Africa. The association of malaria and hypoglycemia and acidosis can be especially dangerous to children. The association of nutrition with other important parasitic protozoans such as trichomoniasis, African trypanosomiasis, Chagas disease, leishmaniasis, and toxoplasmosis is less clear, but the weight of evidence suggests the suboptimal anti-protozoal immune responses that are associated with undernutrition will exacerbate disease pathogenesis.

Chapter 7 presents the interface of nutrition and helminth infections [36]. Geary and Haque remind us that parasitic helminths in the phyla Nematoda and Platyhelminthes have coevolved with humans for millennia. While once ubiquitous in human populations, helminths are now far more likely to occur in the 1.5–2 billion residents of tropical regions that experience limited sanitation and public health infrastructures. The chronic nature of helminth infections together with high parasite burden contributes to greater pathogenicity and adverse clinical outcomes including impaired growth and development and potential cognitive deficits. The long-lasting immunity typical of viral and bacterial infections is elusive for helminths; hence, reinfection is common. Thus, although mass drug administration is an anchor of control campaigns, the direct benefit is short term. More work on the effectiveness of anthelmintic drugs and the population dynamics of transmission in the face of mass drug administration is needed [37, 38]. A syndemic of helminth parasites, malnutrition, and coinfections is linked to poverty and suboptimal potable water and food hygiene, poor disposal of human waste, and suboptimal public health and medical care infrastructures.

## Part III: Nutrition Issues During Major Infections: Case Studies of Nutrition and Infectious Disease

Part III includes five in-depth case studies on specific infectious diseases where nutrition-infection interactions have been extensively explored: diarrheal and enteric disease, HIV and tuberculosis, arboviruses, malaria, and soil-transmitted helminths. A case study on influenza is included in the virology primer (Chap. 5) [30].

Chapter 8 addresses one of the most compelling interactions in global child health, namely nutrition and intestinal pathogens causing diarrheal diseases [39]. Authors Siddiqui, Belayneh, and Bhutta focus on low- and middle-income countries and the role of protein-calorie and micronutrient deficiencies in exacerbating the risk of exposure to pathogens in high-risk communities and institutional environments like hospitals or clinics. Nutritional deficiencies diminish the effectiveness of immune mechanisms, compromising the ability of the child to block pathogen entry and mount an effective immune response. The diminished capacity of an undernourished host to maintain an effective gut mucosal barrier leads to accelerated pathogenicity with more severe clinical consequences. Treatments may be less effective in undernourished compared to well-nourished children. Antibiotics are effective in reducing bacterial burdens but may also disrupt the gut microbiome and its inherent protective capacities. Rare instances when malnutrition may reduce the pathogenicity of gut pathogens are highlighted, notably that the risk of amoebic infection declines with host iron deficiency. Nutritional deficiencies and gut bacterial perturbations that reduce effective host immune responses have been posited for decades as a reason that eradication of global polio virus type 1, an enteric infection, has been hard to achieve [40, 41].

Chapter 9 presents the specific nutritional issues inherent in single and concurrent human immunodeficiency virus (HIV) and tuberculosis (TB) infections [42]. Authors Baum, Tamargo, and Wanke highlight the nutritional compromises in resource-limited settings and among individuals who have advanced, untreated HIV or TB disease. Individuals who are malnourished have an increased risk of infection and those infected with HIV or TB are likely to develop nutritional abnormalities. Throughout the history of HIV and TB, nutritional issues have been prominent. TB was termed consumption, indicating the devastating nutritional impact of terminal disease. TB was also more common in the poor with compromised diets. In the more modern era of HIV infection, wasting syndrome has been a common primary manifestation and selected antiretroviral drugs like protease inhibitors have been associated with lipodystrophies. The advent of antiretroviral therapy (ART) with fewer side effects has allowed people in higher income settings to live with HIV, but now they cope with overweight and/or metabolic abnormalities. The TB/HIV example highlights the challenge of teasing apart cause and effect in assessing nutrition and infection interactions [43].

Chapter 10 highlights the special circumstances whereby nutrition interacts with arthropod-borne viral interactions, known as arboviruses [44]. Villamor and Villar highlight potential role of host nutritional in arboviral disease risks and outcomes, especially dengue. Risk of exposure to infectious insect bites can be increased or decreased by selected diets. Nutrition can alter the robustness of immune/inflammatory responses against viral infection. In turn, arboviral infections can increase metabolic demands and diminish host appetite, thus altering host nutritional status. Pediatric obesity has been associated with an increased risk of adverse dengue-related outcomes, although causality is uncertain. Dengue severity may be altered with low levels of specific fatty acids and amino acids, vitamin D, and some minerals, though it is possible that nutritional deficiencies were caused by severe dengue infection itself. Interventions with vitamin E and zinc in patients with dengue fever show promise to limit disease severity. For Chikungunya virus, overweight and obesity in pregnancy have been associated with increased seropositivity, but again, directionality of the association is unknown. An important frontier is the nature of nutrition and Zika virus interactions.

Chapter 11 presents the complexities of nutrition and malaria interactions [45]. Authors Kim, Goheen, and Bei highlight the huge dual burden of malaria and undernutrition, particularly among children and pregnant women in Sub-Saharan Africa. Public health interventions and surveillance methods remain imperfect, as the range, extent, and magnitude of interactions between the two diseases remain unclear. While there are many antecedents to both malaria and malnutrition, they are largely interrelated. A systems biology approach that considers the influences of both malnutrition and malaria simultaneously will allow us to move beyond a "single disease, single solution" strategy possibility to design more effective, targeted, and integrated interventions in areas where both conditions co-occur.

Chapter 12 considers associations between nutrition and soil-transmitted helminths (STHs), the most common human parasites [46]. Scott and Koski explore epidemiological and experimental evidence that diet and nutritional status influence the risk of exposure to infective stages, and the ability of larval stages to cross tissue barriers, mature, and reproduce. They examine how specific macronutrients and micronutrients affect the innate and adaptive immunity to STHs, and the consequences of nutrient deficiencies for STH-induced pathology. STH-driven anti-inflammatory responses may down-modulate the severity of chronic nutrition-related diseases. Evidence that nutritional interventions reduce STH infection and that deworming improves nutritional status is reviewed. A complex context exists for interactions among coexisting infections, coexisting nutrient deficiencies, and the micro-biome [47].

## Part IV: Integration of Cross-Cutting Issues in Nutrition/ Infection Interactions

Section Four considers cross-cutting issues that affect the intersection of nutrition and infectious disease, including nutrition and drug interactions, coinfections that coexist with multiple forms of malnutrition, and the impact of climate change in the context of nutrition and infectious disease. Part IV ends by consolidating relevant clinical and public health approaches to addressing infection in the context of nutrition, and thus providing a sharp focus on the clinical relevance of the intersection between nutrition and infection.

Chapter 13 is a detailed review of drug interactions with nutritional factors in infectious diseases [48]. Author Boullata highlights the many interactions between drugs and nutrition that can affect health outcomes. He details routes of influence and categorizes subtypes of drug-nutrition interactions based on inherent properties of the drugs, nutrients or food matrix, and similarities in physiologic disposition. For each, he delineates pharmaceutical, pharmacokinetic, and pharmacodynamic interactions. After providing a framework for classifying drug-nutrition interactions and their clinical relevance and mechanistic structures, he illustrates various types of drug-nutrition interactions using examples of available antimicrobial agents. This chapter illuminates the complexity and clinical importance that emerges from intentional consideration of nutrition and pharmaceutical interactions.

Chapter 14 seeks an integrated ecological and epidemiological perspective of coinfection and nutrition [49]. Author Ezenwa notes that concurrent infection (or coinfection) is the norm rather than the exception in real-world populations. Likewise, nutritional deficiencies are also common and coinfection and multiple nutritional deficiencies frequently co-occur in the same populations. Despite the coincidence of these two phenomena, however, only a small fraction of studies on infection and malnutrition address the issue of coinfection or co-deficiency. This chapter explores whether applying an ecological framework that accounts for feeding or "trophic" relationships between species can help advance our understanding of how nutrition affects coinfection (e.g., helminths and tuberculosis), and reciprocally, how coinfection affects nutrition (e.g., helminths and malaria). Applying a trophic approach to studying coinfection and nutrition involves specific methods that can be incorporated into epidemiological studies.

Chapter 15 addresses an urgent modern crisis, namely the pathways inherent in global warming and other climate change that intersect with future nutrition and infection risks [50]. Rocklöv, Ahlm, Scott, and Humphries use the twenty-first-century climate change projections to illustrate the inevitable effects on both nutrition and infection. Based on a systems perspective that incorporates past global health and climate associations and that uses scenario-based assessment and model results, they conclude that action on all three challenges (climate change, malnutrition, and infectious diseases) is time-critical. Understanding already observed and projected impacts requires a multidisciplinary approach, including agriculture, grazing behavior, human migration, medical entomology, hydrology, oceanography/limnology and fisheries, and many other themes. The interface of climate change, undernutrition, and infections are intertwined within the United Nations 2030 Sustainable Development Goals.

Chapter 16 synthesizes the implications for public health and clinical practitioners as they address issues of public health and infection. Vermund, Scott, and Humphries extract the clinical implications of the previous chapters, highlighting the clinical and public health relevance of nutritional status for infectious disease prevention, diagnostics, and treatment [51]. They review the causal paradigm for infection and nutrition and highlight the 1968 WHO monograph just after its half-century anniversary.

Thanks to new tools in biological and social sciences, understanding of the complex roots of global nutritional status is growing rapidly. The synergies resulting from changing diets, increasingly sedentary lifestyles, the recently recognized epidemic of overnutrition, genetic predispositions, and environmental influences are better understood. Yet the global epidemic of undernutrition has not yet been fully addressed. In today's world, with almost a billion people suffering from undernutrition and almost a billion people experiencing overweight and obesity, and billions suffering from infectious diseases, this book provides a fresh look at the intersection of nutrition and infectious diseases.

We present this book as a resource for clinical, research, public health, and educational settings. We are consolidating knowledge on the complexity of the nutrition-infection axis in the hope that improved knowledge will lead to improved health through less malnutrition and infectious diseases, better preventative and curative medicine, and more appropriate public health strategies. While the 1968 WHO monograph sought to exhaustively reference relevant articles, that task is no longer achievable. Over the last 50 years advances in the field of nutrition and infection has clearly identified some mechanisms and relationships, while other areas are still struggling to understand apparently conflicting and contradictory results. New analytic and diagnostic tools, the advent of more advanced human microbiome research, and new –omics and bioinformatics approaches are opening new horizons in understanding the complex dyad of nutrition-infection interactions. What will the next 50 years bring?

New Haven, CT, USA                                                  Debbie L. Humphries
Ste-Anne de Bellevue, QC, USA                                           Marilyn E. Scott
New Haven, CT, USA                                                     Sten H. Vermund

# References

1. UNICEF. The state of food security and nutrition in the world 2018. 2018 [updated 2018-09-11T10:53:32+00:00.
2. World Health Organization. Obesity and overweight 2018 Geneva. Switzerland: World Health Organization; 2018. https://www.who.int/news-room/fact-sheets/detail/obesity-and-overweight. Accessed 2 July 2020.
3. World Health Organization. Obesity: preventing and managing the global epidemic: World Health Organization; 2000.
4. James PT, Rigby N, Leach R. International Obesity Task F. The obesity epidemic, metabolic syndrome and future prevention strategies. Eur J Cardiovasc Prev Rehabil. 2004;11(1):3–8.
5. James WP. WHO recognition of the global obesity epidemic. Int J Obes (Lond). 2008;32(Suppl 7):S120–6.
6. Mayne ST, Ferrucci LM, Cartmel B. Lessons learned from randomized clinical trials of micronutrient supplementation for cancer prevention. Annu Rev Nutr. 2012;32:369–90.
7. Mayne ST, Playdon MC, Rock CL. Diet, nutrition, and cancer: past, present and future. Nat Rev Clin Oncol. 2016;13(8):504–15.
8. Collaboration NCDRF. Worldwide trends in body-mass index, underweight, overweight, and obesity from 1975 to 2016: a pooled analysis of 2416 population-based measurement studies in 128.9 million children, adolescents, and adults. Lancet. 2017;390(10113):2627–42.
9. Morris NP. The neglect of nutrition in medical education: a firsthand look. JAMA Intern Med. 2014;174(6):841–2.
10. Nestle M, Baron RB. Nutrition in medical education: from counting hours to measuring competence. JAMA Intern Med. 2014;174(6):843–4.
11. Kris-Etherton PM, Pratt CA, Saltzman E, Van Horn L. Introduction to nutrition education in training medical and other health care professionals. Am J Clin Nutr. 2014;99(5 Suppl):1151S–2S.
12. Collaborators GBDDD. Estimates of the global, regional, and national morbidity, mortality, and aetiologies of diarrhoea in 195 countries: a systematic analysis for the Global Burden of Disease Study 2016. Lancet Infect Dis. 2018;18(11):1211–28.
13. World Health Organization. World malaria report. Geneva: World Health Organization; 2018. Contract No.: Licence: CC BY-NC-SA 3.0 IGO.
14. Jourdan PM, Lamberton PHL, Fenwick A, Addiss DG. Soil-transmitted helminth infections. Lancet. 2018;391(10117):252–65.
15. Food in a time of COVID-19. Nat Plants. 2020;6(5):429.
16. Dunn CG, Kenney E, Fleischhacker SE, Bleich SN. Feeding low-income children during the Covid-19 pandemic. N Engl J Med. 2020;382(18):e40.
17. Okonofua FE, Eimuhi KE, Omonkhua AA. COVID-19: perspectives and reflections from Africa. Afr J Reprod Health. 2020;24(1):10–3.
18. Oliveira TC, Abranches MV, Lana RM. Food (in)security in Brazil in the context of the SARS-CoV-2 pandemic. Cad Saude Publica. 2020;36(4):e00055220.
19. Duchateau FX, Ramin G, Lepetit A. COVID-19: response plan for International Medical Assistance companies. Eur J Emerg Med. 2020;27(3):158–60.
20. The Lancet Global H. Food insecurity will be the sting in the tail of COVID-19. Lancet Glob Health. 2020;8(6):e737.
21. Shah GH, Shankar P, Schwind JS, Sittaramane V. The detrimental impact of the COVID-19 crisis on health equity and social determinants of health. J Public Health Manag Pract. 2020;26(4):317–9.
22. Laviano A, Koverech A, Zanetti M. Nutrition support in the time of SARS-CoV-2 (COVID-19). Nutrition. 2020;74:110834.
23. Scrimshaw NS, Taylor CE, Gordon JE. Interactions of nutrition and infection. Monogr Ser World Health Organ. 1968;57:3–329.
24. Scrimshaw NS, Taylor CE, Gordon JE. Interactions of nutrition and infection. Am J Med Sci. 1959;237(3):367–403.
25. Humphries DL, Scott ME, Vermund SH. Pathways linking nutritional status and infectious disease. In: Humphries DL, Scott ME, Vermund SH, editors. Nutrition and infectious disease: shifting the clinical paradigm: Humana Press; 2020.

26. Barffour MA, Humphries DL. Core principles: infectious disease risk in relation to macro and micronutrient status. In: Humphries DL, Scott ME, Vermund SH, editors. Nutrition and infectious disease: shifting the clinical paradigm: Humana Press; 2020.

27. Stephensen CB. Primer on immune response and interface with malnutrition. In: Humphries DL, Scott ME, Vermund SH, editors. Nutrition and infectious disease: shifting the clinical paradigm: Humana Press; 2020.

28. National Institute of Allergy and Infectious Diseases. Overview of the immune system. National Institute of Health; updated Dec 30, 2013. https://www.niaid.nih.gov/research/immune-system-overview. Accessed 2 July 2020.

29. Berkley JA. Bacterial infections and nutrition – a primer. In: Humphries DL, Scott ME, Vermund SH, editors. Nutrition and infectious disease: shifting the clinical paradigm: Humana Press; 2020.

30. Green WD, Karlsson EA, Beck MA. Viral infections and nutrition: influenza virus as a case study. In: Humphries DL, Scott ME, Vermund SH, editors. Nutrition and infectious disease: shifting the clinical paradigm: Humana Press; 2020.

31. Uyeki TM. Influenza. Ann Intern Med. 2017;167(5):ITC33–48.

32. Kash JC, Walters KA, Davis AS, Sandouk A, Schwartzman LM, Jagger BW, et al. Lethal synergism of 2009 pandemic H1N1 influenza virus and Streptococcus pneumoniae coinfection is associated with loss of murine lung repair responses. MBio. 2011;2(5)

33. Fedson DS. Influenza, evolution, and the next pandemic. Evol Med Public Health. 2018;2018(1):260–9.

34. Cilek L, Chowell G, Ramiro FD. Age-specific excess mortality patterns during the 1918–1920 influenza pandemic in Madrid, Spain. Am J Epidemiol. 2018;187(12):2511–23.

35. Wiser MF. Nutrition and protozoan pathogens of humans -- a primer. In: Humphries DL, Scott ME, Vermund SH, editors. Nutrition and infectious diseases: shifting the clinical paradigm: Humana Press; 2020.

36. Geary TG, Haque M. Human helminth infections. In: Humphries DL, Scott ME, Vermund SH, editors. Nutrition and infectious disease: shifting the clinical paradigm: Humana Press; 2020.

37. Humphries DL, Nguyen S, Kumar S, Quagraine JE, Otchere J, Harrison LM, et al. Effectiveness of albendazole for hookworm varies widely by community and correlates with nutritional factors: a cross-sectional study of school-age children in Ghana. Am J Trop Med Hyg. 2017;96(2):347–54.

38. Humphries DL, Nguyen S, Boakye D, Wilson M, Cappello M. The promise and pitfalls of mass drug administration to control intestinal helminth infections. Curr Opin Infect Dis. 2012;25(5):584–9.

39. Siddiqui F, Belayneh G, Bhutta ZA. Nutrition and diarrheal disease and enteric pathogens. In: Humphries DL, Scott ME, Vermund SH, editors. Nutrition and infectious disease: shifting the clinical paradigm: Humana Press; 2020.

40. Lasch EE, Abed Y, Abdulla K, El Tibbi AG, Marcus O, El Massri M, et al. Successful results of a program combining live and inactivated poliovirus vaccines to control poliomyelitis in Gaza. Rev Infect Dis. 1984;6(Suppl 2):S467–70.

41. Saleem AF, Mach O, Quadri F, Khan A, Bhatti Z, Rehman NU, et al. Immunogenicity of poliovirus vaccines in chronically malnourished infants: a randomized controlled trial in Pakistan. Vaccine. 2015;33(24):2757–63.

42. Baum M, Tamargo JA, Wanke C. Nutrition in HIV and tuberculosis. In: Humphries DL, Scott ME, Vermund SH, editors. Nutrition and infectious disease: shifting the clinical paradigm: Humana Press; 2020.

43. Camp WL, Allen S, Alvarez JO, Jolly PE, Weiss HL, Phillips JF, et al. Serum retinol and HIV-1 RNA viral load in rapid and slow progressors. J Acquir Immune Defic Syndr Hum Retrovirol. 1998;18(4):401–6.

44. Villamor E, Villar LA. Nutrition and arboviral infections. In: Humphries DL, Scott ME, Vermund SH, editors. Nutrition and infectious disease: shifting the clinical paradigm: Humana Press; 2020.

45. Kim HH, Bei AK. Nutritional frameworks in malaria. In: Humphries DL, Scott ME, Vermund SH, editors. Nutrition and infectious disease: shifting the clinical paradigm; 2020.

46. Scott ME, Koski K. Soil-transmitted Helminths – does nutrition make a difference? In: Humphries DL, Scott ME, Vermund SH, editors. Nutrition and infectious disease: shifting the clinical paradigm: Humana Press; 2020.

47. Yang I, Woltemate S, Piazuelo MB, Bravo LE, Yepez MC, Romero-Gallo J, et al. Different gastric microbiota compositions in two human populations with high and low gastric cancer risk in Colombia. Sci Rep. 2016;6:18594.

48. Boullata JI. Drug-nutrition interactions in infectious diseases. In: Humphries DL, Scott ME, Vermund SH, editors. Nutrition and infectious disease: shifting the clinical paradigm: Humana Press; 2020.

49. Ezenwa VO. Co-infection and nutrition: integrating ecological and epidemiological perspectives. In: Humphries DL, Scott ME, Vermund SH, editors. Nutrition and infectious disease: shifting the clinical paradigm: Springer; 2020.

50. Rocklov J, Ahlm C, Scott ME, Humphries DL. Climate change pathways and potential future risks to nutrition and infection. In: Humphries DL, Scott ME, Vermund SH, editors. Nutrition and infectious disease: shifting the clinical paradigm: Humana Press; 2020.

51. Vermund SH, Scott ME, Humphries DL. Public health and clinical implications of nutrition-infection interactions. In: Humphries DL, Scott ME, Vermund SH, editors. Nutrition and infectious disease: shifting the clinical paradigm: Humana Press; 2020.

# Series Editor Page

The great success of the Nutrition and Health Series is the result of the consistent overriding mission of providing health professionals with texts that are essential because each includes: (1) a synthesis of the state of the science, (2) timely, in-depth reviews by the leading researchers and clinicians in their respective fields, (3) extensive, up-to-date fully annotated reference lists, (4) a detailed index, (5) relevant tables and figures, (6) identification of paradigm shifts and the consequences, (7) virtually no overlap of information between chapters, but targeted, inter-chapter referrals, (8) suggestions of areas for future research, and (9) balanced, data-driven answers to patient as well as health professionals questions which are based upon the totality of evidence rather than the findings of any single study.

The series volumes are not the outcome of a symposium. Rather, each editor has the potential to examine a chosen area with a broad perspective, both in subject matter and in the choice of chapter authors. The international perspective, especially with regard to public health initiatives, is emphasized where appropriate. The editors, whose trainings are both research and practice oriented, have the opportunity to develop a primary objective for their book, define the scope and focus, and then invite the leading authorities from around the world to be part of their initiative. The authors are encouraged to provide an overview of the field, discuss their own research, and relate the research findings to potential human health consequences. Because each book is developed de novo, the chapters are coordinated so that the resulting volume imparts greater knowledge than the sum of the information contained in the individual chapters.

*Nutrition and Infectious Diseases: Shifting the Clinical Paradigm*, edited by Debbie L Humphries, PhD, MPH; Marilyn E Scott, PhD; and Sten H. Vermund, MD, PhD, the 90th volume published in this Series, is a very welcome and most timely addition to the Nutrition and Health Series and fully exemplifies the Series' goals. As we learn more about the pandemic-causing virus, COVID-19, it becomes clearer that nutritional status, specific nutrient intake levels (especially for essential nutrients), and nutritionally related health factors such as obesity significantly affect the risk of contracting this viral disease as well as surviving the infection. Certainly, these are not inconsistent findings as the historic review presented in this volume recounts the consistent findings of low micronutrient status and increased risk of morbidity and mortality for infected individuals, as well as coinfection from more than one pathogenic infectious disease. The over-arching goal of the volume is to provide clinically relevant and timely, objective guidance to health professionals and advanced students who are involved in public health research and/or provide nutrition care for patients at all life stages and health status. The editors have fulfilled the need for a text that can expand the clinical framework for responding to infectious diseases by highlighting the important, under-recognized role that nutritional status plays in altering the risk of exposure and susceptibility to infection, severity of disease, and effectiveness of treatments. The book has been developed to serve as a reference for curriculum development in courses such as Nutrition and Infectious Disease, Global Health, and related topics.

# Editors

The editors of this informative text are international experts in their fields and have been recognized by their peers as outstanding contributors as evidenced by their degrees, affiliations and honors.

Debbie L Humphries is an instructor of Public Health Practice (Microbial Diseases) at the Yale School of Public Health, where she has been since 2007. Her PhD in nutrition at Cornell University also included a focus on infectious diseases, and field research in Vietnam on the complex causes of anemia in women and children. As a nutritionist, she studies the intersection of nutritional status and infection disease, with research addressing the impact of infection on anemia, and the role of nutritional status in susceptibility to hookworm infection and response to drug treatment through ongoing epidemiological research in Ghana. As part of her teaching responsibilities, Dr. Humphries has taught a course on Global Nutrition since 1999, including an explicit focus on nutrition and infection since 2009. She has mentored over 60 MPH students, in addition to several medical students, physicians' assistants, and graduate nursing students. Through her nutrition course, Dr. Humphries has worked closely with public health undergraduate and graduate students to help them conceptualize and assess potential interactions between nutritional status and infectious disease. Dr. Humphries has a strong commitment to interdisciplinary and transdisciplinary thinking and work. She has worked with students on studies addressing the impact of food choices in driving and adapting to climate change and community public health research. Growing out of her interest in the ways human sanitation systems affect environmental health, public health and food systems, she has codeveloped, with an environmental engineer and environmental scientist, a course on rethinking urban sanitation. This book grows out of her interest in increasing understanding and knowledge of the multidisciplinary issues at the intersection of nutrition and infectious disease.

Marilyn E. Scott is a Professor of Parasitology at McGill University in Montreal, Canada. After receiving her PhD from the Institute of Parasitology at Macdonald Campus of McGill University, she did postdoctoral research at Imperial College, London, UK, in experimental parasite epidemiology. She returned to McGill as an Assistant Professor in 1982. She was Director of the Institute of Parasitology from 1990 to 2000 and Director of the McGill School of Environment from 2008 to 2013. She is currently Associate Dean (Academic) for the Faculty of Agricultural and Environmental Sciences. A major focus of Dr. Scott's work over the past 30 years has been on nutrition-infection interactions both in human and laboratory mouse populations. In collaboration with Kristine Koski (Human Nutrition, McGill) and a network of collaborators in Panama and Guatemala, she has examined interactions among a wide range of coexisting infections and micronutrient deficiencies, as well as their associations with host immunity and health. In the laboratory, she has used a mouse-nematode model to explore the impact of zinc, protein, and energy restriction on infection and immunity. More recently, her students have investigated impaired fetal and neonatal growth and development in off-spring of infected and protein deficient pregnant and lactating mice, including consequences of the maternal infection on the pup microbiome and the pup brain. Through her career, she has trained 50 graduate students and 6 postdoctoral fellows, and has published 1 book, 16 review articles and book chapters, and over 125 original articles. She was the 1991 recipient of the Henry Baldwin Ward Medal from the American Society of Parasitologists for her contributions to the field by a researcher under the age of 40. In 2006, she received the Robert Wardle Award from the Canadian Society of Zoologists (Parasitology Section) for outstanding contributions by a Canadian to parasitology. She was the recipient of both the Macdonald Campus and the Principal's Prize for Teaching Excellence in 2011.

Sten H. Vermund is Dean of the Yale School of Public Health, the Anna M.R. Lauder Professor of Public Health, and Professor of Pediatrics at the Yale School of Medicine. He is a pediatrician and infectious disease epidemiologist focused on diseases of low and middle income countries, and on health disparities in the USA. His work on HIV-HPV interactions among women in a Bronx methadone program motivated a change in the 1993 CDC AIDS case surveillance definition and inspired cervical cancer screening programs launched within global HIV/AIDS programs. Dr. Vermund's research has focused on health-care access, adolescent medicine, prevention of mother-to-child HIV transmission, and reproductive health. He has founded two nongovernmental organizations: Centre for Infectious Disease Research in Zambia (CIDRZ) and Friends in Global Health in Mozambique and Nigeria. Dr. Vermund is a member of the National Academy of Medicine and a Fellow of the AAAS. He has authored over 600 papers and chapters and serves on several journal editorial boards, and on multiple international and US advisory committees.

# Objectives and Organization of the Volume

The objectives of this comprehensive volume are to provide health professionals including clinicians, dietitians, nutritionists, and related students, both graduate and advanced undergraduates, with a broad review of the major pathogens that infect humans and the role of nutritional status, nutritional consequences, and the nutritional needs of infected patients during the various life stages as well as during the stages of infection. The emphasis of many of the chapters is on the adverse effects of undernutrition in young children and its consequences especially when the pathogen causes chronic, progressive disease. Malnutrition that results in obesity is also discussed at length, and this topic is especially timely during the COVID-19 pandemic as the world's population is getting more overweight; obesity, diabetes, and cardiovascular diseases are major risk factors for infection, greater morbidity, and death due to this viral pathogen. The volume contains four parts and logically begins with reviews of the basics of nutrition research as well as the basics of the field of clinical immunology. Part I provides an overarching framework for critically examining the relevant studies that evaluate complex, multiple interactions.

## Part I – The Foundations of the Nutrition-Infection Nexus

Part I contains three introductory chapters that provide the framework for examining the two-way interactions between nutritional status and pathogen success. Chapter 1, written by the volume's editors, describes in detail the complex of factors that occur in order for a pathogen to infect a host, and the added complexities of overall nutritional status at different life stages of the host and pathogen, further, real-world effects of multiple infective agents as well as multiple specific nutritional excesses/deficiencies. Of equal importance are the two-way interactions at all phases of disease progression including asymptomatic infection that we are now seeing in many of the COVID-infected. In order for the reader to have a firm understanding of the nutrient/infectious disease interactions, all terms are defined in detail beginning with the term, nutritional status. The chapter presents an historical analysis of the growth in awareness of the links seen between nutritional factors and infectivity, be it synergistic or the rarer antagonistic, or the few incidences when it appears that there is no interaction between these factors. All of these factors become important challenges to successful clinical studies and these challenges are examined in all of the book's chapters. Finally, this chapter includes numerous targeted examples of interactions that describe the framework used throughout the rest of the chapters.

Chapter 2 reviews the history of research that defined the role of dietary intake and generation of immune responses to infections. The chapter includes over 400 key primary and more recent references as well as seven valuable tables and reviews the role of each of the major food components – protein, carbohydrates, and fats, their food sources, requirements in health and with infection, as well as their importance to the functioning of the immune system. Essential nutrients are also reviewed and other dietary components that have a role in the development of immune responses to infection are also examined. Chapter 3 describes in detail, the organization of the immune system's responses to infection. There is an examination of the initial and rapid innate immune response compared to the slower, more specific and long-lasting adaptive immune response. The components of each of these responses are discussed; the types of pathogens that may be encountered are examined and the consequences of initial malnutrition on the response to infection are reviewed especially in light of the nutritional costs of the immune system's responses to infections. Additionally, the response of the individual's immune system to its microbiome is examined. The chapter includes in-depth discussions of the types of immune cells and factors and describes their functions with regard to local and systemic inflammatory responses, Types 1, 2, and 3 and regulatory immune responses. Each of the key nutrients, most of which are essential micronutrients, is discussed in detail as deficiencies in these have been documented to significantly reduce immune responses to pathogens; likewise adequate and/or supplemental intake levels can prevent certain infections and/or reduce the infection rate and duration.

## Part II: Types of Infectious Diseases and Influences of Nutrition

Chapter 4 examines the broad array of bacteria that the human immune system interacts with on a daily basis as well as the bacteria that cause infection. The chapter examines the effects of both undernutrition and overnutrition on these responses and concentrates on clinical data mainly from studies in undernourished children. The chapter includes a review of the classification of bacteria and the major members of these classes including both pathogenic and beneficial examples. Antimicrobial resistance and hospital acquired infections, mainly bacterial, and the adverse effects of malnutrition in this setting are described. Undernutrition is linked to decreased efficacy of the innate immune system that permits pathogenic bacteria entry through the skin, mucous membranes, and GI tract where gastric acidity may be decreased. Reduced intake of key essential micronutrients including vitamins A and D, zinc, and iron is reviewed with regard to increased risk of bacterial infections. Nutritional interventions have had mixed effects, and there is a paucity of large-scale double-blind intervention studies that examine the effects of nutrients in patients with serious bacterial infections.

Chapter 5 is of special interest now as the COVID-19 pandemic rages across the world. This chapter, containing over 250 relevant references, reviews basic virology, several well-known viruses including measles, herpes, Ebola, HIV and provides a number of up-to-date references with regard to the data concerning COVID-19 and obesity available in September, 2020. The chapter concentrates on the complex interactions between influenza virus infection, nutritional status, and specific nutrient deficiencies. The chapter reviews the cycle of viral replication and causes of infectivity as well as the annual development of flu vaccines. The data clearly indicate that poor nutritional status is a strong risk factor for viral infections and that infection severity as well as robust response to vaccination are dependent upon nutritional adequacy especially in young children. There is an in-depth discussion of the "triple burden of malnutrition" in resource poor nations where undernutrition, essential micronutrient deficiencies, and obesity are seen in the population. There is a bidirectional interaction between viral infection and nutritional status; of interest, undernutrition of key micronutrients can foster virus mutation that then reduces the efficacy of vaccines. Also, obesity has been shown to independently and significantly increase morbidity and mortality from H1N1 infection. There is a detailed review of the roles of vitamins A and D in the maintenance of epithelial tissue integrity and thus the essentiality in reducing the risk of lung epithelial viral infections including influenza. Vitamin E and C's unique roles in enhancing immune responses and affecting the flu virus directly are reviewed. Minerals associated with enhancing the immune system and/or affecting the virulence of viruses are reviewed. Additionally, there is a discussion of the different life stages, immune function, and nutritional status.

Chapter 6 comprehensively discusses the protozoan pathogens that infect humans and the role of nutrition in the acquisition, development, treatment, and clearance of both intestinal and blood-borne pathogens. The chapter, including the 16 excellent tables and figures, reviews the biology of the nine most common protozoan pathogens in humans and describes their life cycles and route of transmission. Most of the intestinal pathogens cause diarrhea and lead to an immediate loss of nutrients without absorption into the blood. This state of undernutrition is most common in young children who live in economically compromised conditions. Systemic infections increase the metabolic rate and thus increase the requirement for energy-rich foods that are often in short supply. The protozoan pathogen also requires energy and related nutrients from the host, and if the host's immune system is not optimal, the pathogen will grow and replicate at the expense of the host. Protein/energy malnutrition adversely affects host responses to most pathogens, and the chapter includes data as well on specific nutrients including iron, glucose, vitamins A, $B_{12}$, and E that are reviewed with regard to the requirements of specific pathogenic protozoa.

Chapter 7 looks at the effects of helminth infections on nutritional status. These infections are chronic and are mainly seen in tropical environments that are resource constrained and affect those at nutritional risk especially children. Childhood growth, cognitive function, and physical strength are all impacted negatively by helminth infection. The chapter reviews in detail the major roundworm, flatworm, and tapeworm parasites, their life cycles, and the results of their infection on the digestive circulatory and other relevant body systems.

As with protozoa, there is the dual relationship between infection and nutritional status with helminths resulting in a vicious circle that chronically weakens the host. Control programs and treatment strategies are reviewed. Of interest, there is a discussion of the potential for beneficial effects of nematode infestation on the host's microbiome – further research is warranted.

## Part III: Nutrition Issues During Major Infections: Case Studies of Nutrition and Infectious Disease

Chapter 8 concentrates on the serious effects of diarrheal-causing pathogens and their adverse effects on the nutritional status of children living in reduced resource areas around the globe. There is a review of the definitions of different types of diarrhea, its epidemiology, and extensive discussion of major risk factors for infection. The chapter also looks at the effects of malnutrition prior to infection as a serious risk factor for diarrhea in these children; factors reviewed include reduced gut immunity and overall immune responses at the body entry points. The relatively new clinical disorder, Environmental Enteric Dysfunction, described in 2014, is reviewed. Mechanisms of immune and microbiome dysfunction and the effects of impaired and/or chronic inflammation on the GI tract resulting in nutrient malabsorption and increased risk of enteric infections are described.

Chapter 9 provides an updated picture of the current HIV patient who is receiving antiretroviral therapy and is now considered in chronic remission. However, HIV chronic treatment is associated with a lipodystrophy syndrome that can result in obesity in the patient. We learn that the patient often has other health issues that may include illegal drug use and is often malnourished with micronutrient deficiencies but not energy deficient. HIV patients who are not treated and often reside in resource deficient countries are also at increased risk of tuberculosis, and this double burden of infections can result in further immunocompromise, diarrhea, and malnutrition. The chapter includes 422 references that provide the reader with an accurate historical perspective of HIV, its etiology, profiles of the infected individuals, and a comprehensive review of all nutritionally related intervention studies. I am very pleased that Dr. Baum, who I first met more than 30 years ago when we both worked in the new field of nutritional immunology, has contributed this chapter. She was the first investigator to examine the nutritional status in HIV-infected patients and evaluated nutrition's role in determining the potential for adequate immune responses. Dr. Baum continues to contribute as the expert investigator in this field and has expanded her research to include tuberculosis' effect in HIV-infected patients. With regard to tuberculosis, resurgence in Africa is mainly in HIV-infected untreated persons. Tuberculosis is a greater risk to the undernourished and causes malnutrition in the relatively well-nourished HIV-infected individual. The chapter includes a comprehensive review of nutritional assessment tools including anthropometric, biochemical, and nutritional assessments in specific populations including those with HIV with or without tuberculosis.

Chapter 10 concentrates on the three major arboviral diseases (arthropods as the virus vector; mosquitoes and ticks) that adversely affect human health.

The chapter outlines all of the currently known arboviruses that infect humans and characteristics of these viruses and identifies the key diseases that have been studied. There is a comprehensive review of risk factors for developing any of these diseases that include factors in the environment, from climate change to the level of immunomodulators produced by the host. All of the factors can affect and/or be affected by nutritional status. Dengue disease is the most significant mosquito-borne viral infection worldwide. There is a description of the phenomenon that has been seen to arise when there is secondary infection with a related but not identical serotype of the virus, and the host has an "antibody-dependent enhancement" of the first infection, but a weakened response to the second infection and becomes severely infected by this related secondary infection. This phenomenon can also occur if a vaccine to dengue or any other virus that has different serotypes, or the piece of the virus used to develop the vaccine raises a weakened response. As vaccines are developed for COVID-19, research to determine the potential risk of "antibody-dependent enhancement" must be well understood and avoided. The study of effects of nutritional status on arboviral infections is a relatively new field of investigation, and the most research has been conducted on the nutritional determinants of the severity and progression of dengue fever. Observational studies suggest that pediatric obesity increases the risk of severe disease. The chapter comprehensively reviews the data available concerning macro- and micronutrient status and risk of these infections as well as reviewing the preliminary intervention studies mainly using one or more of the essential vitamins and minerals. The two other arboviruses examined include Chikungunya seen in Africa and Zika virus infections. The few studies that have examined nutritional factors in Chikungunya are discussed; no studies to date have addressed the interactions between nutrition and Zika virus infection in humans. The authors suggest that relationship between nutritional factors and arboviral diseases is an open, promising area of research with potentially highly relevant public health and clinical applications.

Chapter 11 provides the reader with a broad overview of the epidemiology, pathogen lifecycle, infectivity, and clinical nutrition aspects of malaria, a febrile, debilitating, and painful illness caused by a species of the Plasmodium protozoan parasite that is carried in mosquitoes and injected into human skin. Malaria is a major killer in Sub-Saharan Africa where there continues to cause more than 400,000 deaths/year. Undernourished children and pregnant women in this region are at greatest risk. The chapter, containing over 200 targeted references, provides frameworks for examining the complex roles of nutritional and other environmental influences on all aspects of malarial disease. The chapter reviews the types of nutritional studies that are published including different types of observational as well as clinical intervention studies. Novel findings are examined including the studies showing that there is increased attraction of infected mosquitoes to human hosts, and of uninfected mosquitoes to infected hosts as well as subtle metabolic interactions between infected and noninfected host red blood cells. There is an in-depth review of the role of anemia and iron status in the severity of malaria. As seen in virtually all of the pathogenic infections described in this volume, undernutrition, especially of essential nutrients, adversely affects the immune system and thus may increase the risk of a weak immune response to the malarial protozoan; these effects are also described. The complex interactions between malarial infection, drug therapies, micronutrient status, especially iron, zinc, and folate, and pregnancy are reviewed in detail. The chapter concludes by enumerating research opportunities and key gaps in current data.

Chapter 12 describes the effects of infection with intestinal worms, commonly grouped together as soil-transmitted helminths. This group of helminths contains the most common human parasites globally. The chapter, containing more than 250 relevant references, reviews the stages of development of the pathogen, means of contact and modes of transmission, and the role that undernutrition/adequate nutrition play at each stage as the parasite has developed genetically to thrive or die based upon the nutritional status of the host. Laboratory animal studies and clinical data are reviewed. Specific effects of essential micronutrient deficiencies on the life stages of the helminth are outlined. In addition to in-depth examination of potential host defenses at all stages of infection and their nutritional dependences, the new, unique area of the unexpected protective effects of soil-transmitted helminth infection against nutrition-related chronic diseases including obesity and diabetes are examined mainly in animal models and small clinical trials. The beneficial effects of deworming, treatment of concomitant infections, and nutritional interventions are discussed and highly recommended based upon the literature review. The chapter includes boxed areas containing helpful key "take home messages" for each section.

## Part IV: Integration of Cross-Cutting Issues in Nutrition/ Infection Interactions

Chapter 13 examines the critical drug-nutrient interactions that can affect the patient infected with any of the pathogens discussed in the previous chapters. The chapter's author, Dr. Joseph Boullata has coedited two editions of the very well-received volumes entitled *Handbook of Drug-Nutrient Interactions* that are also a part of the Nutrition and Health Series. The chapter reviews the types of antimicrobials that are used in therapy and their pharmacological modes of action as well as the potential for their interactions with the patient's overall nutritional status. Three major mechanisms of actions of antimicrobials are described and the relevant drugs are classified according to these criteria. Additionally, drug-nutrient interactions are examined with regard to effects on absorption, distribution, metabolism, and excretion of the drug and/or the nutrient or nutritional status. The complexity of these interactions are discussed in detail with regard to pharmacokinetic and pharmacodynamics interactions. Each type of reaction is reviewed in light of specific findings from studies of antimicrobial drugs used in field studies where nutritional factors are also examined. The general adverse effects of many drugs can also affect nutritional status via nausea, fatigue, loss of appetite, etc. and these effects are also described. The chapter also includes a detailed description of the currently know strategies to treat COVID-19 including all pharmaceuticals in clinical study as of May 2020. Additionally, there is a comprehensive review of the nutrition effects of these drugs and other modalities that remain in clinical use. The chapter includes over 250 up-to-date, valuable references and 7 critically important tables and figures. The drug/nutrient tables are of particular importance as currently there are no comprehensive databases for drug-nutrient interactions that are available electronically.

Chapter 14 reviews the complexities of determining the role(s) of diet, overall nutritional status, and specific nutrient status when a patient has more than one pathogenic infection. As indicated by the author, concurrent infection is the norm rather than the exception in real-world populations where most host individuals are infected by more than one parasite species simultaneously. Likewise, nutritional deficiencies are also common and coinfection and multiple nutritional deficiencies frequently co-occur in the same economically depressed populations. The chapter includes most of the recent epidemiological survey studies that have reported on the significant increased risk of adding to already well-established nutrient deficiencies with multiple infections; iron is an important example. The chapter's objective is to draw insights from ecological studies combined with epidemiological data to guide future research. Examples of ecological approaches to host/parasite interactions are described and illustrated in the excellent figures included in the chapter. The chapter also includes case studies that examine the availability of host nutritional resources, resource use by parasites, host immune defenses, and the inter-connections among these processes simultaneously; this trophic approach can help us understand the numerous complexities associated with coinfection-nutrition interactions.

Chapter 15, which reviews the overarching area of climate change, adds further complexity to the interactions that affect nutrition/infection interactions. The chapter describes the current climate challenges and assessment frameworks and then presents an overview of ways in which climate is linked to nutrition and infections. Climate change, undernutrition, and infections are each individually reviewed, and the chapter concludes by highlighting how climate change, nutrition, and infection are all intertwined in the United Nations 2030 Sustainable Development Goals. The major focus of controlling the adverse effects of climate change is via $CO_2$ emissions reduction. These emissions are linked to warming of our planet resulting in ice melt that cause increased water in the oceans and warming of ocean waters, as but two examples. Current climate changes will affect the choices for food production. Parasite success has been linked to climate warming and other environmental changes; these are reviewed in detail. Moreover, food production's major role in increasing $CO_2$ is detailed as are the interactions both positive and negative between climate change and infection rates. The potential interactions of climate change and viral infections remind us that the COVID-19 pandemic may have been enhanced by our current climate conditions. As mentioned above, nutritional risk factors, such as obesity, have already been identified as increasing adverse effects seen with COVID-19 infection. This comprehensive and timely chapter contains 10 valuable figures and tables as well as over 100 targeted references.

Chapter 16, written by the volume's editors, concentrates on the clinical research aspects of nutritional requirements and provides the reader with a clear and data-driven synthesis of the key learning from the book's chapters. The editors indicate that the totality of the evidence points to the generalizable finding that improved nutrition, including adequate, but not excessive intake of needed macro- and micronutrients, can reduce infectious risks by augmenting vigorous immune responses. There is an excellent, detailed analysis of the process of "Causal Analysis" which is used in the place of data from placebo-controlled trials. Based upon this type of analysis, global public health strategies can be further developed and implemented that disregard social prejudices in favor of improving the population's overall health. The goal of reducing the risk of infection by enhancing immune responses is of equal value to the healthy person and the patient who is ill. The goal is the same across the lifespan and for all sexual identities, races, and ethnic communities. As we see today, with the emergence of a pandemic-causing virus, COVID19, a robust immune response is essential, and initial findings are reporting links to worsening viral effects in obesity as well as lower than normal levels of certain micronutrients. Of equal importance is an appreciation of the nutritional consequences of infection and the increased need to know the nutritional requirements during infection as well as a preventative measure in the face of, for example, a pandemic.

## Conclusions

The above description of the volume's 16 chapters attests to the depth of information provided by the 25 highly respected chapter authors and volume editors. Each chapter includes complete definitions of terms with the abbreviations fully defined and consistent use of terms between chapters. Key features of the comprehensive volume include over 90 detailed tables and informative figures; an extensive, detailed index; and more than 3,600 up-to-date references that provide the reader with excellent sources of worthwhile practice-oriented information that will be of great value to health providers, specialized nutrition practitioners as well as clinical researchers, and graduate and medical students. In addition to specific data on foods and diets, the volume contains important sensitive chapters related to the multiple interactions, both positive and negative, between overall nutritional status, essential nutrient availability, body weight, age, sex, pregnancy, growth, and the impact of one or more pathogenic infections. Unique chapters include ones that examine drug-nutrient interactions with a section that describes drug-nutrient interactions in the COVID-infected patient; review the effects of climate change on both nutritional status and potential for new infectious agents; and examine the development of immune responses and the role of the life cycle of almost every significant human pathogen in the infection of the host, whether nutritionally adequate or malnourished. This comprehensive volume is of great value to health professionals in the fields of nutrition, nursing, public health, infectious diseases, and clinical medicine and has been developed to serve as the primary text for graduate and medical students studying nutrition and infectious diseases.

In conclusion, *Nutrition and Infectious Diseases: Shifting the Clinical Paradigm*, edited by Debbie L Humphries, PhD, MPH; Marilyn E Scott, PhD; and Sten H. Vermund, MD, PhD, provides health professionals in many areas of nutrition and infectious disease research and practice with the most current and well-referenced volume on the importance of evidence-based interventions to assure the overall health of the individual. The volume serves the reader as the benchmark for integrating the complex interrelationships between nutritionally related risk factors such as obesity, micronutrient deficiencies and undernutrition, and pathogenic infection or infections in pregnancy, young childhood, in growth years, in the labor forces, seniors, and others at risk populations. The novel chapters, concerning climate change, causal analysis, and risks of new infections from many pathogens, add further to this valuable volume by providing relevant, timely, and concise data. The broad scope as well as in-depth reviews found in each chapter makes this excellent volume a very welcome addition to the Nutrition and Health Series.

Adrianne Bendich, PhD, FACN, FASN<br>
Series Editor

# Acknowledgments

We are grateful for the support of outstanding editors and others who have made this book possible. Samantha Lonuzzi, from Springer, responded encouragingly to the initial query asking if Springer might be interested in such a volume. Adrianne Bendich helped to shape the book proposal into the structure and content you see here. Michael Wilt has been an outstanding publishing editor, providing clear guidelines and rapid feedback as we navigated the complex process of permissions and formatting for previously published tables and figures. Brittany Connolly helped to create the space and encouragement needed to fit the work on this book into an already over-full schedule. We are grateful to all of the authors of the chapters who said yes to this project, and enthusiastically and thoroughly tackled the complex subject matter.

# Contents

# About the Series Editors

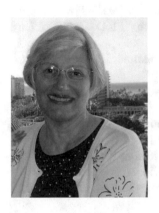

**Adrianne Bendich** has served as the Nutrition and Health Series **Editor** for more than 20 years and has provided leadership and guidance to more than 200 editors that have developed the 90 well-respected and highly recommended volumes in the Series.

In addition to *Nutrition and Infectious Diseases: Shifting the Clinical Paradigm*, edited by Debbie L Humphries, PhD, MPH; Marilyn E Scott, PhD; and Sten H. Vermund, MD, PhD, major new editions published in 2012–2019 include:

1. *Nutritional and Medical Management of Kidney Stones*, edited by Haewook Han, Walter Mutter and Samer Nasser, 2019
2. *Vitamin E in Human Health*, edited by Peter Weber, Marc Birringer, Jeffrey B. Blumberg, Manfred Eggersdorfer, Jan Frank, 2019
3. *Handbook of Nutrition and Pregnancy, Second Edition*, edited by Carol J. Lammi-Keefe, Sarah C. Couch and John P. Kirwan, 2019
4. *Dietary Patterns and Whole Plant Foods in Aging and Disease*, edited as well as written by Mark L. Dreher, Ph.D., 2018
5. *Dietary Fiber in Health and Disease*, edited as well as written by Mark L. Dreher, Ph.D., 2017
6. *Clinical Aspects of Natural and Added Phosphorus in Foods*, edited by Orlando M. Gutierrez, Kamyar Kalantar-Zaden\h and Rajnish Mehrotra, 2017
7. *Nutrition and Fetal Programming*, edited by Rajendram Rajkumar, Victor R. Preedy and Vinood B. Patel, 2017
8. *Nutrition and Diet in Maternal Diabetes*, edited by Rajendram Rajkumar, Victor R. Preedy and Vinood B. Patel, 2017
9. *Nitrite and Nitrate in Human Health and Disease, Second Edition*, edited by Nathan S. Bryan and Joseph Loscalzo, 2017
10. *Nutrition in Lifestyle Medicine*, edited by James M. Rippe, 2017
11. *Nutrition Guide for Physicians and Related Healthcare Professionals, Second Edition*, edited by Norman J. Temple, Ted Wilson and George A. Bray, 2016

35. *Bioactive Dietary Factors and Plant Extracts in Dermatology*, edited by Dr. Ronald Ross Watson and Dr. Sherma Zibadi, 2013
36. *Omega 6/3 Fatty Acids*, edited by Dr. Fabien De Meester, Dr. Ronald Ross Watson and Dr. Sherma Zibadi, 2013
37. *Nutrition in Pediatric Pulmonary Disease*, edited by Dr. Robert Dumont and Dr. Youngran Chung, 2013
38. *Nutrition and Diet in Menopause*, edited by Dr. Caroline J. Hollins Martin, Dr. Ronald Ross Watson and Dr. Victor R. Preedy, 2013.
39. *Magnesium and Health*, edited by Dr. Ronald Ross Watson and Dr. Victor R. Preedy, 2012.
40. *Alcohol, Nutrition and Health Consequences*, edited by Dr. Ronald Ross Watson, Dr. Victor R. Preedy, and Dr. Sherma Zibadi, 2012
41. *Nutritional Health, Strategies for Disease Prevention, Third Edition*, edited by Norman J. Temple, Ted Wilson, and David R. Jacobs, Jr., 2012
42. *Chocolate in Health and Nutrition*, edited by Dr. Ronald Ross Watson, Dr. Victor R. Preedy, and Dr. Sherma Zibadi, 2012
43. Iron Physiology and Pathophysiology in Humans, edited by Dr. Gregory J. Anderson and Dr. Gordon D. McLaren, 2012

Earlier books included *Vitamin D, Second Edition*, edited by Dr. Michael Holick; *Dietary Components and Immune Function* edited by Dr. Ronald Ross Watson, Dr. Sherma Zibadi, and Dr. Victor R. Preedy; *Bioactive Compounds and Cancer* edited by Dr. John A. Milner and Dr. Donato F. Romagnolo; *Modern Dietary Fat Intakes in Disease Promotion* edited by Dr. Fabien De Meester, Dr. Sherma Zibadi, and Dr. Ronald Ross Watson; *Iron Deficiency and Overload* edited by Dr. Shlomo Yehuda and Dr. David Mostofsky; *Nutrition Guide for Physicians* edited by Dr. Edward Wilson, Dr. George A. Bray, Dr. Norman Temple, and Dr. Mary Struble; *Nutrition and Metabolism* edited by Dr. Christos Mantzoros; and *Fluid and Electrolytes in Pediatrics* edited by Leonard Feld and Dr. Frederick Kaskel. Recent volumes include *Handbook of Drug-Nutrient Interactions* edited by Dr. Joseph Boullata and Dr. Vincent Armenti; *Probiotics in Pediatric Medicine* edited by Dr. Sonia Michail and Dr. Philip Sherman; *Handbook of Nutrition and Pregnancy* edited by Dr. Carol Lammi-Keefe, Dr. Sarah Couch, and Dr. Elliot Philipson; *Nutrition and Rheumatic Disease* edited by Dr. Laura Coleman; *Nutrition and Kidney Disease* edited by Dr. Laura Byham-Grey, Dr. Jerrilynn Burrowes, and Dr. Glenn Chertow; *Nutrition and Health in Developing Countries* edited by Dr. Richard Semba and Dr. Martin Bloem; *Calcium in Human Health* edited by Dr. Robert Heaney and Dr. Connie Weaver; and *Nutrition and Bone Health* edited by Dr. Michael Holick and Dr. Bess Dawson-Hughes.

Dr. Bendich served as President of Consultants in Consumer Healthcare LLC, and has edited ten books including *Preventive Nutrition: The Comprehensive Guide for Health Professionals, Fifth Edition* coedited with Dr. Richard Deckelbaum (www.springer.com/series/7659). Dr. Bendich serves on the Editorial Boards of the *Journal of Nutrition in Gerontology and Geriatrics* and *Antioxidants* and has served as Associate Editor for *Nutrition* the International Journal, served on the Editorial Board of the *Journal of Women's Health and Gender-Based Medicine*, and served on the Board of Directors of the American College of Nutrition.

Dr. Bendich was Director of Medical Affairs at GlaxoSmithKline (GSK) Consumer Healthcare and provided medical leadership for many well-known brands including TUMS and Os-Cal. Dr. Bendich had primary responsibility for GSK's support for the Women's Health Initiative (WHI) intervention study. Prior to joining GSK, Dr. Bendich was at Roche Vitamins Inc. and was involved with the groundbreaking clinical studies showing that folic acid-containing multivitamins significantly reduced major classes of birth defects. Dr. Bendich has coauthored over 100 major clinical research studies in the area of preventive nutrition. She is recognized as a leading authority on antioxidants, nutrition and immunity and pregnancy outcomes, vitamin safety, and the cost-effectiveness of vitamin/mineral supplementation.

Dr. Bendich received the Roche Research Award, is a *Tribute to Women and Industry* Awardee, and was a recipient of the Burroughs Wellcome Visiting Professorship in Basic Medical Sciences. Dr. Bendich was given the Council for Responsible Nutrition (CRN) Apple Award in recognition of her many contributions to the scientific understanding of dietary supplements. In 2012, she was recognized for her contributions to the field of clinical nutrition by the American Society for Nutrition and was elected a Fellow of ASN (FASN). Dr. Bendich served as an Adjunct Professor at Rutgers University. She is listed in Who's Who in American Women.

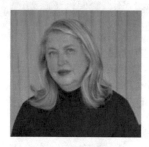

**Connie W. Bales** is Professor of Medicine in the Division of Geriatrics, Department of Medicine, Duke School of Medicine, and Senior Fellow in the Center for the Study of Aging and Human Development at Duke University Medical Center. She is also Associate Director for Education/Evaluation of the Geriatrics Research, Education, and Clinical Center at the Durham VA Medical Center. Dr. Bales is a well-recognized expert in the field of nutrition, chronic disease, function, and aging. Over the past two decades, her laboratory at Duke has explored many different aspects of diet and activity as determinants of health during the latter half of the adult life course. Her current research focuses primarily on enhanced protein as a means of benefiting muscle quality, function, and other health indicators during geriatric obesity reduction and for improving perioperative outcomes in older patients. Dr. Bales has served on NIH and USDA grant review panels and is Past-Chair of the Medical Nutrition Council of the American Society for Nutrition. She has edited three editions of the *Handbook of Clinical Nutrition and Aging*, is Editor-in-Chief of the *Journal of Nutrition in Gerontology and Geriatrics*, and is a Deputy Editor of *Current Developments in Nutrition*.

# About the Editors

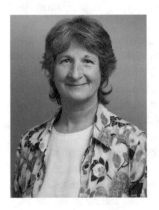

**Debbie L. Humphries** is an instructor of Public Health Practice (Microbial Diseases) at the Yale School of Public Health, where she has been since 2007. Her PhD in nutrition at Cornell University also included a focus on infectious diseases, and field research in Vietnam on the complex causes of anemia in women and children. As a nutritionist, she studies the intersection of nutritional status and infection disease, with research addressing the impact of infection on anemia, and the role of nutritional status in susceptibility to hookworm infection and response to drug treatment through ongoing epidemiological research in Ghana. As part of her teaching responsibilities, Humphries has taught a course on Global Nutrition since 1999, including an explicit focus on nutrition and infection since 2009. She has mentored over 60 MPH students, in addition to several medical students, physicians' assistants, and graduate nursing students. Through her nutrition course Dr. Humphries has worked closely with public health and graduate students to help them conceptualize and assess potential interactions between nutritional status and infectious disease.

Dr. Humphries has a strong commitment to interdisciplinary and transdisciplinary thinking and work. She has worked with students on studies addressing the impact of food choices in driving and adapting to climate change, community public health research, and cogeneration of knowledge in community settings. Growing out of her interest in the ways human sanitation systems affect environmental health, public health and food systems, she has codeveloped, with an environmental engineer and environmental scientist, a course on rethinking urban sanitation. This book grows out of her interest in increasing understanding and knowledge of the multidisciplinary issues at the intersection of nutrition and infectious disease.

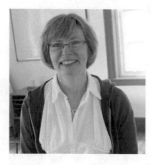

**Marilyn E. Scott** is a Professor of Parasitology at McGill University in Montreal, Canada. After receiving her PhD from the Institute of Parasitology at Macdonald Campus of McGill University, she did postdoctoral research at Imperial College, London, UK, in experimental parasite epidemiology. She returned to McGill as an Assistant Professor in 1982. She was Director of the Institute of Parasitology from 1990 to 2000 and Director of the McGill School of Environment from 2008 to 2013. She is currently Associate Dean (Academic) for the Faculty of Agricultural and Environmental Sciences.

A major focus of her work over the past 30 years has been on nutrition-infection interactions both in human and laboratory mouse populations. In collaboration with Dr. Kristine Koski (Human Nutrition, McGill) and a network of collaborators in Panama and Guatemala, she has examined interactions among a wide range of coexisting infections and micronutrient deficiencies, as well as their associations with host immunity and health. In the laboratory, she has used a mouse-nematode model to explore the impact of zinc, protein, and energy restriction on infection and immunity. More recently, her students have investigated impaired fetal and neonatal growth and development in offspring of infected and protein deficient pregnant and lactating mice, including consequences of the maternal infection on the pup microbiome and the pup brain.

Through her career, she has trained 50 graduate students and 6 postdoctoral fellows and has published 1 book, 16 review articles and book chapters, and over 125 original articles. She was the 1991 recipient of the Henry Baldwin Ward Medal from the American Society of Parasitologists for her contributions to the field by a researcher under the age of 40. In 2006, she received the Robert Wardle Award from the Canadian Society of Zoologists (Parasitology Section) for outstanding contributions by a Canadian to parasitology. She was the recipient of both the Macdonald Campus and the Principal's Prize for Teaching Excellence in 2011.

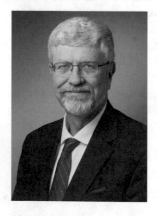

**Sten H. Vermund** is Dean of the Yale School of Public Health, the Anna M.R. Lauder Professor of Public Health, and Professor of Pediatrics at the Yale School of Medicine. He is a pediatrician and infectious disease epidemiologist focused on diseases of low- and middle-income countries, and on health disparities in the USA. His work on HIV-HPV interactions among women in a Bronx methadone program motivated a change in the 1993 CDC AIDS case surveillance definition and inspired cervical cancer screening programs launched within global HIV/AIDS programs. Dr. Vermund's research has focused on health-care access, adolescent medicine, prevention of mother-to-child HIV transmission, and reproductive health. He has founded two nongovernmental organizations: Centre for Infectious Disease Research in Zambia (CIDRZ) and Friends in Global Health in Mozambique and Nigeria. Dr. Vermund is a member of the National Academy of Medicine and a Fellow of the AAAS. He has authored over 600 papers and chapters and serves on several journal editorial boards and on multiple international and US advisory committees.

# Contributors

**Clas Ahlm, PhD** Department of Clinical Microbiology, Infection and Immunology, Umeå University, Umeå, Sweden

**Maxwell A. Barffour, MPH, PhD** McQueary College of Health and Human Services, Missouri State University, Springfield, MO, USA

**Marianna K. Baum, PhD** Florida International University, Miami, FL, USA

**Melinda A. Beck, PhD** Department of Nutrition, Gilling's School of Global Public Health, University of North Carolina at Chapel Hill, Chapel Hill, NC, USA

**Amy Kristine Bei, PhD** Department of Epidemiology of Microbial Diseases, Yale School of Public Health, New Haven, CT, USA

**Grace Belayneh, BSc, MSc** Duke-NUS Medical School, Singapore, Singapore

**James A. Berkley, FRCPC H FMedSci** Centre for Tropical Medicine and Global Health, Nuffield Department of Clinical Medicine, University of Oxford, Oxford, UK

Kenya Medical Research Institute/Wellcome Trust Research Programme, Kilifi, Kenya

Childhood Acute Illness & Nutrition (CHAIN) Network, Nairobi, Kenya

**Zulfiqar A. Bhutta, MBBS, FRCPC H, FAAP, PhD** Robert Harding Chair in Global Child Health & Policy, SickKids Centre for Global Child Health, The Hospital for Sick Children, Toronto, ON, Canada

Departments of Paediatrics, Nutritional Sciences and Public Health, University of Toronto, Toronto, ON, Canada

**Joseph I. Boullata, PharmD, RPh, CNS-S, FASPEN, FACN** Clinical Nutrition Support Services, Hospital of the University of Pennsylvania, Philadelphia, PA, USA

**Vanessa O. Ezenwa, PhD** Odum School of Ecology & Department of Infectious Diseases, College of Veterinary Medicine, University of Georgia, Athens, GA, USA

**Timothy G. Geary, PhD** Institute of Parasitology, McGill University, Ste-Anne de Bellevue, QC, Canada

School of Biological Sciences, Queen's University Belfast, Belfast, UK

**Morgan M. Goheen, MD, PhD** Department of Internal Medicine, Yale School of Medicine, New Haven, CT, USA

**William David Green, PhD, MS** Department of Nutrition, Gilling's School of Global Public Health, University of North Carolina at Chapel Hill, Chapel Hill, NC, USA

**Manjurul Haque, PhD** Institute of Parasitology, McGill University, Ste-Anne de Bellevue, QC, Canada

**Debbie L. Humphries, PhD, MPH** Department of Epidemiology of Microbial Disease, Yale School of Public Health, Yale University, New Haven, CT, USA

**Erik A. Karlsson, PhD** Virology Unit, Institut Pasteur du Cambodge, Phnom Penh, Cambodia

**Harry Hyunteh Kim, MPH, BSc** Department of Epidemiology of Microbial Diseases, Yale School of Public Health, New Haven, CT, USA

**Kristine G. Koski, PhD** School of Human Nutrition, McGill University (Macdonald Campus), Ste-Anne de Bellevue, QC, Canada

**Joacim Rocklöv, BSc, MSc, PhD** Department of Public Health and Clinical Medicine, Section of Sustainable Health, Umeå University, Umeå, Sweden

Heidelberg Institute of Global Health, Heidelberg University, Heidelberg, Germany

**Marilyn E. Scott, PhD** Institute of Parasitology, McGill University (Macdonald Campus), Ste-Anne de Bellevue, QC, Canada

McGill University, Macdonald Campus, Sainte-Anne de Bellevue, QC, Canada

**Fahad Javaid Siddiqui, MBBS, MSc** SickKids Centre for Global Child Health, The Hospital for Sick Children, Toronto, ON, Canada

Duke-NUS Medical School, Singapore, Singapore

**Charles B. Stephensen, PhD** Immunity and Disease Prevention Research Unit, USDA Western Human Nutrition Research Center, University of California, Davis, Davis, CA, USA

Nutrition Department, University of California, Davis, CA, USA

**Javier A. Tamargo, MS** Florida International University, Miami, FL, USA

**Sten H. Vermund, MD, PhD** Department of Epidemiology of Microbial Disease, Yale School of Public Health, Yale University, New Haven, CT, USA

Yale School of Public Health, Yale University, New Haven, CT, USA

**Eduardo Villamor, MD, DrPH** Department of Epidemiology, University of Michigan School of Public Health, Ann Arbor, MI, USA

**Luis A. Villar, MD, MSc** Departamento de Ciencias Basicas, Universidad Industrial de Santander, Facultad de Medicina, Centro de Investigaciones Epidemiológicas, Bucaramanga, Colombia

**Christine Wanke, MD** Professor Emeritus Tufts University School of Medicine, Boston, MA, USA

**Mark F. Wiser, PhD** Department of Tropical Medicine, Tulane University School of Public Health and Tropical Medicine, New Orleans, LA, USA

# Part I
# The Foundations of the Nutrition-Infection Nexus

# Chapter 1
# Pathways Linking Nutritional Status and Infectious Disease: Causal and Conceptual Frameworks

Debbie L. Humphries, Marilyn E. Scott, and Sten H. Vermund

## Abbreviations

| | |
|------|------------------------------|
| AGP  | Alpha glycoprotein           |
| BCG  | Bacille Calmette-Guerin      |
| CYP  | Cytochrome P450              |
| HIV  | Human immunodeficiency virus |
| Ig   | Immunoglobulin               |
| IL   | Interleukin                  |
| PEM  | Protein-energy malnutrition  |
| RCT  | Randomized controlled trial  |
| TB   | Tuberculosis                 |
| Th   | T helper                     |
| Treg | Regulatory T cells           |
| WAZ  | Weight-for-age               |

### Key Points
- Many criteria have been developed for demonstrating causality, but few have been refined for application to the design or analysis of nutrition-infection interactions.
- A conceptual framework for exploring the impact of host nutritional status on infectious disease needs to consider the impact of nutrition on both the host and the pathogen.
- Infection alters nutritional status through a variety of mechanisms.
- Establishing causation in a context of multiple nutrient deficiencies and infections is challenging, especially given the difficulty of directly extrapolating mechanisms identified under controlled experimental conditions to natural populations.

D. L. Humphries (✉)
Department of Epidemiology of Microbial Disease, Yale School of Public Health, Yale University, New Haven, CT, USA
e-mail: debbie.humphries@yale.edu

S. H. Vermund
Yale School of Public Health, Yale University, New Haven, CT, USA
e-mail: sten.vermund@yale.edu

M. E. Scott
Institute of Parasitology, McGill University, Ste-Anne de Bellevue, QC, Canada
e-mail: marilyn.scott@mcgill.ca

© Springer Nature Switzerland AG 2021
D. L. Humphries et al. (eds.), *Nutrition and Infectious Diseases*, Nutrition and Health,
https://doi.org/10.1007/978-3-030-56913-6_1

There are varying combinations of infectious diseases and micronutrient and macronutrient deficiencies in the different ecological settings around the world. Even within a community, the combination of infectious agents and nutritional deficiencies varies among individuals. Pathogens can be affected by nutritional status through multiple pathways that may have distinct consequences depending on the host and environment. Host nutritional status can affect success of a pathogen, beginning with exposure to the infectious agent through to the resolution of the infection, either naturally or through response to interventions. Some of the pathways may result from changes in host behavior and others through biochemical and metabolic changes in the host or pathogen. Given the multiple potential pathways, exploring causal relationships between a specific nutritional disorder or combination of disorders and single or multiple infections poses challenges.

To better frame the exploration of these complex relationships, we lay out key definitions, theories of causality, types of causal relationships, and criteria for assessing causal associations between nutrition and infection. To better understand the relationships between nutrition and infectious disease, we follow the classification system used by Scrimshaw et al. [1] of synergism, antagonism, or no effect. These terms are used to reflect the net combination of effects as even within a single nutrient-infection combination, it is conceivable that, at a mechanistic level, there may be a mix of both synergistic and antagonistic relationships. In presenting an overarching conceptual framework of potential pathways of interaction, we seek a unifying construct that helps frame the other chapters in this book and guides conceptualization of future multidisciplinary research into nutrition-infection interactions.

## Background: Definitions and Tools for Understanding Relationships Between Nutrition and Infection

### Definitions

To set the stage, we clarify the meaning and usage of our central themes: nutritional status and infection.

### Nutritional Status

Nutritional status reflects the body's store of available nutrients and is measured using anthropometry (e.g., height, weight, mid upper arm circumference) and biochemical indicators (e.g., hemoglobin) and concentrations of specific nutrients (e.g., serum retinol) compared against recognized standards or cutoffs. Macronutrients include proteins, lipids (fats), and carbohydrates (sugars), while micronutrients include water-soluble or fat-soluble vitamins, macrominerals, and trace minerals. Nutritional status is an indicator of the balance between nutrient needs and nutrient consumption. Undernutrition includes both micronutrient malnutrition, where intake or absorption of single or multiple micronutrients is inadequate to meet physiological needs for good health, and protein-energy malnutrition, where consumption of macronutrients (protein, carbohydrates, lipids) is insufficient (see Chap. 2); overnutrition often includes both an excess of macronutrients and deficiencies of micronutrients [2].

### Infection

This book focuses on infections of relevance to humans caused by viruses, bacteria, protozoans, and helminths. We distinguish between an infection (i.e., the presence of a pathogen) and disease (i.e., signs, symptoms, and pathology [disease progression]). We note that disease severity is a function of pathogen virulence (see Box 1.1), host tolerance, and pathogen load. The chapters address infections

**Box 1.1  Definition of Terms**

- Susceptibility – the set of complementing genetic or environmental causes sufficient to make a person contract a disease after being exposed to the specific causes [7, 8]
- Vulnerability – contextual factors that influence the likelihood of exposure of individuals and communities
- Virulence – the ability of a specific strain of a microorganism to produce disease [9], often related to the rate of replication of the infectious agent or its intrinsic invasive capacity
- Tolerance – the process whereby the body becomes increasingly resistant through continued exposure [9] or produces less pathology for a given infection load
- Pathogenicity – the ability of a pathogen to produce disease [9] or symptoms, often as a consequence of an overactive immune or inflammatory response
- Resistance – the ability of the host to limit infection or disease [10], typically through effective barriers or immune responses that have a genetic component

that are harmful, but also highlight situations where pathogens may have beneficial effects (e.g., Shea-Donohue et al. [3]), such as within the microbiome [4, 5]. Limited attention is given to infections that cause disease directly within the vector, unless the impact on the vector is also associated with altered impact on human hosts. Both asymptomatic and symptomatic infections are addressed where relevant, particularly as there is a growing awareness of pathological changes that may be happening in the asymptomatic stage of infections, such as in infections with the human immunodeficiency virus (HIV), where asymptomatic infection is associated with a 10% increase in resting energy expenditure [6]. Where helpful in understanding underlying mechanisms, we make reference to studies in livestock as well as rodent models.

## Theories of Causality

Prior to exploring criteria for assessing causal relationships, it is important to characterize the kind of causality being explored. Historically, understanding causality has been both a philosophical and a natural science pursuit. Aristotle was an influential early proposer of theories of causality, unpacking the theoretical cause of an "object" [11]. More recent representations of causal relationships have reflected on multiple potential meanings of the phrase "A causes B". Parascandola and Weed concluded that an epidemiological perspective is best served by a counterfactually based[1] probabilistic definition of causality that uses probability statistics to assess the impact of a condition when it is present compared to when it is absent [12]. Thygesen and colleagues utilized two theories of causality: regularity and generative. The regularity theory proposes that we can say "A causes B" when we observe a statistical pattern indicating that A is followed by B. The generative theory proposes that we can say "A causes B" when we have identified pathways and biological mechanisms that could lead from A to B [13], independent of epidemiological evidence. In the usage by Thygesen and colleagues, regularity theory is similar to probabilistic causality, while generative theory is focused on biological mechanisms and has no clear counterpart in the Parascandola and Weed framework [13].

From a nutritional epidemiological perspective, both regularity and generative causality can be used as possible pathways to evaluate cause and effect, and their joint use is ideal. Generative causality occurs in nutrition when a specific nutritional deficiency leads to specific physiological conditions in human populations, and we have a mechanistic understanding of the relationship. Vitamin A defi-

---

[1] Counterfactual probabilistic approaches assess the statistical association of presence and absence of a potential risk factor with the condition of concern.

ciency causing xerophthalmia (abnormally dry conjunctiva and cornea of the eyes) is a good example. The larger focus of nutritional epidemiology has been on whether deficiencies or excesses of nutrients (such as vitamin A) could affect the acquisition and/or the progression of other diseases, even when mechanisms are not yet well understood. In this second context, causality is understood as either "regular" when the association is solely epidemiological or "generative" [12] when mechanisms are understood.

## Criteria for Assessing Relationships Between Infections and Malnutrition

Identifying and characterizing patterns of association and relationships between two events are fundamental to the history of science. In the field of infectious diseases, theories of causality began from detecting the presence of an infectious agent. Koch's postulates (Table 1.1) were a key conceptual innovation that allowed researchers to demonstrate with scientific precision that a specific agent caused a specific infection. This was revolutionary and led to rapid identification of interventions to reduce infectious diseases such as cholera. With the development of the science of epidemiology over the last century, there has been a growing understanding of causality as more than a single factor leading to a single outcome and an increasing awareness of the importance of nonpathogenic influences on infectious diseases. With this changing understanding, analyses of probabilistic associations and potentially causal relationships rely on much more than Koch's postulates. In particular, emerging understanding of asymptomatic disease, cofactors in the manifestation of infectious pathology, and other complexities that were not known in Koch's nineteenth century all inform current understandings of causality.

To give a noninfectious-/non-nutrient-focused example of determining causality, in the 1960s, the growing epidemic of lung cancer motivated scientists to look for causal theories and criteria that were relevant in assessing emerging patterns in medicine and public health. The principal focus was on the role of tobacco in lung cancer, and this contributed to the development of a more probabilistic and epidemiologically focused set of criteria for assessing potentially causal relationships [14]. Bradford Hill (Table 1.1) identified seven criteria, only one of which he considered essential: temporality [15]. Building on the Bradford Hill criteria, and specifically addressing issues that arise in considering causality in the field of nutritional epidemiology, Potischman and Weed [16] focused on a subset of the Bradford Hill criteria (Table 1.1) with the addition of biological plausibility, a criterion reflecting the generative theory of causality of Thygesen [13].

Monteiro and colleagues combined both sets of criteria and added one more: analogies from similar conditions (Table 1.1) [17]. They then used each criterion separately to assess evidence of a causal relationship between a species of malaria, *Plasmodium vivax*, and subsequent undernutrition [17]. One of the most challenging criteria, temporality, was addressed through multiple cohort stud-

**Table 1.1** Criteria for causal inference, drawn from several sources

| Koch's postulates (1890) [129] infection focus | Bradford Hill (1964) [15] cancer/tobacco | Potischman and Weed (1999) [16] nutrition | Monteiro et al. (2016) [17] |
|---|---|---|---|
| Pathogen present in every case of disease<br>Pathogen isolated from host with disease<br>Symptoms/disease reproduced when pure culture of pathogen inoculated into healthy susceptible host<br>Pathogen recoverable from experimentally infected host | Strength<br>Consistency<br>Specificity<br>Temporality<br>Biological gradient<br>Coherence<br>Experimental design | Strength<br>Consistency<br>Temporality<br>Dose response (biological gradient)<br>Biological plausibility | Strength<br>Consistency<br>Specificity<br>Temporality<br>Biological gradient<br>Coherence<br>Experiment(al design)<br>Plausibility (biological)<br>Analogy |

ies in *P. vivax*-endemic areas that assessed nutritional status prior to infection with *P. vivax* [17]. They concluded that current evidence is consistent with *P. vivax* contributing to undernutrition in endemic settings, demonstrating the applicability of clearly stated causal analysis to situations of nutritional and infectious disease epidemiology. Their analysis offers a compelling example of using rigorous causal analysis from a breadth of criteria to assess the strength of the evidence for a given relationship.

## Types of Relationships

From a theoretical perspective, poor nutritional status could have a direct association with infection in three ways. Poor nutritional status could have a synergistic effect on an infection where it promotes the infection in some way, it could diminish the infection with an antagonistic effect, or it could have no impact on the infection, either because of independence of the two conditions or because the synergistic aspects cancel out the antagonistic dimensions of the association.

### Synergistic Relationships Between Nutrition and Infection

A number of nutritional deficiencies can reduce the ability of a host to resist a pathogen, and a number of infections can impair nutritional status. This kind of causality is said to be synergistic in that both the infection and malnutrition exert negative effects on host health. There is an extensive literature documenting synergistic relationships between malnutrition and infections, and the public health significance has become evident [18–20]. In the mid-1990s, several researchers developed an approach for estimating population-level effects of malnutrition (low weight-for-age) on risk of infant and child mortality [21, 22]. Pelletier and colleagues estimated population attributable risks from data on mortality rates from specific childhood infections for children with differing nutritional status [22]. Thus, they estimated that 56% of all child deaths from 53 developing countries were due to underlying malnutrition, as malnourished children had a higher mortality rate for diarrhea, malaria, and pneumonia than well-nourished children [21]. This analysis of the synergistic relationship between malnutrition and childhood mortality has clear implications at the population level in terms of the broader clinical and public health efforts needed to address malnutrition in order to reduce childhood mortality.

The impact of undernutrition on transmission of tuberculosis (TB) in the central-eastern Indian states has been explored using modeling [23]. The authors modeled several different scenarios of future undernutrition, based on reductions in undernutrition achieved over the past 20–30 years by countries such as Bangladesh (5.0% annual decrease in the proportion of their population with inadequate caloric intake), Vietnam (8.0% annual decrease), and Ghana (11.7% annual decrease) [23]. The models suggested that a modest improvement in caloric intake (in range of that achieved in Bangladesh) could avert 4.8 million TB cases and 1.6 million TB deaths in Central and Eastern India over 20 years [23]. In this example, the synergistic relationship was inferred by the association between improvements when caloric intake increased and a proportional reduction in TB cases observed across regions, though the ecologic association may or may not hold in real-world circumstances.

Combined diarrhea and malnutrition provide another example of a synergistic relationship. Severely undernourished children (weight for age z score (WAZ) < −3.0) had an odds ratio of 9.5 for mortality from diarrhea when compared with children with a WAZ > −1.0 [24].

Both macronutrient deficiencies such as protein-energy malnutrition and deficiencies of specific micronutrients can lead to increased severity of infections. Vitamin A deficiency increases the severity of measles to the point that vitamin A supplementation is recommended for children with measles [25–27]. Iron deficiency can also interact synergistically with infections. For example, progression to gastric cancers was increased if Mongolian gerbils infected with *Helicobacter pylori*, a bacterial infection that causes stomach ulcers, were fed an iron-depleted diet instead of an iron-replete diet [28, 29].

## Antagonistic Relationships Between Nutrition and Infection

An antagonistic relationship is less frequent but can be vitally important. One example is when a nutritional deficiency reduces infection-induced pathology more than it reduces the host immune response; a second example is when an infection reduces severity of malnutrition [1]. One early report of the negative effects of malnutrition on the host being countered by a benefit of reduced infection emerged in a feeding camp in Ethiopia during a 1970s famine in Somalia where iron repletion was used. The odds ratio for positive malaria blood smears was 13.4 among those who received supplemental iron, relative to nomads who were iron deficient and who did not receive iron [30]. The antagonistic relationship between malaria and iron continues to be documented, with a recent longitudinal study showing increased risk of a positive malaria smear among infants in the highest quartile of iron status [31]. In a mouse model of urinary tract infections with uropathogenic *Escherichia coli* (UPEC), animals on a low-iron diet had a significantly lower bacterial burden [32]. Dietary iron has also been suggested to have an antagonistic relationship in hookworm infections, with both iron deficiency and iron excess reducing hookworm egg output in hamsters and normal levels of iron significantly increasing hookworm egg output and decreasing hamster survival [33]. This latter example emphasizes the nonlinear relationship between iron supplementation and hookworm infection, with antagonistic effects at extremes of the spectrum of iron status and synergistic effects in the normal range of iron status [33]. In an attempt to strengthen the case for causality, recent studies have focused on potential biological mechanisms underlying antagonistic relationships between iron and infections [34].

## No Relationship Between Nutrition and Infection

There are some infections where mild to moderate malnutrition does not appear to affect risk of infection or disease, and infection does not appear to affect nutritional status. However, a critical assessment must consider the consistency of conclusions among studies, the number of studies/subjects, and whether a given relationship may hold for more extreme nutritional status, as with anemia/low iron and hookworm [33]. In a review of 13 studies of dengue fever and nutrition, there was no consistent pattern between malnutrition measured solely by anthropometry and the three forms of dengue. Interestingly, however, subgroup analyses suggested that more severe dengue (dengue shock syndrome) might be increased in underweight individuals (i.e., synergistic relationship), whereas less severe dengue may be more prevalent in mildly malnourished individuals. Finding no association between nutritional status and disease severity may indicate that a particular pathogen is not affected by host nutritional state or may reflect a heterogeneity of impacts under differing nutritional conditions and/or study populations [35].

# A Conceptual Framework for the Infection-Malnutrition Interface

One of the challenges in clarifying the influences of nutritional status on infection is the ongoing host-pathogen "negotiation" during an infection (Fig. 1.1). At each stage of an infection, the host seeks to block the spread of the pathogen, and the pathogen seeks to overcome the host defenses [36]. Building

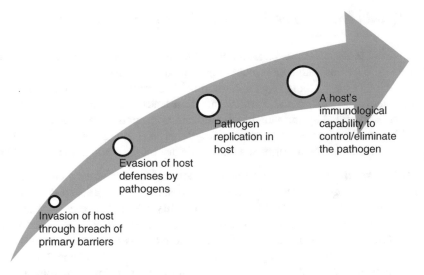

**Fig. 1.1** Classification of host-pathogen interactions. (Reprinted by permission from Springer Nature: Sen et al. [36])

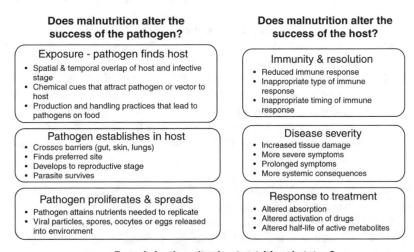

**Fig. 1.2** Pathways by which nutritional status may alter (**a**) pathogen success and (**b**) host success at all stages of infection, through influences on behavior and immune function. Framework for designing, categorizing, and reporting research questions and evidence at the interface of nutrition and infectious diseases. We note that different research designs and evidence are needed to address the questions in each box

on the stages of an infection, we have developed a framework guided by plausible biological mechanisms that delineates phases during the progression of an infection, to enable a more thorough exploration of the potential pathways of influence of nutritional status on infectious diseases. Six stages are identified, three focused on impacts of nutrition on the pathogen and three focused on impacts on the host. Pathways related to the pathogen include (1) finding the host; (2) establishment, maturation, and survival within the host; and (3) division or reproduction of the pathogen and subsequent release of infectious stages to the environment or to another host. Pathways related to the host include (1) immunological or inflammatory responses that may lead to resolution of infection, (2) progression of disease symptoms that may be due to pathogen-induced damage or immunopathology, and (3) response to treatments (Fig. 1.2).

## Exposure (Spatial and Temporal Overlap of Host and Pathogen)

Preventing exposure to an infectious pathogen is one of the primary approaches to preventing infections. Examples of individual behavioral interventions include the use of bednets to prevent mosquito bites and malaria infection, washing vegetables thoroughly to remove potential pathogens, or wearing long pants and sleeves to prevent the *Borrelia* infection leading to Lyme disease. Population-level interventions are exemplified by spraying to kill potential arthropod disease vectors, pasteurization of milk, or fluoridation of a water supply to reduce *Streptococcus mutans*-mediated dental caries. There are multiple pathways by which nutritional status or dietary intake could affect risk of exposure.

**Behavioral Pathways** Both protein-energy malnutrition and iron deficiency can lead to fatigue and limited energy [37], and an early study on human starvation found that reduced mobility compensated for much of the unmet energy needs [38]. Reduced mobility may reduce exposure to outdoor pathogens such as helminths or sylvatic leishmaniasis. In contrast, increased time indoors may increase exposure to airborne respiratory pathogens [39] or exposure to peri-domestic insect vectors that transmit vector-borne diseases such as Chagas disease (see Chap. 6) [40]. A modeling study exploring transmission of mosquito-borne diseases under conditions of varying levels of human mobility found that both low mobility and high mobility populations were predicted to have lower prevalence of infection, with moderately mobile populations having higher rates of transmission [41].

**Diet-Related Pathways** Many pathogens are transmitted through food, either because this is a typical route of exposure, or because of accidental contamination. Thus, dietary choices together with decisions about washing or cooking foods can influence exposure to infectious agents, and food choices and styles of food preparation may themselves be influenced by nutritional status. Both zinc and iron deficiency are strongly associated with pica, defined as the craving and consumption of non-food items such as chalk, ice, paint chips, and soil [42, 43]. A study published in 2010 analyzed 88 samples of soils sold for consumption in markets in Africa, Europe, and the United States and identified bacterial and fungal contamination in almost all of the samples, suggesting that consumption of such non-food items could lead to exposure to pathogens [44].

**Chemical Cues to the Pathogen** A more hypothetical pathway between nutritional status and exposure is the possibility that a malnourished individual emits volatiles that increase or decrease the attractiveness of the host to particular vectors. Vector biting behavior, including choice of humans over livestock and other nonhuman mammals, is strongly influenced by volatile organic compound scents, and there is increasing evidence that volatiles are influenced by diet and metabolism [45]. Vertebrates are known to rely on chemical cues to detect (and choose) prey and to warn of approaching predators. For example, fish release a chemical alarm signal that warns other fish of the presence of predators [46], and both parasite-infected fish and tadpoles have been shown to release alarm signals [47]. Mosquito vectors detect hosts by recognition of volatile compounds [48, 49], visual cues, $CO_2$, human odors, body heat, and other nonvolatile compounds (Fig. 1.3) [50].

While evidence is strong that vectors are influenced by visual and olfactory cues, evidence on the impacts of nutritional status on host odors, $CO_2$ release, and nonvolatiles is still nascent. Restriction of vitamin E intake has been shown to reduce chemical signaling in lizards [51]. If nutritional status affects human emissions in any way, it could alter the ability of parasites or vectors to find a suitable host. Where transmission occurs via active penetration by the pathogen, such as in hookworm, or biting by a vector such as in malaria, volatiles may also attract (or deter) infectious stages and vectors to (from) the host. Malnutrition can also decrease the basal metabolic rate [52], which would lower body heat, thus changing another important vector cue.

**Fig. 1.3** Graphic illustrating the sensory cues used by mosquito vectors to target human hosts depicting visual cues, $CO_2$, odors, body heat, and nonvolatiles. (Reprinted with permission from Elsevier: Montell and Zwiebel [50])

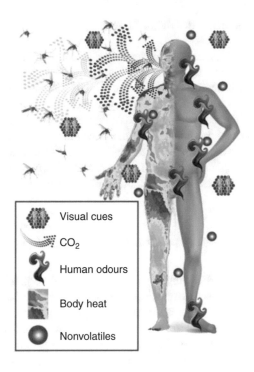

Visual cues

$CO_2$

Human odours

Body heat

Nonvolatiles

## *Establishment of Infection (Pathogen Successfully Crosses Host Barriers, Establishes at Appropriate Tissue Location, and Matures)*

A successful infection requires that infectious agents establish and reach a hospitable final location. This typically involves two steps – (a) breaching protective physical, biological, and chemical barriers, such as epithelial membranes, microbial biofilms, and stomach enzymes, and (b) transitioning (sometimes changing through developmental stages) during migration to a suitable site where replication or reproduction can occur.

### Breaching the Barriers

The integrity and health of barriers can be directly (and indirectly) affected by host nutritional status. Humans have three primary barriers – the gut (gastrointestinal), skin (integumentary), and lung (pulmonary) barriers. With the gut barrier, relationships between nutritional status and epithelial integrity have been demonstrated for vitamin A deficiency and protein-energy malnutrition. Vitamin A deficiency leads to increased intestinal permeability in animal and in vitro models [53, 54], and child malnutrition in general has been closely associated with altered structure and function of the intestinal mucosa [55, 56]. A general thinning of the skin with protein-energy malnutrition in a mouse model has been reported [57]. Several studies have identified a role for vitamin D in pulmonary epithelial integrity [58–60]. However, research on the impact of nutritional status on barrier functions to pathogens is limited primarily to the gut.

**Migration to Target Tissues**

As the pathogen migrates through the host, it faces additional physical barriers such as cell walls, blood vessels, and lung tissue, whose integrity and physical or immunological competence may be affected by macro- or micronutrient deficiencies. During migration, pathogens typically undergo morphological, physiological, biochemical, and molecular transitions that have evolved to enable them to exploit their host. Any of these transitions can be sensitive to host nutritional status, as pathogens are dependent on the host for providing essential nutrients. Once the pathogen reaches its destination, it needs to remain in the site and this often involves adherence to target tissues. Nutrients may play a role in this adherence, as with iron in the case of the vaginal pathogen, *Trichomonas vaginalis*, where iron induces synthesis of key adhesion molecules [61, 62]. Nutrient-dependent mechanisms such as this may be necessary for survival of many pathogens.

## *Pathogen Proliferation (Pathogen Reproduction and Release of Infectious Stages)*

Critical to the ongoing presence of infections in a population is the ability of the pathogen to propagate and then to release infective stages so that the infection can be transmitted to others. Propagation happens in a variety of ways, including viral replication, binary fission, and production of spores or gametes or eggs. As pathogens rely on host nutrients (see Chaps. 4, 5, 6, 7, and 14) [40, 63–66], deficiencies of essential nutrients can have a direct negative impact on pathogen propagation unless the pathogen is able to outcompete the host for the limited nutrients. Research using an avian model has shown that fleas on nestlings that received dietary supplementation laid more eggs than fleas on unsupplemented nestlings [67].

Once a pathogen has reproduced, it is transmitted to new hosts by direct contact; by release of transmission forms into the environment through bodily fluids, feces, or airborne particles; or by transfer into vectors or intermediate hosts. Host nutritional status may reduce movement of the transmission stage out of the host. For example, if peripheral blood flow is reduced, malaria gametocytes may not be available to mosquitoes when they bite. Host nutritional status may alter the interval between infection and transmission, the duration of release of transmission forms from the host, the longevity of infectious stages outside the host, their infectivity to the next host, or the geographical range over which infection is spread. For example, in a randomized controlled trial (RCT) of adults with moderate selenium deficiency, those who received selenium supplements shed poliovirus in the feces for a shorter period after polio vaccination [68]. This could mean that selenium-deficient individuals might transmit the virus for a longer period of time. If nutritional status alters gut transit time through diarrhea or constipation, infective stages might be released prematurely or, alternatively, might be retained in the gut, thus compromising their viability.

Furthermore, through coevolutionary processes, host nutritional status may change pathogen genetics. This has been demonstrated in an experimental model where repeated passage of coxsackievirus B3 virus through several generations of vitamin E-deficient or selenium-deficient mice led to a viral phenotype with increased virulence [69]. In this case, vitamin E and selenium deficiencies increased the pathogenicity of the virus.

## *Immune Responses to Natural Infection and to Vaccines Lead to Resolution of Infection*

When a host kills or expels an established pathogen, this is referred to as natural recovery. Nutritional deficiencies are well known to impair the ability of the host to respond effectively to an infection, allowing persistence of infections that are usually cleared rapidly (see Chap. 3) [70–74]. Nutritional status is accepted as an important modifier of immune response to vaccines, although the specifics of the impacts are less clear [75]. Studies in the 1980s explored particular dimensions of immune response such as B-cell versus T-cell responses to measles vaccination [76, 77]. Protein-energy malnutrition has been associated with a decreased response to tuberculin sensitivity skin tests following BCG vaccination against tuberculosis in children [78], and a third of protein-deficient pigs that were vaccinated with the attenuated human rotavirus vaccine developed diarrhea after subsequent exposure to rotavirus, but none of the vaccinated protein-sufficient pigs did [79]. In an RCT of newborns in Pakistan, zinc deficiency was shown to reduce the efficacy of oral poliovirus vaccine, but surprisingly zinc supplementation did not improve vaccine efficacy [80]. Demonstration of the causal connection between vaccine efficacy and nutritional status has been limited by the low number of studies, poor quality of data, and heterogeneity in variables across studies that make comparisons very challenging [81]. More recently, it seems the gut microbiome may modulate the interaction between nutritional status and vaccine efficacy, at least for oral vaccines [82]. While there are a number of studies assessing impact of malnutrition on immune function (see Chap. 3), studies are still needed to better unpack how nutritional status affects vaccine efficacy [83, 84].

## Disease Severity (Pathogen Leads to Symptoms and/or Immunopathology)

In human populations, infections that are rapidly resolved often go undetected. However, when natural mechanisms of clearance (self-regulation by the infection or immune-mediated processes) are interrupted, infections may become pathogenic, and disease severity may increase. In an observational study of the intestinal protozoan infection *Cryptosporidium parvum*, the prevalence of clinical complications in Jamaican children was higher in children with low weight-for-height compared to well-nourished children [85]. This situation can be seen as an example where malnutrition may have permitted ongoing parasite replication and in turn increased infection-induced disease severity.

Many pathogens have virulence factors that contribute to their ability to cause disease. Nutrient-dependent virulence factors have been identified in numerous pathogens, such as *Entamoeba histolytica* [86], *T. vaginalis* [61], and *H. pylori* [28]. For example, with host iron deficiency, *H. pylori* upregulates high iron affinity transporters in order to obtain the iron it needs, and these high affinity transporters are associated with increased pathogenicity [28]. HIV has also been implicated in nutrition-infection pathogenic interactions (see Chap. 9) [87]. Selenium is one micronutrient where deficiency has been linked to poor HIV clinical outcomes, while selenium supplementation has been shown to improve HIV clinical outcomes and to reduce the incidence of TB among HIV-infected persons [88–91]. Serum retinol has been studied as a risk factor for adverse HIV outcomes, but it is difficult to assess cause and effect, as persons with advancing HIV disease may have altered food intakes and temporality is difficult to determine [92, 93].

The ability of the host to tolerate or limit infection-induced damage can be influenced by nutritional status. Vitamin A/retinoic acid plays a key role in the development of mucosal tolerance through its role in induction of regulatory T cells (Tregs), which are an important downregulator of the immune response. Vitamin A/retinoic acid is an important stimulator of differentiation and proliferation of Tregs, T helper Type 2 (Th2), T helper 17 (Th17), and IgA plasma cells [94]. Appetite is another pathway by which nutrition may affect tolerance to a pathogen. A recent analysis of the impact of fasting behaviors on viral and bacterial infections concluded that fasting was protective against disease progression for a bacterial infection, *Listeria monocytogenes*, in mice, whereas glucose supplementation helped protect mice from influenza virus [95]. With the *L. monocytogenes* infection, anorexia led to ketogenesis which helped to reduce antibacterial inflammation and release of antibacterial reactive oxygen species. In contrast, with influenza, glucose supplementation helped prevent initiation of stress-mediated apoptosis [95]. Nutritional status and dietary intake are important mediators of disease, through pathways affecting both pathogen virulence and host tolerance.

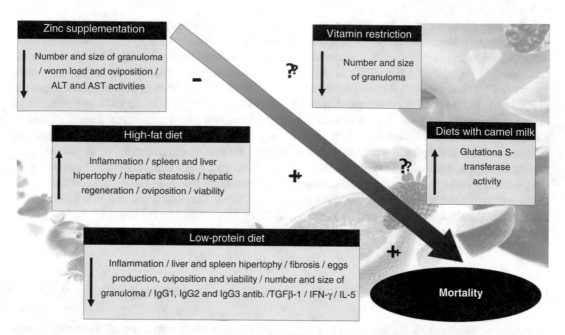

**Fig. 1.4** In vivo preclinical evidence of the impact of different dietary strategies on parasitological, immunological, biochemical, and histopathological parameters in animals infected by *Schistosoma mansoni*. The main diagonal arrow indicated the primary measure of outcome. Black arrows in each box indicate the effect direction for each accessory outcome. (−) mitigates and (+) stimulates mortality. (?) uncertain impact on parasitemia and mortality (insufficient data). (Used with permission from Cambridge University Press: Marques et al. [100])

The severity of many infectious diseases results from an over aggressive immune response that itself causes pathology, as dramatized by the COVID-19 pandemic. In such situations, diet and nutritional status may alter the degree of immunopathology [96–99]. A recent systematic review of preclinical evidence shows that hepatic granulomas in mice infected with the trematode parasite, *Schistosoma mansoni*, were fewer in number and/or size in mice fed low-protein or vitamin-restricted diets and in zinc-supplemented mice, but higher in mice fed a high-fat diet (Fig. 1.4) [100].

## *Response to Treatment (Pathogen Cleared or Symptoms Reduced)*

When an infected individual receives drug treatment, nutritional status may affect the host ability to use the pharmaceuticals effectively. Nutritional status can affect drug distribution, drug absorption, plasma binding of drugs, drug activation, and drug clearance [55, 101–106]. Protein-energy malnutrition alters gut integrity and gastric emptying, which can affect drug absorption. Drug activation, the conversion of an inactive form to the active form, and drug clearance are both important steps for a number of drugs. Cytochrome P450 (CYP) enzymes are the dominant pathway by which drugs are metabolized for both activation and clearance [107, 108]. Both protein-calorie malnutrition and iron deficiency have been shown to affect cytochrome P450 3A4 (CYP3A4) activity. Rats on a protein- and calorie-restricted diet had less CYP generally [109, 110] and CYP3A specifically [109]. In addition, rats with protein-calorie malnutrition had decreased hepatic metabolism via CYP3A [111]. The decrease in activation may affect drug dosage, leading to a need for higher doses in malnourished individuals. One study in patients on hemodialysis with low CYP3A4 found an increase in CYP3A4 after receiving intravenous iron supplementation [112]. These examples emphasize the importance of this often-overlooked area. Chapter 13 provides an in-depth review of drug-nutrient interactions relevant to infectious diseases (see Chap. 13) [113].

## Pathogen Affects Nutritional Status

In terms of the reverse pathway, namely, the pathogen affecting the host's nutritional status, multiple biological pathways have been delineated. Persons with infections can lose their appetites and suffer from gastrointestinal disturbances and many other manifestations that compromise optimal nutrition. Pathogens damage host tissues, they may compete with the host for nutrients, and they induce and maintain energy-intensive immune responses [19, 114]. A vigorous immune response can place extraordinary nutritional demands on a host, and even immune surveillance is nutritionally demanding. Persons with chronic or severe infections may become malnourished unless intakes are adjusted to cover increased demand. Hunger and food insecurity contribute to delayed initiation and nonadherence to antiretroviral therapy for HIV in Africa, especially if patients recognize that the medicines stimulate their appetite and food is unavailable [130]. Damage of host tissue in the gut can impair nutrient absorption and lead to malnutrition, as in the case of environmental enteropathy [115, 116]. Damage to host tissue can also lead to increased physiological demand for nutrients to repair the damage, and if the increased demand cannot be met through available diets, the body may draw down other physiological stores, thus limiting physiological functioning [114]. Bartelt and colleagues have developed a model of protein-deficient mice coinfected with *Giardia lamblia* and enteroaggregative *Escherichia coli* for exploring impacts of coinfection on malnutrition and vice versa [117]. The authors demonstrated that the combined infection and protein deficiency led to a greater weight loss and alterations in metabolic functioning than the combined infection and an isocaloric complete diet, although both protocols led to weight loss [117].

Infection-induced immune responses can result in release of pyrogens such as prostaglandin $E_2$ that triggers an increased basal metabolic rate and fever. Counter to the old adage "feed a cold and starve a fever," fever increases the nutrient need of the host. A small study of 12 healthy volunteers demonstrated that fasting facilitated a humoral immune response, whereas eating fostered more of a cell-mediated response [118]. Perhaps infections that are resolved by a humoral response (like many helminth infections) would benefit from fasting, whereas those that are cleared by a cell-mediated response (many bacterial and protozoan infections that induce a fever) would be exacerbated by fasting.

There is a growing awareness of the complex ways that pathogens, diet, and the microbiota of a host interact, and a comprehensive understanding of the impacts of such interactions is still nascent. A recent study highlighting the influences of diet on the microbiome found that two groups of mice with the same initial microbiome composition had different microbial communities 8 weeks after being fed a low-fat and high-plant polysaccharide diet (similar to rural limited resource settings) compared with a high-fat high-sugar diet (Western) [119]. Research on the microbiome as a potential mediator of nutrition-infection interactions is important to consider going forward [120].

## Challenges in Investigating Nutrition and Infectious Disease

Once mechanisms by which nutritional status affect infections have been demonstrated, there are several challenges in estimating the impact in human populations: (1) heterogeneity of nutritional status; (2) heterogeneity of infections; (3) a historical research emphasis on the role of infections in causing malnutrition rather than the opposite; and (4) difficulty in extrapolating from controlled lab studies to human populations.

Nutritional status can vary at the level of macronutrient and/or micronutrient concentration within individuals (i.e., high level of one nutrient, low or moderate levels of other nutrients) and also among individuals within communities and between communities. Identifying relatively homogeneous populations that differ in nutritional variables of interest but that are similar for other nutritional variables is challenging. Deficiencies or excesses of macro- or micronutrients seldom occur apart from other nutritional perturbations. Thus measurements of multiple nutrients are essential for accurately characterizing nutritional status, with significant associated clinical or public health research costs [121]. In addition, individual nutritional status is difficult to measure, both at the macro- and micronutrient levels. High-quality biomarkers of nutritional status are expensive to obtain and challenging to interpret, as nutrient levels in bodily fluids can shift as nutrients are shuttled to different locations in the body, despite no changes in overall nutrient status. For example, serum biomarkers of nutritional status are highly variable, depending on multiple factors including time since the most recent meal, infection status, hydration, diurnal variation, varying metabolic demands, and perhaps host genetics [122]. A field study of children in Zambia found alterations in biomarkers of iron and vitamin A that varied by stage of the acute phase response (incubation, early convalescence, convalescence, and healthy) as measured by C-reactive protein and $\alpha_1$-acid glycoprotein (AGP) [123, 124]. Given the multiple potential influences on such biomarkers, identifying optimum cutoffs as indicative of deficiency is challenging.

Similarly, individuals, communities, and regions can vary in terms of the number and variety of infections [125]. In human populations, infections vary in terms of the time since exposure to the pathogen, the exposure dose, or intensity of infection, whether it is an initial infection or a secondary infection with the same agent, and what other pathogens and microbiome the host harbors. Each of these factors can affect immune response and potentially also the interaction between nutrition and infection.

An additional challenge is that a multiplicity of factors can affect nutrition and, similarly, that a large number of factors can affect infection. This complexity makes it challenging to generalize from highly controlled laboratory models to free-living situations (see Box 1.2), even though laboratory models are very helpful in identifying generative causal relationships. The field of ecology is replete with examples where a scientist can demonstrate a clear pattern in the laboratory that is not apparent under more natural conditions. The profile of infection dynamics of an intestinal nematode of mice, *Heligmosomoides polygyrus*, differed markedly between an inbred susceptible and inbred resistant strain of mouse under controlled laboratory infections. However, when the two strains lived together in a large indoor enclosure where natural transmission occurred, the infection profile was undistin-

---

**Box 1.2  Impact of Variations in Pathogen Virulence and Host Susceptibility**

Scrimshaw et al. (citing H.S. Schneider, 1950, *Strategic concepts in Epidemiology*) note that laboratory studies generally use homogeneous animal and disease models, where virulence of the pathogen and susceptibility of the host are known. Schneider used an experimental 3 × 3 study design with three host characteristics (1) inbred resistant, (2) outbred mixed (mix of susceptible and resistant), and (3) inbred susceptible as well as three pathogen characteristics (a) uniformly virulent, (b) mixed virulent and avirulent, and (c) uniformly avirulent, to explore the impact of nutritional status. Schneider found that nutritional status only played a role in the outbred host group that was infected with the mixed virulence pathogen, a situation most likely found in humans. Thus, highly controlled laboratory models may actually *underestimate* the impact of nutrition in real-world settings [1].

guishable between the two strains [126]. Similarly, resistance of C57BL/6 inbred lab mice to the intestinal nematode, *Trichuris muris*, was not evident when the mice were moved into a seminatural outdoor enclosure prior to, or after experimental infection, as evidenced by higher number of worms and worm biomass relative to mice infected in the lab [127]. This contextual element for infection extends to nutrition-infection interactions, where laboratory conditions and conclusions may not be generalizable even to natural infections in the mouse. This makes it even harder to extrapolate lab findings to humans.

## Conclusions

Taken together, this overview highlights the myriad pathways by which host nutritional status may influence all aspects of the host-pathogen interaction. It also highlights the challenges in both design and analysis faced by researchers whose goal is to demonstrate causality, and by inference the challenges faced by clinical and public health sectors charged with preventing and controlling infectious diseases. Through the examples provided in the subsequent chapters of this book, we hope to highlight not only the need for more rigorous application of causality analysis especially during epidemiological research and in systematic reviews and meta-analyses on infection-nutrition interactions but also the importance of laboratory research that identifies plausible mechanisms that may be relevant in human populations. Given the influence of nutritional status on infections and vice versa, effective global control of infectious disease will require addressing the relationships between malnutrition and infections [128], and the conceptual framework proposed in this chapter may be useful in this context.

## References

1. Scrimshaw NS, Taylor CE, Gordon JE. Interactions of nutrition and infection. Monogr Ser World Health Organ. 1968;57:3–329.
2. Barffour MA, Humphries DL. Core principles: infectious disease risk in relation to macro and micronutrient status. In: Humphries DL, Scott ME, Vermund SH, editors. Nutrition and infectious disease: shifting the clinical paradigm. Totowa: Humana Press; 2020.
3. Shea-Donohue T, Qin B, Smith A. Parasites, nutrition, immune responses and biology of metabolic tissues. Parasite Immunol. 2017;39(5). https://doi.org/10.1111/pim.12422.
4. Biesalski HK. Nutrition meets the microbiome: micronutrients and the microbiota. Ann N Y Acad Sci. 2016;1372(1):53–64.
5. Valdes AM, Walter J, Segal E, Spector TD. Role of the gut microbiota in nutrition and health. BMJ. 2018;361:k2179.
6. Kosmiski L. Energy expenditure in HIV infection. Am J Clin Nutr. 2011;94(6):1677S–82S.
7. Diderichsen F, Hallqvist J, Whitehead M. Differential vulnerability and susceptibility: how to make use of recent development in our understanding of mediation and interaction to tackle health inequalities. Int J Epidemiol. 2019;48(1):268–74.
8. Khoury MJ, Flanders WD, Greenland S, Adams MJ. On the measurement of susceptibility in epidemiologic studies. Am J Epidemiol. 1989;129(1):183–90.
9. Mosby's Medical Dictionary. 2009. https://medical-dictionary.thefreedictionary.com/susceptibility. Accessed 12 Aug 2019.
10. McGraw-Hill concise dictionary of modern medicine. New York: McGraw-Hill; 2002.
11. Falcon A. Aristotle on causality. The Stanford encyclopedia of philosophy. Stanford: The Metaphysics Research Lab, Center for the Study of Language and Information, Stanford University; 2019.
12. Parascandola M, Weed DL. Causation in epidemiology. J Epidemiol Community Health. 2001;55(12):905–12.
13. Thygesen LC, Andersen GS, Andersen H. A philosophical analysis of the Hill criteria. J Epidemiol Community Health. 2005;59(6):512–6.

14. Doll R, Peto R. The causes of cancer: quantitative estimates of avoidable risks of cancer in the United States today. J Natl Cancer Inst. 1981;66(6):1191–308.

15. Hill AB. The environment and disease: association or causation? J R Soc Med. 2015;108(1):32–7.

16. Potischman N, Weed DL. Causal criteria in nutritional epidemiology. Am J Clin Nutr. 1999;69(6):1309S–14S.

17. Monteiro WM, Alexandre MA, Siqueira A, Melo G, Romero GA, d'Avila E, et al. Could Plasmodium vivax malaria trigger malnutrition? Revisiting the Bradford Hill criteria to assess a causal relationship between two neglected problems. Rev Soc Bras Med Trop. 2016;49(3):274–8.

18. Scrimshaw NS, SanGiovanni JP. Synergism of nutrition, infection, and immunity: an overview. Am J Clin Nutr. 1997;66(2):464S–77S.

19. Bourke CD, Berkley JA, Prendergast AJ. Immune dysfunction as a cause and consequence of malnutrition. Trends Immunol. 2016;37(6):386–98. https://doi.org/10.1016/j.it.2016.04.003.

20. Walson JL, Berkley JA. The impact of malnutrition on childhood infections. Curr Opin Infect Dis. 2018;31(3):231–6.

21. Pelletier DL, Frongillo EA Jr, Schroeder DG, Habicht JP. The effects of malnutrition on child mortality in developing countries. Bull World Health Organ. 1995;73(4):443–8.

22. Pelletier DL, Frongillo EA Jr, Schroeder DG, Habicht JP. A methodology for estimating the contribution of malnutrition to child mortality in developing countries. J Nutr. 1994;124(10 Suppl):2106S–22S.

23. Oxlade O, Huang CC, Murray M. Estimating the impact of reducing under-nutrition on the tuberculosis epidemic in the central eastern states of India: a dynamic modeling study. PLoS ONE. 2015;10(6):e0128187.

24. Black RE, Allen LH, Bhutta ZA, Caulfield LE, de Onis M, Ezzati M, et al. Maternal and child undernutrition: global and regional exposures and health consequences. Lancet. 2008;371(9608):243–60.

25. D'Souza RM, D'Souza R. Vitamin A for treating measles in children. Cochrane Database Syst Rev. 2002;(1):CD001479.

26. Coutsoudis A, Broughton M, Coovadia HM. Vitamin A supplementation reduces measles morbidity in young African children: a randomized, placebo-controlled, double-blind trial. Am J Clin Nutr. 1991;54(5):890–5.

27. Coutsoudis A, Kiepiela P, Coovadia HM, Broughton M. Vitamin A supplementation enhances specific IgG antibody levels and total lymphocyte numbers while improving morbidity in measles. Pediatr Infect Dis J. 1992;11(3):203–9.

28. Haley KP, Gaddy JA. Nutrition and Helicobacter pylori: host diet and nutritional immunity influence bacterial virulence and disease outcome. Gastroenterol Res Pract. 2016;2016:3019362.

29. Noto JM, Gaddy JA, Lee JY, Piazuelo MB, Friedman DB, Colvin DC, et al. Iron deficiency accelerates Helicobacter pylori-induced carcinogenesis in rodents and humans. J Clin Invest. 2013;123(1):479–92.

30. Murray MJ, Murray AB, Murray MB, Murray CJ. The adverse effect of iron repletion on the course of certain infections. Br Med J. 1978;2(6145):1113–5.

31. Moya-Alvarez V, Cottrell G, Ouedraogo S, Accrombessi M, Massougbodgi A, Cot M. High iron levels are associated with increased malaria risk in infants during the first year of life in Benin. Am J Trop Med Hyg. 2017;97(2):497–503.

32. Bauckman KA, Matsuda R, Higgins CB, DeBosch BJ, Wang C, Mysorekar IU. Dietary restriction of iron availability attenuates UPEC pathogenesis in a mouse model of urinary tract infection. Am J Physiol Renal Physiol. 2019;316(5):F814–22.

33. Held MR, Bungiro RD, Harrison LM, Hamza I, Cappello M. Dietary iron content mediates hookworm pathogenesis in vivo. Infect Immun. 2006;74(1):289–95.

34. Spottiswoode N, Duffy PE, Drakesmith H. Iron, anemia and hepcidin in malaria. Front Pharmacol. 2014;5:125.

35. Trang NTH, Long NP, Hue TTM, Hung LP, Trung TD, Dinh DN, et al. Association between nutritional status and dengue infection: a systematic review and meta-analysis. BMC Infect Dis. 2016;16:172.

36. Sen R, Nayak L, De RK. A review on host-pathogen interactions: classification and prediction. Eur J Clin Microbiol Infect Dis. 2016;35(10):1581–99.

37. Yokoi K, Konomi A. Iron deficiency without anaemia is a potential cause of fatigue: meta-analyses of randomised controlled trials and cross-sectional studies. Br J Nutr. 2017;117(10):1422–31.

38. Keys A, Brozek J, Henschel A, Mickelson A, Taylor H. The biology of human starvation. Minneapolis: University of Minnesota Press; 1950.

39. Sze To GN, Chao CY. Review and comparison between the Wells-Riley and dose-response approaches to risk assessment of infectious respiratory diseases. Indoor Air. 2010;20(1):2–16.

40. Wiser MF. Nutrition and protozoan pathogens of humans—a primer. In: Humphries DL, Scott ME, Vermund SH, editors. Nutrition and infectious diseases: shifting the clinical paradigm. Totowa: Humana Press; 2020.

41. Acevedo MA, Prosper O, Lopiano K, Ruktanonchai N, Caughlin TT, Martcheva M, et al. Spatial heterogeneity, host movement and mosquito-borne disease transmission. PLoS ONE. 2015;10(6):e0127552.

42. Miao D, Young SL, Golden CD. A meta-analysis of pica and micronutrient status. Am J Hum Biol. 2015;27(1):84–93. https://doi.org/10.1002/ajhb.22598.

43. Borgna-Pignatti C, Zanella S. Pica as a manifestation of iron deficiency. Expert Rev Hematol. 2016;9(11):1075–80.

44. Kutalek R, Wewalka G, Gundacker C, Auer H, Wilson J, Haluza D, et al. Geophagy and potential health implications: geohelminths, microbes and heavy metals. Trans R Soc Trop Med Hyg. 2010;104(12):787–95.
45. Spanel P, Smith D. Volatile compounds in health and disease. Curr Opin Clin Nutr Metab Care. 2011;14(5):455–60.
46. Brown GE, Elvidge CK, Macnaughton CJ, Ramnarine I, Godin JGJ. Cross-population responses to conspecific chemical alarm cues in wild Trinidadian guppies, Poecilia reticulata: evidence for local conservation of cue production. Can J Zool. 2010;88(2):139–47.
47. Poulin R, Marcogliese DJ, McLaughlin JD. Skin-penetrating parasites and the release of alarm substances in juvenile rainbow trout. J Fish Biol. 1999;55(1):47–53.
48. Majeed S, Hill SR, Birgersson G, Ignell R. Detection and perception of generic host volatiles by mosquitoes modulate host preference: context dependence of (R)-1-octen-3-ol. R Soc Open Sci. 2016;3(11):160467.
49. Majeed S, Hill SR, Dekker T, Ignell R. Detection and perception of generic host volatiles by mosquitoes: responses to $CO_2$ constrains host-seeking behaviour. R Soc Open Sci. 2017;4(5):170189.
50. Montell C, Zwiebel LJ. Mosquito sensory systems. In: Raikhel AS, editor. Advances in insect physiology, vol. 51. London: Elsevier; 2016.
51. Garcia-Roa R, Saiz J, Gomara B, Lopez P, Martin J. Dietary constraints can preclude the expression of an honest chemical sexual signal. Sci Rep. 2017;7(1):6073.
52. McCue MD. Starvation physiology: reviewing the different strategies animals use to survive a common challenge. Comp Biochem Physiol A Mol Integr Physiol. 2010;156(1):1–18.
53. Li Y, Gao Y, Cui T, Yang T, Liu L, Li T, et al. Retinoic acid facilitates toll-like receptor 4 expression to improve intestinal barrier function through retinoic acid receptor beta. Cell Physiol Biochem. 2017;42(4):1390–406.
54. de Medeiros PHQS, Pinto DV, de Almeida JZ, Rego JMC, Rodrigues FAP, Lima AAM, et al. Modulation of intestinal immune and barrier functions by vitamin a: implications for current understanding of malnutrition and enteric infections in children. Nutrients. 2018;10(9):1128.
55. Rytter MJ, Kolte L, Briend A, Friis H, Christensen VB. The immune system in children with malnutrition—a systematic review. PLoS ONE. 2014;9(8):e105017.
56. Attia S, Feenstra M, Swain N, Cuesta M, Bandsma RHJ. Starved guts: morphologic and functional intestinal changes in malnutrition. J Pediatr Gastroenterol Nutr. 2017;65(5):491–5.
57. Sugiyama A, Fujita Y, Kobayashi T, Ryu M, Suzuki Y, Masuda A, et al. Effect of protein malnutrition on the skin epidermis of hairless mice. J Vet Med Sci. 2011;73(6):831–5.
58. Gorman S, Buckley AG, Ling KM, Berry LJ, Fear VS, Stick SM, et al. Vitamin D supplementation of initially vitamin D-deficient mice diminishes lung inflammation with limited effects on pulmonary epithelial integrity. Physiol Rep. 2017;5(15):e13371.
59. Li W, Dong H, Zhao H, Song J, Tang H, Yao L, et al. 1,25-Dihydroxyvitamin D3 prevents toluene diisocyanate-induced airway epithelial barrier disruption. Int J Mol Med. 2015;36(1):263–70.
60. Shi YY, Liu TJ, Fu JH, Xu W, Wu LL, Hou AN, et al. Vitamin D/VDR signaling attenuates lipopolysaccharide induced acute lung injury by maintaining the integrity of the pulmonary epithelial barrier. Mol Med Rep. 2016;13(2):1186–94.
61. Figueroa-Angulo EE, Rendon-Gandarilla FJ, Puente-Rivera J, Calla-Choque JS, Cardenas-Guerra RE, Ortega-Lopez J, et al. The effects of environmental factors on the virulence of Trichomonas vaginalis. Microbes Infect. 2012;14(15):1411–27.
62. Moreno-Brito V, Yanez-Gomez C, Meza-Cervantez P, Avila-Gonzalez L, Rodriguez MA, Ortega-Lopez J, et al. A Trichomonas vaginalis 120 kDa protein with identity to hydrogenosome pyruvate:ferredoxin oxidoreductase is a surface adhesin induced by iron. Cell Microbiol. 2005;7(2):245–58.
63. Berkley JA. Bacterial infections and nutrition—a primer. In: Humphries DL, Scott ME, Vermund SH, editors. Nutrition and infectious disease: shifting the clinical paradigm. Totowa: Humana Press; 2020.
64. Green WD, Karlsson EA, Beck MA. Viral infections and nutrition: influenza virus as a case study. In: Humphries DL, Scott ME, Vermund SH, editors. Nutrition and infectious disease: shifting the clinical paradigm. Totowa: Humana Press; 2020.
65. Geary TG, Haque M. Human Helminth infections. In: Humphries DL, Scott ME, Vermund SH, editors. Nutrition and infectious disease: shifting the clinical paradigm. Totowa: Humana Press; 2020.
66. Ezenwa VO. Co-infection and nutrition: integrating ecological and epidemiological perspectives. In: Humphries DL, Scott ME, Vermund SH, editors. Nutrition and infectious disease: shifting the clinical paradigm. Totowa: Springer; 2020.
67. Tschirren B, Bischoff LL, Saladin V, Richner H. Host condition and host immunity affect parasite fitness in a bird-ectoparasite system. Funct Ecol. 2007;21(2):372–8.
68. Broome CS, McArdle F, Kyle JA, Andrews F, Lowe NM, Hart CA, et al. An increase in selenium intake improves immune function and poliovirus handling in adults with marginal selenium status. Am J Clin Nutr. 2004;80(1):154–62.

69. Beck MA. Increased virulence of coxsackievirus B3 in mice due to vitamin E or selenium deficiency. J Nutr. 1997;127(5 Suppl):966S–70S.

70. Stephensen CB. Primer on immune response and interface with malnutrition. In: Humphries DL, Scott ME, Vermund SH, editors. Nutrition and infectious disease: shifting the clinical paradigm. Totowa: Humana Press; 2020.

71. Maares M, Haase H. Zinc and immunity: an essential interrelation. Arch Biochem Biophys. 2016;611:58–65.

72. Avery JC, Hoffmann PR. Selenium, selenoproteins, and immunity. Nutrients. 2018;10(9):1203.

73. Bono MR, Tejon G, Flores-Santibanez F, Fernandez D, Rosemblatt M, Sauma D. Retinoic acid as a modulator of T cell immunity. Nutrients. 2016;8(6):349.

74. Spinas E, Saggini A, Kritas SK, Cerulli G, Caraffa A, Antinolfi P, et al. Crosstalk between vitamin B and immunity. J Biol Regul Homeost Agents. 2015;29(2):283–8.

75. Zimmermann P, Curtis N. Factors that influence the immune response to vaccination. Clin Microbiol Rev. 2019;32(2):e00084–18.

76. Idris S, El Seed AM. Measles vaccination in severely malnourished Sudanese children. Ann Trop Paediatr. 1983;3(2):63–7.

77. Powell GM. Response to live attenuated measles vaccine in children with severe kwashiorkor. Ann Trop Paediatr. 1982;2(3):143–5.

78. Udani PM. BCG vaccination in India and tuberculosis in children: newer facets. Indian J Pediatr. 1994;61(5):451–62.

79. Miyazaki A, Kandasamy S, Michael H, Langel SN, Paim FC, Chepngeno J, et al. Protein deficiency reduces efficacy of oral attenuated human rotavirus vaccine in a human infant fecal microbiota transplanted gnotobiotic pig model. Vaccine. 2018;36(42):6270–81.

80. Habib MA, Soofi S, Sheraz A, Bhatti ZS, Okayasu H, Zaidi SZ, et al. Zinc supplementation fails to increase the immunogenicity of oral poliovirus vaccine: a randomized controlled trial. Vaccine. 2015;33(6):819–25.

81. Savy M, Edmond K, Fine PE, Hall A, Hennig BJ, Moore SE, et al. Landscape analysis of interactions between nutrition and vaccine responses in children. J Nutr. 2009;139(11):2154S–218S.

82. Bhattacharjee A, Hand TW. Role of nutrition, infection, and the microbiota in the efficacy of oral vaccines. Clin Sci (Lond). 2018;132(11):1169–77.

83. Smailnejad Ganji K, Mohammadzadeh I, Mohammadnia-Afrouzi M, Ebrahimpour S, Shahbazi M. Factors affecting immune responses to vaccines. Gazz Med Ital. 2018;177(5):219–28.

84. Parker EP, Ramani S, Lopman BA, Church JA, Iturriza-Gomara M, Prendergast AJ, et al. Causes of impaired oral vaccine efficacy in developing countries. Future Microbiol. 2018;13:97–118.

85. MacFarlane DE, Horner-Bryce J. Cryptosporidiosis in well nourished and malnourished children. Acta Paediatr. 1987;76(3):474–7.

86. Gastelum-Martinez A, Leon-Sicairos C, Plata-Guzman L, Soto-Castro L, Leon-Sicairos N, de la Garza M. Iron-modulated virulence factors of Entamoeba histolytica. Future Microbiol. 2018;13:1329–41.

87. Wanke C, Baum M. Nutrition in HIV and tuberculosis. In: Humphries DL, Scott ME, Vermund SH, editors. Nutrition and infectious disease: shifting the clinical paradigm. Totowa: Springer; 2020.

88. Baum MK, Shor-Posner G, Lai S, Zhang G, Lai H, Fletcher MA, et al. High risk of HIV-related mortality is associated with selenium deficiency. J Acquir Immune Defic Syndr Hum Retrovirol. 1997;15(5):370–4.

89. Campa A, Baum MK, Bussmann H, Martinez SS, Farahani M, van Widenfelt E, et al. The effect of micronutrient supplementation on active TB incidence early in HIV infection in Botswana. Nutr Diet Suppl. 2017;9:37–45.

90. Campa A, Shor-Posner G, Indacochea F, Zhang G, Lai H, Asthana D, et al. Mortality risk in selenium-deficient HIV-positive children. J Acquir Immune Defic Syndr Hum Retrovirol. 1999;20(5):508–13.

91. Hurwitz BE, Klaus JR, Llabre MM, Gonzalez A, Lawrence PJ, Maher KJ, et al. Suppression of human immunodeficiency virus type 1 viral load with selenium supplementation: a randomized controlled trial. Arch Intern Med. 2007;167(2):148–54.

92. Kassu A, Andualem B, Van Nhien N, Nakamori M, Nishikawa T, Yamamoto S, et al. Vitamin A deficiency in patients with diarrhea and HIV infection in Ethiopia. Asia Pac J Clin Nutr. 2007;16(Suppl 1):323–8.

93. Camp WL, Allen S, Alvarez JO, Jolly PE, Weiss HL, Phillips JF, et al. Serum retinol and HIV-1 RNA viral load in rapid and slow progressors. J Acquir Immune Defic Syndr Hum Retrovirol. 1998;18(4):401–6.

94. Sirisinha S. The pleiotropic role of vitamin A in regulating mucosal immunity. Asian Pac J Allergy Immunol. 2015;33(2):71–89.

95. Wang A, Huen SC, Luan HH, Yu S, Zhang C, Gallezot JD, et al. Opposing effects of fasting metabolism on tissue tolerance in bacterial and viral inflammation. Cell. 2016;166(6):1512–25.e12.

96. Zabetakis I, Lordan R, Norton C, Tsoupras A. COVID-19: the inflammation link and the role of nutrition in potential mitigation. Nutrients. 2020;12(5):1466.

97. Ciavarella C, Motta I, Valente S, Pasquinelli G. Pharmacological (or synthetic) and nutritional agonists of PPAR-gamma as candidates for cytokine storm modulation in COVID-19 disease. Molecules. 2020;25(9):2076.

98. Grant WB, Lahore H, McDonnell SL, Baggerly CA, French CB, Aliano JL, et al. Evidence that vitamin D supplementation could reduce risk of influenza and COVID-19 infections and deaths. Nutrients. 2020;12(4):988.
99. Cena H, Chieppa M. Coronavirus disease (COVID-19-SARS-CoV-2) and nutrition: is infection in Italy suggesting a connection? Front Immunol. 2020;11:944.
100. Marques DVB, Felizardo AA, Souza RLM, Pereira AAC, Goncalves RV, Novaes RD. Could diet composition modulate pathological outcomes in schistosomiasis mansoni? A systematic review of in vivo preclinical evidence. Parasitology. 2018;145(9):1127–36.
101. Oshikoya KA, Sammons HM, Choonara I. A systematic review of pharmacokinetics studies in children with protein-energy malnutrition. Eur J Clin Pharmacol. 2010;66(10):1025–35.
102. Murray M. Altered CYP expression and function in response to dietary factors: potential roles in disease pathogenesis. Curr Drug Metab. 2006;7(1):67–81.
103. Murray M, Marden NY, Lee AC. Altered CYP expression and function by dietary factors: potential roles in disease pathogenesis. Drug Metab Rev. 2006;38:19–20.
104. Mehta S, Nain CK, Sharma B, Mathur VS. Disposition of four drugs in malnourished children. Drug Nutr Interact. 1982;1(3):205–11.
105. Walker O, Dawodu AH, Salako LA, Alvan G, Johnson AO. Single dose disposition of chloroquine in kwashiorkor and normal children—evidence for decreased absorption in kwashiorkor. Br J Clin Pharmacol. 1987;23(4):467–72.
106. Boullata JI, Hudson LM. Drug-nutrient interactions: a broad view with implications for practice. J Acad Nutr Diet. 2012;112(4):506–17.
107. Walter-Sack I, Klotz U. Influence of diet and nutritional status on drug metabolism. Clin Pharmacokinet. 1996;31(1):47–64.
108. Cederbaum AI. Molecular mechanisms of the microsomal mixed function oxidases and biological and pathological implications. Redox Biol. 2015;4:60–73.
109. Lee PC, Struve MF, Bezerra JA, Duncan B. Effects of protein malnutrition on liver cytochrome P450s. Nutr Res. 1997;17(10):1577–87.
110. Lee JH, Suh OK, Lee MG. Pharmacokinetic changes in drugs during protein-calorie malnutrition: correlation between drug metabolism and hepatic microsomal cytochrome P450 isozymes. Arch Pharm Res. 2004;27(7):693–712.
111. Lee YK, Yoon I, Lee MG, Choi YH. Effects of cysteine on the pharmacokinetics of tamoxifen in rats with protein-calorie malnutrition. Xenobiotica. 2012;42(12):1225–34.
112. Pai AB, Norenberg J, Boyd A, Raj D, Chan LN. Effect of intravenous iron supplementation on hepatic cytochrome P450 3A4 activity in hemodialysis patients: a prospective, open-label study. Clin Ther. 2007;29(12):2699–705.
113. Boullata JI. Drug-nutrition interactions in infectious diseases. In: Humphries DL, Scott ME, Vermund SH, editors. Nutrition and infectious disease: shifting the clinical paradigm. Totowa: Humana Press; 2020.
114. Stephensen CB. Burden of infection on growth failure. J Nutr. 1999;129(2S Suppl):534S–8S.
115. Guerrant RL, Oria RB, Moore SR, Oria MO, Lima AA. Malnutrition as an enteric infectious disease with long-term effects on child development. Nutr Rev. 2008;66(9):487–505.
116. Korpe PS, Petri WA Jr. Environmental enteropathy: critical implications of a poorly understood condition. Trends Mol Med. 2012;18(6):328–36.
117. Bartelt LA, Bolick DT, Mayneris-Perxachs J, Kolling GL, Medlock GL, Zaenker EI, et al. Cross-modulation of pathogen-specific pathways enhances malnutrition during enteric co-infection with Giardia lamblia and enteroaggregative Escherichia coli. PLoS Pathog. 2017;13(7):e1006471.
118. van den Brink GR, van den Boogaardt DE, van Deventer SJ, Peppelenbosch MP. Feed a cold, starve a fever? Clin Diagn Lab Immunol. 2002;9(1):182–3.
119. Turnbaugh PJ, Ridaura VK, Faith JJ, Rey FE, Knight R, Gordon JI. The effect of diet on the human gut microbiome: a metagenomic analysis in humanized gnotobiotic mice. Sci Transl Med. 2009;1(6):6ra14.
120. Goulet O. Potential role of the intestinal microbiota in programming health and disease. Nutr Rev. 2015;73(Suppl 1):32–40.
121. Gonzalez-Fernandez D, Pons ED, Rueda D, Sinisterra OT, Murillo E, Scott ME, et al. C-reactive protein is differentially modulated by co-existing infections, vitamin deficiencies and maternal factors in pregnant and lactating indigenous Panamanian women. Infect Dis Poverty. 2017;6(1):94.
122. Gibson R. Principles of nutritional assessment. 2nd ed. Oxford: Oxford University Press; 2005.
123. Bresnahan KA, Chileshe J, Arscott S, Nuss E, Surles R, Masi C, et al. The acute phase response affected traditional measures of micronutrient status in rural Zambian children during a randomized, controlled feeding trial. J Nutr. 2014;144(6):972–8.
124. Bresnahan KA, Tanumihardjo SA. Undernutrition, the acute phase response to infection, and its effects on micronutrient status indicators. Adv Nutr. 2014;5(6):702–11.

125. Gonzalez-Fernandez D, Koski KG, Sinisterra OT, Del Carmen PE, Murillo E, Scott ME. Interactions among urogenital, intestinal, skin, and oral infections in pregnant and lactating Panamanian Ngabe women: a neglected public health challenge. Am J Trop Med Hyg. 2015;92(6):1100–10.
126. Scott ME. Heligmosomoides polygyrus (Nematoda): susceptible and resistant strains of mice are indistinguishable following natural infection. Parasitology. 1991;103(Pt 3):429–38.
127. Leung JM, Budischak SA, Chung The H, Hansen C, Bowcutt R, Neill R, et al. Rapid environmental effects on gut nematode susceptibility in rewilded mice. PLoS Biol. 2018;16(3):e2004108.
128. Bhutta ZA, Berkley JA, Bandsma RHJ, Kerac M, Trehan I, Briend A. Severe childhood malnutrition. Nat Rev Dis Primers. 2017;3:17067.
129. Evans AS. Causation and disease: a chronological journey. The Thomas Parran lecture. Am J Epidemiol. 1978;108(4):249–58.
130. Chop E, Duggaraju A, Malley A, Burke V, Caldas S, Yeh PT et al. Food insecurity, sexual risk behavior, and adherence to antiretroviral therapy among women living with HIV: A systematic review. Health Care Women Int. 2017; 38(9):927.

# Chapter 2
# Core Principles in Nutrition: Nutrient Needs, Metabolism, and Potential Influences on Infectious Diseases

**Maxwell A. Barffour and Debbie L. Humphries**

## Abbreviations

| | |
|---|---|
| Ab | Antibody |
| AGP | Alpha glycoprotein |
| ALA | Alpha linolenic acid |
| AMDR | Acceptable macronutrient distribution range |
| ATP | Adenosine triphosphate |
| CoA | Coenzyme A |
| CRBP | Cellular retinol binding protein |
| CRP | C-reactive protein |
| DCytB | Duodenal cytochrome B |
| DIT | Diiodotyrosine |
| DMTI | Divalent metal transporter |
| DNA | Deoxy-ribonucleic acid |
| EAR | Estimated average requirement |
| EPA | Eicosapentaenoic Acid |
| EPO | Erythropoietin |
| FAO | Food and Agriculture Organization |
| GLUT | Glucose transporter |
| GPX | Glutathione peroxidase |
| HCP | Heme carrier protein |
| HDL | High-density lipoprotein |
| ID | Iron deficiency |
| IDD | Iodine deficiency disorders!!! |
| IgG | Immunoglobulin |
| IZiNCG | International Zinc Nutrition Consultative Group |

M. A. Barffour (✉)
McQueary College of Health and Human Services, Missouri State University, Springfield, MO, USA

University of Missouri School of Medicine, Columbia, MO, USA
e-mail: maxwellabarffour@missouristate.edu

D. L. Humphries
Epidemiology of Microbial Disease, Yale School of Public Health, Yale University, New Haven, CT, USA
e-mail: debbie.humphries@yale.edu

© Springer Nature Switzerland AG 2021
D. L. Humphries et al. (eds.), *Nutrition and Infectious Diseases*, Nutrition and Health,
https://doi.org/10.1007/978-3-030-56913-6_2

| | |
|---|---|
| LDL | Low-density lipoprotein |
| MIT | Mono-diiodotyrosine |
| mRNA | Messenger ribonucleic acid |
| PEM | Protein energy malnutrition |
| PTH | Parathyroid hormone |
| PUFA | Polyunsaturated fatty acid |
| RBP | Retinol binding protein |
| RDA | Recommended dietary allowance |
| RNA | Ribonucleic acid |
| ROS | Reactive oxygen species |
| $T_3$ | Triiodothyronine |
| $T_4$ | Thyroxine |
| TAG | Tri-acyl glycerol |
| TMAO | Trimethylamine N-oxide |
| VAD | Vitamin A deficiency |
| VLDL | Very low-density lipoprotein |
| WHO | World Health Organization |

**Key Points**
- There are several overlapping pathways through which macro- and micronutrients affect the immune systems and infections.
- Adequate nutritional status is important for normal proliferation and differentiation of all immune cell types.
- Adequate nutritional status is important for normal functioning of all immune cell types, including antibody and cytokine production.
- Several micronutrients (e.g., iron, vitamin A, etc.) are involved in pro-inflammatory responses to infection, providing an early resistance against invading pathogens.
- Several nutrients (e.g., vitamin A, vitamin K, thiamin) moderate the strength of the inflammatory responses, preventing or limiting autoimmune reactions.
- Antioxidant vitamins, minerals, and amino acids protect the integrity of immune cell membranes from free radical attacks.

# Introduction

The framework for understanding the interactions between nutrition and infections has evolved over time to accommodate trends in the diagnosis of both nutritional status and disease. Historically, malnutrition has often been defined by anthropometric indices (including weight for age, and height for age z-scores). By this metric, undernutrition (defined as stunting or underweight) has been consistently shown to elevate the risk of disease and death, with especially grave consequences for child survival in resource-limited communities. A systematic review of evidence accrued in the last two decades estimated that undernutrition was the underlying causes of ~50% of child mortality in low- and middle-income countries, mostly from pneumonia, diarrhea, and malaria [1]. Over time, estimates were revised to include the effects of specific micronutrient deficiencies on childhood mortality. A publication in the 2008 Lancet series on Maternal Child Health and Nutrition reviewing the causes of childhood mortality estimated that deficiencies of iron, vitamin A, and zinc may be responsible for about a third of childhood deaths [2]. More recent estimates are based on pooled analyses of controlled studies in which children were supplemented with specific micronutrients, and overall, the evidence supports the conclusion that improving nutritional status is associated with improved infectious disease outcomes. Several systematic reviews have concluded that zinc supplementation can reduce the incidence of diarrhea by ~20% and duration by ~12 hours [3]; and vitamin A supplementation has been associated with ~30% reduction in malaria morbidity [4] although the evidence base for this appears inconsistent and very context-specific. As more data become available, the discussion on nutrition-infection interactions has evolved to put a greater emphasis on potential adverse effects of micronutrient supplementation on infection. For the most part, discussions of adverse effects have centered on iron, which has been associated with increased risk of morbidity, including an elevated risk for malaria, gastrointestinal and respiratory illnesses. Evidence is emerging that iron-containing supplements adversely affect the gut microbiome by decreasing the abundance of non-pathogenic commensal bacterial such as bifidobacteria, while increasing the abundance of pathogenic *Escherichia coli* [5–7]. Iron deficiency has also been shown to compromise cytokine production, a critical component of both innate and adaptive immunity. Thus for nutrients like iron and selenium, for which evidence of both benefit and harm exists, additional studies are needed to shed light on the contexts and doses necessary to maximize benefits while minimizing potential harm.

In exploring the role of nutrients in disease, it is important to understand that nutrients do not work in isolation and that deficiencies or supplementation of one or multiple nutrients may affect the physiological role of other nutrients. For instance, vitamin C is critical for iron absorption, and deficiency of this vitamin may lead to functional iron deficiency and with that, impairment of iron-dependent functional outcomes. Similarly, copper (acting through ceruloplasmin) is involved in the conversion of iron from the ferrous to the ferric state and therefore enhances iron absorption. Such nutrient-nutrient interactions also occur among nutrients which share common absorption pathways, as is the case with copper, zinc, and iron, all of which use the divalent metal ion transporter during absorption in the enterocytes [8, 9]. These nutrient-nutrient interactions are supported by community-based trials; for example, zinc supplementation alone has been shown to improve diarrhea outcomes, but this effect is compromised when zinc is administered together with other micronutrients, especially those containing iron. Understanding the nature of nutrient-nutrient interactions is important in populations where multiple nutritional deficiencies exist.

Finally, it is important to also recognize the effects of infection on nutrition. Since the 1968 World Health Organization (WHO) monograph on the interactions between nutrition and infections, scientists have known that both acute and especially persistent infections are associated with worsening nutrition status, whether defined by anthropometry or by biochemical indicators of specific micronutrients. Chronic or persistent diarrhea episodes are associated with elevated risk of linear growth faltering, and clinical infections are often accompanied by anorexia, which leads to a decrease in food intake. In addition, infections (especially when accompanied by systemic inflammation) are associated with impaired absorption, impaired utilization, and increased urinary excretion in some cases. The acute phase response, the host's attempt to reduce tissue damage, initiate repair, and limit the growth of pathogens [10–13], is characterized by an increase in positive acute phase proteins (and associated metabolites) and a concurrent reduction in negative acute phase proteins (and their associated metabolites). This has been strongly demonstrated for several key micronutrients, including iron, zinc and vitamin A. Following invasion by pathogens, macrophages and monocytes, acting via cytokines, up- or downregulate the synthesis of specific proteins which are associated with absorption, mobilization, and transport of key micronutrients. For instance, in the case of zinc and vitamin A, the acute phase response is associated with downregulation of hepatic synthesis of albumin and retinol binding protein, whereas in the case of iron, the synthesis of ferritin is upregulated to aid intracellular iron sequestration. For acute infections, effects of the acute phase response are generally considered transient and benign. With repeated infections, however, the effects of the alterations in micronutrient metabolism driven by the acute phase response may accumulate, especially for nutrients that are actively excreted and for those whose absorption is heavily impacted by infections. This pattern is reflected in the adverse effect of recurrent diarrhea on linear growth and may also underlie the fact that exposure to infections, such as malaria, during gestation, is associated with elevated risk for low birthweight.

This chapter discusses the sources, needs, and metabolic functions of macronutrients (carbohydrates, proteins, and lipids) and micronutrients (essential minerals, fat-soluble vitamins, and water-soluble vitamins) as well as putative mechanisms through which they impact the immune system and infectious disease outcomes. The chapter also touches on other nutrients (fluorine, phosphorous, choline, carnitine, and bioflavenoids) for which less evidence exists regarding their role in the etiology of infections. Overall, this chapter is written as a primer for more detailed discussion in the following chapters about the links between specific nutrients and specific diseases in clinical and public health practice. A synthesis table summarizing current recommended biomarkers for each nutrient is provided (Table 2.1).

**Table 2.1** Recommended biomarkers

| Nutrient | Possible biomarkers | Current preferred markers | Limitations of preferred biomarkers | References |
|---|---|---|---|---|
| Macronutrients | | | | |
| Protein | Serum albumin, serum pre-albumin, urinary creatinine, 3-methylhistidine, serum Insulin-like Growth Factor-1 (IGF-1) | Serum pre-albumin | Affected by GI disease, hepatic and kidney disease, surgical trauma, stress, inflammation and infection | Keller [382], Gibson [383] |
| Energy intake | BMI, HAZ, WAZ, WHZ, MUAC, skin fold thicknesses | Children: WHZ; HAZ; Adults: BMI | Best for use at population level | Gibson [383] |
| Essential fatty acids | n-6:n-3 ratio; Omega-3 Index: RBC EPA + DHA content as a percent of membrane FAs | n-3:n-6 ratio most common | n-6 FAs vary in harm; n-3 FAs vary in benefit, so ratio doesn't capture impact | Harris [384] |
| Essential and trace minerals | | | | |
| Iron | Serum ferritin, serum iron, serum transferrin receptor (sTfR); free erythrocyte protoporphyrin (FEP) | Serum ferritin together with C-reactive protein (CRP) and $\alpha_1$-acid-glycoprotein (AGP) in cases of infection/inflammation; also with serum transferrin receptor | Serum ferritin is an acute phase protein and affected by infection; interpret serum ferritin in combination with AGP and CRP | WHO 2011 – Serum Ferritin for assessment of iron [385] |
| Calcium | Free calcium; total calcium; albumin-adjusted total calcium | Free calcium; total calcium | Free calcium is closely regulated in the blood; patients with abnormal albumin may have normal free calciumdespite abnormal calcium status | Lian and Asberg [386] |

**Table 2.1**  (continued)

| Nutrient | Possible biomarkers | Current preferred markers | Limitations of preferred biomarkers | References |
|---|---|---|---|---|
| Zinc | Plasma zinc; urinary zinc excretion; hair zinc; platelet zinc, polymorphonuclear cell zinc; mononuclear cell zinc; erythrocyte zinc | Dietary zinc, plasma zinc concentration and height for age z score of infants and children | Plasma Zn responded in a dose-dependent manner to dietary manipulation; lower response to dietary Zn than to Zn supplements delivered between meals | King et al. [387] |
| Iodine | Urinary iodine; thyroglobulin; serum thyroxine; serum thyroid stimulating hormone; triiodothyronine | Urinary iodine (children, adolescents and those with low/moderate baseline status); thyroglobulin (children & adolescents but not pregnant or lactating women); serum thyroxine (not pregnant and lactating women); serum thyroid stimulating hormone (pregnant and lactating women); | Iodine status during pregnancy and lactation is difficult to measure | Ristic-Medic et al. [388] |
| Selenium | Plasma, erythrocyte, and whole-blood selenium; plasma selenoprotein P; plasma, platelet and whole-blood glutathione peroxidase; urinary selenium; plasma triiodothyroxine:thyroxine ratio; plasma thyroxine; plasma total homocysteine; hair and toenail selenium; erythrocyte and muscle glutathione peroxidase activity | Plasma, erythrocyte and whole-blood selenium; plasma selenoprotein P, plasma, platelet and whole-blood glutathione peroxidase activity | Limited data is available for all of the potential biomarkers; more information is needed on strengths and limitations of each in different populations and with varying intakes | Ashton et al. [389] |
| Copper | Serum copper, Cu/Zn superoxide dismutase; total ceruloplasmin protein; plasma copper; Erythrocyte copper; Platelet copper; Leukocyte superoxide dismutase; Erythrocyte glutathione peroxidase; Platelet glutathione peroxidase; Plasma glutathione peroxidase; Platelet or leukocyte cytochrome-c oxidase; total glutathione; diamine oxidase; urinary pyridinoline | Serum copper (population level); total ceruloplasmin protein | Limited data affects all of the potential biomarkers; total ceruloplasmin protein only reflects changes when individuals are very depleted | Harvey et al. [390] |

(continued)

**Table 2.1** (continued)

| Nutrient | Possible biomarkers | Current preferred markers | Limitations of preferred biomarkers | References |
|---|---|---|---|---|
| Magnesium | Serum or plasma Mg; RBC Mg; WBC Mg; 24 h urine Mg; non-24 h urine Mg; fecal Mg; muscle Mg; other tissue Mg; Mg balance studies; Mg challenge and retention studies; sublingual cell Mg; stable isotope balance studies | Serum magnesium; 24 hr. urine Mg | Serum Mg fluctuates based on diet, albumin levels, kidney excretion of Mg, and only represents 0.8% of total body stores. Current calls to update "normal" range from when it was set in the 1970s. Urine Mg doesn't correlate with body stores or dietary intake | Workinger etal. [391] |
| Fat-soluble vitamins | | | | |
| Vitamin A & carotenoids | Liver reserves; clinical eye signs (xerophthalmia and night blindness); serum retinol; retinol binding protein; dose-response tests; isotope dilution assays | Serum retinol; retinol binding protein | Serum retinol and RBP don't necessarily respond to supplementation; RBP is an acute phase protein influenced by inflammation | Tanumihardjo [392] |
| Vitamin D | Serum 25-hydroxyvitamin D [25(OH)D]; Markers of bone turnover: whole-body or lumbar spine bone mineral density; circulating parathyroid hormone | 25(OH)D | 25(OH)D is currently seen as a robust and reliable biomarker | Seamans and Cashman [393] |
| Vitamin E | Plasma α-tocopherol; tissue α-tocopherol; urinary excretion of α-carboxy-ethyl-hydroxychromanol | Plasma α-tocopherol | Dependent on plasma lipoprotein and cholesterol concentrations; low levels are considered 'specific', but normal levels may not represent adequacy | Traber [394] |
| Vitamin K | Plasma phylloquinone; plasma menaquinone; prothrombin time; undercarboxylated prothrombin; urine Y-Carboxyglutamic acid | Fasting plasma phylloquinone corrected for triglyceride levels | Influenced by triglyceride levels; peaks 6-10 h after meals | Shea and Booth [395] |
| Water-soluble vitamins | | | | |
| Vitamin C | Plasma vitamin C (VC) | Plasma VC | Correlation between dietary intake and plasma VC is ~0.41; influenced by dietary intake so fasting samples are needed; affected by smoking, age, sex, chronic use of aspirin | Dehghan et al. [396] |

**Table 2.1** (continued)

| Nutrient | Possible biomarkers | Current preferred markers | Limitations of preferred biomarkers | References |
|---|---|---|---|---|
| B-complex vitamins | | | | |
| $B_1$ – Thiamine | Erythrocyte transketolase; erythrocyte thiamine pyrophosphate (TPP); whole blood TPP; thiamine urinary thiamine excretion; | Whole blood or erythrocyte TPP | Cutoff levels are not available | Gibson [383] |
| $B_2$ – Riboflavin | Erythrocyte glutathione reductase activity coefficient (EGRAC); urinary riboflavin excretion | EGRAC | Influenced by age, RBC age, Fe deficiency, thresholds for adequacy not yet clear | Gibson [383] |
| $B_3$ – Niacin | Urinary excretion of niacin and niacin metabolites; niacin and niacin enzymes in whole blood and plasma | Urinary excretion of niacin and niacin metabolites | Not sufficiently sensitive for marginal deficiencies | Gibson [383] |
| $B_5$ – Pantothenic Acid | Urinary excretion | Urinary excretion | Limited research on relevant biomarkers | Fukuwatari and Shibata [397] |
| $B_6$ – Pyridoxine | Serum or plasma B6; serum or urinary 4PA; PAr index; 3-hydroxykynurenine:xanthurenic acid ratio; oxoglutarate:glutamate ratio | Erythrocyte pyridoxal 5′-phosphate; urinary 4-pyridoxic acid | Influenced by inflammation, low serum albumin, renal function, pregnancy, age, sex, BMI, oral contraceptives, alcohol consumption, smoking, exercise | Ueland et al. [398] |
| $B_7$ – Biotin | Lymphocyte biotinylated carboxylases; biotin metabolism genes; urinary excretion of biotin | Biotinylated 3-methylcrotonyl-CoA carboxylase (holo-MCC); propionyl-CoA carboxylase (holo-PCC) | Normal levels not yet defined; limitations still being assessed | Eng et al. [399] |
| $B_9$ – Folate | serum and RBC folate; folate protein binding; mass spectrometry to assess total folate | Total plasma folate | Traditional laboratory measurement method is a bacterial growth assay | Shane [400] |
| $B_{12}$ – Cobalamin | serum total $B_{12}$; plasma total $B_{12}$; methylmalonic acid (MMA); total homocysteine response; plasma holotranscobalamin | Plasma & total $B_{12}$; methylmalonic acid, total homocysteine; Combine >2 tests (e.g., plasma cobalamin & MMA) | Unexplained heterogeneity in total $B_{12}$ | Hoey et al. [401], Carmel [402] |

# Macronutrients

## *Carbohydrates*

### Carbohydrate and Sugar Needs, Sources, and Risk of Deficiency

Carbohydrates (molecular formula $(CH_2O)_n$), also known as simple and complex sugars, are a class of biomolecules derived from plant sources [14]. In animals, carbohydrates are the primary source of biochemical energy. Within cells, carbohydrates are oxidized to produce adenosine triphosphate (ATP) (the major source of energy for physiological processes) [15]. The energy released from the removal of one or two phosphate groups from ATP is used to drive major physiological processes, including nutrient absorption, synthesis of macromolecules, muscle contraction, and cell division. The basic unit of carbohydrates is the monosaccharide, with glucose, fructose and galactose being the principal monosaccharides in the human diet (see Table 2.2). Sugars are normally present in the diet as polysaccharides, which must be broken down during digestion before absorption [16]. Glucose and fructose occur in free, non-polymerized units in sources such as dried fruits, honey, and raw fruits and vegetables. Sucrose, a disaccharide composed of one monomer each of glucose and fructose (linked by 1–2 β-glycosidic bonds), occurs commonly in fruits and vegetables; lactose, a disaccharide composed of one glucose monomer and one galactose monomer (linked by 1–2 β glycosidic bonds), occurs commonly in milk. Carbohydrates with 3–9 monomer units are known as oligosaccharides, and those with 10 or more monomer units are called polysaccharides.

Dietary fiber is a term generally used to describe the components of carbohydrates which are relatively resistant to intestinal digestion [16]. Consumption of foods with a high fiber content is believed to reduce the risk for chronic diseases, including heart diseases and some cancers [17]. Dietary fiber may be soluble or insoluble depending on the pH of the medium. Carbohydrates are also commonly characterized by their glycemic potential, defined as the ability to supply glucose for metabolism to energy. Glycemic carbohydrates have a high content of mono-, di-, and oligosaccharides and therefore

**Table 2.2** Dietary carbohydrates based on degree of polymerization

| Number of monomers in chain | Examples | Sources |
|---|---|---|
| Monosaccharides (1) | Glucose, galactose, fructose | Glucose and fructose occur freely in honey and dry fruits and in smaller concentration in raw fruits, berries and vegetables. Glucose is available in corn syrup and fructose is commercially available in high-fructose corn syrup. Galactose is produced from the hydrolyses of lactose present in milk |
| Disaccharides (2) | Maltose (glucose + glucose) Sucrose (glucose + fructose) Lactose (glucose +galactose) | Maltose is starch-derived and occurs in wheat and barley Sucrose is the principal sugar in fruits Lactose is the main sugar in milk |
| Oligosaccharides (3–9) | Malto-dextrins, inulin, polydextrin; | Peas, beans, lentils, wheat, rye, onion, asparagus |
| Polysaccharide (>9) | Starch (α-glucans): amylose and amylopectin Non-starch polysaccharides: cellulose, pectin, plant gums | Cereals, root tubers, and vegetables |

supply glucose readily, whereas non-glycemic carbohydrates have a high amount of non-digestible polysaccharides.

The energy value of dietary carbohydrates is about 4 kcal/g. A minimum of 50 g of daily carbohydrate intake is recommended to avoid breakdown of body fat (ketosis). The Food and Agriculture Organization (FAO) and the World Health Organization (WHO) recommend that ~55% of total energy be supplied by carbohydrates, with no more than 10% coming from free sugars (see Table 2.3). Chronic consumption of low carbohydrate diets can precipitate clinical symptoms such as marasmus. On the other hand, overconsumption of carbohydrates, especially food rich in refined sugars, is linked to chronic diseases such as obesity, diabetes, and health disease.

---

**Box 2.1 Key Facts: Carbohydrates**
- Carbohydrates are derived from plant sources and are the primary source of biochemical energy in animals.
- Monosaccharides, including glucose, fructose and galactose, are the basic unit of carbohydrates.
- Glycemic carbohydrates have a high content of mono, di- and oligosaccharides and therefore supply glucose readily.

---

**Carbohydrate and Sugar Metabolism**

Carbohydrate digestion and absorption occurs in the small intestine. Carbohydrates are hydrolyzed to monomers before absorption into enterocytes [18]. Carbohydrate digestion begins in the mouth where salivary amylase hydrolyzes the glycosidic bonds. The acidic condition in the stomach inhibits this process. However, once the chyme moves into the small intestine, the secretion of bicarbonates restores the alkaline pH needed for amylase action. In the small intestine, pancreatic amylase takes over the role of carbohydrate hydrolysis. The products of amylase activity are mainly disaccharides and a few monosaccharides. The disaccharides must subsequently be broken down by brush border enzymes into monosaccharides, before absorption into enterocytes. At the brush border, three enzymes, namely, gluco-amylase (α-glucosidase), sucrase-isomaltase, and lactase, hydrolyze the disaccharides maltose, sucrose, and lactose, respectively, into their monomer units. Glucose and galactose are absorbed by secondary active transport into enterocytes via the sodium glucose cotransporter. This involves the movement of sodium ions down its concentration gradient. The energy generated is used in the co-transport of glucose and galactose into the cell [19]. The sodium gradient is reestablished by the action of Ssodium-potassium ATPase, which pumps sodium out of the cells using ATP. Glucose and galactose exit the enterocytes and cross the basolateral membrane via facilitated diffusion through a glucose transporter (GLUT) 2 [19]. Fructose enters and exits the enterocytes by facilitated diffusion using GLUT5. Glucose is homeostatically maintained at concentrations in the range of 4.0–5.5 mmol/L through processes such as glycolysis (glucose breakdown), glycogenesis (glycogen formation from glucose units), glycogenolysis (mobilization glucose from glycogen stores), and gluconeogenesis (formation of glucose from non-carbohydrate precursors including amino acids and lactic acid) [20, 21].

Glucose, the major monosaccharide used by cells, is stored as glycogen after absorption. In a state of glucose deprivation and glycogen depletion, limited amounts of glucose can be synthesized in humans by gluconeogenesis, using intermediate products such as lactate, produced from the metabolism of proteins and fatty acids [21]. After a high carbohydrate meal, or in a disease condition such as diabetes which elevates blood glucose levels, glycolysis and glycogenesis are upregulated to clear the excess plasma glucose, restoring glucose to the normal range [20, 21].

**Table 2.3** Characteristics of macronutrients

| Nutrient | Dietary sources | Recommended nutrient intake (WHO/FAO) | Factors influencing absorption & metabolism | Physiological functions | Role in immune function | Conditions and treatments[a] associated with imbalances |
|---|---|---|---|---|---|---|
| Carbohydrates | Fruit, vegetables, grains, dairy products, snack foods; whole grains, legumes | Recommendations for variety, w/intake of fruits & vegetables, pulses, nuts & seeds | Types of food sources, insulin sensitivity, blood glucose levels | Energy source for all organ and tissue systems | Cell signaling systems, cell adhesion, energy source for cellular respiration and synthesis pathways | Adult-onset diabetes, insulin resistance; obesity and comorbidities (hypertension, dyslipidemia, heart disease); interventions: Exercise, reduce simple sugar consumption; taxes on sugar-sweetened beverages and high-sugar snack foods |
| Protein | Meat, dairy products, nuts, legumes, some grains | Safe level in g/kg body weight/d: 6–11 m (1.31); 12–17 m (1.14); 18–23 m (1.03); 24–35 m (0.97); 36–47 m (0.90); 4–6y (0.87); 7–10y (0.92); male 11–14y (0.90); female 11–14y (0.89); male 14–18y (0.87); female 14–18y (0.84); >18y (0.83) | Appetite, protein concentration in diet, high dietary starch/fiber may make consumption of sufficient protein difficult | Structure and enzymes; present in all tissues, all systems | See Table 2.3 for roles of specific amino acids in immune function | Insufficient intake —PEM, decreased functioning of enzymes and body system; interventions: Increase animal source foods; increase consumption of protein-dense foods |
| Lipids | Meats, organ meats, vegetable oils, nuts and seeds | 0–6 m acceptable macronutrient distribution range (AMDR) 40–60% of energy; 6–24 m gradual reduction to 35% of energy; >2y AMDR 20–35% of energy | Availability and functioning of digestive enzymes | Major source of energy; insulates and protects organs; components of plasma membranes; lipid-based signaling molecules | Regulation of membrane fluidity, lipid peroxide formation, signaling molecules (e.g., eicosanoids); associated with gene expression | Dry and bleeding skin; fatty liver; interventions: Increase consumption of dietary fats, attending to best available knowledge of relative merits of different fat sources |
| Essential Fatty Acids: Linoleic acid (n-6); α-Linolenic acid (n-3) | ALA in walnuts, canola, flaxseeds, soybeans; linoleic acid in sunflower seeds, oils from safflower, soybean, corn and canola, nuts and seeds | Adults n-6 AMDR 2.5–9% of Energy; n-3 AMDR 0.5–2% of Energy | ALA is an important precursor for other PUFAs; too much arachidonic acid inhibits conversion of ALA to DHA (IOM macronutrients report) | Regulate gene expression; cytokine messengers both pro-inflammatory (ω-6) and anti-inflammatory (ω-3) | ALA is a precursor for eicosapentaenoic acid (EPA); EPA is the precursor of n-3 eicosanoids, which affect inflammation | Decreased growth; susceptibility to infection; neurological abnormalities; interventions: supplementation with ω-3 s; incorporation of fish into diet |

[a]Supplementation is considered to be an appropriate response for all nutrient deficiencies

## Carbohydrate and Sugar Pathways to Infections

All physiological processes, including the differentiation and proliferation of immune cells, are powered by metabolic energy. Thus carbohydrate deficits, unless compensated for by excess of fat or protein, can be expected to compromise the function of the immune system. Chronic malnutrition is associated with an increased risk for infectious disease morbidity and mortality [22]. In animal models, acute starvation has been associated with a suppression in the number and function of T cells [23]. There is also evidence that calorie restriction in mice increases the risk of death from sepsis [24]. Carbohydrates, as part of the glycoproteins and glycolipids of cell membranes, are essential to the functioning of signaling molecules for different aspects of the immune system, although the mechanisms are not completely characterized [25]. Cell surface carbohydrates may be targets for antigen presenting cells, which are critical in stimulating the maturation of both B and T lymphocytes and the functions of these cells, including antibody and cytokine production [26]. Cell surface carbohydrates are also important in cell adhesion, an important step in pathogen clearance (see Table 2.2) [27].

## *Proteins*

### Protein Needs, Sources, and Risk of Deficiency

Proteins, also known as peptides, are a class of macromolecules composed of amino acids linked by peptide bonds [28]. Amino acids, the basic unit of proteins, are a class of compounds with a nitrogen-containing amino group, a carboxylic acid group, and a side chain, with the side chain differing from one amino acid to the next. Proteins are made up of different combination of ~20 amino acids [29] of which 9 are not produced in sufficient amounts by humans and are therefore considered essential (see Table 2.3). In adult humans, proteins constitute 16% of body weight and are involved in myriad of functions including movement and support (e.g., collagen, actin and myosin), oxygen transport and storage (e.g., hemoglobin and myoglobin), and absorption and transport of nutrients (e.g., transmembrane proteins and pumps; see Table 2.2) [30]. Proteins are the major structural component of enzymes involved in metabolism, and the primary constituent of peptide hormones, as well as the structural component of several signaling molecules, such as the cytokines of the immune system [29].

The common proteins involved in human metabolism are made up of α-amino acids, in which an amino group is connected to the α-carbon atom. Of the more than 300 amino acids found in nature, only ~20 are encoded by the human genome [28]. A few non-protein amino acids, including ornithine, citrulline, and homocysteine, have important roles in mammalian physiology [31, 32]. The catabolism of protein and amino acids yields a wide variety of products including ammonia, carbon dioxide, hydrogen sulfide, urea, nitric oxide, and ketone bodies [28]. Under some conditions, amino acids may be oxidized to generate acetyl coenzyme (Co)A, which is fed into the Krebs cycle and electron transport chain to generate biochemical energy (ATP) to support other metabolic activities [33].

Historically, protein needs have been estimated either by measuring the obligatory nitrogen losses from persons consuming protein-deficient (but otherwise adequate) diets or by estimating the nitrogen balance (i.e., the difference between the amount of nitrogen consumed and the amount excreted in urine, feces, and other tissue fluids) [34–36]. Recommendations take into account estimates of daily losses, which, for adults, include ~37 mg/kg in urine, ~12 mg/kg in feces, ~3 mg/kg through the skin, and an additional 2 mg for other losses (see Table 2.2). The protein supply from a food type is defined by its digestibility, which is the proportion of ingested nitrogen absorbed (i.e., amount of nitrogen consumed minus the amount in feces expressed as percentage of the total amount of nitrogen consumed). Animal food sources generally have the highest protein digestibility and these include eggs (~97% protein digestibility), milk and cheese (~95%), and meat and fish (~94%). Plant sources with high protein digestibility include refined wheat (~96%), peanut butter (~95%), and soy flour (~86%). Protein deficiency is more common in young children because of the high protein requirements for rapid growth and in the elderly because of changes in muscle protein synthesis with aging [37].

## Protein Metabolism

The amount and type of amino acid in portal circulation reflects digestion and absorption of dietary protein. Protein metabolism is homeostatically regulated to ensure that there are sufficient amounts of key amino acids to support physiological needs while preventing the pathogenic effects of excess protein. When in excess, protein may promote the development of neurological disorders and oxidative stress and may adversely affect cardiovascular health [38, 39].

Dietary protein is first broken down in the stomach by the enzyme pepsin [40]. In the acidic medium of the stomach (pH < 4), pepsin hydrolyzes whole proteins in the diet into large polypeptides with the C-terminus occupied by tyrosine, phenylalanine, tryptophan, leucine, glutamine, or glutamic acid [41]. When the acidic chyme enters the small intestine, protein digestion continues with enzymes produced by the duodenal cells and the pancreas. Enterokinase, produced by intestinal mucosa cells, activates the hydrolytic enzymes produced by the pancreas, including trypsin and chymotrypsin. Trypsin hydrolyzes peptide bonds containing basic amino acids at the C-terminus, whereas chymotrypsin hydrolyzes the bonds with neutral amino acids at the C-terminus. Other enzymes involved in the digestion of proteins in the small intestine include carboxypeptidases, aminopeptidases and exopeptidase. Proteins are absorbed into enterocytes mainly in the form of amino acids, dipeptides, and a few oligopeptides. These are taken into the circulation and distributed to the tissues. Amino acids from the degradation of proteins, and those absorbed from the diet, enter amino acid pools in cells throughout the body [42]. From this pool, new proteins are formed when needed. Protein synthesis (translation) is regulated at the levels of gene transcription. Transcription involves the formation of a messenger ribonucleic acid (mRNA) from deoxy-ribonucleic acid (DNA). The mRNA then encodes for specific amino acids, which are joined together via peptide linkages on the ribosomes [43–46]. Unlike carbohydrates and lipids, proteins are not stored. Hence, if protein is consumed in excess of body requirement, the excess is metabolized and the amino groups are excreted as urea. Functional amino acids, including arginine, cysteine, glutamine, leucine, and proline, are now increasingly recognized as necessary nutrients in the maintenance of growth, reproduction, and immunity. In addition to protein synthesis, individual amino acids are involved in specific metabolic reactions as detailed in Tables 2.3 and 2.4.

> **Box 2.2 Protein: Key Facts**
> - Digestion of dietary protein begins in the stomach and continues in the small intestine.
> - Amino acids are absorbed into an amino acid pool, and later used in protein synthesis, but are not stored.
> - During prolonged starvation certain amino acids can be oxidized to acetyl CoA, to generate biochemical energy (ATP).

## Potential Pathways to Infections: Protein

PEM has been shown to exacerbate the severity of several diseases, including pneumonia, especially in children [47]. However, because studies of PEM typically do not disentangle the specific effects of protein versus other energy sources, these studies largely do not shed light on the mechanism involved

**Table 2.4**  Known Functions of α-amino acids

| Amino acid | Function | Role in immune function |
|---|---|---|
| Non-essential amino acids | | |
| Alanine | Protein synthesis; regulation of hormone secretion, gene expression, and cell signaling | Inhibition of apoptosis; stimulation of lymphocyte proliferation; and enhancement of Ab production probably through cellular signaling mechanism |
| Asparagine | Regulation of gene expression and immune function; ammonia detoxification; function of the nervous system | |
| Aspartate | Purine, pyrimidine, asparagine, and arginine synthesis; transamination; urea cycle; activation of NMDA receptors; synthesis of inositol and b-alanine | |
| Cysteine | Disulfide linkage in protein (necessary for correct protein conformation); transport of sulfur | Antioxidant; regulation of cellular redox state |
| Glutamate | Glutamine, citrulline, and arginine synthesis; bridging the urea cycle with the Krebs cycle; transamination; ammonia assimilation; activation of NMDA receptors; NAG synthesis. Excitatory neurotransmitter; inhibition of T cell response and inflammation | Neurotransmitter; inhibition of T cell response and inflammation |
| Glutamine | Regulation of protein turnover through cellular mTOR signaling, gene expression, and immune function; a major fuel for rapidly proliferating cells; inhibition of apoptosis; syntheses of purine, pyrimidine, ornithine, citrulline, arginine, proline, and asparagines; N reservoir; synthesis of NAD(P) | Neurotransmitters; components of the malate shuttle; cell metabolism |
| Glycine | Calcium influx through a glycine-gated channel in the cell membrane; purine and serine synthesis; synthesis of porphyrins; inhibitory neurotransmitter in CNS; co-agonist with glutamate for NMDA receptors; Hemoproteins (e.g., hemoglobin, myoglobin, catalase, and cytochrome c); production of CO (a signaling molecule) | |
| Proline | Collagen structure and function; neurological function; osmoprotectan | Killing pathogens; intestinal integrity; a signaling molecule; immunity; cellular redox state; DNA synthesis; lymphocyte proliferation; ornithine and polyamine formation; gene expression |
| Serine | One-carbon unit metabolism; syntheses of cysteine, purine, pyrimidine, ceramide and phosphatidylserine; synthesis of tryptophan in bacteria; gluconeogenesis; protein phosphorylation; activation of NMDA receptors in brain | Inhibition of apoptosis; stimulation of lymphocyte proliferation; and enhancement of Ab production probably through cellular signaling mechanism |
| Tryptophan | Neurotransmitter-inhibiting production of inflammatory cytokines and superoxide via the actions of serotonin Antioxidant-inhibition of the production of inflammatory cytokines and superoxide via the action of melatonin | Neurotransmitter; inhibition of the production of inflammatory cytokines and superoxide |
| Essential Amino Acids | | |
| Arginine | Activation of mTOR signaling; antioxidant; regulation of hormone secretion; allosteric activation of NAG synthase; ammonia detoxification; regulation of gene expression; immune function; activation of BH4 synthesis; N reservoir; methylation of proteins | Signaling molecule; killing of pathogens; regulation of cytokine production; and mediator of autoimmune diseases |

(continued)

**Table 2.4** (continued)

| Amino acid | Function | Role in immune function |
|---|---|---|
| Histidine | Protein methylation; hemoglobin structure and function; antioxidative dipeptides; one-carbon unit metabolism; allergic reaction; vasodilator; central acetylcholine secretion; regulation of gut function; modulation of the immune response in skin | Allergic reactions; vasodilator; and central acetylcholine secretion; modulation of the immune response in skin |
| Isoleucine | Synthesis of glutamine and alanine; balance among BCAA | |
| Leucine | Regulation of protein turnover through cellular mTOR signaling and gene expression; activator of glutamate dehydrogenase; BCAA balance; flavor enhancer. Regulation of immune responses | |
| Lysine | Regulation of nitric oxide synthesis; antiviral activity (treatment of Herpes simplex); protein methylation (e.g., trimethyllysine in calmodulin), acetylation, ubiquitination, and O-linked glycosylation | Regulation of NO synthesis; antiviral activity |
| Methionine | oxidant; independent risk factor for CVD; inhibition of nitric synthesis; methylation of homocysteine to methionine; one-carbon unit metabolism; methylation of proteins and DNA; polyamine synthesis; gene expression | |
| Phenylalanine | Activation of BH4 (a cofactor for NOS) synthesis; synthesis of tyrosine; neurological development and function | |
| Threonine | Synthesis of the mucin protein that is required for maintaining intestinal integrity and function; immune function; protein phosphorylation and O-linked glycosylation; glycine synthesis | Involved in mucin protein synthesis, which helps maintain intestinal immune function |
| Tyrosine | Protein phosphorylation, nitrosation, and sulfation Neurotransmitter; regulation of immune response through the action of dopamine | |
| Valine | Synthesis of glutamine and alanine; balance among BCAA. | Neurotransmitter; inhibition of the production of inflammatory cytokines and superoxide |

Adapted from Wu [29] and Li Peng et al. (2007)

in protein or amino acid-dependent immunomodulation. Recent studies have shown that gluconeogenic amino acids, such as alanine, are critical for the proper functioning of leucocytes, as they supply the energy substrate for these immune cells. Involvement of specific amino acids in immune function, where known, are detailed in Table 2.3.

## Lipids

### Lipid Needs, Sources, and Risk of Deficiency

Lipids are a group of organic compounds, generally insoluble in aqueous media, that are important energy sources and function in insulating and protecting visceral organs. They are also the major component of plasma membranes, without which cells lose their integrity and ability to function [48, 49]. Long-term storage of lipids occurs in the adipose tissue, and lipids are mobilized from there in times of need. Lipids that are solid at room temperature are called fats, whereas oils are liquid at room temperature. Dietary lipids include triacylglycerol (TAG), steroids, phospholipids, and fat-soluble vitamins (A, D, E, and K). TAG, formed by the esterification of glycerol (a three-carbon triol) with three fatty acid molecules, is the major constituent (~95%) of dietary lipids in humans. The fatty acid components of TAG are even-numbered carbon chains with carboxylic acid functional groups. Fatty acids can be saturated or unsaturated. In saturated fatty acids, each carbon atom (other than the carboxylic carbon) is attached to four hydrogen atoms and hence has no double or triple bonds. Unsaturated fatty acids have one or more double bonds. Polyunsaturated fatty acids (PUFAs) have two or more double bonds, whereas monounsaturated fatty acids have a single double bond. The presence of a double bond reduces the number of hydrogen atoms, the molecular weight, and hence the melting point. For this reason, fats, which are solid at room temperature, are composed largely of saturated fatty acids, and oils have a higher relative composition of polyunsaturated fatty acids. Unsaturated fatty acids are classified by the location of the first double bond in relation to the omega carbon atom (the last carbon atom counting from the carboxylic carbon), as omega-3 (ω-3), omega-6 (ω-6), or omega-9 (ω-9) fatty acids [49].

---

**Box 2.3 Lipids: Key Facts**
- Lipids, such as TAGs and steroids, are generally insoluble in aqueous medium.
- Polyunsaturated fatty acids (PUFA) have two or more double bonds.
- Members of the omega-3 (ω-3) and omega-6 (ω-6) fatty acid family are essential fatty acids that cannot be produced by biosynthetic pathways in humans and must be obtained from the diet.
- Cholesterol is the dominant steroid in humans and is an important component of plasma membranes and a precursor for steroid hormones.

---

Members of the ω-3 and ω-6 fatty acid family are essential fatty acids because humans lack the enzymes which are necessary to insert a cis double bond at the n-6 or the n-3 position of a fatty acid [50]. Two fatty acids are essential, alpha-linolenic acid (ALA, an ω-3) and linoleic (an ω-6) fatty acid, and these are commonly found in plant oils [50]. Omega-9 fatty acids can be produced from linoleic acid. Essential fatty acid deficiency is not common but may present in people who have problems with fatty acid absorption. Symptoms of essential fatty acid deficiency may include dry and bleeding skin and fatty liver (caused by accumulation of other fatty acids) [51]. Essential fatty acid deficiencies are also associated with decreased growth and vulnerability to infections. Essential fatty acids are an integral part of plasma membranes and are also required for the synthesis of eicosanoids, including prostaglandins and leukotrienes. Eicosanoids are signaling molecules involved in regulating physiological activities such as inflammation, immunity, and cell growth. The process of converting essential fatty acids into other fatty acid compounds involves a process of desaturation (in which additional double bonds are added by removing hydrogen atoms) and elongation (in which the chain length is extended by adding extra carbon atoms). Through this process, other important PUFAs can be synthesized. These include arachidonic acid, eicosapentaenoic acid and docosahexaenoic acid, which are important in lowering blood pressure and improving prognosis for heart and other chronic diseases [52]. Outside the endogenous synthesis, PUFAs are supplied in the diet primarily from fish oils. Phospholipids and steroids constitute the other types of lipids. Phospholipids are similar in structure to the TAGs, except that one of the fatty acid chains in the TAG is replaced with a phosphate group. The phosphate group is typically attached to one of four other groups, namely, choline, serine, inositol, and ethanolamine. Phospholipids occur naturally in both animal and plant food sources, and major dietary sources include eggs, soybeans, liver, and peanuts. Steroids are another class of lipid compounds with four rings attached to each other. The dominant steroid in humans, cholesterol, is an important component of plasma membranes. In cell membranes, cholesterol serves as a buffer in regulating membrane fluidity. Cholesterol is also a precursor for steroid hormones, which are important in regulating gene expression.

Requirements for fats are influenced by the levels of other nutrients in the diet and are much higher in infants and young children then adults (see Table 2.2). Vitamin E is essential in preventing oxidation of polyunsaturated fatty acids, so diets higher in PUFAs would need a higher vitamin E intake [53, 54].

---

**Box 2.4 Essential Fatty Acids Sources and Needs**
- Essential fatty acids are found in plant oils from cottonseed, soybean, mustard, walnut, linseed, evening primrose, corn, and safflower.
- Essential fatty acid deficiency is uncommon, except in people with impaired fatty acid absorption.

---

## Lipid Metabolism

Ingested TAGs are digested and absorbed, primarily in the small intestine [55, 56]. In order to be absorbed, fatty acids must first be broken down into mono- and di-acyl glycerol. In the small intestine, the bicarbonate component of bile helps to neutralize the acid in the chyme exiting the stomach. This is necessary to provide the optimal pH for the pancreatic enzymes, such as lipase, which hydrolyze the fatty acids. Bile acids facilitate the emulsification of fat, the mechanical process by which larger fat globules are split into smaller globules, creating a larger surface area for enzymatic action. In children and adults, pancreatic lipase hydrolyzes the TAG into two fatty acid molecules and one monoglyceride. In newborns, however, lipase secretion is low and fat digestion is aided by breastmilk lipase and by lingual lipase produced by the glands of tongue [57, 58]. Monoglycerides, fatty acids, and the product of phospholipid and cholesterol ester hydrolyses are complexed together with fat-soluble vitamins to form micelles. The micelles are absorbed by diffusion across the enterocyte membrane. Glycerol and short-chain fatty acids (with carbon length < 12) can diffuse directly into enterocytes and then into circulation, while longer-chain fatty acids go through several processes in the enterocytes prior to release into circulation. In the enterocytes, the TAG, phospholipids, and cholesterol esters are regenerated from their hydrolyzed components and then incorporated into chylomicrons and transported to the liver via the lymphatic system [59]. Transport of these non-polar lipids through a polar plasma medium is facilitated by complexing to polar protein molecules know as lipoproteins [60]. The lipoprotein forms a hydrophilic surface layer around a hydrophobic core of lipid (including cholesterol esters, TAGs, and phospholipids). The major classes of lipoprotein involved in lipid transport are chylomicrons, very low-density lipoproteins (VLDL), low-density lipoproteins (LDL), and high-density lipoproteins (HDL) [60]. Chylomicrons transport TAG and fat-soluble vitamins. The composition of chylomicrons strongly reflects recent food intake. In the capillaries, the TAGs disassociate from the chylomicron (following the action of lipoprotein lipase). The TAGs then diffuse into cells of the heart and muscles, where they are metabolized as energy. The free chylomicrons (i.e., chylomicrons remnants) are cleared from circulation by hepatocytes [60]. The fat-soluble vitamins are also delivered to tissues as part of chylomicrons. In the liver, cholesterol, cholesterol esters, and a high amount of TAGs are packed into VLDLs [59]. Like chylomicrons, VLDLs also deliver TAGs to the heart and muscle cells [60]. In addition, VLDLs deliver TAGs to adipose tissues for long-term storage. In the tissues, the TAGs are released by the action of lipoprotein lipase. With the gradual release of TAGs, the VLDLs become LDLs and are transported back to the liver and recycled again into VLDLs [59, 61]. HDLs are produced in both the liver and enterocytes and are especially important for delivering lipoprotein C and E, which enhance the actions of lipoprotein lipase, in metabolizing the TAG content of chylomicrons. A high plasma content of LDLs is associated with increased risk for cardiovascular disease, whereas HDLs lower the risk.

## Potential Pathways to Infections: Lipids

There is abundant scientific evidence linking dietary fat to alterations in the structure and functioning of immune system. Lipids influence the immune system through membrane fluidity, lipid peroxide formation, and production of signaling molecules (e.g., eicosanoids) which are critical in inflammation (see Table 2.2) [62]. Lipids are associated with gene expression, including the expressing of genes encoding for vital proteins in the immune system. In vitro studies also suggest that lipids may be critical in initiating apoptosis of infected cells, enhancing their clearance from circulation. Fatty acids have been shown to stimulate the proliferation of lymphocytes [63] and cytokine production [64]. In particular, long-chain ω-3 PUFAs have been shown to prevent excessive inflammatory responses [65]. Consistent with this, supplementation with eicosapentaenoic acid and docosahexaenoic acid is associated with decreases in cytokine concentrations in patients with systemic inflammation [65]. A study in voles and hamsters showed that a reduction in total body fat (induced by the surgical removal of white adipose tissue corresponding to usual winter loss of fat) was associated with a decrease in humoral immune responses, characterized by a reduction in serum immunoglobulin G (IgG) [66]. Additional evidence is needed on the extent to which these results are generalizable to humans.

# Essential Minerals and Trace Elements

## *Iron*

### Iron Needs, Sources, and Risk of Deficiency

Iron is a critical component of every living being and is the fourth most abundant element in the earth's crust. Yet iron remains one of the most widespread nutritional deficiencies, mainly because in its most prevalent oxidized states, it is not readily absorbed and is less bioavailable to most living systems [67]. Iron is an important component of the principal oxygen transport proteins, hemoglobin and myoglobin, and is essential for the process of oxidative phosphorylation, the primary supply of energy for most cells (see Table 2.5) [68]. In this role, iron is critical for most catabolic and anabolic reactions and is therefore necessary for the survival and growth of living cells. In addition, iron is a component of several enzymes involved in redox reactions, including the enzymes of the electron transport system and enzymes involved in nucleic acid biosynthesis, such as ribonucleotide reductase. Iron deficiency (ID) is especially prevalent in young children and vulnerable groups including pregnant and lactating women.

> **Box 2.5 Key Facts: Iron (See Table 2.5)**
> - Iron is an important component of the principal oxygen transport proteins hemoglobin and myoglobin.
> - Iron deficiency (ID) is the most widespread micronutrient deficiency worldwide.
> - ID is especially prevalent in young children and vulnerable groups including pregnant and lactating women.

**Table 2.5** Characteristics of essential and trace minerals

| Nutrient | Dietary sources | Recommended nutrient intake (WHO/FAO) | Factors influencing absorption & metabolism | Physiological functions | Role in immune function | Conditions and interventions[a] associated with imbalances |
|---|---|---|---|---|---|---|
| Iron (Fe) | Heme iron: meat, poultry, fish; non-heme iron: legumes, nuts, seeds, dried fruits, dark green leafy vegetables, egg yolks | 10% bioavailability: 7–12 m (9.3 mg/d); 1–3y (5.8 mg/d); 4–6y (6.3 mg/d); 7–9y (8.9 mg/d); F11–14[b] (14.0 mg/d); F11–14[c](32.7 mg/d); F15–17y (31.0 mg/d); M11–14y (14.6 mg/d); M15–17y (18.8 mg/d); F19–50y (29.4 mg/d); F51+ (11.3 mg/d); M19+ (13.7 mg/d)[d] | Absorption via active, carrier-mediated transport; enhanced by presence of heme iron and vitamin C; inhibited by phytates, polyphenols and tannins [374] | Critical co-factor for enzymes throughout the body, e.g., oxygen transport and oxidative phosphorylation (energy supply to cells); electron transport system; nucleic acid biosynthesis (ribonucleotide reductase) | Low iron: reduction in production of cytokine and reactive oxygen intermediates, impaired lymphocyte development; high iron: increased generation of ROS, secretion of pro-inflammatory cytokines | Iron deficiency associated with anemia, risk of infection, pregnancy complications; iron excess associated with increased risk of harmful gut microbes; interventions: fortification |
| Calcium (Ca) | Milk and dairy products; some vegetables, grains, fruits, legumes, nuts and eggs | 0–6 m (300 mg/d); 7–12 m (400 mg/d); 1–3y (500 mg/d); 4–6y (600 mg/d); 7–9y (700 mg/d); 10–18y (1300 mg/d); 19–50y (1000 mg/d); Female 51–65y (1300 mg/d); male 51y + (1300 mg/d) | Absorption via two pathways – one active and vitamin D dependent, the other passive diffusion; 20–50% of dietary Ca is absorbed [374] | 99% in skeletal system; also in signaling pathways (gene transcription, muscle contraction, cellular secretion, synaptic transmission) | Involved in intracellular signaling and regulation of gene transcription | Deficiency—low bone density, bone fractures, spasms, muscle twitching, numbness or tingling |
| Zinc (Zn) | Meats, seafood (oysters), bran of whole grains, legumes, nuts and seeds, dairy products (milk, yogurt, cheese) | Moderate bioavailability: 0–6 m 2.8 mg/d; 7–12 m 4.1 mg/d; 1–3y 4.1 mg/d; 4–6y 4.8 mg/d; 7–9y 5.6 mg/d; F10–18y 7.2 mg/d; M10–18y 8.6 mg/d; F19+ 4.9 mg/d; M19+ 7.0 mg/d[d] | Absorbed both by passive diffusion and active, carrier-bound transport; phytates inhibit absorption; plant-based diets increase risk of deficiency; Vitamin D enhances Zn uptake [374] | Critical co-factor for enzymes throughout the body, including zinc fingers (DNA transcription) and superoxide dismutase (catalyzes breakdown of superoxide); used for cell signaling (salivary glands, intestine, prostate, immune system) | Role in cell replication, transcription, translation, catalysis and maintenance of mucosal barriers; proliferation of immune cells | Growth retardation, impaired immune function, loss of appetite; interventions: fortification, dietary diversification; food processing techniques to reduce phytates (fermentation, soaking, germination) |

| Iodine (I) | Marine products; iodized salt; milk and milk products | 0–5y (90 ug/d); 6–12y (120 ug/d); >13y (150 ug/d)[d] | In healthy adults absorption is >90%. Deficiencies of selenium, iron, and vitamin A can exacerbate the effects of iodine deficiency | Essential for thyroid functioning, growth, development, mental functioning | Hypo and hyperthyroidism associated with pro-inflammatory responses | Thyroid enlargement (goiter); iodine deficiency during pregnancy associated with stillbirths, abortions, and congenital abnormalities; interventions: fortification (iodization of salt or oil) |
|---|---|---|---|---|---|---|
| Selenium (Se) | Animal products, whole grains, seafood, organ meats and mushrooms | 0–6 months (6 μg); 7–12 m (10 μg); 1–3y(17 μg); 4–6y (22 μg); 7–9y (21 μg); F 10–65y (26 μg); M 10–18y (32 μg); M 19–65y (34 μg); F > 65y (25 μg); M > 65y (33 μg)[d] | Readily absorbed, transported from gut bound to low and very-low density lipoproteins; excess actively excreted in urine [374]. | Glutathione peroxidases are the best studied; involved in deiodination of thyroid hormones, gene expression, levels of reactive oxygen species, brain function, glucose metabolism, reproduction | Regulates levels of reactive oxygen species; involved in activation, proliferation and differentiation of phagocytes and lymphocytes. | Keshan disease (cardiomyopathy) |
| Copper (Cu) | Animal source foods; nuts and legumes | AI for <1y, RDA for >1y: 0–6 months (200 μg); 7–12 m (220 μg); 1–3y (340 μg); 4–8y (440 μg); 9–13y (700 μg); 14–18y (890 μg); 19 + y (900 μg) [403] | Absorption via divalent metal transporter; enhanced by low Cu status; possibly enhanced by L amino acids; diets high in Zn and fiber, and low in protein may have increased Cu need [374] | Co-factor or regulator of several oxidation-reduction enzymes (e.g., cytochrome-c-oxidase – copper/zinc superoxide dismutase I); important for iron metabolism, antioxidant defense, neuropeptide synthesis | Deficiency associated with reduction in thymus size and enlargement of spleen, suppression of monocyte activity, compromised T cell proliferation via reduced IL2 production | In utero deficiency associated with neurological and immunological abnormalities, bone malformation, impaired cardiovascular development; deficiency in adulthood associated with impaired cholesterol metabolism and increased risk of osteoporosis |

(continued)

**Table 2.5** (continued)

| Nutrient | Dietary sources | Recommended nutrient intake (WHO/FAO) | Factors influencing absorption & metabolism | Physiological functions | Role in immune function | Conditions and interventions[a] associated with imbalances |
|---|---|---|---|---|---|---|
| Magnesium (Mg) | Green leafy vegetables, legumes and cereals | 0–6 m (26 mg/d); 7–12 m (54 mg/d); 1–3y (60 mg/d); 4–6y (76 mg/d); 7–9y (100 mg/d); F10–65y (220 mg/d); M10–18y (230 mg/d); M19–65y (260 mg/d); F65+ (190 mg/d); M65+ (224 mg/d)[d] | Both calcium and phosphate reduce bioavailability of magnesium; diarrhea may reduce absorption | Co-factor for hydrolysis of ATP; also co-factor for ATP-dependent reactions involved in DNA replication, gene transcription and translation | Mg deficiency in laboratory studies is associated with an increased pro-inflammatory response, accelerated thymus involution and splenomegaly | Deficiency rare at population level, more common in hospitalized individuals; may be common during pregnancy |

[a]Supplementation is considered to be an appropriate response for all nutrient deficiencies
[b]Requirements pre-menarche
[c]Requirements post-menarche
[d]Requirements vary during pregnancy and lactation

It is believed that ID is the most widespread micronutrient deficiency worldwide [69], although the exact burden is unknown, primarily because of limitations in the current biomarkers for defining population iron status. Hence, the burden of ID is typically projected from prevalence estimates of anemia. The WHO estimates that about 40% of children below 5 years and about half of children between 5 and 14 years are anemic [70]. In general, it is assumed that the burden of ID is about 2.5 times the burden of anemia in developing countries [70]. In malaria-endemic regions, it is estimated that about 50% of all anemias are attributable to ID, whereas in non-malaria-endemic regions, the proportion of all anemias attributable to ID is estimated to be 60% [2].

Causes of Iron Deficiency: ID among women of child-bearing age and children is attributable to inadequate dietary intake during the periods of highest growth, namely, pregnancy, lactation, and early life [71]. Impoverished populations generally consume low levels of highly bioavailable iron sources such as meat, fish, or poultry, coupled with a plant-based diet containing less absorbable forms of iron [72–75]. Animal sources contain the more absorbable heme iron, whereas plant sources of iron are predominantly non-heme and less absorbable [76, 77]. A high consumption of grains increases the intake of inhibitors like phytates and polyphenols, which reduce iron absorption [78–80]. Physiological demands for iron increase during infancy and childhood, and in resource-limited settings, this demand is often unmatched by intake [81, 82]. In full-term, fully breastfed newborns, iron stores are usually adequate to last for about 6 months [82]. However, after 6 months, an external iron supply is necessary to maintain adequate iron status [82]. Blood losses due to infections (malaria, hookworm, schistosomiasis) contribute to ID in endemic regions [83, 84]. Inflammation-inducing infections may also reduce iron absorption from diet [85] and may cause the redistribution of absorbed iron, leading to anemia of inflammation [86–88].

Dietary intake recommendations for iron set by the WHO take into account high, medium, and low bioavailability diets (see Table 2.5). Interest in potential toxicity has grown in the past two decades in light of a growing body of evidence suggesting that supplemental iron may have adverse consequences for health [89, 90]. Iron overload may result from the acute or chronic ingestion of quantities of iron that exceed both the ability to regulate absorption and the intracellular storage capacity. There is no universal threshold for defining systemic iron overload.

## Iron Metabolism

The homeostatic control of iron at the points of absorption, transport, mobilization from stores, and recycling is critical in determining how the iron-dependent pathways interact to influence health outcomes. Under normal physiological conditions, circulatory levels of iron are regulated at the point of absorption and mobilization from major storage sites such as the enterocytes, hepatocytes, and macrophages [91, 92]. Absorption of dietary iron occurs in the duodenal enterocytes [93]. The proteins involved in iron absorption depend on whether heme or non-heme iron is ingested [86, 94]. Absorption of non-heme iron requires the divalent metal transporter (DMTI) [86, 94]. Since most of the ingested iron is in the +3 oxidation state ($Fe^{+3}$), dietary iron must first be converted to $Fe^{+2}$ using the duodenal cytochrome B (DcytB), a process that is enhanced by ascorbic acid [95], before it can be transported by DMT1. Although the absorption of heme iron is not completely understood, it is believed that the heme carrier protein (HCP)1 is involved in importing heme iron from the gut into the enterocytes [96]. Absorbed iron, whether heme or non-heme, is either stored as ferritin, or exported into plasma through the basolateral membrane-bound protein, ferroportin. Iron may be released into the circulation bound to transferrin or may be lost when the enterocytes are sloughed off [86]. Hepcidin is the major regulatory protein involved in the maintenance of iron homeostasis [97–99]. The hepatic synthesis of hepcidin, a 25-amino acid peptide hormone, is upregulated by high extracellular iron concentrations and inflammation [100] and downregulated by erythropoiesis [88, 99]. Upon synthesis, hepcidin binds to ferroportin in the storage cells, causing its internalization and degradation, and hence prevents the release of iron into circulation [101]. Hepcidin synthesis is decreased during ID anemia and in other conditions that upregulate the rate of red blood cell formation. Suppression of hepcidin is associated with an increase in levels of erythropoietin (EPO) which ultimately ensures that there is enough iron for erythropoietic activities [102]. The adult human contains 3–5 g of iron. Between 60 and 75% of total body iron is stored in hemoglobin and about 25% is stored as ferritin in hepatocytes and macrophages.

### Potential Pathways to Infections: Iron

The bulk of the scientific literature on the role of iron in infection disease etiology focuses on the potential adverse effects of both supplemental iron [89, 90] and endogenous iron obtained through routine diet [103]. Global interest in understanding the role of iron in the pathology of infections gained momentum in 2006, following the publication of a large community-based trial [90] which concluded that children in a malaria-endemic region in Zanzibar receiving 12.5 mg of iron were about 12% more likely to die or need treatment at a hospital and about 15% more likely to be admitted to a hospital compared to the control group. Because a parallel trial in southern Nepal, a non-malaria-endemic region, found no adverse effect of iron supplementation on severe morbidity or mortality [104], the initial global reaction was that this adverse effect was driven by malaria. More recent evidence from both experimental and observational studies appears to suggest that iron intake or status, beyond the absorptive and storage capacity, may precipitate adverse outcomes for infections [103]. Although not clearly understood, possible mechanisms include the increased availability of non-transferrin bound iron [85, 105–107] and therefore increased accessibility of iron to invading parasites [108], the increased generation of reactive oxygen species (ROS) [107, 109–112], iron redistribution, and dyserythropoiesis through the hormonal activities of hepcidin [91, 113–118], enhancement of co-infections by iron [106, 116, 119–121], delayed parasite clearance and sequestration [122–125], enhanced hemolysis [126, 127], and an exaggerated acute phase response through the secretion of high levels of pro-inflammatory cytokines [107, 119, 128, 129]. Excessive iron loading in the gut, especially when it overlaps with a concurrent reduction in absorption (owing to the presence of systemic inflammation and other factors), may enhance the growth of harmful gut microbes, increasing the risk for gastrointestinal infections, such as diarrhea [106, 130].

On the other end of the spectrum of iron-immune system interactions, some evidence suggests ID may compromise innate immune responses via a reduction in production of cytokine and reactive oxygen intermediates, which are critical for phagocytic clearance [131, 132]. Iron deficiency may also impair lymphocyte development and therefore the adaptive immune response [133].

## *Calcium*

### Calcium Needs, Sources, and Risk of Deficiency

Historically, the essentiality of calcium has been linked to the attainment of peak bone mass and health conditions resulting in low bone density and bone fractures. Calcium exists in nature as a divalent metal with atomic weight of 40. Nearly all (~99%) of the calcium in the body is found in the skeletal system, where it is stored complexed to phosphate groups in the form of hydroxyapatite. As part of the skeletal system, calcium provides support and protection for the visceral organs. Calcium is present in small amounts in intracellular compartments (the sarcoplasmic reticulum found in muscle cells) and is also involved in several signaling pathways linked to key cellular processes such as gene transcription, cellular secretion, and muscle contraction (see Table 2.5) [134, 135]. In the nervous system, calcium is critical for synaptic transmission, triggering the release of the neurotransmitter acetylcholine from the pre-synaptic neuron into the synaptic cleft. This process ensures the transmission of neuronal signals to target organs, regulating downstream physiological processes such as digestion, respiration, and systemic circulation. Because of its role in transmission of nerve impulses and muscle contraction, low calcium levels are associated with irregular spasms and numbness or tingling.

---

**Box 2.6 Key Facts: Calcium (See Table 2.5)**
- Nearly all (~99%) of the body calcium is found in the skeletal system.
- Calcium is critical for several signaling pathways and affects key cellular processes such as gene transcription, cellular secretion and muscle contraction.
- Low calcium levels are associated with irregular spasms, muscle twitching (as in tetanus), and numbness or tingling.

---

Milk and dairy products (such as yoghurt and cheese) constitute the major source (>70%) of dietary calcium [136]. Calcium may also be obtained from some vegetables, grains, fruits, legumes, nuts, and eggs [137]. Calcium needs are set to reflect the amount generally considered adequate to prevent negative calcium balance and resulting bone loss. Recommended intake does not change for pregnant or lactating women (see Table 2.5). Calcium status is linked to vitamin D status in that vitamin D regulates the intestinal absorption of calcium [138]. Absorption of calcium in the intestinal mucosa cell requires the action of the vitamin D-dependent protein transient receptor potential vanilloid subfamily member 6 and calmodulin-D [138].

In adults, osteoporosis, characterized by a low bone mineral mass, is the most common outcome of calcium deficiency. Osteoporosis was historically considered a major public health issue among postmenopausal women in high-income countries, but is now known to be a global health problem, also affecting low- and middle-income countries [139]. Low bone mass, and the development of osteoporosis, is common in both postmenopausal women and men over 50 years of age. In children, calcium deficiency increases the risk for nutritional rickets, especially when it overlaps a deficiency in vitamin D [140].

## Calcium Metabolism

Regulation of plasma calcium is controlled by three primary hormones, namely parathyroid hormone (PTH, secreted by the parathyroid glands), calcitonin (secreted by the thyroid gland), and calcitriol (1,25-dihydroxy vitamin $D_3$ (1,25$(OH)_2D_3$), secreted by the kidney in response to PTH) [141]. PTH is produced when plasma calcium levels are low. Within the nephrons in the kidney, PTH stimulates increased reabsorption of calcium from the filtrate and concurrently increases the excretion of phosphates. Also in the kidney, PTH stimulates the conversion of 25-OH-$D_3$ to 1,25$(OH)_2D_3$, which mediates the action of PTH on the kidney by increasing the reabsorption of calcium in the nephron [142]. PTH also has an effect on bones, where it stimulates osteoclasts to break down bones, releasing both calcium and phosphate into circulation. Calcitonin is produced by the thyroid gland in response to high plasma calcium levels and primarily lowers blood calcium levels by inhibiting bone resorption [143]. Mechanisms of bone deposition, and the movement of calcium into bone, are not yet fully understood [144]. Within cells, calcium is highly compartmentalized, and its release is tightly regulated. Nearly all of the intracellular calcium is found in the nucleus (>50%), mitochondria (~20%) and in endoplasmic or sarcoplasmic reticulum (~20%) [145, 146]. Only about 0.5% of intracellular calcium is available in the cytoplasm where it can bind to high affinity proteins to stimulate or inhibit specific physiological processes. Calcium may be lost via urine (~40–200 mg/d) and feces (80–120 mg/d). During stages of growth and development, calcium is concentrated into the skeletal system at a rate of about 150 mg/d [147]. However, once growth ceases, the body maintains a calcium equilibrium through the process of bone remodeling and by the homeostatic regulation of calcium absorption and renal reabsorption or excretion.

### Potential Pathways to Infections: Calcium

Because of its role in intracellular signaling, and in particular, because of its involvement in the regulation of gene transcription, calcium may be critical in the process of immune response (see Table 2.5) [148]. It has been hypothesized that calcium may play a role in regulating antibody production and the pro-inflammatory responses in some disease conditions [149]. The potential involvement of calcium in immune responses is also supported by the discovery of a calcium-dependent gene in T lymphocytes [150]. Additional evidence is needed regarding the role of calcium in the immune responses to infection in human population.

## Zinc

### Zinc Needs, Sources, and Risk of Deficiency

Zinc deficiency, affecting >30% of the world population, is a leading cause of morbidity and mortality, particularly in low-income settings [151]. Zinc is the second most abundant trace element in the human body, constituting 2–4 g in the adult human. Zinc is an essential trace mineral involved in several catalytic, structural, and regulatory roles in humans. Plasma zinc, commonly used to assess zinc status, represents only ~1% of the total body zinc and is not a reliable indicator of an individual's zinc status (see Table 2.1). In light of the absence of specific and sensitive biomarkers of zinc status, the current dietary recommendation for zinc is based on an approach which considers both the physiological requirement by age and gender and the minimum amount required to offset daily losses occurring primarily via feces and urine (see Table 2.5). In addition, this approach considers the additional amount of zinc required to promote and support a state of healthy growth, pregnancy, and lactation, as well as a consideration for the factors that influence the absorption and bioavailability of dietary zinc sources. The WHO estimates the total endogenous zinc losses at 1.40 mg/d for males and 1.00 mg/d for females, and daily physiological zinc requirements at 0.84 mg for 6–12 month infants, 0.83 mg for 1–3 year old children, 0.97 mg for 3–6 years, and ~ 1.12–1.54 mg from 6–18 years, depending on age and gender (see Table 2.5) [152, 153].

Zinc is available in several food groups. Rich sources of zinc include red meat, whole grains, and some seafood. The bioavailability of zinc from animal-source foods is higher than plant sources because phytates and other non-digestible plant ligands bind to, and therefore inhibit, zinc absorption. Therefore, zinc deficiency is very prevalent in settings where staples or routine diets are predominantly plant-based. In grains, zinc is present at higher concentration in the germ and bran, making refined grains a poor dietary source for zinc. Zinc deficiency is especially high during the period of complementary feeding. During this period, adequate supply through optimal complementary feeding is necessary to replace breastmilk zinc and to meet the demands for rapid growth occurring at this time.

---

**Box 2.7 Sources and Needs: Zinc (See Table 2.5)**
- Red meat, whole grains, and some seafoods are rich sources of zinc.
- Phytates in plants bind to and inhibit zinc absorption.
- Zinc deficiency is especially high during complementary feeding of young children.

---

## Zinc Metabolism

The fraction of zinc absorbed depends on the amount present in the diet and the amount of inhibitors consumed. Although up to 70% of zinc administered in aqueous forms may be absorbed, the fractional zinc absorption decreases when consumed as part of a meal [154]. Dietary zinc is released into the small intestine and absorbed into the enterocytes by a family of zinc transporters that also regulate the efflux of absorbed zinc from the enterocytes into circulation. The expression of these transporters is believed to be regulated by the total zinc content of the diet. Zinc absorption also involves the divalent metal transporter DMT1. There is inconsistent evidence on how the presence of other cations, such as iron and copper, may affect the absorption of zinc via DMT1 [155–157]. Zinc absorption is increased in individuals that are zinc deficient [158]. Dietary zinc is absorbed in the duodenum and transported to the liver bound to albumin. Approximately 70% of circulatory zinc is bound to albumin, so any physiological processes which affect the synthesis or mobilization of albumin will also lower plasma zinc concentrations. Homeostatic regulation zinc is achieved mainly by regulating intestinal absorption and excretion, and these processes are often synergistic [159, 160].

## Potential Pathways to Infections: Zinc

Adequate zinc status may boost immune response via multiple pathways, several of which are due to the role of zinc in cell replication, transcription, translation, catalysis [161], and maintenance of mucosal and barrier immunity [162, 163]. Zinc plays an essential role in both innate and adaptive immune responses. It is important for proliferation of immune cells, including macrophages and neutrophils, required for the initial defense against invading pathogens. Zinc's role in the enhancement of mucosal repair is the basis for recommending zinc treatment for gastrointestinal and respiratory illnesses. In particular, the WHO and UNICEF recommend that therapeutic zinc (20 mg) be given daily for 10–14 days during diarrhea episodes as adjunctive treatment for diarrhea, along with oral rehydration solution [164, 165]. There is currently no consensus or recommendations regarding the use of zinc during respiratory tract infections, as the body of scientific evidence is inconsistent and inconclusive [3, 166]. There is emerging evidence suggesting that zinc may enhance adaptive immunity [167] by increasing antibody responses to some infections [168] and by increasing the proliferation of B and T lymphocytes [169]. However, the results have not been consistent across studies [170]. Evidence also suggests zinc may reduce the generation of ROS and, therefore, may reduce the severity of the pro-inflammatory responses to certain infections [171].

## *Iodine*

### Iodine Needs, Sources, and Risk of Deficiency

Iodine was first discovered as a violet vapor released by the combustion of seaweed. In historical Chinese medicine, seaweeds were used in the treatment of goiter (enlargement of the thyroid gland) [172]. It is now known that seaweeds and other seafoods are rich sources of iodine, a critical component of thyroid hormones produced by the thyroid glands (see Table 2.5) [173]. The thyroid gland produces two important hormones, triiodothyronine ($T_3$) and thyroxine ($T_4$), both of which are involved in regulating basal metabolism. Through the action of these hormones, iodine promotes normal physical and cognitive growth [174]. Iodine deficiency disorders (IDD) include a spectrum of disorders characterized by impairment of thyroid hormone biosynthesis [175]. Because the thyroid hormone is critical for growth and metabolism, iodine deficiency is associated with physical and neurological growth impairment and, in severe forms, may increase the risk of death in children. The classic symptoms of iodine deficiency are goiter and cretinism (severe growth retardation and developmental delays) [175]. Other physical manifestations of iodine deficiency include congenital abnormalities and stillbirths. Because the iodine content of typically consumed foods is low (< 80 ug/serving), many countries now have universal iodine supplementation programs, achieved primarily via use of iodized salts [176].

---

**Box 2.8 Key Facts: Iodine**
- In historical Chinese medicine, seaweeds (now known to contain a high amount of iodine) were used in the treatment of goiter.
- Iodine is a component of thyroid hormones.
- Thyroid hormones regulate basal metabolism and physical and cognitive growth.
- Goiter and cretinism are the classic symptoms of iodine deficiency.
- In many countries, universal salt iodization has been established to reduce IDD.

---

### Iodine Metabolism

Iodine is highly absorbable, with around 90% of dietary iodine absorbed via active transport in the small intestine [177]. Circulatory iodine is removed from the blood by the kidney and thyroid gland. Up to 80% of the body's iodine is stored in the thyroid gland. Iodine uptake by the thyroid may range from as low as 10% (during states of adequacy) to as high as 90% during states of severe deficiency [178, 179]. This homeostatic control is believed to be regulated at the level of gene transcription, such that the expression of genes for the iodine transport protein, sodium-iodide symporter, is up- or down-regulated to meet the body's needs [180, 181]. In the thyroid, the protein thyroglobulin is converted to mono-diiodotyrosine (MIT) and diiodotyrosine (DIT) by the addition of one or two units of iodine to tyrosine residues [182]. These reactions are catalyzed by the enzyme thyroperoxidase, in the presence of hydrogen peroxide. The hormones $T_3$ and $T_4$ are the end products, formed by the combination of one DIT with one MIT (to produce $T_3$) or by combing two DIT polymers (to produce $T_4$) [182]. Both $T_3$ and $T_4$ behave like steroid hormones, by binding to nuclear receptors and activating the transcription of several genes.

**Potential Pathways to Infections: Iodine**

Studies have shown that immune cells have the genes for the transcription of mRNA for thyroglobulin and thyroxine peroxidase, two proteins required for the synthesis of the thyroid hormones [183]. It is plausible that iodine plays a role in immune responses, although the evidence for this is limited. Because thyroid hormones are involved in general metabolism and growth, it is conceivable that iodine, acting through these hormones, may be involved in the proliferation and differentiation of immune cells, or in regulating the products of immune cells, including cytokine and antibody production. Animal studies have shown that administration of iodine can result in an increase in proliferation of T lymphocytes and natural killer cells [184]. There is also some evidence than both hypo- and hyperthyroidism, defined by changes in $T_3$ and $T_4$ levels, are associated with changes in proinflammatory activities and changes in levels of ROS [185].

# Selenium

**Selenium Needs, Sources, and Risk of Deficiency**

Research on the role of selenium in human nutrition has evolved rapidly over the last few decades from an initial focus on potential selenium toxicity [186] to a focus on potential health benefits of trace amounts of selenium [187]. Limited evidence in the first half of the twentieth century suggested selenium was associated with alkali disease and blind staggers in animals [188]. In the second half of the twentieth century, strong evidence emerged linking selenium intake to prevention of necrosis of the liver in rat models consuming a vitamin E deficient diet [189]. Around the same time, selenium deficiency was also linked to Keshan disease, a fatal disease affecting heart muscle (cardiomyopathy) and endemic in certain regions of China [190]. Recent evidence suggests that selenium is essential in proper brain functioning [191], glucose metabolism [192], and reproduction [193, 194]. The biological activity of selenium occurs through its association with selenoproteins, a class of proteins capable of forming complexes with selenium. The primary sources of selenium in the diet are animal products and grains such as wheat and corn [195]. Selenium may also come from fungi sources like mushrooms and yeast. Selenium intake guidelines consider both safety and needs (see Table 2.5). Regardless of the source, dietary selenium is typically in the form of seleno-amino acids. In animal source foods, selenium may exist as either selenocysteine (cysteine residues with selenium replacing the sulfur in the side group) or as selenomethionine (methionine residues with selenium replacing the sulfur in the side group). In plant sources, selenium exists solely as selenomethionine. Both forms of selenium are efficiently absorbed (>80%) via active transport by duodenal enterocytes.

Although the spectrum of selenium deficiencies is not well characterized, it appears that the major cause of low plasma selenium is living in regions with low levels of selenium in soil [196, 197]. Historically, evidence of selenium deficiency came from studies demonstrating the responsiveness of certain disease conditions to selenium supplementation. Notably, selenium deficiency was first linked to Keshan disease because patients with symptoms consistent with this disease responded positively to selenium supplementation [198]. However, even for Keshan disease, it remains debatable whether selenium deficiency is the underlying cause, as several recent studies have linked factors independent of selenium status, such as family history and specific genetic polymorphisms [199], to Keshan disease. Hence the health outcomes associated with selenium deficiency remain poorly characterized [200]. Evidence from country-level food balance sheets suggests a high prevalence of selenium deficiency in sub-Saharan Africa [201] and South Asia [202, 203]. Selenium deficiency has also been reported in vulnerable groups such as patients on parenteral nutrition and preterm newborns [204–206]. In most studies selenium deficiency is defined by the activity of glutathione peroxidase 3 (GPX3) <86.9 ng m/L) or iodothyronine deiodinase (IDI) <64.8 ng m/L (see Table 2.1). In a recent study in Malawi, selenium deficiency was diagnosed in 63% of Malawian women of reproductive age [196].

## Selenium Metabolism

Absorbed selenium is transported bound to protein in plasma. The biologic activities of selenium rely on its incorporation into selenoproteins. In selenoproteins, the 21st amino acid position is occupied by selenocysteine, a derivative of cysteine in which the sulfur in the side chain is replaced with selenium [207]. There are several known selenoproteins, and these are generally considered to have the ability to localize in both the nucleus and cytoplasm, suggesting their involvement in intracellular signaling and transcription. Glutathione peroxidases (GPXs) are the most studied selenoproteins. These proteins catalyze the breakdown of hydroperoxides, a process critical to maintaining the integrity of cells [208, 209]. The catalytic activities of GPXs are aided by glutathione. GPX proteins have different forms, such as cytosol GPX, gastrointestinal GPX, plasma GPX, phospholipid hydroperoxide GPX, and olfactory system GPX. A second group of selenoproteins catalyzes the deiodination of thyroid hormones, and regulates downstream cellular processes such as gene expression [210, 211].

---

**Box 2.9 Sources and Needs: Selenium (See Table 2.5)**
- Major sources of selenium include animal products, grains, and mushrooms.
- Selenocystein (found in animal products) and selenomethione (found in both plants and animal products) are the major dietary forms of selenium.

---

## Potential Pathways to Infections: Selenium

Selenium's role in regulating levels of ROS provides a basis for its role in reducing inflammation [212]. The regulation of ROS is believed to be achieved through the action of the GPX family of selenoproteins [213]. Optimal selenium levels are necessary in both the initiation of the immune response, as well as in downregulation of the immune response [214]. It is believed that adequate selenium status is necessary for optimal activation of phagocytes and lymphocytes and in the proliferation and differentiation of these immune cells [213]. Limited evidence also suggests that selenium may be involved in regulating the action of interleukin (IL)2, by increasing the expression of receptors for IL2 by lymphocytes [215]. Selenium may also be involved in the switch from the T helper (Th)1 pro-inflammatory response to the less inflammatory Th2 type of immune response [216].

## *Copper*

### Copper Needs, Sources, and Risk of Deficiency

The essentiality of copper was demonstrated in the first half of the twentieth century, in a study where copper was shown to be critical for hematopoiesis in rats [217]. In humans, the earliest evidence of the essentiality of copper came from studies conducted in the late twentieth century and thereafter, which showed a strong association between low plasma copper concentrations and anemia [218, 219]. The adult human contains ~100 mg copper, mostly concentrated in tissues of the skeletal system (muscles and bones), the brain, and the liver. Copper is a transition metal, which exists in two oxidation states ($Cu^{2+}$ and $Cu^{1+}$). In biological systems, the $Cu^{2+}$ state is the predominant form [220]. Copper acts as a cofactor or allosteric regulator of several oxidation-reduction enzymes. Enzymes requiring copper include cytochrome-c-oxidase (involved in the electron transport chain in the inner mitochondrial membrane), copper/zinc superoxide dismutase I (catalyzes the conversion of free radicals to hydrogen peroxides), and ceruloplasmin (major copper-carrying protein in the body) (see Table 2.5) [221]. Ceruloplasmin is a ferroxidase, involved in the conversion of ferrous to ferric iron [222], thereby enhancing iron transport in plasma via binding to transferrin. Emerging evidence primarily from animal models also suggests that copper is involved in the expression of several genes [223].

---

**Box 2.10 Sources and Needs: Copper**
- Animal products, nuts and legumes are major sources of copper in the diet.
- In adults, 900 µg/day is recommended.
- Risk of copper deficiency increases in settings with a high burden of malnutrition.

---

Copper deficiency has been reported in malnourished children, highlighting its essentiality for growth [224–226]. Animal foods constitute the major sources of dietary copper. Other food sources of copper include nuts and legumes.

**Copper Metabolism**

Absorption of copper from the gut into enterocytes is via DMT1, the same protein used in the absorption of iron, zinc, and other mineral cations. Absorbed copper is transported in the blood bound to albumin, and upon reaching the liver, it is complexed to the protein ceruloplasmin. Most (~90%) of the copper in circulation is bound to ceruloplasmin and transported to target tissues and organs. Within cells, copper is an essential cofactor for enzymatic reactions including reactions catalyzed by ceruloplasmin, superoxide dismutase, and cytochrome C oxidase. In this role, copper serves as an antioxidant nutrient and may protect the integrity of cells from attack by free radicals [227]. In particular, copper-zinc superoxide dismutase is localized in the cytosol and intermembrane space where it catalyzes the conversion of free oxygen radicals to hydrogen peroxides, which can subsequently be broken down by the catalase enzyme.

---

**Box 2.11 Key Facts: Copper**
- Essentiality of copper was established in the twentieth century as a nutrient critical for the formation of cellular components of blood.
- The adult human has ~100 mg of copper distributed in muscles, bones, the brain, and the liver.
- Copper is a cofactor for several enzyme-catalyzed reactions.
- Copper facilitates iron absorption by the conversion of ferrous to ferric iron; copper deficiency increases risk of anemia.

---

**Potential Pathways to Infections: Copper**

There are several theoretical pathways by which copper may affect the immune system, some of which are supported by recent evidence from in vitro studies and animal models. Copper is believed to affect both structural and functional components of the innate and adaptive immune systems. Copper deficiency (defined by plasma ceruloplasmin) has been associated with a reduction in thymus size and an enlargement of the spleen in copper-deficient mice relative to controls [228]. In vitro studies using copper chelators showed that the induction of copper deficiency suppressed the activities of monocytes [229]. Evidence from in vitro studies and animal models also suggests that copper deficiency compromises T cell proliferation via a reduction in cytokine production, particularly IL2, which serves as a trigger for T cell proliferation [230]. It is believed that this reduction in T cell proliferation may be partly due to a copper-dependent reduction in mitogenic response, although the mechanisms are not clear [231]. Copper may also enhance phagocytosis, modulation of neutrophil functioning, and differentiation of several immune cell types [232]. There is limited evidence from human studies regarding the role of copper in immunity and infections. In one small study of 19 copper deficient, marasmic children in Chilé, copper supplementation had no impact on several immuno-globulins in both blood and saliva, despite improvement in the phagocytic index [233]. Other more recent studies have shown that a copper-sufficient diet may potentially decrease the proliferation of peripheral blood mononuclear cells, although these studies were small and the evidence generally inconclusive [234]. Therefore, additional evidence from human studies regarding the role of copper in the immune response is needed.

## *Magnesium*

**Magnesium Needs, Sources, and Risk of Deficiency**

It is estimated that the human body contains ~23 g of magnesium and about half of this is concentrated in the bones [235]. There is a high concentration of intracellular magnesium, especially in cells with a high energy need. Magnesium acts as a cofactor in muscle cells for all metabolic reactions involving the hydrolysis of ATP (see Table 2.5) [235]. Phosphorylation of enzymes results in their activation or inactivation and thus regulates the downstream physiological pathways. Magnesium, in its role as a cofactor for ATP-dependent reactions, is also critical for DNA replication, gene transcription and translation [236]. About 1% of magnesium is available in the extracellular fluids, bound to specific proteins.

---

**Box 2.12 Key Facts: Magnesium**
- Magnesium is the second most abundant divalent cation in the human body, after calcium.
- Energy-dependent reactions require magnesium for the hydrolysis of ATP.
- About 27% of magnesium in the human body is found in muscle.

---

Magnesium is supplied in the diet from both plant and animal sources, although plants constitute the major sources of dietary magnesium [237]. Green leafy vegetables, legumes, and cereals are all good sources of magnesium [238]. Animal sources, because of the high concentrations of calcium and phosphate, tend to have a low amount of bioavailable magnesium. Magnesium requirements increase with age and are generally higher in adult men relative to women (see Table 2.5). Requirements increase during pregnancy (~400 mg) but not during lactation [239].

Although magnesium deficiency is uncommon at the population level, deficiencies can be high in hospital patients, especially in patients with diseases which interfere with gut and renal functions. Magnesium deficiency is estimated at ~10% in hospital patients [240]. Magnesium deficiency during pregnancy is especially high in low-income settings, and hypomagnesia during pregnancy may increase the risk for poor fetal development and mortality [241, 242]. Magnesium deficiency can also result from familial hypomagnesia, an inherited disorder [243]. Magnesium deficiency may also result from diseases such as diarrhea, which reduce the transit time of food through the intestines and decrease absorption, although the evidence for this mechanism is limited [244].

## Magnesium Metabolism

In normal adults, up to 50% of dietary magnesium is absorbed in the small intestine via both simple diffusion and facilitated transport requiring transmembrane proteins. Body magnesium levels are regulated mainly in the kidney [245]. When concentrations are higher than normal, renal reabsorption of magnesium is decreased, increasing the amount excreted in the urine [246]. In the kidney, the proximal tubule, the ascending limb of the loop of Henle and the distal convoluted tubule reabsorb approximately 15%, 70%, and 10%, respectively, of magnesium in the glomerular filtrate [245]. About 65% of the body's magnesium is mineralized as part of bones, and an additional 32% is complexed to biomolecules, including nucleic acids and proteins [247]. Within cells, approximately 80% of the magnesium is bound to protein and nucleic acids, and it is believed that the binding of magnesium provides stability for these molecules [247].

## Potential Pathways to Infections: Magnesium

Experimentally induced magnesium deficiency in animal models has been associated with changes in several aspects of the immune response (see Table 2.5). In rat models, magnesium deficiency was associated with an increased pro-inflammatory response [248, 249], characterized by increased production of several cytokines [250]. It is believed that this action may in part be mediated by an increase in polymorphonuclear cells and neutrophils [251]. Magnesium deficiency has also been linked to anatomical changes in key immune system organs. In particular, magnesium deficiency in rats is associated with accelerated thymus involution and splenomegaly [252]. In thymus cells, magnesium is known to influence gene expression, and this process may affect the production of some cytokine receptors. There is limited evidence regarding the role in magnesium in immune response in humans.

# Fat Soluble Vitamins

## Vitamin A and Carotenoids

### Vitamin A and Carotenoids Needs, Sources, and Risk of Deficiency

Vitamin A refers to retinol and related molecules and may be pre-formed or derived from pro-vitamin A carotenoids. Pre-formed vitamin A, commonly found in animal source foods such as liver, egg, fish liver oils, and dairy products, includes all trans retinol, all trans retinal and 3-dehydroretinol. The pro-vitamin A carotenoids include β-carotene, α-carotene, and β-cryptoxanthin and are commonly found in yellow fruits and vegetables and green leafy vegetables. These carotenoids constitute the major supply of vitamin A in the diet. Upon consumption, pro-vitamin A carotenoids are cleaved to form vitamin A derivatives (see Table 2.6) [253].

**Table 2.6** Characteristics of fat-soluble vitamins

| Nutrient | Dietary sources | Recommended nutrient intake (WHO/FAO) | Factors influencing absorption & metabolism | Physiological functions | Role in immune function | Conditions and interventions[a] associated with imbalances |
|---|---|---|---|---|---|---|
| Vitamin A & carotenoids | Colorful plants containing carotenoids, liver, fish oils, butter, cheese, milk fat, other dairy products, and egg yolk, fortified cereals | In µg retinol equivalents (RE)/day 0–6 m (375); 7–12 m (400); 1–3y (400); 4–6y (450); 7–9y (500); 10–18y (600); F19–65y (500); M19–65y (600); 65y + (600)[b] | Pre-formed vitamin A absorbed via active transport; dietary fat (5–10 g in a meal) and bile salts required for proper absorption; carotenoids absorbed via diffusion, cleaved and converted to forms of retinol; stored in the liver | Cellular differentiation and proliferation; enables vision in dim light; regulates gene transcription | Key regulators of epithelial cell differentiation and growth; reduces secretion of pro-inflammatory cytokines; supplementation is associated with increased eryptosis | Xeropthalmia (night blindness), anemia, immune dysfunction, poor growth and maturation; interventions: high-dose vitamin A supplementation, dietary diversification, food fortification, biofortification |
| Vitamin D | Dietary: oily fish, cod liver oil, dairy. Absorption through skin with sunlight | 0–50y (5 µg/d); 51–65y (10 µg/d); 65y + (15 µg/d) | Absorbed in intestine by passive diffusion together with long chain fatty acids; carried in chylomicrons; requires dietary fat and bile salts for absorption | Regulates blood calcium levels; also involved in reproduction and immune function | Linked to several autoimmune diseases | Deficiency historically associated with rickets in children |
| Vitamin E | Vegetable oils (soybean, sunflower, corn and palm oil) | 0–12 m (2.7 mg α-Tocopherol Equivalents (TE)/day); 1–6y (5.0 mg α-TE/day); 7–9y (7.0 mg α-TE/day); F10y + (7.5 mg α-TE/day); M10y + (10.0 mg α-TE/day) | Absorbed through passive diffusion in duodenum; enhanced by dietary fat and particularly saturated fats; decreased by polyunsaturated fats; carried in blood and lymph bound to lipid-carrying proteins | Antioxidant, protects integrity of plasma membranes by preventing oxidation of polyunsaturated fatty acids by free radicals | Adequacy associated with increased proliferation of lymphocytes; interacts synergistically with selenium in enhancing the production of immunoglobulin (IgG) and splenic cytokine expression | Deficiency first associated with reproduction and fetal growth; now associated with atherosclerosis and hemolytic anemia |
| Vitamin K | Green leafy vegetables, oils, dairy, some cereals; gut microbes | 0–6 m (5 µg/d); 7–12 m (10 µg/d); 1–3y (15 µg/d); 4–6y (20 µg/d); 7–9y (25 µg/d); 10–18y (35–55 µg/d); F19y + (55 µg/d); M19y + (65 µg/d) | Absorbed during process of fat digestion and absorption; requires a protein carrier; disease conditions affecting fat digestion may reduce absorption [374] | Important co-factor for blood coagulation | Phylloquinone and menaquinone associated with reduced pro-inflammatory response during chronic disease | Hemorrhage |

[a]Supplementation and/or fortification is considered to be an appropriate response for all nutrient deficiencies
[b]Requirements vary during pregnancy and lactation

About 2.8 million children are at risk for vitamin A deficiency (VAD) and about 250 million others are at risk of other functional disorders of vitamin A deficiency [254]. VAD is defined as serum or plasma retinol concentration below 0.7 μmol/L [255]. VAD is considered a public health problem in about 122 countries [255] and is associated with adverse health outcomes including increased morbidity and mortality risk. In young children, the major causes of VAD are low vitamin A content of breast milk [256], low intake of vitamin A from dietary sources, and high prevalence of infectious diseases [257, 258]. Poor maternal nutritional status during pre-gestation, gestation, and early postpartum periods is associated with low vitamin A content of breast milk [259, 260]. Newborns typically have very low vitamin A stores at birth and thus rely on the vitamin A status of the mother to improve their vitamin A stores. Unfortunately, women in undernourished regions of the world may not consume sufficient quantities of foods containing bioavailable vitamin A [261–264], and, as a result, infants born under these conditions are at an increased risk of VAD [258]. Although the vitamin A requirement for women increases only slightly during pregnancy, requirements increase substantially during lactation (from 700 μg/d in the non-pregnant, non-lactating woman to 1300 μg/d during lactation) [265]. In low-income countries, meals served to children typically contain very little animal source foods such as liver, egg, and dairy products and thus contain limited quantities of bioavailable preformed vitamin A (retinyl esters) [266].

---

**Box 2.13 Key Facts: Vitamin A**
- Pro-vitamin A carotenoids (β-carotene, α-carotene, and β-cryptoxanthin) are commonly found in yellow fruits and vegetables and green leafy vegetables.
- VAD is especially common among young children in low-income countries.
- Semi-annual high-dose vitamin A supplementation is a global strategy for reducing burden of VAD.
- VAD is associated with impaired vision and elevated risk of morbidity and mortality.
- Vitamin A (and other fat-soluble vitamins) is absorbed during the digestion and absorption of dietary lipids.
- In the intestine, pro-vitamin A is converted to retinal and then to retinol.
- The physiological activity of vitamin A is mainly in its retinoic acid form.

---

A third factor increasing risk of VAD in developing countries is the high prevalence of infectious diseases such as malaria, measles, diarrhea, and pneumonia [267–272]. Infections in children are associated with anorexia, malabsorption, impaired nutrient transportation, and increased losses [267–272]. When compared to healthy children, in a small trial, absorption of isotope-labeled retinyl acetate was reduced by about 30% during both diarrhea and respiratory illnesses [269]. Some evidence from animal studies suggests that malaria parasites are able to incorporate host vitamin A and may deprive the host of essential vitamin A [273]. During severe infections, up to 6.0 μmol of retinol (representing over 18% of liver stores in young children) may be lost daily via urine [268]. Inflammation-induced hyporetinolemia has been demonstrated under multiple disease conditions including diarrhea, pneumonia, HIV, and malaria [274, 275].

### Vitamin A and Carotenoid Metabolism

Much of the retinol obtained from the diet comes from the digestion of retinyl esters and esters of pro-vitamin A carotenoids. As part of lipid digestion in the small intestine, retinol and carotenoids are released from their esters and absorbed into enterocytes [276]. In the enterocytes, retinol is re-esterified and incorporated into chylomicrons to be transported to the liver. Some absorbed β-carotene is metabolized to retinal and then to retinol before being esterified and incorporated in chylomicrons. β-carotene may also be incorporated directly into chylomicrons. After incorporation into chylomicrons, retinol and carotenoids are transported in the lymphatic system, which drains into the systemic circulation via the jugular vein, before being transported to the liver for storage as retinol palmitate. When needed, retinol is released from the liver bound to a complex of retinol binding protein (RBP) and transthyretin. Bound retinol is delivered via the systemic circulation to target cells, where RBP binds to its receptor on the target cell, allowing for the diffusion of retinol into the cell. Once inside the cell, retinol binds an intracellular RBP, cellular retinol binding protein (CRBP). The CRBP-retinol complex is the dominant form of retinol available within cells [277], where it is involved in the conversion of retinol to retinoic acid, which binds to nuclear receptors to modulate replication and transcription of key genes (see Table 2.6) [278].

The metabolic roles of vitamin A are typically accomplished through its retinoic acid derivative. Via this metabolite, vitamin A regulates physiological processes that affect growth, vision, reproduction, and immunity. The up-regulation of immune pathways by vitamin A is achieved through the binding of retinoic acid to nuclear receptors and the subsequent activation of these receptors, effectively up-regulating transcription and translation, cell proliferation and differentiation (see Table 2.6) [279, 280].

### Potential Pathways to Infections: Vitamin A and Carotenoids

Vitamin A is involved in several physiological pathways connected to several disease etiologies. Adequate vitamin A status has been associated with enhancement of both innate and adaptive immune responses (see Table 2.6) [270, 281–284]. Vitamin A metabolites are key regulators of epithelial cell differentiation and growth [285] and are therefore critical in promoting epithelial tissue integrity, an important component of the innate defense system. Vitamin A has adjuvant potential and may enhance antibody responses to secondary infections [286]. Vitamin A also affects anti-inflammatory responses, characterized by a reduction in the secretion of pro-inflammatory cytokines [287, 288]. In infections such as malaria, which are accompanied by inflammation, this anti-inflammatory potential of vitamin A may be especially important in preventing the progression to severe outcomes. Vitamin A supplementation is associated with increased eryptosis (the suicidal death of red blood cells) [289] and may therefore expedite the clearance of parasitized red blood cells during malaria infection [287, 288]. Vitamin A may also enhance the potency of some drugs [290–292] and may improve erythropoiesis [293].

## *Vitamin D*

### Vitamin D Needs, Sources, and Risk of Deficiency

Vitamin D is best known for its role in regulating blood calcium levels, along with the hormones calcitonin and PTH [294]. In this role, vitamin D maintains calcium balance by regulating calcium absorption, reabsorption in renal tubules, and release from bone cells (see section "Proteins"). In addition. More recent literature has shed light on the role of vitamin D in other physiological processes including reproduction [295] and immunity [296]. Only a small amount (10–20%) of vitamin D is supplied by the diet [297]. The remaining 80–90% is obtained through the skin following exposure to sunlight. Consequently, there is high seasonal variation in the regional burden of vitamin D deficiency. In industrialized nations, vitamin D supplements are available over the counter in doses ranging from 400 to 50,000 IU of vitamin $D_2$ or $D_3$.

Historically, it has been assumed that people in the tropics, because of prolonged exposure to sunlight, will make enough vitamin D to meet their needs. However, recent studies have documented a high prevalence of vitamin D deficiency globally, including a high prevalence in both tropical and non-tropical countries [298] and in countries with and without widespread vitamin D fortified foods. About 1 billion people globally are estimated to be vitamin D deficient, and the prevalence is high in all age groups [298]. Assessment of vitamin D status is challenging because the metabolically active form does not correlate strongly with health outcomes and because assays for the metabolites which correlate better with health outcomes are not adequately standardized. The assessment of vitamin D is typically based on the plasma concentration of the 25(OH)D (see Table 2.1). Although there is no consensus on what constitutes an optimal 25(OH)D, current cut-offs are set by considering the levels of the metabolites below which downstream metabolic processes may be affected, including levels that lead to highest suppression of PTH levels, highest absorption of dietary calcium, and highest bone mineralization [299]. In general 25(OH)D levels below 25 nmol/L are associated with metabolic disorders [299], including disorders affecting both the skeletal and non-skeletal systems. Levels between 25 and 50 nmol/L are considered marginal deficiency and levels >50 nmol/L are considered sufficient to meet physiological needs.

---

**Box 2.14 Sources and Needs: Vitamin D**
- 80–90% of the body's vitamin D is obtained through the skin following exposure to sunlight.
- 10–20% of vitamin D is supplied by the diet, from food sources such as oily fish.
- In general plasma 25(OH)D levels below 25 nmol/L are considered as vitamin D deficiency.
- An estimated 1 billion people may be vitamin D deficient globally.
- Vitamin D deficiency is associated with rickets in children.

---

**Vitamin D Metabolism**

Vitamin D, being a fat-soluble vitamin, is incorporated into micelles and then absorbed into enterocytes. In the epidermis of the skin, 7-dehydrocholesterol is converted to vitamin D upon exposure to sunlight, which is then transported to the liver for conversion to other vitamin D metabolites (see Table 2.6) [300]. Cutaneous ($D_2$) or dietary ($D_3$) vitamin D is transported in circulation bound to an $\alpha_2$-globulin vitamin-D binding protein. The metabolically active form of vitamin D, calcitriol (also known as 1,25(OH)$D_2$), is produced after hydroxylation of vitamin $D_2$/$D_3$ first in the liver (to form 25(OH)D) and then in the kidney by 1-$\alpha$-hydroxylase enzyme to form 1,25(OH)$D_2$) [301, 302]. Calcitriol, by binding to vitamin D receptors, is known to regulate calcium metabolism, cell differentiation, and cell division. When calcium levels are low, the parathyroid gland produces PTH, which then stimulates production of calcitriol by the kidney. Peripheral tissues respond to calcitriol by expressing the vitamin D receptor [300]. Upon binding to vitamin D, the receptor acts as a transcription factor [303], regulating the expression of several genes, including those responsible for the uptake of calcium and phosphate in the gut, and proteins involved in bone remodeling [304].

**Potential Pathways to Infections: Vitamin D**

Several immune cells possess the cellular machinery needed for the conversion of 25(OH)D to 1,25(OH)$_2$D [305], and immune cells are able to express the vitamin D receptor necessary for the signaling function of vitamin D [306]. Vitamin D is involved in both innate and adaptive immune responses [305]. Vitamin D may modulate immune responses to infection by promoting the development of antigen presenting cells, which are necessary for humoral immunity [305]. This is consistent with in vitro studies which showed that vitamin D exerts an antibacterial effect on monocytes in patients with tuberculosis [307, 308]. In the adaptive immune system, vitamin D may enhance the development of T suppressor cells, which are critical in shutting off the immune response following the clearance of an invading pathogen [309]. Vitamin D deficiency has been linked to an increased risk of several autoimmune diseases, including type 1 diabetes and multiple sclerosis [296].

## *Vitamin E*

### **Vitamin E Needs, Sources, and Risk of Deficiency**

Vitamin E is the general term used to describe a group of compounds, including four tocopherols (α, β, γ, and δ) and their respective toco-trienols (α, β, γ, and δ). Vitamin E was discovered in the early twentieth century as a fat-soluble factor critical for reproduction and fetal growth in vitamin E-deficient rats fed a highly oxidizable lard [310]—hence the name tocopherol (which means an alcohol-containing molecule responsible for childbirth). Vitamin E is now known to be involved in other physiological processes beyond reproduction. Most of the biological activities of vitamin E revolve around preventing the oxidation of polyunsaturated fatty acids by free radicals, an important factor in maintaining integrity of plasma membranes (see Table 2.6) [311]. All naturally occurring vitamin E compounds have the chromanol ring, bearing a hydroxyl group, which can donate an electron to free radicals, and as a result, reduce the oxidative potential of the free radicals. Of the vitamin E metabolites, α-tocopherols are the predominant form in humans and the isoform which exhibits the most anti-oxidant activity [311]. It is believed that the antioxidant role of vitamin E is implicated in disease conditions such as atherosclerosis and hemolytic anemia as well as in promoting resistance to infections [312]. While dietary sources are important contributors to vitamin E intake, supplements are increasingly becoming a major source of vitamin E in both developed and developing counties [313].

Vitamin E deficiency has been associated with loss of cell life, and this is believed to be the primary factor responsible for vitamin E deficiency-induced anemia (in the case of red blood cells), neuronal dysfunction (in nerve cells), and myopathies (in cardiac and vascular tissues) [314]. Vitamin E status is typically defined by plasma or serum concentrations (see Table 2.1). In adults, vitamin E deficiency is defined as plasma α-tocopherol concentration below 12 µmol/L. Vitamin E status in children is not well characterized, although it has been suggested that serum concentrations between 7 and 24 µmol/L may reflect normal variations [315]. Studies investigating vitamin E deficiency have often used different cut-offs, resulting in wide variations in the estimated prevalence of vitamin E deficiency. In low- and middle-income countries, where the burden is believed to be greatest, the estimated prevalence of vitamin E deficiency has ranged from as low as 20% to a high of 90% depending on region and target population [313]. In general, the evidence seems to suggest that in populations with a high burden of vitamin E deficiency, young children and the elderly are the most likely to be deficient [313, 316].

## Vitamin E Metabolism

An estimated 68% of dietary vitamin E is absorbed in duodenal enterocytes [317]. Alpha-tocopherol esters are thought to be hydrolyzed by gut esterase before incorporation into micelles. Alpha-tocopherol passively diffuses across cell membranes and into enterocytes. Vitamin E from dietary intake is absorbed in the intestines as part of fatty acid digestion and absorption and is then incorporated into chylomicrons and transported via the lymphatic system [314]. Vitamin E is ultimately transported to the liver, where it is primarily stored in parenchyma cells. When needed, vitamin E (mainly α-tocopherol) is released by the liver into circulation as part of VLDLs [318]. In the body, vitamin E is incorporated into tissues or cellular components which have a high fatty acid composition, such as cell membranes, the liver, the brain, erythrocytes, and adipose cells. In particular, adipose cells have stores of vitamin E, although these are not typically mobilized during deficiency states. It is in the adipose cells that the antioxidant properties of vitamin E are exploited. Free radicals (i.e., biochemical species with unpaired electrons) react readily with the PUFA component of cell membranes. The double bonds in PUFAs are a rich source of electrons for the highly reactive free radicals. By donating electrons to stabilize the free radicals, vitamin E protects the integrity of cell membranes. In the antioxidant reactions involving vitamin E, a vitamin E radical intermediate is formed. It is believed that this intermediate is subsequently converted back to vitamin E by the actions of ascorbic acid [319] and glutathione [320, 321].

## Potential Pathways to Infections: Vitamin E

Evidence from both animal and human studies suggests that the antioxidant role of vitamin E is exploited in the immune response [322]. Vitamin E adequacy has been associated with increased proliferation of cells involved in immune defense, which may result in increased production of antibodies and lymphocytes (see Table 2.6) [322]. In animal models, it has been shown that vitamin E interacts synergistically with selenium in enhancing the production of IgG and splenic cytokine expression [323, 324]. This is consistent with several other studies in animal models demonstrating the role of vitamin E in the immune response to specific disease conditions, including viral and bacterial infections [325, 326]. In mouse models, Bou et al. showed that α-tocopherol supplementation may reduce the severity of pneumonia by reducing the pathogen load, in a process involving altered expression of several adhesion molecules required for neutrophil mobility [325]. In humans, vitamin E supplementation has been associated with a lower incidence of pneumonia and other respiratory illnesses [327], although other studies found no evidence of benefits of vitamin E supplementation on pneumonia [328]. There is some evidence suggesting a potentially adverse effect of vitamin E supplementation, as vitamin E supplementation was associated with an increase in malaria parasitemia in HIV-infected Tanzanian women [329]. Additional evidence is needed to assess the benefits versus harm of vitamin E supplementation on the incidence and prognosis of specific infections in humans.

## *Vitamin K*

### Vitamin K Needs, Sources, and Risk of Deficiency

Vitamin K is best known for its role in blood clotting (see Table 2.6). The vitamin was first discovered in 1929 as a factor essential for blood coagulation [330]. Hence the early use of vitamin K in clinical practice focused on the treatment of hemorrhagic diseases, including hemorrhagic disease of the newborn [331]. Recent advances in research have shed further light on the essential role of vitamin K in living systems. Vitamin K comes in two forms, the $K_1$-vitamins (phylloquinone), which are synthesized in plants and algae, and the $K_2$-vitamins (menaquinones), synthesized by bacteria [332]. Phylloquinone forms the major dietary source of vitamin K [332]. Vitamin K is especially abundant in green leafy vegetables, oils, meat products, and to a lesser degree cereals. It is thought that vitamin K may be produced via endogenous synthesis of menaquinone by certain species of gut microbes [332]. However, the evidence is inconsistent regarding how much vitamin K is actually procured by this mechanism [333, 334]. Consumption of diets containing fiber (which is known to reduce the abundance of vitamin-K producing bacteria) is associated with reduced liver stores of vitamin K [335]. This suggests that gut microbes may be important in maintaining adequate vitamin K stores. However, vitamin K deficiency is easily induced by limiting the consumption of vitamin K in the diet, without necessarily affecting the gut microbes, and this suggests that the contribution from gut microbes to the total vitamin K needs may be minimal [336, 337]. Additional evidence is needed to more accurately characterize the relative supply of vitamin K from diet versus gut microbes.

---

**Box 2.15 Key Facts: Vitamin K**
- Vitamin K is involved in blood clotting.
- The two forms of Vitamin K are $K_1$-vitamins (phylloquinone), which are synthesized in plants and algae, and the $K_2$-vitamins (menaquinones), synthesized by bacteria.

---

## Vitamin K Metabolism

Vitamin K is a fat-soluble vitamin and is absorbed in the intestine as part of the process of fat digestion and absorption. Following incorporation into micelles vitamin K is absorbed into enterocytes. Individuals with any disease condition that affects any component of fat digestion, such as pancreatic insufficiency, are at increased risk for vitamin K deficiency. Vitamin K (as part of chylomicrons) in the intestinal mucosa are released into the lymph and transported to the liver bound to lipoproteins. In the liver, vitamin K is involved in carboxylation reactions with amino acid residues known as gamma-carboxyglutamic acid (Gla) [338]. Gla residues are formed via the addition of a third carboxylic acid group to the gamma carbon of glutamic acid, using an enzyme which requires vitamin K as a cofactor [339]. Gla residues are a major component of several blood clotting proteins, including prothrombin. The Gla residues allow the clotting factors to bind to phospholipid surfaces in reactions involving calcium and iron [332].

## Potential Pathways to Infections: Vitamin K

Evidence regarding the role of vitamin K in immune responses to infections is limited. In vitro studies suggest that both phylloquinone (vitamin K from plant and algae sources) and menaquinone (vitamin K from bacteria) are associated with reduced pro-inflammatory responses during chronic disease (see Table 2.6) [340]. A study by Reddi et al. showed that production of IL-6 from fibroblast cultures correlated negatively with the concentration of vitamin K compounds, including $K_1$ and $K_2$, added to the cell culture [340]. Additional evidence from animal studies suggests that vitamin K may moderate pro-inflammatory responses by suppressing lipopolysaccharide-induced inflammation [341]. It is uncertain whether these mechanisms are applicable to humans. More importantly, it is unknown whether these mechanisms are involved in down-regulating pro-inflammatory responses to infectious diseases. In a clinical study of acute and intractable diarrhea in children, Bay et al. concluded that, among children with bloody diarrhea, coagulation parameters may be improved by administering vitamin K [342].

# Water-Soluble Vitamins

## Vitamin C

### Vitamin C Needs, Sources, and Risk of Deficiency

In the mid-eighteenth century, James Lind, a surgeon in the Royal British Navy, conducted one of the earliest dietary clinical trials, which showed that citrus fruits were efficacious in treating scurvy [343, 344]. This followed earlier accounts in the sixteenth century, which indicated that potions made from the leaves of a particular tree were effective in curing a disease condition during which patients presented with symptoms consistent with scurvy [344]. We now know that scurvy results from a lack of proper folding of structural proteins, a process that requires vitamin C [343, 345]. Although many animals can synthesize vitamin C endogenously from glucose or galactose precursors, humans and other primates, because of the lack of the enzyme L-gulonolactone oxidase, are not able to produce vitamin C [346]. Thus adequate intake of vitamin C in humans is essential. In addition to preventing scurvy, vitamin C plays a role in the synthesis of several signaling hormones and neurotransmitters, including norepinephrine (see Table 2.7) [347]. Vitamin C deficiency has been associated with impaired brain development and may compromise memory formation or retrieval through its negative effects on the hippocampus [348, 349]. Fruit and vegetables are the major sources of vitamin C, and citrus fruits (including oranges, grapefruits, and lemons), kiwifruit, potatoes, melon, cauliflower, and broccoli are particularly rich sources [350, 351].

Because fruits and vegetables are widely consumed, vitamin C deficiency is uncommon. Vitamin C deficiency (defined as plasma concentrations <11 μM) [352] affects an estimated 5–10% of adults in upper-income countries [353]. In lower and middle income countries, recent reports of scurvy have come from refugee populations where food aid did not include foods rich in vitamin C [354, 355]. Predominately formula-fed infants may be at increased risk for vitamin C deficiency [356]. Vitamin C toxicity is uncommon, likely because excess intake is regulated by the homeostatic control of urinary vitamin C [357, 358].

### Vitamin C Metabolism

Up to 90% of dietary vitamin C is absorbed [349], and vitamin C is absorbed in the small intestine as ascorbate (the ionized form of vitamin C) and dehydroascorbic acid (the oxidized form of vitamin C). Vitamin C is absorbed by passive diffusion, facilitated diffusion [359, 360] and active transport [361, 362]. Because of its polar nature, vitamin C is transported in the blood without a transport protein. Plasma vitamin C levels are maintained at an upper limit of ~15 mg/L, and this upper limit is maintained by urinary excretion in the event of excess intake [349]. Vitamin C concentrations inside target cells are typically higher than circulating levels in plasma, and this disparity is maintained by an ATP-dependent mechanism which pumps ascorbic acid into cells against the concentration gradient. Vitamin C is distributed widely in tissues, including the brain (2–10 mM), liver (~1 mM) and lungs (~1 mM) [357]. The heart, muscle, and kidney each contain ~0.2–0.5 mM of vitamin C [357]. In cells, ascorbic acid participates in oxidation and reduction reactions. It is these redox reactions which form the basis for most physiological processes involving vitamin C. Vitamin C is particularly known for

**Table 2.7** Characteristics of water-soluble vitamins

| Nutrient | Dietary sources | Recommended nutrient intake (WHO/FAO) | Pathways of absorption & metabolism | Physiological functions | Role in immune function | Conditions and interventions[a] associated with deficiencies |
|---|---|---|---|---|---|---|
| Vitamin C | Fruit and vegetables, particularly citrus | 0–6 m (25 mg/d); 7 m–6y (30 mg/d); 7–9y (35 mg/d); 10–18y (40 mg/d); 19+ (45 mg/d)[b] | Absorption via carrier-mediated active transport into cells and released into cytosol; excess excreted in urine [374] | Cofactor in collagen and other proteins; enhances Fe absorption; synthesis of norepinephrine, neurotransmitters and other signaling hormones | May enhance antibody production and T cell proliferation and differentiation | Scurvy; impaired memory and brain development |
| B-complex vitamins | | | | | | |
| B₁ – Thiamine | Pork, liver, whole grains, meat, legumes | 0–6 m (0.2 mg/d); 7–12 m (0.3 mg/d); 1–3y (0.5 mg/d); 4–6y (0.6 mg/d); 7–9y (0.9 mg/d); F10+ (1.1 mg/d); M10+ (1.2 mg/d) | Absorbed by active transport, not stored in the body | Coenzyme in energy metabolism | Deficiency may exacerbate the pro-inflammatory responses and oxidative stress [404] | Beriberi; Wernicke's |
| B₂ – Riboflavin | Milk, liver, whole grains, dark green vegetables | 0–6 m (0.3 mg/d); 7–12 m (0.4 mg/d); 1–3y (0.5 mg/d); 4–6y (0.6 mg/d); 7–9y (0.9 mg/d); F10–18y (1.0 mg/d); M10+ (1.3 mg/d); F19+ (1.1 mg/d)[b] | Absorbed by an active carrier, facilitated by bile salts; little net storage | Coenzyme in energy production | Enhance neutrophil migration [405] and macrophage viability [406] | Growth faltering, dermatitis, alopecia and cornea vascularization |
| B₃ – Niacin | Liver, fish, poultry, meat, whole grain, peanuts | 0–6 m (2 mg niacin equivalents (NE)/d); 7–12 m (4 mg NE/d); 1–3y (6 mg NE/d); 4–6y (8 mg NE/d); 7–9y (12 mg NE/d); 10–18y (16 mg NE/d); F19y + (14 mg NE/d); M19y + (16 mg NE/d)[b] | Absorbed by simple and facilitated diffusion; circulates in blood in free form, can be synthesized from tryptophan | Coenzyme in fatty acid synthesis; Electron acceptor in glucose catabolism | Moderates production of pro-inflammatory cytokines [407, 408]; may activate immune responses in immune-suppressed individual [409] | Pellagra (characterized by Casal's collar), diarrhea, skin disorders |

| | Sources | Requirements | Absorption/metabolism | Function | Immune/infection role | Deficiency |
|---|---|---|---|---|---|---|
| B₅ – Pantothenic Acid | Lliver, whole grain, meats, kidney, fresh vegetable, egg yolk, made by intestinal bacteria | 0–6 m (1.7 mg/d); 7–12 m (1.8 mg/d); 1–3y (2.0 mg/d); 4–6y (3.0 mg/d); 7–9y (4.0 mg/d); 10y + (5.0 mg/d)[b] | Absorbed by facilitated diffusion; transported in blood within erythrocytes and plasma; rapidly excreted, limited storage only in fat cells | Lipid synthesis and chain elongation | Suppresses bacteria growth by stimulating both innate and adaptive immune response [410] | Rare |
| B₆ – Pyridoxine | Pork, liver, whole grains, meat, legumes | 0–6 m (0.1 mg/d); 7–12 m (0.3 mg/d); 1–3y (0.5 mg/d); 4–6y (0.6 mg/d); 7–9y (1.0 mg/d); F10–18y (1.2 mg/d); M10–18y (1.3 mg/d); F19–50y (1.3 mg/d); M19–50y (1.3 mg/d); F50y + (1.5 mg/d); M50y + (1.7 mg/d)[b] | Absorbed by passive diffusion; carried by erythrocytes, bound primarily to hemoglobin and albumin, to all cells; significant amounts found in liver, brain, spleen, kidney and heart; no appreciable stores [374]. | Synthesis of non-essential amino acids, neurotransmitters; glucose metabolism | Enhances apoptosis, reduces proliferation of CD4+ T cells and inhibits TH1 cytokine production [411] | Skin disorders, anemia, dermatitis |
| B₇ – Biotin | | 0–6 m (5 μg/d); 7–12 m (6 μg/d); 1–3y (8 μg/d); 4–6y (12 μg/d); 7–9y (20 μg/d); 10–18y (25 μg/d); >18y (30 μg/d)[b] | Only free biotin is absorbed (via facilitated diffusion) | Carboxyl carrier; energy synthesis | Unknown | Skin disorders, hair loss, developmental delay |
| B₉ – Folate | Dark green leafy vegetables, liver, kidney, meats, fish, whole grains | μg dietary folate equivalents (DFE) 0–12 m (80 μg DFE/d); 1–3y (150 μg DFE/d); 4–6y (200 μg DFE/d); 7–9y (300 μg DFE/d); >13y (400 μg DFE/d)[b] | Absorption is primarily active, carrier-mediated and pH dependent; metabolites circulate in plasma, cellular uptake by highly specific folate-binding protein | DNA synthesis; Protein synthesis | Regulates synthesis of cytokines by monocytes [412] | Megaloblastic anemia, diarrhea |
| B₁₂ – Cobalamin | Animal source foods | 0–6 m (0.4 μg/d); 7–12 m (0.7 μg/d); 1–3y (0.9 μg/d); 4–6y (1.2 μg/d); 7–9y (1.8 μg/d); 10y + (2.4 μg/d)[b] | GI functioning; absorbed via receptor in terminal ileum (REF 3 in Hoey); small amount of passive diffusion | Coenzyme in biosynthesis and catabolism; development of red blood cells | Deficiency up-regulates TNF-alpha synthesis by macrophages [413]; Supplementation associated with increased production of IL-6 [416] | Macrocytic anemia, neurological and cognitive impairments, cardiovascular disease, bone fractures |

[a]Supplementation and fortification are considered to be appropriate responses for all nutrient deficiencies in this table

[b]Requirements vary during pregnancy and lactation

its role in maintaining the three-dimensional structure of collagen, the most abundant protein in the human body [345]. Hydroxylation of proline and lysine residues is a critical step in collagen folding, and requires vitamin C (see Table 2.7) [343]. This property of vitamin C underscores its role in the etiology of scurvy [343], which is characterized by symptoms including poor wound healing, bleeding of gums and skin, anemia and body pain. As an antioxidant, vitamin C is also involved in the reduction of iron in the ferric state (+3) to the ferrous (+2) state. This step is necessary for iron absorption by the divalent metal iron transporter in enterocytes [95].

---

**Box 2.16 Sources and Needs: Vitamin C**
- Scurvy is classic symptom of vitamin C deficiency.
- Humans and other primates, because of the lack of the enzyme L-gulonolactone oxidase, are not able to produce vitamin C.
- Fruit and vegetables comprise the major source of vitamin C.
- Vitamin C deficiency is uncommon because fruits and vegetables are widely consumed.
- Vitamin C toxicity is also uncommon because excess intake is regulated by the homeostatic control of urinary vitamin C.
- Plasma vitamin C levels are maintained at an upper limit of ~15 mg/L.

---

### Potential Pathways to Infections: Vitamin C

The role of vitamin C in immunity against specific infections has been an area of intense research and debate over the last 60 years. Several plausible pathways have been suggested. These include the enhancement of T cell proliferation and differentiation [363] and enhancement of antibody production [364, 365], although the support for the latter hypothesis has been inconsistent [366, 367]. Vitamin C deficiency in experimental subjects was associated with impaired delayed-type hypersensitivity, recovered with supplementation, highlighting the role of vitamin C in T cell function (see Chap. 3) [368]. Levels of ascorbate in immune cells, particularly leucocytes, decrease quickly following an infection, and then return to normal after the infections resolve [369, 370]. Some consider vitamin C to be especially important in staving off viral infections although the evidence base has not been consistent [371–373]. While some studies have shown that vitamin C is efficacious in reducing both incidence and severity of common colds, other clinical studies found no such effect [371, 372]. A recent meta-analyses of trials delivering 200 mg daily vitamin C found no impact on incidence of colds and only a small but statistically significant reduction in duration of colds in both children (by ~13%) and adults (by ~8%) [373].

## The B-Complex Vitamins

### B-Complex Needs, Sources, and Risk of Deficiency

The B-complex vitamins are group of eight water-soluble compounds typically present in the same food sources. The B-complex vitamins are thiamin ($B_1$), riboflavin ($B_2$), niacin ($B_3$), pantothenic acid ($B_5$), pyridoxine ($B_6$), biotin ($B_7$), folate ($B_9$), and cobalamin ($B_{12}$). In general, these vitamins functions as coenzymes or cofactors in the synthesis and degradation of biomolecules. B-complex vitamins are critical in energy metabolism and are especially critical in tissues and systems with high energy demand, such as the brain, nervous system, and muscles. Because of their role in DNA and protein metabolism, B-complex vitamins are also critical for growth (especially during fetal and early childhood stages). They are also important in maintaining structural integrity of cells (including red blood cells) and proteins such as hemoglobin. Some B-complex vitamins are rarely deficient (e.g., pantothenic acid) and others such as folate are frequently deficient in low-income settings and in hospitalized patients. Deficiencies of B-complex vitamins are associated with degenerative diseases, growth stunting, anemia, and skin disorders. Risk of folate deficiency increases during pregnancy and has been associated with neural tube defects. Recommendations for intake of B-complex vitamins are typically tied to daily energy intake, although recommendations for biotin are tied to the total intake of protein (see Table 2.7).

## B-Complex Absorption and Transport

The absorption and transport of water-soluble B-complex vitamins are similar, in part because of the shared hydrophilic characteristics (see Table 2.7). Some B-complex vitamins, including thiamine, riboflavin, folate, and $B_{12}$, are absorbed by active transport, while others, such as niacin, utilize facilitated diffusion at lower concentrations and passive diffusion at higher concentrations. Still others, such as pyridoxine, rely primarily on passive diffusion for absorption. Biotin is an important exception, as less than 50% of bound biotin from plant sources is hydrolyzed and available for absorption. Binders such as avidin in raw egg whites can prevent hydrolysis, unless the avidin has been denatured by cooking [374]. The B-complex vitamins may be transported freely in blood (e.g., niacin) or bound to albumin in the case of riboflavin and pyridoxine ($B_6$). Pharmacological interactions can inhibit active folate transport (see Chap. 14). As they are water-soluble, the B-complex vitamins are not stored in the body.

## B-Complex Metabolism

B-complex vitamins are essential coenzymes in catabolism and biosynthesis and precursors for molecules involved in biosynthesis (see Table 2.7). Several are coenzymes for energy and glucose metabolism; thiamine is a coenzyme in glycolysis and the Krebs's cycle, generating cellular energy in the form of ATP. Riboflavin is a coenzyme for oxidation-reduction reactions, including the generation of energy in the electron transport chain. Niacin is a coenzyme in fatty acid synthesis, as an electron acceptor in glucose catabolism. $B_{12}$ is a co-factor for two important enzymes: methylmalonyl CoA mutase, which is involved in the degradation of cholesterol, some fatty acids, and amino acids for use in tricarboxylic acid cycle, and methionine synthase, which is involved in remethylation of homocysteine to methionine (see Table 2.7).

---

**Box 2.17 Sources and Needs: B Vitamins**
- Because of their role in energy, DNA and protein metabolism, deficiencies of B-complex vitamins are associated with degenerative diseases, growth stunting and anemia.
- Animal source foods (including liver, poultry, meat and fish), whole grains, and legumes are good sources of B-complex vitamins.
- Folate is abundant in dark green leafy vegetables.

**Potential Pathways to Infection: B-Complex**

The B-complex vitamins have been shown to modulate several components of both innate and adaptive immune responses. Several of the B-complex vitamins, including niacin and thiamin have antioxidant properties and may therefore be important in moderating the pro-inflammatory responses to infections. Folate and vitamin $B_{12}$ regulate the synthesis of cytokines, whereas vitamin $B_6$ is involved in inducing apoptosis. Specific examples of immune-modulatory roles are summarized in Table 2.7 [374].

## Other Nutrients

The previously covered macro- and micronutrients are those most likely to be deficient or excessive in humans. There are additional nutrients with varying levels of evidence for roles in nutrition and infection. We will touch briefly on a few—fluorine, phosphorus, choline and carnitine. Interested readers are referred to the Institute of Medicine Dietary Reference Intake guides for more information about additional essential nutrients [375–378].

## *Fluorine Overview*

Fluorine is an essential mineral with roles in bone formation and prevention and treatment of dental caries [375]. When intake is insufficient to maintain necessary levels, fluoride is mobilized from calcified tissues, and excretion may exceed ingestion [375]. A protective effect of fluoride on both early childhood caries and oral *Streptococcus mutans* (a principal cause of caries) has been demonstrated [194]. Fluoride is not the only relevant micronutrient for dental caries, as both caries and periodontitis can be exacerbated by micronutrient deficiencies of vitamin C, vitamin D, or vitamin $B_{12}$ [195]. Fluoride-containing toothpaste/dentifrice, low sugar intakes, and excellent oral hygiene are a trifecta of practices that can reduce both caries and periodontal disease [196–198]. There is a growing awareness of the importance of the relationship between oral and systemic health. Severe dental caries is a serious infectious disease whose bacteriological components can drive disease progression in other organ systems. Periodontitis, also of infectious and inflammatory origin, can seed the blood stream with gum-derived microorganisms, increasing risk of multiple chronic diseases and conditions, including cardiovascular disease [199–202]. Periodontitis has also been implicated in preterm birth, rheumatoid arthritis, and even diminished cognitive function, though the quality and consistency of evidence is not adequate to make definitive causal statements (205–208).

## *Phosphorus Overview*

Phosphorus is as essential to life as oxygen, carbon, and nitrogen [374] and is generally found in its phosphate form ($PO_4^{3-}$). It is an essential component of bones, phospholipids, adenine and guanine nucleotides, and ATP [375]. Phosphates are highly prevalent in foods, and processed foods, soft drinks and animal source foods are good sources of dietary phosphorus. Deficiency is seen only in rare situations such as premature infants fed insufficient phosphorus in formula [374].

## *Choline Overview*

Choline is a water-soluble molecule widely distributed in foods, highly unstable and thus difficult to measure accurately in foods, although humans on a choline-free parenteral diet show signs of deficiency [374]. As a component of lecithin (phosphatidylcholine), choline is found in many foods and is also frequently used as a stabilizer and emulsifying agent in processed foods [374]. Symptoms of deficiency include deficits in central nervous system functioning and a fatty liver, and symptoms of excess include hypotension [376]. Choline is a precursor for membrane phospholipids, lipid and cholesterol transport proteins and acetylcholine, an important neurotransmitter [376]. Evidence is emerging of a potential role for choline in synthesis of metabolites such as trimethylamine N-oxide that are associated with risk of CVD [379].

## *Carnitine Overview*

Carnitine is a water-soluble molecule that can be synthesized in the body, except in extreme conditions such as premature infants and individuals suffering from extreme trauma [374]. Meat and particularly organ meats are good dietary sources, while dairy products, whole grains, and some legumes and vegetables contain moderate amounts [374]. Carnitine is an essential component in fatty acid oxidation particularly in the mitochondrial membrane. Deficiencies are only seen under extreme conditions, and carnitine is generally recycled in the body quite efficiently, with approximately 90% of the carnitine reaching the kidneys being reabsorbed and returned to circulation [374]. L-carnitine is being investigated as a potential supplement to reduce inflammation. A 2019 systematic review concluded that regular supplementation with L-carnitine was significantly associated with lower levels of inflammatory markers such as CRP, IL6, and TNFα [380].

## Emerging Nutrients

Bioflavonoids are polyphenolic compounds found throughout the plant kingdom. While characteristics of deficiency have not been identified, there is a growing interest in the potential antioxidant capacity of flavonoids for reducing inflammation [381]. Flavonoid content may be an important mediator for the reduced risk of inflammatory conditions of diets rich in fruits and vegetables [381].

## Conclusions

Both epidemiologic and mechanistic evidence support the role of specific nutrients in protecting against infectious disease. For instance, adjunctive zinc therapy is recommended by the WHO for managing complications of acute diarrhea in low- and middle-income countries, based on evidence from systematic reviews indicating a protective effect of zinc on the duration of diarrhea. Similarly, high-dose vitamin A supplementation remains a global public health intervention against childhood morbidity and mortality from infections. Several other micronutrients, including vitamin D, calcium, magnesium, and copper, have been shown to have potentially protective effects against infections, although the evidence is generally insufficient or too inconsistent to drive policy changes. For other nutrients such as iron, there is population-level evidence of both beneficial and adverse outcomes, and additional data are needed to ascertain the contexts where supplementation may be optimal. Mechanistic evidence, relying on in vitro studies and animal models, indicates that nutrition influences immune functioning through multiple pathways, including proliferation and differentiation of immune cells, regulation of production of immune modulators, and the strength and duration of the inflammatory responses to infections. When present in adequate concentrations, nutrients important for cell division, transcription, and translation, such as zinc, vitamins A, and D, and iodine, promote proliferation and differentiation of several types of immune cells and enhance mucosal immunity, therefore helping to reduce the incidence and severity of disease of the lungs and gut. Nutrients such as copper and magnesium, which are critical in energy metabolism, support the growth and function of the thymus and enhance biosynthetic activities of immune cells, including the production of cytokines critical to immune cell signaling. The antioxidant minerals and vitamins (vitamins A, E, C, copper, and selenium) are thought to prolong the lifespan of immune cells by preventing the attack of cellular membranes by free radicals and downregulating the production of pro-inflammatory cytokines. Thus, whether nutrients are acquired through routine dietary intake or via supplementation programs, nutritional status may influence the risk of exposure and susceptibility to infections, the progression from subclinical to clinical infections, and the duration or recovery from clinical manifestation of infections.

*Key Gaps and Challenges*. While extensive laboratory work has gone into broadly characterizing the mechanisms by which nutrients affect immune function, additional evidence is needed to elucidate the specific pathways by which nutrients directly affect specific pathogens and their transmission. Such research might be used to identify particular relationships between host nutritional status and pathogens that could provide complementary and supportive interventions for traditional pharmaceutical approaches and also be of value in a preventative context.

Challenges for in vitro studies and animal studies:

- Often nutrients are used at pharmacological rather than physiological concentrations. A database that recommends physiologically relevant concentrations for use in vitro would aid laboratory scientists in designing their studies.
- Defining a clear pipeline from proof of concept (e.g., cells produce a specific molecule in response to in vitro stimulation), to a more realistic in vitro set up (e.g., including multiple nutrients), to an in vivo animal model with various combinations of nutrient deficiencies and infections might remind the research community of the importance of incorporating more of the real-world complexity.

Challenges for human studies:

- The benefits and limitations of available biomarkers of nutritional status need to be more clearly developed, especially for micronutrients. Several of the currently used nutritional biomarkers are acute phase proteins or respond to acute phase reactions. As a result, levels of these biomarkers are altered during systemic inflammation, often leading to mischaracterization of nutritional status. This phenomenon has been widely demonstrated in settings with acute infections. Less well understood is the impact of chronic infections or of multiple infections on nutrient biomarkers. More holistic studies that measure a wider range of infections, immune status, and nutrients will provide databases from which the impact of multiple co-existing conditions on nutrient biomarkers can be assessed. This will be extremely important in ensuring that biomarkers are accurately interpreted both in epidemiological and clinical settings.
- There are considerable challenges to reaching a consensus on the relative risks and benefits of specific nutritional interventions, due to heterogeneity among studies in context, age of the study population, dose and formulation of nutrients, presence and severity of other nutrient deficiencies and of co-existing infections, and differences among studies in the outcomes measured. One of the

consequences of this heterogeneity may be the apparently contradictory conclusions often emerging from research studies. Prioritization of study and population characteristics to be tested and measured, as well as expert consideration of when evidence from other populations may be appropriate for analogy of exploration, could help address this challenge.

- We have come to rely on systematic reviews and meta-analyses. Yet many of the studies included in these analyses were conducted over a decade ago. Globally, the prevalence of undernutrition is declining, and health systems are generally improving. Consistent with this transition, it is conceivable that future nutritional interventions, particularly those targeting undernutrition, may have a more limited impact at the population level than previously reported. However, such interventions may still have a significant impact in clinical settings where the most severe cases are likely to present. By controlling for this changing context, it may be possible to recommend public health and clinical situations where specific nutritional inventions are appropriate, as well as contexts where particular interventions may not be appropriate.

Expansion of the scientific body of knowledge on nutrition-infection interactions would be aided by more human studies and a clear consensus on strategies and biomarkers for defining nutritional status at the individual and population level. With increased attention to the complexity of research study design, and increased collaboration between disciplines, we are confident that the challenges facing research at the interface of nutrition and infection can be met.

# References

1. Pelletier DL, Frongillo EA Jr, Schroeder DG, Habicht JP. The effects of malnutrition on child mortality in developing countries. Bull World Health Organ. 1995;73(4):443–8.
2. Black RE, Allen LH, Bhutta ZA, Caulfield LE, de Onis M, Ezzati M, et al. Maternal and child undernutrition: global and regional exposures and health consequences. Lancet. 2008;371(9608):243–60.
3. Brown KH, Peerson JM, Baker SK, Hess SY. Preventive zinc supplementation among infants, preschoolers, and older prepubertal children. Food Nutr Bull. 2009;30(1 Suppl):S12–40.
4. Shankar AH, Genton B, Semba RD, Baisor M, Paino J, Tamja S, et al. Effect of vitamin A supplementation on morbidity due to Plasmodium falciparum in young children in Papua New Guinea: a randomised trial. Lancet. 1999;354(9174):203–9.
5. Paganini D, Uyoga MA, Kortman GAM, Cercamondi CI, Winkler HC, Boekhorst J, et al. Iron-containing micronutrient powders modify the effect of oral antibiotics on the infant gut microbiome and increase post-antibiotic diarrhoea risk: a controlled study in Kenya. Gut. 2019;68(4):645–53.
6. Tang M, Frank DN, Hendricks AE, Ir D, Esamai F, Liechty E, et al. Iron in micronutrient powder promotes an unfavorable gut microbiota in Kenyan infants. Nutrients. 2017;9(7):776.
7. Paganini D, Zimmermann MB. The effects of iron fortification and supplementation on the gut microbiome and diarrhea in infants and children: a review. Am J Clin Nutr. 2017;106(Suppl 6):1688s–93s.
8. Espinoza A, Le Blanc S, Olivares M, Pizarro F, Ruz M, Arredondo M. Iron, copper, and zinc transport: inhibition of divalent metal transporter 1 (DMT1) and human copper transporter 1 (hCTR1) by shRNA. Biol Trace Elem Res. 2012;146(2):281–6.
9. Sharp P. The molecular basis of copper and iron interactions. Proc Nutr Soc. 2004;63(4):563–9.
10. Steel DM, Whitehead AS. The major acute phase reactants: C-reactive protein, serum amyloid P component and serum amyloid A protein. Immunol Today. 1994;15(2):81–8.
11. Borregaard N, Theilgaard-Monch K, Cowland JB, Stahle M, Sorensen OE. Neutrophils and keratinocytes in innate immunity--cooperative actions to provide antimicrobial defense at the right time and place. J Leukoc Biol. 2005;77(4):439–43.
12. Wan JM, Haw MP, Blackburn GL. Nutrition, immune function, and inflammation: an overview. Proc Nutr Soc. 1989;48(3):315–35.
13. Kushner I. The phenomenon of the acute phase response. Ann N Y Acad Sci. 1982;389:39–48.
14. Cummings JH, Stephen AM. Carbohydrate terminology and classification. Eur J Clin Nutr. 2007;61(Suppl 1):S5–18.
15. Elia M, Cummings JH. Physiological aspects of energy metabolism and gastrointestinal effects of carbohydrates. Eur J Clin Nutr. 2007;61(Suppl 1):S40–74.

16. Mann J, Cummings JH, Englyst HN, Key T, Liu S, Riccardi G, et al. FAO/WHO scientific update on carbohydrates in human nutrition: conclusions. Eur J Clin Nutr. 2007;61(Suppl 1):S132–7.

17. Kunzmann AT, Coleman HG, Huang WY, Kitahara CM, Cantwell MM, Berndt SI. Dietary fiber intake and risk of colorectal cancer and incident and recurrent adenoma in the prostate, lung, colorectal, and ovarian cancer screening trial. Am J Clin Nutr. 2015;102(4):881–90.

18. Gray GM. Carbohydrate digestion and absorption. Gastroenterology. 1970;58(1):96–107.

19. Levin RJ. Digestion and absorption of carbohydrates--from molecules and membranes to humans. Am J Clin Nutr. 1994;59(3 Suppl):690s–8s.

20. Kitabchi AE. Hormonal control of glucose metabolism. Otolaryngol Clin N Am. 1975;8(2):335–44.

21. Ruderman NB, Toews CJ, Shafrir E. Role of free fatty acids in glucose homeostasis. Arch Intern Med. 1969;123(3):299–313.

22. Caulfield LE, de Onis M, Blossner M, Black RE. Undernutrition as an underlying cause of child deaths associated with diarrhea, pneumonia, malaria, and measles. Am J Clin Nutr. 2004;80(1):193–8.

23. Wing EJ, Magee DM, Barczynski LK. Acute starvation in mice reduces the number of T cells and suppresses the development of T-cell-mediated immunity. Immunology. 1988;63(4):677–82.

24. Alonso-Alvarez C, Tella JL. Effects of experimental food restriction and body-mass changes on the avian t-cell-mediated response. Can J Zool. 2001;79(1):101–5.

25. Cobb BA, Kasper DL. Coming of age: carbohydrates and immunity. Eur J Immunol. 2005;35(2):352–6.

26. Weir DM. Carbohydrates as recognition molecules in infection and immunity. FEMS Microbiol Immunol. 1989;1(6–7):331–40.

27. Brandley BK, Schnaar RL. Cell-surface carbohydrates in cell recognition and response. J Leukoc Biol. 1986;40(1):97–111.

28. Massey KA, Blakeslee CH, Pitkow HS. A review of physiological and metabolic effects of essential amino acids. Amino Acids. 1998;14(4):271–300.

29. Wu G. Amino acids: metabolism, functions, and nutrition. Amino Acids. 2009;37(1):1–17.

30. Wu G. Functional amino acids in growth, reproduction, and health. Adv Nutr. 2010;1(1):31–7.

31. Moinard C, Cynober L. Citrulline: a new player in the control of nitrogen homeostasis. J Nutr. 2007;137(6 Suppl 2):1621s–5s.

32. Wu G, Bazer FW, Dai Z, Li D, Wang J, Wu Z. Amino acid nutrition in animals: protein synthesis and beyond. Ann Rev Anim Biosci. 2014;2:387–417.

33. Wagenmakers AJ. Muscle amino acid metabolism at rest and during exercise: role in human physiology and metabolism. Exerc Sport Sci Rev. 1998;26:287–314.

34. Millward DJ. Metabolic demands for amino acids and the human dietary requirement: Millward and rRvers (1988) revisited. J Nutr. 1998;128(12 Suppl):2563s–76s.

35. Pillai RR, Kurpad AV. Amino acid requirements in children and the elderly population. Br J Nutr. 2012;108(Suppl 2):S44–9.

36. Pencharz PB, Ball RO. Different approaches to define individual amino acid requirements. Annu Rev Nutr. 2003;23:101–16.

37. Paddon-Jones D, Rasmussen BB. Dietary protein recommendations and the prevention of sarcopenia. Curr Opin Clin Nutr Metab Care. 2009;12(1):86–90.

38. Smith CD, Carney JM, Starke-Reed PE, Oliver CN, Stadtman ER, Floyd RA, et al. Excess brain protein oxidation and enzyme dysfunction in normal aging and in Alzheimer disease. Proc Natl Acad Sci U S A. 1991;88(23):10540–3.

39. Smith CD, Carney JM, Tatsumo T, Stadtman ER, Floyd RA, Markesbery WR. Protein oxidation in aging brain. Ann N Y Acad Sci. 1992;663:110–9.

40. Silk DB, Grimble GK, Rees RG. Protein digestion and amino acid and peptide absorption. Proc Nutr Soc. 1985;44(1):63–72.

41. Silk DB. Digestion and absorption of dietary protein in man. Proc Nutr Soc. 1980;39(1):61–70.

42. Robertson JH, Wheatley DN. Pools and protein synthesis in mammalian cells. Biochem J. 1979;178(3):699–709.

43. Merrick WC. Mechanism and regulation of eukaryotic protein synthesis. Microbiol Rev. 1992;56(2):291–315.

44. Merrick WC. Eukaryotic protein synthesis: an in vitro analysis. Biochimie. 1994;76(9):822–30.

45. Moldave K. Eukaryotic protein synthesis. Annu Rev Biochem. 1985;54:1109–49.

46. Rhoads RE. Regulation of eukaryotic protein synthesis by initiation factors. J Biol Chem. 1993;268(5):3017–20.

47. Chisti MJ, Tebruegge M, La Vincente S, Graham SM, Duke T. Pneumonia in severely malnourished children in developing countries - mortality risk, aetiology and validity of WHO clinical signs: a systematic review. Tropical Med Int Health. 2009;14(10):1173–89.

48. German JB. Dietary lipids from an evolutionary perspective: sources, structures and functions. Matern Child Nutr. 2011;7(Suppl 2):2–16.

49. Hulbert AJ, Turner N, Storlien LH, Else PL. Dietary fats and membrane function: implications for metabolism and disease. Biol Rev Camb Philos Soc. 2005;80(1):155–69.

50. Meyer BJ, Mann NJ, Lewis JL, Milligan GC, Sinclair AJ, Howe PR. Dietary intakes and food sources of omega-6 and omega-3 polyunsaturated fatty acids. Lipids. 2003;38(4):391–8.
51. Simopoulos AP. Omega-3 fatty acids in health and disease and in growth and development. Am J Clin Nutr. 1991;54(3):438–63.
52. Gill I, Valivety R. Polyunsaturated fatty acids, part 1: occurrence, biological activities and applications. Trends Biotechnol. 1997;15(10):401–9.
53. Valk EE, Hornstra G. Relationship between vitamin E requirement and polyunsaturated fatty acid intake in man: a review. Int J Vitam Nutr Res. 2000;70(2):31–42.
54. Zhao Y, Monahan FJ, McNulty BA, Li K, Bloomfield FJ, Duff DJ, et al. Plasma n-3 polyunsaturated fatty status and its relationship with vitamin E intake and plasma level. Eur J Nutr. 2017;56(3):1281–91.
55. Carey MC, Small DM, Bliss CM. Lipid digestion and absorption. Annu Rev Physiol. 1983;45:651–77.
56. Watkins JB. Lipid digestion and absorption. Pediatrics. 1985;75(1 Pt 2):151–6.
57. Lindquist S, Hernell O. Lipid digestion and absorption in early life: an update. Curr Opin Clin Nutr Metab Care. 2010;13(3):314–20.
58. Fredrikzon B, Hernell O, Blackberg L. Lingual lipase. Its role in lipid digestion in infants with low birthweight and/or pancreatic insufficiency. Acta Paediatr Scand Suppl. 1982;296:75–80.
59. Canbay A, Bechmann L, Gerken G. Lipid metabolism in the liver. Z Gastroenterol. 2007;45(1):35–41.
60. Kwiterovich PO Jr. The metabolic pathways of high-density lipoprotein, low-density lipoprotein, and triglycerides: a current review. Am J Cardiol. 2000;86(12a):5L–10L.
61. Nguyen P, Leray V, Diez M, Serisier S, Le Bloc'h J, Siliart B, et al. Liver lipid metabolism. J Anim Physiol Anim Nutr (Berl). 2008;92(3):272–83.
62. de Pablo MA, Alvarez de Cienfuegos G. Modulatory effects of dietary lipids on immune system functions. Immunol Cell Biol. 2000;78(1):31–9.
63. Calder PC. Fatty acids, dietary lipids and lymphocyte functions. Biochem Soc Trans. 1995;23(2):302–9.
64. Soyland E, Lea T, Sandstad B, Drevon A. Dietary supplementation with very long-chain n-3 fatty acids in man decreases expression of the interleukin-2 receptor (CD25) on mitogen-stimulated lymphocytes from patients with inflammatory skin diseases. Eur J Clin Investig. 1994;24(4):236–42.
65. Sijben JW, Calder PC. Differential immunomodulation with long-chain n-3 PUFA in health and chronic disease. Proc Nutr Soc. 2007;66(2):237–59.
66. Demas GE, Drazen DL, Nelson RJ. Reductions in total body fat decrease humoral immunity. Proc Biol Sci. 2003;270(1518):905–11.
67. Hurrell RF. Bioavailability of iron. Eur J Clin Nutr. 1997;51(Suppl 1):S4–8.
68. Abbaspour N, Hurrell R, Kelishadi R. Review on iron and its importance for human health. J Res Med Sci. 2014;19(2):164–74.
69. WHO/CDC. Assessing the iron status of population. Geneva: World Health Organization; 2004.
70. WHO/UNICEF/UNO. Iron deficiency anemia assessment, prevention and control. Geneva: World Health Organization; 2001.
71. Berger J, Dillon JC. Control of iron deficiency in developing countries. Sante. 2002;12(1):22–30.
72. Berglund S, Domellof M. Meeting iron needs for infants and children. Curr Opin Clin Nutr Metab Care. 2014;17(3):267–72.
73. Pasricha SR, Drakesmith H, Black J, Hipgrave D, Biggs BA. Control of iron deficiency anemia in low- and middle-income countries. Blood. 2013;121(14):2607–17.
74. Shander A, Goodnough LT, Javidroozi M, Auerbach M, Carson J, Ershler WB, et al. Iron deficiency Anemia-bridging the knowledge and practice gap. Transfus Med Rev. 2014;28(3):156–66.
75. Rivera S, Liu L, Nemeth E, Gabayan V, Sorensen OE, Ganz T. Hepcidin excess induces the sequestration of iron and exacerbates tumor-associated anemia. Blood. 2005;105(4):1797–802.
76. Davidsson L. Approaches to improve iron bioavailability from complementary foods. J Nutr. 2003;133(5 Suppl 1):1560s–2s.
77. Hallberg L. Iron requirements and bioavailability of dietary iron. Experientia Suppl. 1983;44:223–44.
78. López MA, Martos FC. Iron availability: an updated review. Int J Food Sci Nutr. 2004;55(8):597–606.
79. Stoltzfus RJ, Chway HM, Montresor A, Tielsch JM, Jape JK, Albonico M, et al. Low dose daily iron supplementation improves iron status and appetite but not anemia, whereas quarterly anthelminthic treatment improves growth, appetite and anemia in Zanzibari preschool children. J Nutr. 2004;134(2):348–56.
80. Totino PR, Magalhaes AD, Silva LA, Banic DM, Daniel-Ribeiro CT, Ferreira-da-Cruz MF. Apoptosis of non-parasitized red blood cells in malaria: a putative mechanism involved in the pathogenesis of anaemia. Malar J. 2010;9:350.
81. De-Regil LM, Suchdev PS, Vist GE, Walleser S, Pena-Rosas JP. Home fortification of foods with multiple micronutrient powders for health and nutrition in children under two years of age. Cochrane Database Syst Rev. 2011;(9):Cd008959.

82. Griffin IJ, Abrams SA. Iron and breastfeeding. Pediatr Clin N Am. 2001;48(2):401–13.
83. Stoltzfus RJ, Chwaya HM, Tielsch JM, Schulze KJ, Albonico M, Savioli L. Epidemiology of iron deficiency anemia in Zanzibari schoolchildren: the importance of hookworms. Am J Clin Nutr. 1997;65(1):153–9.
84. Ndyomugyenyi R, Kabatereine N, Olsen A, Magnussen P. Malaria and hookworm infections in relation to haemoglobin and serum ferritin levels in pregnancy in Masindi district, western Uganda. Trans R Soc Trop Med Hyg. 2008;102(2):130–6. Epub 2007 Nov 9.
85. Cercamondi CI, Egli IM, Ahouandjinou E, Dossa R, Zeder C, Salami L, et al. Afebrile Plasmodium falciparum parasitemia decreases absorption of fortification iron but does not affect systemic iron utilization: a double stable-isotope study in young Beninese women. Am J Clin Nutr. 2010;92(6):1385–92.
86. Anderson GJ, Frazer DM, McLaren GD. Iron absorption and metabolism. Curr Opin Gastroenterol. 2009;25(2):129–35.
87. Barisani D, Pelucchi S, Mariani R, Galimberti S, Trombini P, Fumagalli D, et al. Hepcidin and iron-related gene expression in subjects with Dysmetabolic hepatic Iron overload. J Hepatol. 2008;49(1):123–33.
88. Nemeth E. Iron regulation and erythropoiesis. Curr Opin Hematol. 2008;15(3):169–75.
89. Soofi S, Cousens S, Iqbal SP, Akhund T, Khan J, Ahmed I, et al. Effect of provision of daily zinc and iron with several micronutrients on growth and morbidity among young children in Pakistan: a cluster-randomised trial. Lancet. 2013;382(9886):29–40.
90. Sazawal S, Black RE, Ramsan M, Chwaya HM, Stoltzfus RJ, Dutta A, et al. Effects of routine prophylactic supplementation with iron and folic acid on admission to hospital and mortality in preschool children in a high malaria transmission setting: community-based, randomised, placebo-controlled trial. Lancet. 2006;367(9505):133–43.
91. Nweneka CV, Doherty CP, Cox S, Prentice A. Iron delocalisation in the pathogenesis of malarial anaemia. Trans R Soc Trop Med Hyg. 2010;104(3):175–84.
92. Chang KH, Stevenson MM. Malarial anaemia: mechanisms and implications of insufficient erythropoiesis during blood-stage malaria. Int J Parasitol. 2004;34(13–14):1501–16.
93. Muir A, Hopfer U. Regional specificity of iron uptake by small intestinal brush-border membranes from normal and iron-deficient mice. Am J Phys. 1985;248(3 Pt 1):G376–9.
94. Mohan K, Stevenson MM. Dyserythropoiesis and severe anaemia associated with malaria correlate with deficient interleukin-12 production. Br J Haematol. 1998;103(4):942–9.
95. Hallberg L, Brune M, Rossander L. Effect of ascorbic acid on iron absorption from different types of meals. Studies with ascorbic-acid-rich foods and synthetic ascorbic acid given in different amounts with different meals. Hum Nutr Appl Nutr. 1986;40(2):97–113.
96. Shayeghi M, Latunde-Dada GO, Oakhill JS, Laftah AH, Takeuchi K, Halliday N, et al. Identification of an intestinal heme transporter. Cell. 2005;122(5):789–801.
97. Park CH, Valore EV, Waring AJ, Ganz T. Hepcidin, a urinary antimicrobial peptide synthesized in the liver. J Biol Chem. 2001;276(11):7806–10.
98. Ganz T. Hepcidin, a key regulator of iron metabolism and mediator of anemia of inflammation. Blood. 2003;102(3):783–8.
99. Nemeth E, Valore EV, Territo M, Schiller G, Lichtenstein A, Ganz T. Hepcidin, a putative mediator of anemia of inflammation, is a type II acute-phase protein. Blood. 2003;101(7):2461–3.
100. Nemeth E, Rivera S, Gabayan V, Keller C, Taudorf S, Pedersen BK, et al. IL-6 mediates hypoferremia of inflammation by inducing the synthesis of the iron regulatory hormone hepcidin. J Clin Invest. 2004;113(9):1271–6.
101. Nemeth E, Tuttle MS, Powelson J, Vaughn MB, Donovan A, Ward DM, et al. Hepcidin regulates cellular iron efflux by binding to ferroportin and inducing its internalization. Science. 2004;306(5704):2090–3.
102. Pinto JP, Ribeiro S, Pontes H, Thowfeequ S, Tosh D, Carvalho F, et al. Erythropoietin mediates hepcidin expression in hepatocytes through EPOR signaling and regulation of C/EBPalpha. Blood. 2008;111(12):5727–33.
103. Barffour MA, Schulze KJ, Coles CL, Chileshe J, Kalungwana N, Arguello M, et al. High iron stores in the low malaria season increase malaria risk in the high transmission season in a prospective cohort of rural Zambian children. J Nutr. 2017;147(8):1531–6.
104. Tielsch JM, Khatry SK, Stoltzfus RJ, Katz J, LeClerq SC, Adhikari R, et al. Effect of routine prophylactic supplementation with iron and folic acid on preschool child mortality in southern Nepal: community-based, cluster-randomised, placebo-controlled trial. Lancet. 2006;367(9505):144–52.
105. Schumann K, Kroll S, Romero-Abal ME, Georgiou NA, Marx JJ, Weiss G, et al. Impact of oral iron challenges on circulating non-transferrin-bound iron in healthy Guatemalan males. Ann Nutr Metab. 2012;60(2):98–107.
106. Hurrell RF. Safety and efficacy of iron supplements in malaria-endemic areas. Ann Nutr Metab. 2011;59(1):64–6.
107. Hershko C. Mechanism of iron toxicity. Food Nutr Bull. 2007;28(4 Suppl):S500–9.
108. Wilson ME, Britigan BE. Iron acquisition by parasitic protozoa. Parasitol Today. 1998;14(9):348–53.
109. Arese P, Schwarzer E. Malarial pigment (haemozoin): a very active 'inert' substance. Ann Trop Med Parasitol. 1997;91(5):501–16.

110. Lang E, Qadri SM, Lang F. Killing me softly – suicidal erythrocyte death. Int J Biochem Cell Biol. 2012;44(8):1236–43.
111. Lang F, Lang KS, Lang PA, Huber SM, Wieder T. Mechanisms and significance of eryptosis. Antioxid Redox Signal. 2006;8(7–8):1183–92.
112. Lang F, Qadri SM. Mechanisms and significance of eryptosis, the suicidal death of erythrocytes. Blood Purif. 2012;33(1–3):125–30.
113. de Mast Q, Syafruddin D, Keijmel S, Riekerink TO, Deky O, Asih PB, et al. Increased serum hepcidin and altera-tions in blood iron parameters associated with asymptomatic P. falciparum and P. vivax malaria. Haematologica. 2010;95(7):1068–74.
114. Drakesmith H, Prentice AM. Hepcidin and the iron-infection axis. Science. 2012;338(6108):768–72.
115. Howard CT, McKakpo US, Quakyi IA, Bosompem KM, Addison EA, Sun K, et al. Relationship of hepcidin with parasitemia and anemia among patients with uncomplicated Plasmodium falciparum malaria in Ghana. Am J Trop Med Hyg. 2007;77(4):623–6.
116. Johnson EE, Wessling-Resnick M. Iron metabolism and the innate immune response to infection. Microbes Infect. 2012;14(3):207–16.
117. Portugal S, Carret C, Recker M, Armitage AE, Goncalves LA, Epiphanio S, et al. Host-mediated regulation of superinfection in malaria. Nat Med. 2011;17(6):732–7.
118. Portugal S, Drakesmith H, Mota MM. Superinfection in malaria: Plasmodium shows its iron will. EMBO Rep. 2011;12(12):1233–42.
119. Ganz T. Iron in innate immunity: starve the invaders. Curr Opin Immunol. 2009;21(1):63–7.
120. Oppenheimer SJ. Iron and its relation to immunity and infectious disease. J Nutr. 2001;131(2S–2):616S–33S; discussion 33S–35S.
121. Righetti AA, Glinz D, Adiossan LG, Koua AY, Niamke S, Hurrell RF, et al. Interactions and potential implications of Plasmodium falciparum-hookworm coinfection in different age groups in South-Central Cote d'Ivoire. PLoS Negl Trop Dis. 2012;6(11):e1889.
122. Koka S, Foller M, Lamprecht G, Boini KM, Lang C, Huber SM, et al. Iron deficiency influences the course of malaria in Plasmodium berghei infected mice. Biochem Biophys Res Commun. 2007;357(3):608–14.
123. Matsuzaki-Moriya C, Tu L, Ishida H, Imai T, Suzue K, Hirai M, et al. A critical role for phagocytosis in resistance to malaria in iron-deficient mice. Eur J Immunol. 2011;41(5):1365–75.
124. Smith HJ, Meremikwu M. Iron chelating agents for treating malaria. Cochrane Database Syst Rev. 2003;(2):CD001474.
125. Casals-Pascual C, Huang H, Lakhal-Littleton S, Thezenas ML, Kai O, Newton CR, et al. Hepcidin demonstrates a biphasic association with anemia in acute Plasmodium falciparum malaria. Haematologica. 2012;97(11):1695–8.
126. el Hassan AM, Saeed AM, Fandrey J, Jelkmann W. Decreased erythropoietin response in Plasmodium falciparum malaria-associated anaemia. Eur J Haematol. 1997;59(5):299–304.
127. Stevens RD. Anaemia -- the scourge of the third world. Health Millions. 2000;26(2):21–3.
128. O'Donnell A, Fowkes FJ, Allen SJ, Imrie H, Alpers MP, Weatherall DJ, et al. The acute phase response in children with mild and severe malaria in Papua New Guinea. Trans R Soc Trop Med Hyg. 2009;103(7):679–86.
129. Jason J, Archibald LK, Nwanyanwu OC, Bell M, Buchanan I, Larned J, et al. Cytokines and malaria parasitemia. Clin Immunol. 2001;100(2):208–18.
130. Hurrell R. Iron and malaria: absorption, efficacy and safety. Int J Vitam Nutr Res. 2010;80(4–5):279–92.
131. Collins HL, Kaufmann SH, Schaible UE. Iron chelation via deferoxamine exacerbates experimental salmonel-losis via inhibition of the nicotinamide adenine dinucleotide phosphate oxidase-dependent respiratory burst. J Immunol. 2002;168(7):3458–63.
132. Wang L, Harrington L, Trebicka E, Shi HN, Kagan JC, Hong CC, et al. Selective modulation of TLR4-activated inflammatory responses by altered iron homeostasis in mice. J Clin Invest. 2009;119(11):3322–8.
133. Cherayil BJ. Iron and immunity: immunological consequences of iron deficiency and overload. Arch Immunol Ther Exp. 2010;58(6):407–15.
134. Brini M, Carafoli E. Calcium pumps in health and disease. Physiol Rev. 2009;89(4):1341–78.
135. Mata AM, Sepulveda MR. Calcium pumps in the central nervous system. Brain Res Brain Res Rev. 2005;49(2):398–405.
136. Gueguen L, Pointillart A. The bioavailability of dietary calcium. J Am Coll Nutrn. 2000;19(2 Suppl):119s–36s.
137. Fleming KH, Heimbach JT. Consumption of calcium in the U.S.: food sources and intake levels. J Nutr. 1994;124(8 Suppl):1426s–30s.
138. Christakos S, Lieben L, Masuyama R, Carmeliet G. Vitamin D endocrine system and the intestine. Bonekey Rep. 2014;3:496.
139. Pettifor JM. Calcium and vitamin D metabolism in children in developing countries. Ann Nutr Metab. 2014;64(Suppl 2):15–22.

140. Pettifor JM. Vitamin D &/or calcium deficiency rickets in infants & children: a global perspective. Indian J Med Res. 2008;127(3):245–9.

141. DeLuca HF. The role of vitamin D and its relationship to parathyroid hormone and calcitonin. Recent Prog Horm Res. 1971;27:479–516.

142. Rasmussen H, Wong M, Bikle D, Goodman DB. Hormonal control of the renal conversion of 25-hydroxycholecalciferol to 1,25-dihydroxycholecalciferol. J Clin Invest. 1972;51(9):2502–4.

143. Austin LA, Heath H 3rd. Calcitonin: physiology and pathophysiology. N Engl J Med. 1981;304(5):269–78.

144. Blair HC, Larrouture QC, Tourkova IL, Liu L, Bian JH, Stolz DB, et al. Support of bone mineral deposition by regulation of pH. Am J Physiol Cell Physiol. 2018;315(4):C587–C97.

145. Marchi S, Patergnani S, Missiroli S, Morciano G, Rimessi A, Wieckowski MR, et al. Mitochondrial and endoplasmic reticulum calcium homeostasis and cell death. Cell Calcium. 2018;69:62–72.

146. Brini M, Cali T, Ottolini D, Carafoli E. Intracellular calcium homeostasis and signaling. Met Ions Life Sci. 2013;12:119–68.

147. Flynn A. The role of dietary calcium in bone health. Proc Nutr Soc. 2003;62(4):851–8.

148. Crabtree GR. Calcium, calcineurin, and the control of transcription. J Biol Chem. 2001;276(4):2313–6.

149. Singh H, Sen R, Baltimore D, Sharp PA. A nuclear factor that binds to a conserved sequence motif in transcriptional control elements of immunoglobulin genes. Nature. 1986;319(6049):154–8.

150. Negulescu PA, Shastri N, Cahalan MD. Intracellular calcium dependence of gene expression in single T lymphocytes. Proc Natl Acad Sci U S A. 1994;91(7):2873–7.

151. Sandstead HH. Zinc deficiency. A public health problem? Am J Dis Child. 1991;145(8):853–9.

152. Gibson RS, King JC, Lowe N. A review of dietary zinc recommendations. Food Nutr Bull. 2016;37(4):443–60.

153. World Health Organization, Food and Agricultural Organization, International Atomic Energy Association. Trace elements in human health and nutrition. Geneva: World Health Organization; 1996.

154. Roohani N, Hurrell R, Kelishadi R, Schulin R. Zinc and its importance for human health: an integrative review. J Res Med Sci. 2013;18(2):144–57.

155. Scheers N. Regulatory effects of Cu, Zn, and Ca on Fe absorption: the intricate play between nutrient transporters. Nutrients. 2013;5(3):957–70.

156. Whittaker P. Iron and zinc interactions in humans. Am J Clin Nutr. 1998;68(2 Suppl):442s–6s.

157. Brown KH, Wessells KR, Hess SY. Zinc bioavailability from zinc-fortified foods. Int J Vitam Nutr Res. 2007;77(3):174–81.

158. Krebs NF. Overview of zinc absorption and excretion in the human gastrointestinal tract. J Nutr. 2000;130(5S Suppl):1374s–7s.

159. Hambidge M, Krebs NF. Interrelationships of key variables of human zinc homeostasis: relevance to dietary zinc requirements. Annu Rev Nutr. 2001;21:429–52.

160. King JC, Shames DM, Woodhouse LR. Zinc homeostasis in humans. J Nutr. 2000;130(5S Suppl):1360s–6s.

161. Ying AJ, Shu XL, Gu WZ, Huang XM, Shuai XH, Yang LR, et al. Effect of zinc deficiency on intestinal mucosal morphology and digestive enzyme activity in growing rat. Zhonghua Er Ke Za Zhi. 2011;49(4):249–54.

162. Song YM, Kim MH, Kim HN, Jang I, Han JH, Fontamillas GA, et al. Effects of dietary supplementation of lipid-coated zinc oxide on intestinal mucosal morphology and expression of the genes associated with growth and immune function in weanling pigs. Asian-Australas J Anim Sci. 2018;31(3):403–9.

163. Roy SK, Behrens RH, Haider R, Akramuzzaman SM, Mahalanabis D, Wahed MA, et al. Impact of zinc supplementation on intestinal permeability in Bangladeshi children with acute diarrhoea and persistent diarrhoea syndrome. J Pediatr Gastroenterol Nutr. 1992;15(3):289–96.

164. WHO/UNICEF. Zinc supplementation in the management of diarrhoea. World Health Organization; 2004.

165. WHO/UNICEF. Clinical management of acute diarrhoea in children: WHO/UNICEF joint statement. Geneva: World Health Organization; 2004.

166. Tielsch JM, Khatry SK, Stoltzfus RJ, Katz J, LeClerq SC, Adhikari R, et al. Effect of daily zinc supplementation on child mortality in southern Nepal: a community-based, cluster randomised, placebo-controlled trial. Lancet. 2007;370(9594):1230–9.

167. Kruse-Jarres JD. The significance of zinc for humoral and cellular immunity. J Trace Elem Electrolytes Health Dis. 1989;3(1):1–8.

168. Kheirouri S, Alizadeh M. Decreased serum and mucosa immunoglobulin A levels in vitamin A and zinc-deficient mice. Cent Eur J Immunol. 2014;39(2):165–9.

169. Haase H, Rink L. Zinc signals and immune function. Biofactors. 2014;40(1):27–40.

170. Deloria-Knoll M, Steinhoff M, Semba RD, Nelson K, Vlahov D, Meinert CL. Effect of zinc and vitamin A supplementation on antibody responses to a pneumococcal conjugate vaccine in HIV-positive injection drug users: a randomized trial. Vaccine. 2006;24(10):1670–9.

171. Prasad AS, Bao B, Beck FW, Kucuk O, Sarkar FH. Antioxidant effect of zinc in humans. Free Radic Biol Med. 2004;37(8):1182–90.

172. Vanderpas JB, Moreno-Reyes R. Historical aspects of iodine deficiency control. Minerva Med. 2017;108(2):124–35.
173. Zimmermann MB. Research on iodine deficiency and goiter in the 19th and early 20th centuries. J Nutr. 2008;138(11):2060–3.
174. Zimmermann MB, Boelaert K. Iodine deficiency and thyroid disorders. Lancet Diabetes Endocrinol. 2015;3(4):286–95.
175. Delange F. The disorders induced by iodine deficiency. Thyroid. 1994;4(1):107–28.
176. Zimmermann MB. Assessing iodine status and monitoring progress of iodized salt programs. J Nutr. 2004;134(7):1673–7.
177. Alexander WD, Harden RM, Harrison MT, Shimmins J. Some aspects of the absorption and concentration of iodide by the alimentary tract in man. Proce Nutr Soc. 1967;26(1):62–6.
178. DeGroot LJ. Kinetic analysis of iodine metabolism. J Clin Endocrinol Metab. 1966;26(2):149–73.
179. Pedraza PE, Obregon MJ, Escobar-Morreale HF, del Rey FE, de Escobar GM. Mechanisms of adaptation to iodine deficiency in rats: thyroid status is tissue specific. Its relevance for man. Endocrinology. 2006;147(5):2098–108.
180. Smanik PA, Ryu KY, Theil KS, Mazzaferri EL, Jhiang SM. Expression, exon-intron organization, and chromosome mapping of the human sodium iodide symporter. Endocrinology. 1997;138(8):3555–8.
181. Schmutzler C, Kohrle J. Implications of the molecular characterization of the sodium-iodide symporter (NIS). Exp Clin Endocrinol Diabetes. 1998;106(Suppl 3):S1–10.
182. Dunn JT. Thyroglobulin, hormone synthesis and thyroid disease. Eur J Endocrinol. 1995;132(5):603–4.
183. Bilal MY, Dambaeva S, Kwak-Kim J, Gilman-Sachs A, Beaman KD. A role for iodide and thyroglobulin in modulating the function of human immune cells. Front Immunol. 2017;8:1573.
184. Chen X, Liu L, Yao P, Yu D, Hao L, Sun X. Effect of excessive iodine on immune function of lymphocytes and intervention with selenium. J Huazhong Univ Sci Technolog Med Sci. 2007;27(4):422–5.
185. De Vito P, Incerpi S, Pedersen JZ, Luly P, Davis FB, Davis PJ. Thyroid hormones as modulators of immune activities at the cellular level. Thyroid. 2011;21(8):879–90.
186. Schomburg L, Schweizer U, Kohrle J. Selenium and selenoproteins in mammals: extraordinary, essential, enigmatic. Cell Mol Life Sci. 2004;61(16):1988–95.
187. Daniels LA. Selenium metabolism and bioavailability. Biol Trace Elem Res. 1996;54(3):185–99.
188. Moxon AL, Rhian M. Selenium poisoning. Physiol Rev. 1943;23(4):305–37.
189. Schwarz K, Foltz CM. Selenium as an integral part of factor 3 against dietary necrotic liver degeneration. 1951. Nutrition. 1999;15(3):255.
190. Observations on effect of sodium selenite in prevention of Keshan disease. Chin Med J (Engl). 1979;92(7):471–6.
191. Zhang Y, Zhou Y, Schweizer U, Savaskan NE, Hua D, Kipnis J, et al. Comparative analysis of selenocysteine machinery and selenoproteome gene expression in mouse brain identifies neurons as key functional sites of selenium in mammals. J Biol Chem. 2008;283(4):2427–38.
192. Stranges S, Marshall JR, Natarajan R, Donahue RP, Trevisan M, Combs GF, et al. Effects of long-term selenium supplementation on the incidence of type 2 diabetes: a randomized trial. Ann Intern Med. 2007;147(4):217–23.
193. Wu SH, Oldfield JE, Whanger PD, Weswig PH. Effect of selenium, vitamin E, and antioxidants on testicular function in rats. Biol Reprod. 1973;8(5):625–9.
194. Su D, Novoselov SV, Sun QA, Moustafa ME, Zhou Y, Oko R, et al. Mammalian selenoprotein thioredoxin-glutathione reductase. Roles in disulfide bond formation and sperm maturation. J Biol Chem. 2005;280(28):26491–8.
195. Wolf WR, Goldschmidt RJ. Updated estimates of the selenomethionine content of NIST wheat reference materials by GC-IDMS. Anal Bioanal Chem. 2007;387(7):2449–52.
196. Phiri FP, Ander EL, Bailey EH, Chilima B, Chilimba ADC, Gondwe J, et al. The risk of selenium deficiency in Malawi is large and varies over multiple spatial scales. Sci Rep. 2019;9(1):6566.
197. Hurst R, Siyame EW, Young SD, Chilimba AD, Joy EJ, Black CR, et al. Soil-type influences human selenium status and underlies widespread selenium deficiency risks in Malawi. Sci Rep. 2013;3:1425.
198. Chen J. An original discovery: selenium deficiency and Keshan disease (an endemic heart disease). Asia Pac J Clin Nutr. 2012;21(3):320–6.
199. Jiang S, Li FL, Dong Q, Liu HW, Fang CF, Shu C, et al. H558R polymorphism in SCN5A is associated with Keshan disease and QRS prolongation in Keshan disease patients. Genet Mol Res. 2014;13(3):6569–76.
200. Lei C, Niu X, Ma X, Wei J. Is selenium deficiency really the cause of Keshan disease? Environ Geochem Health. 2011;33(2):183–8.
201. Joy EJ, Ander EL, Young SD, Black CR, Watts MJ, Chilimba AD, et al. Dietary mineral supplies in Africa. Physiol Plant. 2014;151(3):208–29.
202. Fordyce F. Selenium geochemistry and health. Ambio. 2007;36(1):94–7.
203. Li C. Selenium deficiency and endemic heart failure in China: a case study of biogeochemistry for human health. Ambio. 2007;36(1):90–3.
204. von Stockhausen HB. Selenium in total parenteral nutrition. Biol Trace Elem Res. 1988;15:147–55.

205. Korpela H, Nuutinen LS, Kumpulainen J. Low serum selenium and glutathione peroxidase activity in patients receiving short-term total parenteral nutrition. Int J Vitam Nutr Res. 1989;59(1):80–4.

206. Abrams CK, Siram SM, Galsim C, Johnson-Hamilton H, Munford FL, Mezghebe H. Selenium deficiency in long-term total parenteral nutrition. Nutr Clin Pract. 1992;7(4):175–8.

207. Kurokawa S, Berry MJ. Selenium. Role of the essential metalloid in health. Met Ions Life Sci. 2013;13:499–534.

208. Cheng WH, Ho YS, Valentine BA, Ross DA, Combs GF Jr, Lei XG. Cellular glutathione peroxidase is the mediator of body selenium to protect against paraquat lethality in transgenic mice. J Nutr. 1998;128(7):1070–6.

209. Fu Y, Cheng WH, Porres JM, Ross DA, Lei XG. Knockout of cellular glutathione peroxidase gene renders mice susceptible to diquat-induced oxidative stress. Free Radic Biol Med. 1999;27(5–6):605–11.

210. Yen PM. Physiological and molecular basis of thyroid hormone action. Physiol Rev. 2001;81(3):1097–142.

211. Fraczek-Jucha M, Kabat M, Szlosarczyk B, Czubek U, Nessler J, Gackowski A. Selenium deficiency and the dynamics of changes of thyroid profile in patients with acute myocardial infarction and chronic heart failure. Kardiol Pol. 2019;77(7-8):674–82.

212. Hoffmann PR, Berry MJ. The influence of selenium on immune responses. Mol Nutr Food Res. 2008;52(11):1273–80.

213. Hoffmann PR. Mechanisms by which selenium influences immune responses. Arch Immunol Ther Exp. 2007;55(5):289–97.

214. Huang Z, Rose AH, Hoffmann PR. The role of selenium in inflammation and immunity: from molecular mechanisms to therapeutic opportunities. Antioxid Redox Signal. 2012;16(7):705–43.

215. Roy M, Kiremidjian-Schumacher L, Wishe HI, Cohen MW, Stotzky G. Selenium supplementation enhances the expression of interleukin 2 receptor subunits and internalization of interleukin 2. Proc Soc Exp Biol Med. 1993;202(3):295–301.

216. Li W, Beck MA. Selenium deficiency induced an altered immune response and increased survival following influenza A/Puerto Rico/8/34 infection. Exp Biol Med (Maywood). 2007;232(3):412–9.

217. Underwood EJ. Trace metals in human and animal health. J Hum Nutr. 1981;35(1):37–48.

218. Sturgeon P, Brubaker C. Copper deficiency in infants. Am J Dis Child. 1956;92:254–65.

219. Cordano A, Baertl J, Graham G. Copper deficiency in infants. Pediatrics. 1964;34:324–36.

220. Arredondo M, Nunez MT. Iron and copper metabolism. Mol Asp Med. 2005;26(4–5):313–27.

221. Uauy R, Olivares M, Gonzalez M. Essentiality of copper in humans. Am J Clin Nutr. 1998;67(5 Suppl):952s–9s.

222. Kaplan J, O'Halloran TV. Iron metabolism in eukaryotes: Mars and Venus at it again. Science. 1996;271(5255):1510–2.

223. Furst P, Hu S, Hackett R, Hamer D. Copper activates metallothionein gene transcription by altering the conformation of a specific DNA binding protein. Cell. 1988;55(4):705–17.

224. Bashar SA, Sharmeen L. Serum levels of trace elements (zinc and copper) in malnourished children in Bangladesh. J Pak Med Assoc. 1983;33(10):251–5.

225. Gautam B, Deb K, Banerjee M, Ali MS, Akhter S, Shahidullah SM, et al. Serum zinc and copper level in children with protein energy malnutrition. Mymensingh Med J. 2008;17(2 Suppl):S12–5.

226. Singla PN, Chand P, Kumar A, Kachhawaha JS. Serum, zinc and copper levels in children with protein energy malnutrition. Indian J Pediatr. 1996;63(2):199–203.

227. McCord JM. Oxygen-derived free radicals in postischemic tissue injury. N Engl J Med. 1985;312(3):159–63.

228. Lukasewycz OA, Prohaska JR. The immune response in copper deficiency. Ann N Y Acad Sci. 1990;587:147–59.

229. Huang ZL, Failla ML. Copper deficiency suppresses effector activities of differentiated U937 cells. J Nutr. 2000;130(6):1536–42.

230. Percival SS. Copper and immunity. Am J Clin Nutr. 1998;67(5 Suppl):1064s–8s.

231. Hopkins RG, Failla ML. Chronic intake of a marginally low copper diet impairs in vitro activities of lymphocytes and neutrophils from male rats despite minimal impact on conventional indicators of copper status. J Nutr. 1995;125(10):2658–68.

232. Bae B, Percival SS. Retinoic acid-induced HL-60 cell differentiation is augmented by copper supplementation. J Nutr. 1993;123(6):997–1002.

233. Heresi G, Castillo-Duran C, Munoz C, Arevalo M, Schlesinger L. Phagocytosis and immunoglobulin levels in hypocupremic infants. Nutr Res. 1985;5:1327–34.

234. Kelley DS, Daudu PA, Taylor PC, Mackey BE, Turnlund JR. Effects of low-copper diets on human immune response. Am J Clin Nutr. 1995;62(2):412–6.

235. Elin RJ. Assessment of magnesium status. Clin Chem. 1987;33(11):1965–70.

236. Bieker JJ, Martin PL, Roeder RG. Formation of a rate-limiting intermediate in 5S RNA gene transcription. Cell. 1985;40(1):119–27.

237. Larsson SC, Orsini N, Wolk A. Dietary magnesium intake and risk of stroke: a meta-analysis of prospective studies. Am J Clin Nutr. 2012;95(2):362–6.

238. Ford ES, Mokdad AH. Dietary magnesium intake in a national sample of US adults. J Nutr. 2003;133(9):2879–82.

239. Seo JW, Park TJ. Magnesium metabolism. Electrolyte Blood Press. 2008;6(2):86–95.

240. Abbott LG, Rude RK. Clinical manifestations of magnesium deficiency. Miner Electrolyte Metab. 1993;19(4–5):314–22.
241. Pathak P, Kapil U. Role of trace elements zinc, copper and magnesium during pregnancy and its outcome. Indian J Pediatr. 2004;71(11):1003–5.
242. Schlegel RN, Cuffe JS, Moritz KM, Paravicini TM. Maternal hypomagnesemia causes placental abnormalities and fetal and postnatal mortality. Placenta. 2015;36(7):750–8.
243. Kausalya PJ, Amasheh S, Gunzel D, Wurps H, Muller D, Fromm M, et al. Disease-associated mutations affect intracellular traffic and paracellular Mg2+ transport function of Claudin-16. J Clin Invest. 2006;116(4):878–91.
244. Hoorn EJ, Zietse R. Disorders of calcium and magnesium balance: a physiology-based approach. Pediatr Nephrol. 2013;28(8):1195–206.
245. Bindels RJ. 2009 Homer W. Smith Award: minerals in motion: from new ion transporters to new concepts. J Am Soc Nephrol. 2010;21(8):1263–9.
246. Quamme GA. Renal magnesium handling: new insights in understanding old problems. Kidney Int. 1997;52(5):1180–95.
247. Romani A. Regulation of magnesium homeostasis and transport in mammalian cells. Arch Biochem Biophys. 2007;458(1):90–102.
248. Weglicki WB, Phillips TM, Freedman AM, Cassidy MM, Dickens BF. Magnesium-deficiency elevates circulating levels of inflammatory cytokines and endothelin. Mol Cell Biochem. 1992;110(2):169–73.
249. Weglicki WB, Phillips TM. Pathobiology of magnesium deficiency: a cytokine/neurogenic inflammation hypothesis. Am J Phys. 1992;263(3 Pt 2):R734–7.
250. Weglicki WB, Dickens BF, Wagner TL, Chmielinska JJ, Phillips TM. Immunoregulation by neuropeptides in magnesium deficiency: ex vivo effect of enhanced substance P production on circulating T lymphocytes from magnesium-deficient mice. Magnes Res. 1996;9(1):3–11.
251. Tam M, Gomez S, Gonzalez-Gross M, Marcos A. Possible roles of magnesium on the immune system. Eur J Clin Nutr. 2003;57(10):1193–7.
252. Malpuech-Brugere C, Nowacki W, Gueux E, Kuryszko J, Rock E, Rayssiguier Y, et al. Accelerated thymus involution in magnesium-deficient rats is related to enhanced apoptosis and sensitivity to oxidative stress. Br J Nutr. 1999;81(5):405–11.
253. von Lintig J. Provitamin A metabolism and functions in mammalian biology. Am J Clin Nutr. 2012;96(5):1234s–44s.
254. World Health Organization, UNICEF. Global prevalence of vitamin A deficiency micronutrient deficiency information system. Geneva: World Health Organization; 1995. Contract no.: working paper no. 2.
255. WHO. Global prevalence of Vitamin A deficiency in populations at risk, 1995–2005. WHO Global Database on vitamin A deficiency. World Health Organization; 2008.
256. Mahalanabis D. Breast feeding and vitamin A deficiency among children attending a diarrhoea treatment centre in Bangladesh: a case-control study. BMJ (Clinical research ed). 1991;303(6801):493–6.
257. Rahmathullah L, Raj MS, Chandravathi TS. Aetiology of severe vitamin a deficiency in children. Natl Med J India. 1997;10(2):62–5.
258. Miller M, Humphrey J, Johnson E, Marinda E, Brookmeyer R, Katz J. Why do children become vitamin a deficient? J Nutr. 2002;132(9 Suppl):2867S–80S.
259. UNICEF. State of the world's children 2000. www.unicef.org/. New York: sowc00 UNICEF; 2000.
260. WHO. Complementary feeding of young children in developing countries: a review of current scientific knowledge. Geneva, Switzerland, World Health Organization; 1998. Contract No.: Pub no. WS 130 98 CO.
261. Fawzi WW, Herrera MG, Willett WC, el Amin A, Nestel P, Lipsitz S, et al. Vitamin A supplementation and dietary vitamin A in relation to the risk of xerophthalmia. Am J Clin Nutr. 1993;58(3):385–91.
262. Filteau SM, Tomkins AM. Promoting vitamin A status in low-income countries. Lancet. 1999;353(9163):1458–9.
263. Solomons NW, Bulux J. Plant sources of provitamin A and human nutriture. Nutr Rev. 1993;51(7):199–204.
264. Solomons NW, Bulux J. Identification and production of local carotene-rich foods to combat vitamin A malnutrition. Eur J Clin Nutr. 1997;51(Suppl 4):S39–45.
265. Institute of Medicine. Dietary reference intakes for Vitamin A, Vitamin K, Arsenic, Boron, Chromium, Copper, Iodine, Iron, Manganese, Molybdenum, Nickel, Silicon, Vanadium, and Zinc. Washington, DC: National Academy Press; 2001.
266. Nemeth E, Roetto A, Garozzo G, Ganz T, Camaschella C. Hepcidin is decreased in TFR2 hemochromatosis. Blood. 2005;105(4):1803–6.
267. Kelly P, Musuku J, Kafwembe E, Libby G, Zulu I, Murphy J, et al. Impaired bioavailability of vitamin A in adults and children with persistent diarrhoea in Zambia. Aliment Pharmacol Ther. 2001;15(7):973–9.
268. Mitra AK, Alvarez JO, Stephensen CB. Increased urinary retinol loss in children with severe infections. Lancet. 1998;351(9108):1033–4.
269. Sivakumar BR. Absorption of labelled vitamin A in children during infection. Br J Nutr. 1972;27:299–304.
270. Stephensen CB. Vitamin A, infection, and immune function. Annu Rev Nutr. 2001;21:167–92.

271. Stephensen CB, Alvarez JO, Kohatsu J, Hardmeier R, Kennedy JI Jr, Gammon RB Jr. Vitamin A is excreted in the urine during acute infection. Am J Clin Nutr. 1994;60(3):388–92.

272. Stephensen CB, Gildengorin G. Serum retinol, the acute phase response, and the apparent misclassification of vitamin A status in the third National Health and Nutrition Examination Survey. Am J Clin Nutr. 2000;72(5):1170–8.

273. Mizuno Y, Kawazu SI, Kano S, Watanabe N, Matsuura T, Ohtomo H. In-vitro uptake of vitamin A by Plasmodium falciparum. Ann Trop Med Parasitol. 2003;97(3):237–43.

274. Velasquez-Melendez G, Okani ET, Kiertsman B, Roncada MJ. Vitamin A status in children with pneumonia. Eur J Clin Nutr. 1995;49(5):379–84.

275. Schulze KJ, Christian P, Wu LS, Arguello M, Cui H, Nanayakkara-Bind A, et al. Micronutrient deficiencies are common in 6- to 8-year-old children of rural Nepal, with prevalence estimates modestly affected by inflammation. J Nutr. 2014;144(6):979–87.

276. D'Ambrosio DN, Clugston RD, Blaner WS. Vitamin A metabolism: an update. Nutrients. 2011;3(1):63–103.

277. Napoli JL. Retinoic acid: its biosynthesis and metabolism. Prog Nucleic Acid Res Mol Biol. 1999;63:139–88.

278. Napoli JL. Biosynthesis and metabolism of retinoic acid: roles of CRBP and CRABP in retinoic acid: roles of CRBP and CRABP in retinoic acid homeostasis. J Nutr. 1993;123(2 Suppl):362–6.

279. Hall JA, Grainger JR, Spencer SP, Belkaid Y. The role of retinoic acid in tolerance and immunity. Immunity. 2011;35(1):13–22.

280. Hall JA, Cannons JL, Grainger JR, Dos Santos LM, Hand TW, Naik S, et al. Essential role for retinoic acid in the promotion of CD4(+) T cell effector responses via retinoic acid receptor alpha. Immunity. 2011;34(3):435–47.

281. Cunningham-Rundles S, McNeeley DF, Moon A. Mechanisms of nutrient modulation of the immune response. J Allergy Clin Immunol. 2005;115(6):1119–28; quiz 29.

282. Field CJ, Johnson IR, Schley PD. Nutrients and their role in host resistance to infection. J Leukoc Biol. 2002;71(1):16–32.

283. Semba RD. Vitamin A and immunity to viral, bacterial and protozoan infections. Proc Nutr Soc. 1999;58(3):719–27.

284. Smith SM, Levy NS, Hayes CE. Impaired immunity in vitamin A-deficient mice. J Nutr. 1987;117(5):857–65.

285. De Luca LM, Darwiche N, Celli G, Kosa K, Jones C, Ross S, et al. Vitamin A in epithelial differentiation and skin carcinogenesis. Nutr Rev. 1994;52(2 Pt 2):S45–52.

286. Desowitz RS. Plasmodium berghei: immunologic enhancement of antigen by adjuvant addition. Exp Parasitol. 1975;38(1):6–13.

287. Serghides L, Kain KC. Peroxisome proliferator-activated receptor gamma-retinoid X receptor agonists increase CD36-dependent phagocytosis of Plasmodium falciparum-parasitized erythrocytes and decrease malaria-induced TNF-alpha secretion by monocytes/macrophages. J Immunol. 2001;166(11):6742–8.

288. Serghides L, Kain KC. Mechanism of protection induced by vitamin A in falciparum malaria. Lancet. 2002;359(9315):1404–6.

289. Niemoeller OM, Foller M, Lang C, Huber SM, Lang F. Retinoic acid induced suicidal erythrocyte death. Cell Physiol Biochem. 2008;21(1–3):193–202.

290. Thriemer K, Wernsdorfer G, Rojanawatsirivet C, Kollaritsch H, Sirichainsinthop J, Wernsdorfer WH. In vitro activity of artemisinin alone and in combination with retinol against Plasmodium falciparum. Wien Klin Wochenschr. 2005;117(Suppl 4):45–8.

291. Parizek M, Sirichaisinthop J, Wernsdorfer G, Noedl H, Kollaritsch H, Wernsdorfer WH. Synergistic interaction between monodesbutyl-benflumetol and retinol in Plasmodium falciparum. Wien Klin Wochenschr. 2007;119(19–20 Suppl 3):53–9.

292. Knauer A, Congpuong K, Wernsdorfer G, Reinthaler FF, Sirichaisinthop J, Wernsdorfer WH. Synergism between quinine and retinol in fresh isolates of Plasmodium falciparum. Wien Klin Wochenschr. 2008;120(19–20 Suppl 4):69–73.

293. Cusick SE, Tielsch JM, Ramsan M, Jape JK, Sazawal S, Black RE, et al. Short-term effects of vitamin A and antimalarial treatment on erythropoiesis in severely anemic Zanzibari preschool children. Am J Clin Nutr. 2005;82(2):406–12.

294. Rolvien T, Krause M, Jeschke A, Yorgan T, Puschel K, Schinke T, et al. Vitamin D regulates osteocyte survival and perilacunar remodeling in human and murine bone. Bone. 2017;103:78–87.

295. Franasiak JM, Lara EE, Pellicer A. Vitamin D in human reproduction. Curr Opin Obstet Gynecol. 2017;29(4):189–94.

296. Adorini L, Penna G. Control of autoimmune diseases by the vitamin D endocrine system. Nat Clin Pract Rheumatol. 2008;4(8):404–12.

297. Holick MF, Chen TC. Vitamin D deficiency: a worldwide problem with health consequences. Am J Clin Nutr. 2008;87(4):1080s–6s.

298. Palacios C, Gonzalez L. Is vitamin D deficiency a major global public health problem? J Steroid Biochem Mol Biol. 2014;144 Pt A:138–45.

299. van Schoor NM, Lips P. Worldwide vitamin D status. Best Pract Res Clin Endocrinol Metab. 2011;25(4):671–80.

300. Lips P. Vitamin D physiology. Prog Biophys Mol Biol. 2006;92(1):4–8.

301. Schuster I. Cytochromes P450 are essential players in the vitamin D signaling system. Biochim Biophys Acta. 2011;1814(1):186–99.
302. Inoue Y, Segawa H, Kaneko I, Yamanaka S, Kusano K, Kawakami E, et al. Role of the vitamin D receptor in FGF23 action on phosphate metabolism. Biochem J. 2005;390(Pt 1):325–31.
303. Haussler MR, Haussler CA, Jurutka PW, Thompson PD, Hsieh JC, Remus LS, et al. The vitamin D hormone and its nuclear receptor: molecular actions and disease states. J Endocrinol. 1997;154(Suppl):S57–73.
304. Jurutka PW, Bartik L, Whitfield GK, Mathern DR, Barthel TK, Gurevich M, et al. Vitamin D receptor: key roles in bone mineral pathophysiology, molecular mechanism of action, and novel nutritional ligands. J Bone Miner Res. 2007;22(Suppl 2):V2–10.
305. Hewison M. Vitamin D and immune function: an overview. Proc Nutr Soc. 2012;71(1):50–61.
306. Liu PT, Stenger S, Li H, Wenzel L, Tan BH, Krutzik SR, et al. Toll-like receptor triggering of a vitamin D-mediated human antimicrobial response. Science. 2006;311(5768):1770–3.
307. Martineau AR, Timms PM, Bothamley GH, Hanifa Y, Islam K, Claxton AP, et al. High-dose vitamin D(3) during intensive-phase antimicrobial treatment of pulmonary tuberculosis: a double-blind randomised controlled trial. Lancet. 2011;377(9761):242–50.
308. Chun RF, Lauridsen AL, Suon L, Zella LA, Pike JW, Modlin RL, et al. Vitamin D-binding protein directs monocyte responses to 25-hydroxy- and 1,25-dihydroxyvitamin D. J Clin Endocrinol Metab. 2010;95(7):3368–76.
309. Hayes CE, Nashold FE, Spach KM, Pedersen LB. The immunological functions of the vitamin D endocrine system. Cell Mol Biol (Noisy-le-Grand). 2003;49(2):277–300.
310. Niki E, Traber MG. A history of vitamin E. Ann Nutr Metab. 2012;61(3):207–12.
311. Wang X, Quinn PJ. Vitamin E and its function in membranes. Prog Lipid Res. 1999;38(4):309–36.
312. Herrera E, Barbas C. Vitamin E: action, metabolism and perspectives. J Physiol Biochem. 2001;57(2):43–56.
313. Dror DK, Allen LH. Vitamin E deficiency in developing countries. Food Nutr Bull. 2011;32(2):124–43.
314. Drevon CA. Absorption, transport and metabolism of vitamin E. Free Radic Res Commun. 1991;14(4):229–46.
315. Farrell PM, Levine SL, Murphy MD, Adams AJ. Plasma tocopherol levels and tocopherol-lipid relationships in a normal population of children as compared to healthy adults. Am J Clin Nutr. 1978;31(10):1720–6.
316. Oldewage-Theron WH, Samuel FO, Djoulde RD. Serum concentration and dietary intake of vitamins a and E in low-income south African elderly. Clin Nutr. 2010;29(1):119–23.
317. Traber MG. Vitamin E regulatory mechanisms. Annu Rev Nutr. 2007;27:347–62.
318. Bjorneboe A, Bjorneboe GE, Drevon CA. Absorption, transport and distribution of vitamin E. J Nutr. 1990;120(3):233–42.
319. McCay PB. Vitamin E: interactions with free radicals and ascorbate. Annu Rev Nutr. 1985;5:323–40.
320. Costagliola C, Libondi T, Menzione M, Rinaldi E, Auricchio G. Vitamin E and red blood cell glutathione. Metabolism. 1985;34(8):712–4.
321. Chow CK. Vitamin E and blood. World Rev Nutr Diet. 1985;45:133–66.
322. Lee GY, Han SN. The role of vitamin E in immunity. Nutrients. 2018;10(11):1614.
323. Dalia AM, Loh TC, Sazili AQ, Jahromi MF, Samsudin AA. Effects of vitamin E, inorganic selenium, bacterial organic selenium, and their combinations on immunity response in broiler chickens. BMC Vet Res. 2018;14(1):249.
324. Khan MZ, Akter SH, Islam MN, Karim MR, Islam MR, Kon Y. The effect of selenium and vitamin E on the lymphocytes and immunoglobulin-containing plasma cells in the lymphoid organ and mucosa-associated lymphatic tissues of broiler chickens. Anat Histol Embryol. 2008;37(1):52–9.
325. Bou Ghanem EN, Clark S, Du X, Wu D, Camilli A, Leong JM, et al. The alpha-tocopherol form of vitamin E reverses age-associated susceptibility to streptococcus pneumoniae lung infection by modulating pulmonary neutrophil recruitment. J Immunol. 2015;194(3):1090–9.
326. Sheridan PA, Beck MA. The immune response to herpes simplex virus encephalitis in mice is modulated by dietary vitamin E. J Nutr. 2008;138(1):130–7.
327. Hemila H. Vitamin E administration may decrease the incidence of pneumonia in elderly males. Clin Interv Aging. 2016;11:1379–85.
328. Graat JM, Schouten EG, Kok FJ. Effect of daily vitamin E and multivitamin-mineral supplementation on acute respiratory tract infections in elderly persons: a randomized controlled trial. JAMA. 2002;288(6):715–21.
329. Olofin IO, Spiegelman D, Aboud S, Duggan C, Danaei G, Fawzi WW. Supplementation with multivitamins and vitamin a and incidence of malaria among HIV-infected Tanzanian women. J Acquir Immune Defic Syndr. 2014;67(Suppl 4):S173–8.
330. Ferland G. The discovery of vitamin K and its clinical applications. Ann Nutr Metab. 2012;61(3):213–8.
331. Brace L. The pharmacology and therapeutics of vitamin K. Am J Med Technol. 1983;49(6):457–63.
332. Shearer MJ. Vitamin K metabolism and nutriture. Blood Rev. 1992;6(2):92–104.
333. Shearer MJ. Vitamin K in parenteral nutrition. Gastroenterology. 2009;137(5 Suppl):S105–18.
334. Mijares ME, Nagy E, Guerrero B, Arocha-Pinango CL. Vitamin K: biochemistry, function, and deficiency. Review. Investig Clin. 1998;39(3):213–29.

335. Mathers JC, Fernandez F, Hill MJ, McCarthy PT, Shearer MJ, Oxley A. Dietary modification of potential vitamin K supply from enteric bacterial menaquinones in rats. Br J Nutr. 1990;63(3):639–52.

336. Conly JM, Stein K. The production of menaquinones (vitamin K2) by intestinal bacteria and their role in maintaining coagulation homeostasis. Prog Food Nutr Sci. 1992;16(4):307–43.

337. Conly JM, Stein K, Worobetz L, Rutledge-Harding S. The contribution of vitamin K2 (menaquinones) produced by the intestinal microflora to human nutritional requirements for vitamin K. Am J Gastroenterol. 1994;89(6):915–23.

338. Wallin R, Martin LF. Vitamin K-dependent carboxylation and vitamin K metabolism in liver. Effects of warfarin. J Clin Invest. 1985;76(5):1879–84.

339. Corrigan JJ Jr. The vitamin K-dependent proteins. Adv Pediatr. 1981;28:57–74.

340. Reddi K, Henderson B, Meghji S, Wilson M, Poole S, Hopper C, et al. Interleukin 6 production by lipopolysaccharide-stimulated human fibroblasts is potently inhibited by naphthoquinone (vitamin K) compounds. Cytokine. 1995;7(3):287–90.

341. Ohsaki Y, Shirakawa H, Hiwatashi K, Furukawa Y, Mizutani T, Komai M. Vitamin K suppresses lipopolysaccharide-induced inflammation in the rat. Biosci Biotechnol Biochem. 2006;70(4):926–32.

342. Bay A, Oner AF, Celebi V, Uner A. Evaluation of vitamin K deficiency in children with acute and intractable diarrhea. Adv Ther. 2006;23(3):469–74.

343. Peterkofsky B. Ascorbate requirement for hydroxylation and secretion of procollagen: relationship to inhibition of collagen synthesis in scurvy. Am J Clin Nutr. 1991;54(6 Suppl):1135s–40s.

344. Bartholomew M. James Lind's treatise of the scurvy (1753). Postgrad Med J. 2002;78(925):695–6.

345. Pullar JM, Carr AC, Vissers MCM. The roles of vitamin C in skin health. Nutrients. 2017;9(8):866.

346. Banhegyi G, Braun L, Csala M, Puskas F, Mandl J. Ascorbate metabolism and its regulation in animals. Free Radic Biol Med. 1997;23(5):793–803.

347. Englard S, Seifter S. The biochemical functions of ascorbic acid. Annu Rev Nutr. 1986;6:365–406.

348. Tveden-Nyborg P, Johansen LK, Raida Z, Villumsen CK, Larsen JO, Lykkesfeldt J. Vitamin C deficiency in early postnatal life impairs spatial memory and reduces the number of hippocampal neurons in Guinea pigs. Am J Clin Nutr. 2009;90(3):540–6.

349. Sotiriou S, Gispert S, Cheng J, Wang Y, Chen A, Hoogstraten-Miller S, et al. Ascorbic-acid transporter Slc23a1 is essential for vitamin C transport into the brain and for perinatal survival. Nat Med. 2002;8(5):514–7.

350. Garcia-Closas R, Berenguer A, Jose Tormo M, Jose Sanchez M, Quiros JR, Navarro C, et al. Dietary sources of vitamin C, vitamin E and specific carotenoids in Spain. Br J Nutr. 2004;91(6):1005–11.

351. Abdullah M, Jamil RT, Attia FN. Vitamin C (ascorbic acid). StatPearls. Treasure Island: StatPearls Publishing LLC; 2019.

352. Smith JL, Hodges RE. Serum levels of vitamin C in relation to dietary and supplemental intake of vitamin C in smokers and nonsmokers. Ann N Y Acad Sci. 1987;498:144–52.

353. Touvier M, Lioret S, Vanrullen I, Bocle JC, Boutron-Ruault MC, Berta JL, et al. Vitamin and mineral inadequacy in the French population: estimation and application for the optimization of food fortification. Int J Vitam Nutr Res. 2006;76(6):343–51.

354. Desenclos JC, Berry AM, Padt R, Farah B, Segala C, Nabil AM. Epidemiological patterns of scurvy among Ethiopian refugees. Bull World Health Organ. 1989;67(3):309–16.

355. Ververs M, Muriithi JW, Burton A, Burton JW, Lawi AO. Scurvy outbreak among South Sudanese adolescents and Young men – Kakuma Refugee Camp, Kenya, 2017-2018. MMWR Morb Mortal Wkly Rep. 2019;68(3):72–5.

356. Francis J, Rogers K, Brewer P, Dickton D, Pardini R. Comparative analysis of ascorbic acid in human milk and infant formula using varied milk delivery systems. Int Breastfeed J. 2008;3:19.

357. Lindblad M, Tveden-Nyborg P, Lykkesfeldt J. Regulation of vitamin C homeostasis during deficiency. Nutrients. 2013;5(8):2860–79.

358. Jacob RA. Classic human vitamin C depletion experiments: homeostasis and requirement for vitamin C. Nutrition. 1993;9(1):74. 85–6

359. Wagner ES, White W, Jennings M, Bennett K. The entrapment of [14C]ascorbic acid in human erythrocytes. Biochim Biophys Acta. 1987;902(1):133–6.

360. Wilson JX, Dixon SJ. High-affinity sodium-dependent uptake of ascorbic acid by rat osteoblasts. J Membr Biol. 1989;111(1):83–91.

361. Welch RW, Bergsten P, Butler JD, Levine M. Ascorbic acid accumulation and transport in human fibroblasts. Biochem J. 1993;294(Pt 2):505–10.

362. Washko P, Rotrosen D, Levine M. Ascorbic acid transport and accumulation in human neutrophils. J Biol Chem. 1989;264(32):18996–9002.

363. Huijskens MJ, Walczak M, Koller N, Briede JJ, Senden-Gijsbers BL, Schnijderberg MC, et al. Technical advance: ascorbic acid induces development of double-positive T cells from human hematopoietic stem cells in the absence of stromal cells. J Leukoc Biol. 2014;96(6):1165–75.

364. Amakye-Anim J, Lin TL, Hester PY, Thiagarajan D, Watkins BA, Wu CC. Ascorbic acid supplementation improved antibody response to infectious bursal disease vaccination in chickens. Poult Sci. 2000;79(5):680–8.
365. Wu CC, Dorairajan T, Lin TL. Effect of ascorbic acid supplementation on the immune response of chickens vaccinated and challenged with infectious bursal disease virus. Vet Immunol Immunopathol. 2000;74(1–2):145–52.
366. Albers R, Bol M, Bleumink R, Willems AA, Pieters RH. Effects of supplementation with vitamins a, C, and E, selenium, and zinc on immune function in a murine sensitization model. Nutrition. 2003;19(11–12):940–6.
367. Hesta M, Ottermans C, Krammer-Lukas S, Zentek J, Hellweg P, Buyse J, et al. The effect of vitamin C supplementation in healthy dogs on antioxidative capacity and immune parameters. J Anim Physiol Anim Nutr (Berl). 2009;93(1):26–34.
368. Stephensen CB. Primer on immune response and Interface with malnutrition. In: Humphries DL, Scott ME, Vermund SH, editors. Nutrition and infectious disease: shifting the clinical paradigm. New York, NY: Humana Press; 2020.
369. Wilson CW, Loh HS. Common cold and vitamin C. Lancet. 1973;1(7804):638–41.
370. Wilson CW, Loh HS, Foster FG. The beneficial effect of vitamin C on the common cold. Eur J Clin Pharmacol. 1973;6(1):26–32.
371. Anderson TW, Reid DB, Beaton GH. Vitamin C and the common cold: a double-blind trial. Can Med Assoc J. 1972;107(6):503–8.
372. Elwood PC, Lee HP, St Leger AS, Baird M, Howard AN. A randomized controlled trial of vitamin C in the prevention and amelioration of the common cold. Br J Prev Soc Med. 1976;30(3):193–6.
373. Douglas RM, Hemila H, D'Souza R, Chalker EB, Treacy B. Vitamin C for preventing and treating the common cold. Cochrane Database Syst Rev. 2004;(4):Cd000980.
374. Berdanier CD, Berdanier LA. Advanced nutrition: macronutrients, micronutrients, and metabolism. Boca Raton, FL: CRC Press; 2015.
375. Institute of Medicine. Dietary reference intakes for calcium, phosphorus, magnesium, vitamin D, and fluoride. Washington, DC: National Academies Press (US); 1997.
376. Institute of Medicine. Dietary reference intakes for thiamin, riboflavin, niacin, vitamin B6, folate, vitamin B12, pantothenic acid, biotin, and choline. Washington, DC: National Academies Press (US); 1998.
377. Institute of Medicine. Dietary reference intakes for water, potassium, sodium, chloride, and sulfate. Washington, DC: National Academy Press; 2005.
378. Institute of Medicine. Dietary reference intakes for vitamin a, vitamin K, arsenic, boron, chromium, Copper, iodine, Iron, manganese, molybdenum, nickel, silicon, vanadium, and zinc. Washington, DC: The National Academies Press; 2001.
379. Wang Z, Klipfell E, Bennett BJ, Koeth R, Levison BS, Dugar B, et al. Gut flora metabolism of phosphatidylcholine promotes cardiovascular disease. Nature. 2011;472(7341):57–63.
380. Haghighatdoost F, Jabbari M, Hariri M. The effect of L-carnitine on inflammatory mediators: a systematic review and meta-analysis of randomized clinical trials. Eur J Clin Pharmacol. 2019;75(8):1037–46.
381. Maleki SJ, Crespo JF, Cabanillas B. Anti-inflammatory effects of flavonoids. Food Chem. 2019;299:125124.
382. Keller U. Nutritional laboratory markers in malnutrition. J Clin Med. 2019;8(6):775.
383. Gibson R. Principles of nutritional assessment. 2nd ed. Oxford: Oxford University Press; 2005.
384. Harris WS. The Omega-6:Omega-3 ratio: a critical appraisal and possible successor. Prostaglandins Leukot Essent Fatty Acids. 2018;132:34–40.
385. World Health Organization. Serum ferritin concentrations for the assessment of iron status and iron deficiency in populations. World Health Organization; 2011. Source: https://www.who.int/vmnis/indicators/serum_ferritin.pdf; Accessed 01/1/2020.
386. Lian IA, Asberg A. Should total calcium be adjusted for albumin? A retrospective observational study of laboratory data from Central Norway. BMJ Open. 2018;8(4):e017703.
387. King JC, Brown KH, Gibson RS, et al. Biomarkers of Nutrition for Development (BOND)-Zinc Review. J Nutr. 2015;146(4):858S–85S. https://doi.org/10.3945/jn.115.220079.
388. Ristic-Medic D, Piskackova Z, Hooper L, Ruprich J, Casgrain A, Ashton K, et al. Methods of assessment of iodine status in humans: a systematic review. Am J Clin Nutr. 2009;89(6):2052S–69S.
389. Ashton K, Hooper L, Harvey LJ, Hurst R, Casgrain A, Fairweather-Tait SJ. Methods of assessment of selenium status in humans: a systematic review. Am J Clin Nutr. 2009;89(6):2025S–39S.
390. Harvey LJ, Ashton K, Hooper L, Casgrain A, Fairweather-Tait SJ. Methods of assessment of copper status in humans: a systematic review. Am J Clin Nutr. 2009;89(6):2009S–24S.
391. Workinger JL, Doyle RP, Bortz J. Challenges in the diagnosis of magnesium status. Nutrients. 2018;10(9):1202.
392. Tanumihardjo SA. Vitamin A: biomarkers of nutrition for development. Am J Clin Nutr. 2011;94(2):658S–65S.
393. Seamans KM, Cashman KD. Existing and potentially novel functional markers of vitamin D status: a systematic review. Am J Clin Nutr. 2009;89(6):1997S–2008S.
394. Traber MG. Vitamin E inadequacy in humans: causes and consequences. Adv Nutr. 2014;5(5):503–14.

395. Shea MK, Booth SL. Concepts and controversies in evaluating vitamin K status in population-based studies. Nutrients. 2016;8(1):8.
396. Dehghan M, Akhtar-Danesh N, McMillan CR, Thabane L. Is plasma vitamin C an appropriate biomarker of vitamin C intake? A systematic review and meta-analysis. Nutr J. 2007;6:41.
397. Fukuwatari T, Shibata K. Urinary water-soluble vitamins and their metabolite contents as nutritional markers for evaluating vitamin intakes in young Japanese women. J Nutr Sci Vitaminol (Tokyo). 2008;54(3):223–9.
398. Ueland PM, Ulvik A, Rios-Avila L, Midttun O, Gregory JF. Direct and functional biomarkers of vitamin B6 status. Annu Rev Nutr. 2015;35:33–70.
399. Eng WK, Giraud D, Schlegel VL, Wang D, Lee BH, Zempleni J. Identification and assessment of markers of biotin status in healthy adults. Br J Nutr. 2013;110(2):321–9.
400. Shane B. Folate status assessment history: implications for measurement of biomarkers in NHANES. Am J Clin Nutr. 2011;94(1):337S–42S.
401. Hoey L, Strain JJ, McNulty H. Studies of biomarker responses to intervention with vitamin B-12: a systematic review of randomized controlled trials. Am J Clin Nutr. 2009;89(6):1981S–96S.
402. Carmel R. Biomarkers of cobalamin (vitamin B-12) status in the epidemiologic setting: a critical overview of context, applications, and performance characteristics of cobalamin, methylmalonic acid, and holotranscobalamin II. Am J Clin Nutr. 2011;94(1):348S–58S.
403. Trumbo P, Yates AA, Schlicker S, Poos M. Dietary reference intakes: vitamin a, vitamin K, arsenic, boron, chromium, copper, iodine, iron, manganese, molybdenum, nickel, silicon, vanadium, and zinc. J Acad Nutr Diet. 2001;101(3):294.
404. de Andrade JAA, Gayer CRM, Nogueira NPA, Paes MC, Bastos V, Neto J, et al. The effect of thiamine deficiency on inflammation, oxidative stress and cellular migration in an experimental model of sepsis. J Inflamm (Lond). 2014;11:11.
405. Verdrengh M, Tarkowski A. Riboflavin in innate and acquired immune responses. Inflamm Res. 2005;54(9):390–3.
406. Mazur-Bialy AI, Buchala B, Plytycz B. Riboflavin deprivation inhibits macrophage viability and activity – a study on the RAW 264.7 cell line. Br J Nutr. 2013;110(3):509–14.
407. Lipszyc PS, Cremaschi GA, Zorrilla-Zubilete M, Bertolino ML, Capani F, Genaro AM, et al. Niacin modulates pro-inflammatory cytokine secretion. A potential mechanism involved in its anti-atherosclerotic effect. Open Cardiovasc Med J. 2013;7:90–8.
408. Zhou E, Li Y, Yao M, Wei Z, Fu Y, Yang Z. Niacin attenuates the production of pro-inflammatory cytokines in LPS-induced mouse alveolar macrophages by HCA2 dependent mechanisms. Int Immunopharmacol. 2014;23(1):121–6.
409. Lebouche B, Jenabian MA, Singer J, Graziani GM, Engler K, Trottier B, et al. The role of extended-release niacin on immune activation and neurocognition in HIV-infected patients treated with antiretroviral therapy – CTN PT006: study protocol for a randomized controlled trial. Trials. 2014;15:390.
410. He W, Hu S, Du X, Wen Q, Zhong XP, Zhou X, et al. Vitamin B5 reduces bacterial growth via regulating innate immunity and adaptive immunity in mice infected with Mycobacterium tuberculosis. Front Immunol. 2018;9:365.
411. Mikkelsen K, Stojanovska L, Prakash M, Apostolopoulos V. The effects of vitamin B on the immune/cytokine network and their involvement in depression. Maturitas. 2017;96:58–71.
412. Au-Yeung KK, Yip JC, Siow YL, Karmin OK. Folic acid inhibits homocysteine-induced superoxide anion production and nuclear factor kappa B activation in macrophages. Can J Physiol Pharmacol. 2006;84(1):141–7.
413. Kuroishi T, Endo Y, Muramoto K, Sugawara S. Biotin deficiency up-regulates TNF-alpha production in murine macrophages. J Leukoc Biol. 2008;83(4):912–20.
414. Scalabrino G, Corsi MM, Veber D, Buccellato FR, Pravettoni G, Manfridi A, et al. Cobalamin (vitamin B(12)) positively regulates interleukin-6 levels in rat cerebrospinal fluid. J Neuroimmunol. 2002;127(1–2):37–43.

# Chapter 3
# Primer on Immune Response and Interface with Malnutrition

Charles B. Stephensen

## Abbreviations

| | |
|---|---|
| AA | Arachidonic acid |
| APC | Antigen-presenting cell |
| CCL | Ligand for CC family chemokines |
| CCR | Receptor for CC family chemokines |
| CRP | C-reactive protein |
| CTL | Cytotoxic T lymphocyte |
| CXCL | Ligand for CXF family chemokines |
| CXCR | Receptor for CXC family chemokines |
| DHA | Docosahexaenoic acid |
| DTH | Delayed-type hypersensitivity |
| EPA | Eicosapentaenoic acid |
| ICAM | Intercellular adhesion molecule |
| IFN | Interferon |
| Ig | Immunoglobulin |
| IL | Interleukin |
| ILC | Innate-lymphoid cell |
| LPS | Lipopolysaccharide |
| LT | Leukotriene |
| MHC | Major histocompatibility complex |
| NF | Nuclear factor |
| NK | Natural Killer |
| PAMP | Pathogen-associated molecular pattern |
| PEM | Protein-energy malnutrition |
| PG | Prostaglandin |
| pIgR | Polymeric immunoglobulin receptor |
| RBP | Retinol binding protein |
| TCR | T-cell receptor |

C. B. Stephensen (✉)
Immunity and Disease Prevention Research Unit, USDA Western Human Nutrition Research Center, University of California, Davis, CA, USA

Nutrition Department, University of California, Davis, CA, USA
e-mail: charles.stephensen@usda.gov

© Springer Nature Switzerland AG 2021
D. L. Humphries et al. (eds.), *Nutrition and Infectious Diseases*, Nutrition and Health,
https://doi.org/10.1007/978-3-030-56913-6_3

| TGF   | Transforming growth factor |
|-------|----------------------------|
| Th1   | T-helper 1 cell            |
| Th17  | T-helper 17 cell           |
| Th2   | T-helper 2 cell            |
| TLR   | Toll-like receptor         |
| TNF   | Tumor Necrosis Factor      |
| Treg  | Regulatory T cell          |

**Key Points**
- Epithelial surfaces, particularly at mucosal sites, are important first-line defenses against pathogens.
- The innate immune system responds rapidly to infection, differentiates among classes of pathogens, and can clear most microbial challenges.
- The adaptive immune system provides pathogen-specific immunity to protect against pathogens that evade the innate system.
- The innate and adaptive systems provide an integrated defense against specific types of pathogens.
- Infections can cause malnutrition by decreasing food intake, decreasing nutrient absorption, increasing nutrient loss, increasing nutrient metabolism, and altering nutrient transport and storage.
- Deficiencies in protein, energy, and specific nutrients can impair host defenses against infection, thus increasing the risk and severity of infections.

## Overview: Hosts, Pathogens, and Commensals

Immunologists and microbiologists, as well as parasitologists, traditionally use the term "host" to refer to humans or other species at risk of developing an infectious disease, and "pathogen" to refer to bacteria, viruses, fungi, and eukaryotic pathogens such as parasites that cause a clinically evident infection. Pathogens have always been the major focus of immunologists who, throughout the twentieth century, have studied how the immune system clears pathogens to resolve an infection. Pathogens may be viruses, bacteria, fungi (or yeast), protozoa, or multicellular parasites including nematodes and flukes. The disease usually occurs when such organisms are specifically adapted to infect humans, the so-called "professional" pathogens. The names of many of these pathogens are well-known: measles virus, the cholera bacterium (*Vibrio cholerae*), the yeast *Candida albicans*, the malaria protozoa (*Plasmodium falciparum* and others of this genus), the hookworm nematodes (*Necator americanus* and *Ancylostoma duodenale*), and the liver fluke (*Schistosoma mansoni*). Most pathogens have evolved methods of evading the innate immune response and must be cleared by adaptive immunity. Some evade, to varying degrees, adaptive immunity as well (e.g., malaria or the human immunodeficiency virus [HIV]).

However, in addition to the microorganisms that cause disease, there has always been an interest in nonpathogenic "commensal" bacteria that "colonize" rather than infect the host, and this area of research is enjoying a major resurgence because of new DNA sequencing and bioinformatic methods to characterize bacterial (and other) communities of microorganisms [1, 2]. Commensals can be beneficial to the host as long as they stay in their specific niche (e.g., the large intestine, skin, nasopharynx), which is usually a body site that is directly exposed to environmental microorganisms. When nonpathogenic (or mildly pathogenic) bacteria encounter a host with a compromised immune system, these "opportunistic" pathogens can cause frank disease. An emerging concept that focuses on the intestinal microbiome (i.e., the community of bacteria that normally colonizes the host gastrointestinal tract, particularly the large intestine) is that this community may be disrupted, a condition termed "dysbiosis" (as opposed to "symbiosis") [3], and then cause diseases such as environmental enteropathy in young children in settings with poor environmental hygiene [4].

Thus immunologists and microbiologists are now considering not only how the immune system deals with frank pathogens but also how it deals with (and does not over-react to) commensal bacteria. This change in the research focus of immunologists is bringing a greater focus to "regulatory" immunity that refers to how the immune system learns to tolerate rather than expel commensal bacteria. The concepts of protective immunity are better developed, and this chapter focuses necessarily on how the host responds to pathogens of different types but also considers how the host immune system may respond but not overrespond to commensal microorganisms.

## Organization of Host Defenses

### *Barrier Defenses*

Many host tissues are exposed to environmental microorganisms, including the skin, conjunctiva, respiratory tract, gut, and urogenital tracts. While these may be appropriate micro-environments for some commensal bacteria, they are also potential "portals of entry" for pathogens adapted to infect the host and cause disease [5]. Tissues at these portals are specifically adapted to prevent access to other body tissues (blood, lungs, submucosal intestinal tissues) via a layered approach, as shown in Fig. 3.1. First, these sites have a surface layer of epithelial cells interspersed with a few lymphoid or myeloid immune cells. Second, the subepithelial tissue provides structure and contains blood vessels that allow immune cells to enter the epithelium when needed, as well as lymphatic drainage that allows egress of antigen-presenting cells (APCs) to the draining lymph node. This access to the epithelium provides for a rapid response by innate immune cells (discussed below) that forms a second level of protection against invasion. The skin and the intestine provide useful examples.

The skin consists of two cellular layers, epidermis and dermis [6]. The epidermis consists of four layers of keratinocytes interspersed with melanocytes and Langerhans cells, a professional APC, and the principal immune cell of the uninfected epidermis. Some commensal microorganisms adhere to the epithelial surface and are adapted to persist in this niche [7]. Pathogens, including strains of *Staphylococcus aureus*, may penetrate the skin using special virulence factors (e.g., enzymes to break down extracellular matrices) to cause deeper infections which, if the local immune response is not sufficient, may become systemic [5, 8]. The dermis contains blood capillaries and lymphatic drainage as well as a variety of immune cells, the number and type varying depending on the immunologic challenge. Such challenges in the skin may be triggered by insects, parasites (e.g., hookworm larvae from soil or *Schistosoma* cercariae released from the aquatic snail intermediate host), or other irritants (e.g., chemicals, ultraviolet light) to which a person may become sensitized (e.g., poison ivy that elicits an adaptive immune response).

The mucosal epithelium of the intestine consists of a single layer of absorptive epithelial cells interspersed with a variety of other cells, including (a) goblet cells that secrete a protective layer of mucus, (b) M cells that collect particulate antigen from the lumen for delivery to mucosa-associated APC in underlying lymphoid aggregates, (c) interdigitating dendritic cells (a type of APC) that send cytoplasmic arms between epithelial cells to directly sample the antigens present in the gut lumen [9], and (d) Paneth cells in intestinal crypts that secrete antifungal α-defensins and other antimicrobial factors including enzymes and lectins [10]. The lamina propria underlying the gut epithelium contains

**Fig. 3.1** Three examples of barrier defenses, the skin (top), bronchial epithelium in the respiratory tract (middle), and the intestinal epithelium (bottom). (From Janeway's Immunobiology 9E by Kenneth Murphy and Casey Weaver. Copyright © 2017 by Garland Science, Taylor & Francis Group, LLC. Used by permission of W. W. Norton & Company, Inc.)

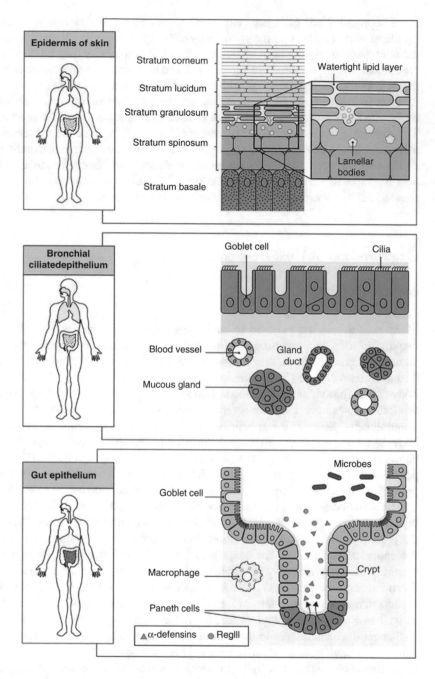

abundant immune cells, particularly macrophages and lymphocytes. Unlike the dermis, there are many lymph nodes in the lamina propria (termed Peyer's patches). A number of factors help protect the epithelial barrier from microorganisms, including peristalsis, the mucus barrier, the relatively rapid turnover of epithelial cells, as well as secreted factors such as immunoglobulin (Ig)A and antimicrobial peptides [11, 12]. IgA and IgM are transported across intestinal epithelial cells and into the gut lumen via the polymeric immunoglobulin receptor (pIgR). In addition to playing a protective role, IgA can also help promote colonization by some commensal bacteria [13]. The extensive network of macrophages and APCs in the lamina propria, in concert with regulatory T (Treg) cells in the lamina propria, helps the body differentiate commensal organisms from pathogens [14].

Other mucosal sites include the mouth, nasopharynx, trachea, esophagus, stomach, and urogenital tracts. These sites have similar organizational features and functions. The lungs present a unique challenge in that alveoli are gas exchange surfaces and due to limits of gas diffusion cannot be organized into multicellular layers. The final line of defense in the lungs is formed by the alveolar macrophages which engulf and clear tiny particles and microorganisms (e.g., *Mycobacterium tuberculosis*).

## Lymphoid Tissues

The immune system in humans and other mammals is made up of primary and secondary organs and tissues located strategically throughout the body to protect against invasion by microorganisms [15], as shown in Fig. 3.2. "Primary" organs, where immune cells develop, include the bone marrow and thymus. All white blood cells (i.e., leukocytes, including lymphocytes, monocytes, and granulocytes which are subdivided into neutrophils, eosinophils, and basophils) originate in the bone marrow, but one subset of lymphocytes, T lymphocytes (also known as "T cells"), needs an additional maturation step in the thymus. In mammals, B lymphocytes (B cells) mature in the bone marrow, but in avian species this step occurs in the bursa of Fabricius. The lymph nodes, spleen, and mucosa-associated lymphoid tissue are "secondary" organs and tissues. These secondary sites are meeting places for immune cells that are connected by the blood and lymphatic systems to allow transmission of information from the innate to the adaptive immune system.

This information transfer occurs when an APC, after an encounter with invading microorganisms, travels via lymphatic vessels from peripheral tissues (e.g., skin, respiratory mucosa, gut) into the closest draining lymph node [15]. As lymph nodes are located regionally along lymphatic vessels, lymphatic vessels drain all tissues of the body; thus this APC-based surveillance system delivers information from any

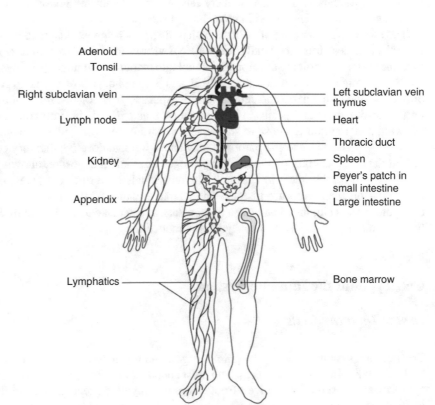

**Fig. 3.2** Organization of primary (shown in yellow) and secondary (shown in blue) lymphoid tissues throughout the body, including the lymphatic draining system. (From Janeway's Immunobiology 9E by Kenneth Murphy and Casey Weaver. Copyright © 2017 by Garland Science, Taylor & Francis Group, LLC. Used by permission of W. W. Norton & Company, Inc.)

site of infection to a regional lymph node. "APC" is a functional definition, and antigen presentation can be made by several cell types, including dendritic cells, macrophages, and B cells (in special cases of soluble antigen that can be internalized via the immunoglobulin on the surface of a B cell). The spleen, like the lymph nodes, provides a site for APCs to transfer information to lymphocytes. The spleen also filters the blood. In the case of a breach of peripheral defenses, blood-borne microorganisms or infected erythrocytes (e.g., in the case of malaria) are removed from the blood by phagocytic cells in the spleen.

## Innate and Adaptive Immunity

The immune system has two components, "innate" and "adaptive" [15], though the two work together as an integrated whole. The cellular constituents of these systems, and their developmental stages, are shown in Fig. 3.3. The innate system is evolutionarily older, and it is fully functional at birth. Innate immune cells (including granulocytes, macrophages, and innate lymphoid cells) use a diverse group of cell-surface or intracellular receptors (e.g., toll-like receptors [TLR]) to recognize molecules containing specific motifs, known as pathogen-associated molecular patterns (PAMP). The TLRs are a well-studied class of receptors, recognizing PAMPs from different classes of bacteria (e.g., flagella), yeast (e.g., cell wall carbohydrate), and viruses (e.g., RNA) [16]. For example, bacterial lipopolysaccharide (LPS) is recognized by TLR4, bacterial flagellin by TLR5, single-stranded RNA (in the cytoplasm of a host cell) by TLR7, and repeated DNA sequences of the bases C and G (common in bacterial but not mammalian genomes) by TLR9. Other receptors perform similar functions. For example, proteins with a nucleotide-binding domain and leucine-rich repeats also recognize PAMPs [17]. These receptors are part of a multi-protein complex in the cytoplasm termed an "inflammasome" that results in cleavage of pro-interleukin (IL)-1β and pro-IL-18 to produce the active cytokines. This pathway can also be activated by nonmicrobial tissue "irritants" such as uric acid crystals, which accumulate in tissues of patients with gout, and the adjuvant alum, which is used in many human vaccines.

The adaptive immune system differs in that the host's response adapts to a specific pathogen (e.g., the RNA measles virus specifically and not RNA viruses in general as would happen within the innate immune system) in order to develop "immunologic memory." Immunologic memory is initiated when the innate immune system interacts with B and T lymphocytes of the adaptive immune system to develop antibody-mediated and cell-mediated responses to pathogens. Immunologic memory depends on the development and persistence of memory T and B cells in lymphoid and other tissues, thus allowing a more rapid response to subsequent exposures to a particular pathogen. While the primary adaptive response to a specific pathogen may take a week to develop, memory cells may then be resident at the portal of entry of a particular pathogen after initial exposure, allowing a nearly immediate response to the subsequent infection. Thus, individuals have different levels of adaptive immunity depending on their exposure history. The adaptive nature of this response explains why the first encounter with a childhood pathogen (e.g., measles) can make a child quite ill, but subsequent infections are rapidly controlled and likely to go unnoticed.

## Cell Types in the Immune System

### Innate Immune Cells

The immune system has many specific lineages, and much new information has been gleaned about these cell types in recent years [15]. The most abundant innate immune cells seen in peripheral blood are of myeloid origin (i.e., derived from a common myeloid precursor cell in the bone marrow) and include monocytes and granulocytes.

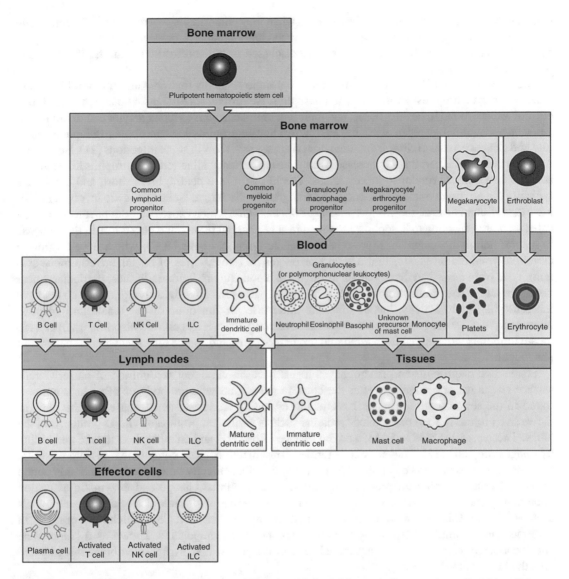

**Fig. 3.3** Lineage of innate immune cells (neutrophil, eosinophil, basophil, mast cell, macrophage, dendritic cell, innate lymphoid cell [ILC], NK cell), adaptive (lymphoid) immune cells (T cell and B cell), platelets, and erythrocytes. (From Janeway's Immunobiology 9E by Kenneth Murphy and Casey Weaver. Copyright © 2017 by Garland Science, Taylor & Francis Group, LLC. Used by permission of W. W. Norton & Company, Inc.)

Monocytes, a homogeneous cell type, exit the bone marrow, circulate in the blood, and differentiate into macrophages following extravasation [18]. Macrophages ingest invading microorganisms into a phagocytic vesicle, the phagosome, using several cell-surface receptors. The phagosome fuses with lysosomes containing antibacterial peptides and enzymes (e.g., lysozyme). Following fusion, a respiratory burst involving NADPH oxidase acidifies the phagolysosome and injects reactive oxygen species which kill ingested microorganisms. While blood-derived monocytes are a major source of tissue macrophages during inflammation, some lineages of tissue-resident macrophages are seeded into tissues before birth, persist through longevity and division, and contribute to tissue-specific defenses as well as repair and homeostasis [19]. Macrophages play a prominent role in responses to intracellular pathogens such as viruses and *M. tuberculosis*. Their cellular transcription machinery allows them to regenerate phagosomes and live for months or even years. Immature dendritic cells, also of myeloid origin, originate in the bone marrow and mature when they enter tissue, where they reside until being stimulated by microorganisms to carry out their principal function of presenting antigen to lymphocytes. Alternatively activated macrophages are discussed in the context of helminth infections and nutrition in Chap. 12 [20].

Granulocytes, named for their prominent cytoplasmic granules that contain antimicrobial molecules, include neutrophils, eosinophils, and basophils. Neutrophils are the most abundant white blood cell but are not found in healthy tissue, and their predominant role is as a phagocytic cell to kill pathogenic bacteria, although recent work has also shown that neutrophils can contribute to adaptive immunity and can have a role in chronic inflammatory diseases as well as in acute infections [21]. Neutrophil numbers at sites of inflammation increase rapidly during bacterial infections. Neutrophils kill engulfed bacteria in a manner similar to macrophages. The life span of a neutrophil is short, and these cells typically die after one round of phagocytosis and granule discharge. Neutrophils are involved in killing extracellular bacteria, such as *Streptococcus pneumoniae*, which cause bacterial pneumonia. Mast cells, similar in function to basophils, are found in subepithelial tissues and play a role in the response to enteric helminth infections. More recently, innate lymphoid cells (ILC), which develop from a common lymphoid progenitor in the bone marrow (as do lymphocytes of the adaptive immune system), have been described that circulate through the blood and are found in tissues, particularly near portals of entry. The primary role of ILCs is not to kill pathogens directly, as lymphocytes do not have inherent phagocytic activity, but to stimulate other effector functions of the innate and adaptive immune system by the production of cytokines. Natural Killer (NK) cells are also important cells in innate immunity, are derived from lymphoid progenitor cells, and can be directly cytocidal but are not phagocytic.

Phagocytic neutrophils and macrophages ingest bacteria via direct recognition of bacterial cell-surface structures or recognition after the bacteria are coated with antibody or other host proteins found in the serum (e.g., lectins such as mannose-binding lectin and acute phase proteins such as C-reactive protein [CRP]) or secretory proteins such as surfactant proteins A and D produced in the lungs. These proteins bind to PAMPs on the surface of bacteria and enhance their uptake and killing by phagocytic cells [22]. This activity is termed "opsonization." The complement system of serum proteins opsonizes bacteria by binding to the bacterial surface directly or to a lectin or antibody bound to the bacteria. Complement proteins undergo a conformational change and enzymatic activation upon binding, and a cascade of such events leads to the formation of biologically active components such as C3a and C5a, which are chemo-attractants for phagocytes, and C3b, which is an opsonin. In addition, the accumulation of several terminal complement components, known as a "membrane attack complex," on the surface of a bacterial cell forms a pore which disrupts membrane integrity and kills the bacteria [15].

## *Lymphocytes and Antigen Specificity in the Adaptive Immune System*

Lymphocytes are the single-cell type of the adaptive immune system, and they produce highly specialized molecules that recognize specific antigens, usually of microbial origin. (In the case of autoimmunity, these molecules may recognize host antigens, causing diseases like type 1 diabetes.) Antigens are generally macromolecules containing one or a few antigenic epitopes, the specific molecular structure recognized during an adaptive immune response. Epitopes are typically subregions of macromolecules such as short sequences of amino acids from a microbial protein or a sequence of monosaccharides on a bacterial polysaccharide. The ability of lymphocytes to recognize the epitopes of antigenic molecules allows the adaptive immune system to identify and target specific microorganisms (e.g., cholera bacteria) or even specific variants of a particular pathogen (e.g., this season's strain of influenza virus). There are two main types of lymphocytes, B and T lymphocytes. The antigen-specificity of B cells is conferred by the production of immunoglobulin (Ig) and of T cells by expression of the T-cell receptor (TCR). While Ig can recognize both peptide and carbohydrate epitopes, the TCR primarily recognizes peptide epitopes. At birth, an infant's B and T cells are naïve to exposure to specific antigens (in utero exposure can induce a memory response in the fetus, however). Naïve B cells develop into antibody-producing plasma cells (as well as memory B cells) during an adaptive immune response. T cells have diverse functions, as they can provide "help" in the development of an adaptive immune response or provide direct, "effector" activity, such as cell-mediated cytotoxicity to eliminate, for example, virus-infected host cells. These roles will be discussed below.

## Adaptive Immune Cells: B Cells

Naïve B cells bear surface immunoglobulin with specificity for a single, unique epitope. Once stimulated, naïve B cells proliferate dramatically and differentiate into both antibody-producing plasma cells and memory B cells. Thus a key element of adaptive immunity is the amplification of a few naïve B cells which recognize one or a few specific epitopes on a microbial pathogen to produce several lineages of highly abundant effector cells (i.e., the plasma cells secreting antibody) and memory cells. The antibody produced by the plasma cells provides protection against pathogens while the longevity of the memory B cells produces immunologic memory to a specific pathogen that allows a more rapid response upon subsequent exposure to the same (or a closely related) pathogen. Plasma cells primarily reside either in the bone marrow, where they secrete antibody that is found in the blood plasma or at sub-mucosal sites, where they secrete antibody specific for mucosal-associated pathogens or commensals. Plasma cells are particularly abundant in the intestine but are also found in the respiratory and urogenital mucosal tissues. Ig molecules have a Y-like molecular structure consisting of two identical heavy (H) and two identical light (L) polypeptide chains. The C-terminus, at the base of the Y, consists of the two heavy chains and denotes the constant (C) region. The two variable (V) regions, forming the two arms above the N-terminal fork of the Y structure, are composed of one heavy and one light chain each. The identical variable regions, at each tip of the Y, are responsible for binding to specific antigens. The diversity of these regions, with regard to recognizing foreign antigens, is driven by somatic (not germline) rearrangement of Ig gene segments, resulting in a highly diverse repertoire of antibody binding capacities.

There are four classes of antibody that play significant roles in response to infections: IgM, IgG, IgA, and IgE. A mature antibody response usually consists of IgG (the primary plasma Ig) and may also include IgE or IgA. IgM is produced early in an immune response, but then wanes, and exists as a pentamer of Ig units held together by a J chain peptide. IgA can form either a monomer or dimer joined by the J chain. Plasma cells at mucosal sites primarily secrete dimeric IgA. Antibodies can bind directly to a soluble antigen (e.g., to "neutralize" bacterial toxins) and to surfaces of microorganisms (as opsonins, to aggregate the microorganisms and to "neutralize" the ability of viruses to enter host cells) via the two antigen-binding sites on each molecule.

## Adaptive Immune Cells: T Cells

T cells are typically divided into two types based on the two surface markers, CD4 and CD8. CD4 T cells provide a variety of effector functions, including "help" in the development of a variety of adaptive immune responses, as discussed below. The primary effector role of CD8 T cells is as a cytotoxic T cell, which kills host cells infected with intracellular pathogens, particularly viruses. Both CD4 and CD8 T cells also develop into memory cells that reside in lymph nodes to provide a more rapid response to subsequent pathogen exposures. As with naïve B cells, naïve CD4 or CD8 T cells proliferate and differentiate into abundant effector and memory T cells, all recognizing the same antigenic epitope (within a lineage derived from a single naïve T cell) via their cell-surface TCR. The TCRs of CD4 and CD8 T cells recognize different epitopes. For example, a viral protein might contain two distinct TCR epitopes, one recognized by a CD4 T cell and the other by a CD8 T cell. CD4 and CD8 T cells have different functions. CD4 T cells are known as T-helper (Th) cells because of their role in helping elicit adaptive immune responses, including the development of CD8 cytotoxic T cells as well as memory B cells and plasma cells. There are currently three widely acknowledged types of effector/memory Th cells, Th1, Th2, and Th17, as shown in Fig. 3.4. These three cell types represent key components of what immunologists now refer to as type 1, type 2, and type 3 immunity, as will be discussed below. Also, among CD4 T cells, there are T-regulatory (Treg) cells and a subset of memory T-helper cells that help elicit antibody responses which are known as T-follicular-helper (Tfh) cells, because of their localization near the B-cell follicles of lymph nodes where they interact with developing memory B cells to promote antibody responses. The majority of T cells express TCRs composed of α and β chains which recognize peptide antigens of nonhost molecules. Diversity in recognition of these foreign antigens is again driven by recombination of TCR gene subregion and somatic mutation, as was the case with the generation of antibody diversity.

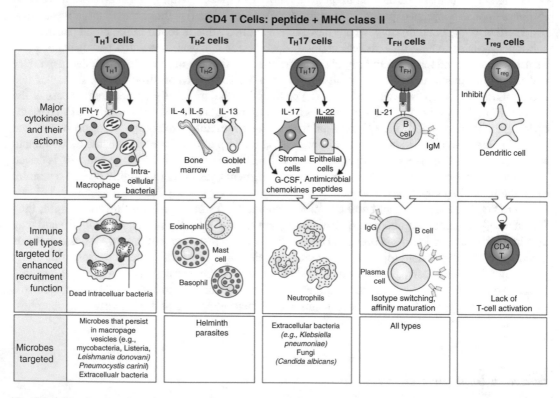

**Fig. 3.4** Major functional groups and activities of memory CD4 T cells which develop after appropriate stimulation (see Fig. 3.5) with antigenic peptide presented via major histocompatibility complex (MHC) class II molecules on the surface of dendritic cells. (From Janeway's Immunobiology 9E by Kenneth Murphy and Casey Weaver. Copyright © 2017 by Garland Science, Taylor & Francis Group, LLC. Used by permission of W. W. Norton & Company, Inc.)

# Functions of the Immune System: Innate Immunity and Inflammation

## *Local Inflammation*

As pathogens disrupt and pass beyond initial barrier defenses, the PAMPs that they carry will stimulate local epithelial cells and immune cells – usually macrophages or dendritic cells – in the tissues underlying the barrier epithelium, to initiate a local inflammatory response. Stimulation of these pattern recognition receptors, such as TLRs, initiates cellular responses including transcription of cytokines, which signal other cells, and chemokines, which can attract more immune cells to this initial site of infection. To give one example, the transcription of many pro-inflammatory cytokines and chemokine genes is regulated by the transcription factor, nuclear factor (NF)-κB [23]. Genes induced by this pathway include genes for the cytokines tumor necrosis factor (TNF)-α and IL-6, as well as genes for two enzymes, cyclooxygenase-2 and 5-lipoxygenase, that produce lipid mediators of infection, including prostaglandin (PG) E2 and leukotriene (LT) B4, respectively. Keratinocytes in the skin express TLRs that are activated during infections causing the production of chemokines that attract T cells (e.g., CCL20 and CXCL9, 10, and 11) and neutrophils (CXCL1 and 8) [6] and cationic antimicrobial peptides such as cathelicidin and β-defensin [24] that mediate killing of invading bacteria and thus protect epithelial surfaces from infection.

The innate immune response can also protect against viral infections. Viral replication in most cells induces transcription of the cytokines interferon (IFN)-α and IFN-β following recognition of double-stranded RNA by TLR3 or other "sensors" such as retinoic acid-inducible gene-1 [25]. These interferons bind to cell-surface receptors on the same and adjacent cells and induce protective factors that degrade viral RNA or otherwise interfere with viral replication. IFN-α and IFN-β also activate NK cells to kill target cells.

These initial responses to infection trigger a local inflammatory response involving cells already at the site and cells recruited to the site by soluble mediators [5, 15]. Many tissues contain resident macrophages that also respond to infection by producing chemokines (CXCL8), cytokines (including IL-12, IL-1β, TNF-α, and IL-6), leukotrienes (including LTB4 and LTE4), prostaglandins (including PGE2), and platelet-activating factor that mediate inflammation. The goal of this inflammation is to eliminate the pathogen or to minimize the spread of the pathogen until adaptive immunity can produce a pathogen-specific response. The key events in inflammation include (a) release of preformed mediators and rapid enzymatic production of mediators followed by transcription and translation of chemokine and cytokine genes; (b) induction of cell adhesion molecules (e.g., intercellular adhesion molecule (ICAM)-1) in the vascular endothelium in adjacent capillaries, which slows the progress of leukocytes; (c) loosening of tight junctions between epithelial cells to allow egress of leukocytes along a chemokine gradient; (d) stimulation of blood clotting by activation of platelets to minimize "escape" of pathogens; and (e) killing of microorganisms or infected cells by the leukocytes attracted to the site. Later, (f) a recovery phase stimulates the repair of damage caused by pathogens or the responding leukocytes.

Innate immune cells such as macrophages, because of their location in tissues throughout the body, are often the first cell to sense the presence of a pathogen via its surface receptors. Epithelial cells at mucosal surfaces can also play a similar role. As mentioned above, different pathogens can elicit different patterns of cytokines from these sensor cells, and these cytokines can elicit different types of immunity directed at particular classes of pathogens, as discussed below. For example, intracellular bacteria and viruses may stimulate dendritic cells and macrophages to produce IL-12, which will stimulate ILC1 and NK cells to produce the effector cytokine IFN-γ which can augment the ability of macrophages to kill intracellular bacteria. NK cells can also kill stressed host cells, which can occur as a result of intracellular infection. Intestinal helminth infections stimulate intestinal epithelial cells

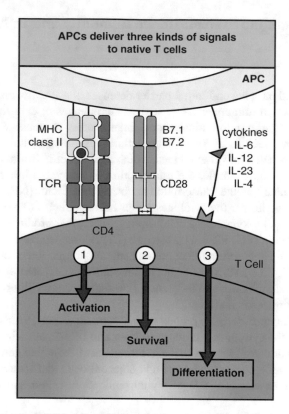

**Fig. 3.5** Antigen-presenting cells (APCs) deliver three signals to naïve T cells to cause activation and allow proliferation and survival and differentiation into memory T cells (which are shown in Fig. 3.5). Step 1, activation, involves antigen-presentation by major histocompatibility (MHC) class II molecules on the surface of an antigen-presenting cell (APC) to a naïve T cell. Step 2, survival, involves the interaction of costimulatory molecules (B7.1 or B7.2) from the APC with CD28 on the T cell. Signal 3, provided by cytokines produced by APC, causes differentiation of naïve T cells into memory T cells with different effector functions. (From Janeway's Immunobiology 9E by Kenneth Murphy and Casey Weaver. Copyright © 2017 by Garland Science, Taylor & Francis Group, LLC. Used by permission of W. W. Norton & Company, Inc.)

to produce cytokines that activate ILC2 cells to produce IL-13, which can enhance mucus production by the intestine to help clear helminths, and IL-5, which attracts eosinophils that are also active in anti-helminth responses. A third example is extracellular bacteria that activate macrophages or dendritic cells may stimulate ILC3 cells to produce IL-17, which attracts neutrophils, and IL-22, which can stimulate the production of antibacterial peptides by epithelial and other cells at a site of infection. These three examples are examples of type 1, type 2, and type 3 immunity, respectively (Table 3.1). Adaptive immune responses with similar effector mechanisms to deal with pathogens (described below) are elicited when this innate response does not clear an infection on its own.

## Systemic Inflammation and the Acute-Phase Response

When production of TNFα, IL-1β, and IL-6 at a site of inflammation is high, serum levels of these cytokines increase, and systemic effects are triggered. These include fever, malaise, muscle aches, and decreased appetite. Fever is induced by PGE2 acting on the hypothalamus. One early name for TNFα was "cachexin" because it decreases appetite, an effect also mediated through the central nervous system. These cytokines also act on hepatocytes to increase the synthesis of positive acute-phase proteins,

**Table 3.1** Typical components of the three types of protective immune responses to pathogens and of inducible Treg (iTreg) cells

| Components | Type 1 | Type 2 | Type 3 | Regulatory |
|---|---|---|---|---|
| Type of pathogens targeted | Viruses, intracellular bacteria | Helminths | Extracellular bacteria | All |
| Innate lymphoid cells (ILC) and their effector cytokines | NK cell, ILC1 IFN-$\gamma$ | ILC2 IL-5, IL-13 | ILC3 IL-17, IL-22 | (Uncertain) |
| Cytokines causing T-helper cell differentiation | IFN-$\gamma$, IL-12 | IL-4 | TGF-$\beta$, IL-6, IL-23 | IL-2, TGF-$\beta$ |
| Adaptive immune cells: T-helper (Th) and cytotoxic T lymphocytes (CTL) and their effector cytokines | Th1 CTL IFN-$\gamma$ | Th2 IL-4, IL-5, IL-13 | Th17 IL-17, IL-22 | iTreg IL-10, TGF-$\beta$ |
| Innate myeloid cells | Macrophage | Eosinophil Basophil Mast cell | Neutrophil | Macrophages may produce IL-10 |
| Antibody response produced by B lymphocytes | IgG, IgA | IgE | IgG, IgA | (No usual, specific role) |
| Role in chronic diseases | Autoimmunity, cardiovascular | Allergy, asthma | Autoimmunity, inflammatory bowel diseases | Dampens chronic responses |

including ferritin, CRP, and mannose-binding lectin, and decrease the synthesis of negative acute-phase proteins, including albumin and retinol-binding protein (RBP), the serum transport protein for vitamin A. The positive acute-phase proteins typically have a protective role in the innate immune response. They increase within a few hours and reach a peak at 10- to >100-fold their initial concentrations within a few days. CRP, for example, increases from about 1 mg/L to >100 mg/L during bacterial pneumonia and binds to cell wall polysaccharides, acting as an opsonin. The reason for decreased levels of negative acute-phase proteins, which may drop by 25–50%, is not clear but may represent a shift of resources to the synthesis of the positive acute-phase proteins. Serum iron, which is bound to the transport protein transferrin, also decreases during the acute phase response as a result of increased hepcidin synthesis [26] (see Chap. 2). Hepcidin blocks normal recycling of transferrin-bound iron through macrophages resulting in increased intracellular and decreased serum iron levels [27]. Increased ferritin synthesis may facilitate intracellular iron storage. This sequestration of iron decreases its availability to opportunistic pathogens. Chronic inflammation may result in the "anemia of chronic disease" by decreasing the availability of iron for erythropoiesis. Serum zinc levels also decrease during the acute phase response to inhibit bacterial zinc acquisition. Macronutrient metabolism is also altered during the acute phase response with elevated levels of serum triglycerides, decreased $\beta$-oxidation of fatty acids, and increased gluconeogenesis. Neutrophils are also mobilized from the bone marrow to increase availability at sites of inflammation, and TNF-$\alpha$ stimulates activation of APC and their migration to lymph nodes.

## Functions of the Immune System: Integration of Innate with Adaptive Immunity

### Antigen-Presenting Cells (APC) Link Innate to Adaptive Immunity

The mission of the APC is to stimulate an adaptive immune response by transferring information about a specific microorganism from the site of infection to the draining lymph node for presentation to T cells [15]. At least three types of "information" are transferred. Figure 3.5 shows the steps in the activation of a naïve T cell.

*First*, unique peptides from microbial protein antigens are displayed on the APC surface by major histocompatibility complex (MHC) molecules for "presentation" to naïve T cells (for recognition via their TCR) in the draining lymph node. This presentation causes the T cell to enter the cell cycle and begin cell division.

*Second*, following antigen-specific stimulation via the TCR, a co-stimulatory signal is required for the naïve T cell to progress through the cell cycle and allow proliferation and survival of daughter cells. Co-stimulatory molecules on the activated APC (e.g., B7-1 and B7-2 molecules, also known as CD80 and CD86) bind to cell-surface receptors on the T cell (e.g., CD28) which enhance cell survival (e.g., by stimulating IL-2 production, an autocrine growth signal for T cells). Such co-stimulation is required for effective development of effector and memory T cells.

*Third*, a differentiation signal is required to steer development of CD4 T cells toward their specific effector/memory phenotype (i.e., Th1, Th2 or Th17) or toward Treg development. This differentiation signal is the keystone of development of the three types of immunity within the adaptive immune system (Table 3.1). This information is provided by cytokines produced by APCs (or other cells in the local environment). IL-12 is the key differentiating cytokine for Th1 cells and type 1 immunity and IL-4 for Th2 cells and type 2 immunity, and three cytokines – TGF-β, IL-6, and IL-23 – initiate development of Th17 cells (so-called because they produce IL-17), a component of type 3 immunity. Specific cytokines steer differentiation toward specific lineages, as discussed below. Treg cell development will be discussed later, and Tfh development occurs in parallel with the Th1, Th2, and Th17 lineages as all of these types of immunity involve antibody production.

## Types of Immunity

During the 1980s, it became clear that different types of pathogens (e.g., viruses, bacteria, helminths) elicited distinct types of responses that integrated components of innate and adaptive immunity into a coordinated response against different types of pathogens. Currently, three main types of immunity (Table 3.1) are widely recognized by immunologists: Type 1 immunity is triggered by viruses and intracellular pathogens, type 2 immunity by helminthic infections, and type 3 by extracellular bacteria and fungi [15]. These types of immunity have both innate components, as discussed above, and adaptive components, which employ similar effector mechanisms. The difference between the two, of course, is the adaptive responses are antigen-specific, while the innate responses rely solely on recognition of classes of pathogens via PAMPS. Each of these types of immunity can also be involved in pathologic responses (Table 3.1). These three types of protective responses have common features that will be described in more detail.

## Type 1 Immunity

Type 1 immunity is directed against viruses and other intracellular pathogens. As discussed above, macrophages and dendritic cells produce IL-12 after exposure to such pathogens, and other innate immune cells, ILC1 and NK cells, respond to this stimulus by producing effector cytokines, particularly IFN-γ. NK cells also target and kill stressed (infected) host cells as part of this response. Activated dendritic cells migrate from the site of infection to a draining lymph node where they present pathogen-specific antigen to naïve CD4 T cells. These cells respond by proliferating, and the IL-12 produced by such dendritic cells stimulates a differentiation program that results in development of an effector and memory Th1 phenotype. The key effector cytokine produced by Th1 cells is IFN-γ, and this cytokine also helps drive naïve T cells toward Th1 development. Effector Th1 cells will leave the draining lymph node within days and be attracted to the site of infection that elicited this response, such as the lung in the case of *M. tuberculosis* infection. At the site of infection, the production of IFN-γ will enhance the antibacterial activity of macrophages, playing a role similar to ILC1 cells. In addition, direct cell-to-cell interactions between Th1 cells and macrophages can deliver survival signals to the macrophage to augment the ability of these macrophages to fight infection. Naïve CD8 T cells can also be stimulated by IL-12-producing dendritic cells during such a response to develop into cytotoxic T lymphocytes (CTLs). Memory Th1 and CTL cells can persist for years and may result in decades-long immunity to pathogens such as measles virus and yellow fever virus. Tfh cells also help elicit development of memory B cells during a type 1 response, resulting in the development of antibody-producing plasma cells that often produce opsonizing and virus-neutralizing IgG to help clear viral infections.

CTLs are the principal type of adaptive immune cells that mediate the killing of host cells infected with viruses (e.g., influenza, hepatitis B, and herpes simplex) and intracellular bacteria (e.g., *M. tuberculosis* and *Salmonella typhimurium*) [28]. CTLs also respond to intracellular protozoan infections caused by *Plasmodium* sp. (malaria), *Toxoplasma gondii* (toxoplasmosis), and *Trypanosoma cruzi* (Chagas disease). CTL kill infected cells (after antigen-specific recognition of the infected cell via the CTL's T-cell receptor for a specific antigen) by the CD95 and perforin/granzyme-mediated lytic pathways [29, 30]. NK cells also kill cells by these mechanisms, but NK recognition is not antigen-specific, relying on the expression of cell-surface markers of infection or stress. Thus NK cells of the innate immune system perform a similar role to CTL of the adaptive immune system. These cytotoxic responses are unique to type 1 immunity. Type 1 immunity can be activated by autoimmune responses and may also be activated during noninfectious damage to tissues, which happens during the development of plaque in coronary arteries, for example, where classically activated macrophages play a role in pathogenesis.

## Type 2 Immunity

Type 2 immunity develops in response to helminthic infections (as well as other antigens such as insect venoms and allergens associated with allergic rhinitis), and the effector mechanisms that develop involve defenses at mucosal, epithelial barriers. These type 2 responses are elicited by the key effector cytokines, including IL-5 and IL-13, and include goblet cell development and resulting mucus accumulation at epithelial surfaces, smooth muscle contractility (e.g., to help eliminate intestinal helminths via enhanced peristalsis), as well as eosinophil and mast cell recruitment to the site of infection where degranulation of eosinophils can kill tissue parasites [31]. IgE antibody also typically develops as part of a type 2 response. IgE can bind via its C-terminus to receptors on the surface of eosinophils, basophils, and mast cells, allowing these cells to be stimulated in an antigen-specific manner. The key differentiating cytokine that drives Th2 development is IL-4. IL-4 is produced by eosinophils, basophils, and mast cells when activated by chitin, a polysaccharide from helminthic parasites (such as the intestinal roundworm *Ascaris lumbricoides* and the hookworms *A. duodenale* and *N. americanus*), as well as from insects and crustaceans. Thus for the development of Th2 cells from naïve T cells, the antigenic stimulus is provided by dendritic cells arriving from the site of infection, but the differentiating signal, IL-4, may come from another cell source within or migrating to the lymph node. Developing Th2 cells also produce IL-4 which helps drive differentiation via autocrine activity.

## Type 3 Immunity

ILC3 cells are found at submucosal sites, and Th17 cells are also commonly elicited by mucosal and skin infections. These type 3 immune cells facilitate responses to a diverse group of extracellular pathogens, including *Klebsiella pneumoniae, Staphylococcus aureus*, and *Candida albicans* [32]. Enteric pathogens, including segmented filamentous bacteria and *Citrobacter rodentium* in mice, elicit strong Th17 responses indicating a role for these cells in enteric infections [33]. Th17 cells are the key memory CD4 T cell involved in type 3 immunity. Their development is stimulated by the cytokines IL-6, IL-23, and transforming growth factor (TGF)-β [34]. TGF-β is constitutively produced at mucosal sites (and is responsible for the development of Treg cells, as discussed below), while IL-6 and IL-23 are elicited during bacterial infections, commonly by macrophages and dendritic cells. The principal effector cytokine produced by ILC3 and Th17 cells is IL-17, which can stimulate epithelial and stromal cells to produce antimicrobial peptides that are effective against extracellular bacteria and chemotactic factors for neutrophils, which are typically recruited to sites of bacterial infection. Th17 cells may be active against nonpathogenic bacteria or opportunistic pathogens under certain circumstances and may thus contribute to chronic inflammation in the gut which may lead to diseases such as irritable bowel disease and, perhaps, to colon cancer [33, 35]. Th17 cells may also play a role in autoimmune disease, perhaps including systemic lupus erythematosus, psoriasis, and rheumatoid arthritis [33].

## Regulatory Immunity

Treg cells play a critical role in the induction of self-tolerance and, thereby, significantly contribute to resistance to autoimmunity [36]. Treg cells are largely CD4+ although CD8+ Treg cells exist and have not yet been extensively characterized [36, 37]. Natural Treg (nTreg) cells develop in the thymus and can dampen responses to self-antigen, while induced Treg (iTreg) cells develop in peripheral lymphoid tissue, including in the intestinal lymphoid tissue. Their differentiation is driven by exposure to TGF-β, retinoic acid, and IL-2 after exposure of a naïve T cell to an antigen. In the intestinal lymphoid tissue, there is a balance between Th17 and Treg development. Both cell types require TGF-β for development. iTreg cells predominate in the absence of inflammation, while Th17 cells develop when IL-6 and IL-23 are produced as a result of local inflammation. iTreg cells play a role in immune homeostasis by suppressing excessive immune responses that may develop in response to infection and may thus be damaging to the host. iTreg cells may also develop with specificity for food antigens or commensal bacteria. Since these responses typically develop in the absence of inflammation, these iTreg cells predominate (and Th17 cells do not develop) and promote tolerance rather than inflammation in response to such antigens. Treg cells comprise 5–10% of peripheral blood CD4 T cells and are characterized and identified by the expression of the signature transcription factor forkhead box P3 (FoxP3) and the surface marker CD25 which is the α chain of the IL-2 receptor. Treg cells have specificity for antigen via a TCR, like other T cells, but the cytokines they produce are typically IL-10 and TGF-β, which downregulate the activity and proliferation of Th1 and Th2 cells and can also dampen production of cytokines by dendritic cells, which may affect the development of Th1, Th2, or Th17 cells. Treg cells also show contact inhibition of CD4 T-cell activation. Thus Treg cells dampen inflammatory responses mediated by Th1, TH2, and Th17 cells and play a role in regulating the extent of immune responses to pathogens or in situations of autoimmunity [38].

# Nutrition-Infection Interactions: Infections Cause Malnutrition

The investment of nutrients into an immune response is of substantial benefit to the host, as the host may die without such a protective response. This survival does come at some nutritional cost, however, and that cost is the topic of this section. The immune response to infection uses nutrients, and this response, via induction of the acute phase response, also makes the host feel ill. Both the immune response and the resulting illness can affect nutritional status via a variety of mechanisms that are reviewed below.

## *Frequency and Severity of Infections*

Common childhood infections increase the risk of malnutrition in children. Lower respiratory tract infections such as pneumonia have a pronounced effect on nutritional status because such severe infections can be clinically severe and substantially decrease food intake, while less severe but more common infections (e.g., mild diarrhea) may also adversely affect infant growth because of their frequency [39]. Opportunistic enteric pathogens or "environmental enteropathy" affecting the intestinal microbiome (and causing immune activation) can also contribute to the development of malnutrition, as evidenced by the negative association of this condition with infant growth [4, 40]. Relatively few studies demonstrate effects of infection on the risk of specific nutritional deficiencies. However, an observational study in Indonesia demonstrated an association between respiratory infections and diarrhea with increased risk for xerophthalmia, the principal clinical manifestation of vitamin A deficiency [41]. In addition, common infections (e.g., chickenpox) have been implicated in the depletion of liver stores or failure of vitamin A intake to maintain liver stores [42].

## *Decreased Food Intake*

Infections increase the risk of malnutrition by a variety of mechanisms that were originally described for vitamin $B_{12}$ [43] and have been reviewed for vitamin A [44]. These mechanisms include decreased food intake, impaired nutrient absorption, direct nutrient loss, increased metabolic requirements, or catabolic losses and altered transport or storage. Acute infections during childhood decrease food intake, the magnitude of the decrease being proportional to illness severity. For example, in community-based studies, the occurrence of acute respiratory infections in children decreased caloric intake by 8% relative to periods when children were asymptomatic [45]. Decreases were 11% for malaria [46] and 18% for diarrhea [45]. Measles generally causes a more severe infection, and one study showed a caloric deficit of 75% compared with intake during recovery [47], although intake during recovery might be slightly higher than normal. Interestingly, a community-based study of infants, employing quantification of breastmilk and food intake, showed that while total energy intake from non-breastmilk sources was decreased by diarrhea and fever, the intake of breastmilk was not affected [48], revealing a previously unrecognized benefit of breastfeeding.

## Decreased Nutrient Absorption

Enteric infections can decrease the absorption of many nutrients. Enteric infections damage the intestinal epithelium and decrease the expression of brush-border enzymes, such as lactase, as shown in a piglet model of neonatal diarrhea [49]. Intestinal barrier damage during mild *Ascaris* infections of children also decreases lactose absorption, which recovers upon anthelminthic treatment [50], as is also true for β-carotene, a fat-soluble nutrient [51]. Absorption of physiological doses of vitamin A is generally quite high (over 90%) but is lower (70–80%) in children with diarrhea, *Ascaris* infection, and non-enteric infections, such as pneumonia [52, 53]. Thus absorption of multiple nutrients can be decreased by enteric infections.

## Increased Nutrient Loss

After absorption, several infections can cause direct nutrient loss, perhaps from intestinal "leakiness" resulting in protein-losing enteropathy, which occurs with post-measles diarrhea [54], or by direct loss of blood, which occurs during hookworm infection leading to iron-deficiency anemia [55]. Nutrients may also be lost through sweating or in urine. Significant amounts of vitamin A can be lost in the urine as a result of proximal tubular dysfunction in the kidney. Low molecular weight plasma proteins, including RBP, filtered through the glomerulus are normally reabsorbed in the proximal tubule [44]. One hospital-based study [56] found adults with severe infections, such as pneumonia or sepsis, excreted substantial amounts of vitamin A (presumably bound to RBP) in the urine, with 24% excreting greater than their recommended daily allowance during a single day. The illness itself may not have been the only cause of this loss, as aminoglycoside antibiotics can impair tubular function and may have been a contributing factor. Children with sepsis also excrete substantial vitamin A in the urine, while children with pneumonia and diarrhea excrete lower amounts [57]. Retinol loss in urine with infections may continue for several days [58] and is often associated with high fever and evidence of kidney tubular dysfunction (e.g., increased urinary levels of β2-microglobulin).

## Increased Nutrient Utilization

During infection, the requirements for some nutrients may increase due to increased utilization or catabolism. For example, resting metabolic rate is increased during HIV infection [59, 60], which demands increased caloric intake to prevent weight loss at equivalent levels of activity. In addition, classical studies of model infections of human volunteers show increased nitrogen loss due to protein catabolism [61]. Some intracellular bacteria manipulate cholesterol metabolism of the host as a means of gaining cholesterol that is needed for synthesis of their own biological membranes [62], which could thus affect the nutrient status of the host.

## Altered Nutrient Transport or Storage

Finally, the plasma levels of several nutrients are decreased during the acute phase response, including iron, zinc, and vitamin A, as recently reviewed [63]. These nutrients are redistributed to tissues, including the liver, during the acute phase response. While transient redistribution of nutrients presumably has some benefits for the host (e.g., decreasing the availability of iron to invading bacteria), chronic inflammation can be detrimental. In the case of iron, chronic inflammation can result in a prolonged increase of hepcidin, which blocks non-heme iron absorption from the gut, decreases recycling of iron from senescent erythrocytes by macrophages, and blocks iron mobilization from liver stores [64], which can result in mild anemia because this altered iron metabolism inhibits erythropoiesis due to this inflammation-induced "deficiency" of iron availability. Whether the redistribution of other nutrients during chronic infection has other adverse effects on the host is not clear.

## Nutrition-Infection Interactions: Malnutrition Impairs Immunity

### Protein-Energy Malnutrition (PEM)

Tuberculosis is an infectious disease that has long been associated with malnutrition, though both cause (malnutrition increasing the risk or severity of tuberculosis) and effect (tuberculosis causing malnutrition) could account for this association. A recent review points out, however, that malnutrition (a low body mass index, essentially low body weight for a given height) was associated with a higher risk of developing the clinically evident disease tuberculosis, though the risk of initial infection is hard to determine [65]. This development of frank disease (as compared to a host controlling the infection and remaining asymptomatic) presumably occurs due to the ability of PEM to impair immune function. A recent, comprehensive review of both animal and human studies indicates that PEM can impair most aspects of innate immunity, including epithelial barriers and the function of neutrophils and macrophages, as well as development of adaptive immunity [63]. Since type 1 immunity is key to controlling tuberculosis, an impaired macrophage or Th1 response could tip the balance from asymptomatic to symptomatic infection. Other T-cell responses are compromised by PEM as well as the function of the thymus itself (the source of T cells). Of particular interest are studies showing that malnutrition is associated with a decrease in the size of the thymus of infants [66] (which can be measured by noninvasive ultrasound). This has significant implications for child health as a small thymus in infancy is associated with an increased risk of death [67, 68]. Fortunately, treatment of malnutrition can reverse changes seen in thymus size and related aspects of T-cell immunity [69].

### Fat-Soluble Vitamins

#### Vitamin A

Vitamin A deficiency can affect nearly all aspects of innate and adaptive immunity, as recently reviewed [63]. Vitamin A deficiency causes squamous metaplasia at epithelial surfaces and thus can impair barrier defenses. Vitamin A deficiency also affects myelopoiesis and granulopoiesis in the bone marrow, thus impairing the activity of monocytes/macrophages and granulocytes [44], and also impairs development and activity of NK cells [70]. APC function is also altered by vitamin A deficiency and can impair antigen presentation [71] as well as enhance the production of IL-12 [72] which may skew some adaptive responses away from the development of Th2 and towards that of Th1 cells. Antibody responses to T-cell-dependent antigens are impaired by vitamin A deficiency [73, 74] with secretory IgA responses being particularly impaired [44]. Retinoic acid produced by some cells of the immune system, including APCs, appears to act in a paracrine manner to promote development of Treg cells in the intestine and may thus play a significant role in maintaining "tolerant" rather than "inflammatory" responses toward gut flora. Retinoic acid also enhances the expression of α4β7 integrin and CCR9 on gut-derived lymphocytes. These molecules allow trafficking back to the gut for mature effector lymphocytes and IgA-producing plasma cells. Vascular endothelium in the gut expresses mucosal vascular addressin cell adhesion molecule 1, to which α4β7 binds thus allowing extravasation. Epithelial and other cells in the gut express CCL25, which attracts CCR9-expressing cells [75].

Vitamin A deficiency increases the risk of death for infants and young children living in areas with a high burden of infectious diseases, and treatment of vitamin A deficiency with high-dose vitamin A capsules has been shown to reduce infant mortality when administered after 6 m of age [76]. Though the use of supplements at younger ages has had variable results, in areas where the risk of maternal vitamin A deficiency is high, decreased child mortality does occur with supplementation [77], suggesting that some interventions may not show benefit because infants may not have been deficient. Vitamin A supplementation can sometimes have adverse effects such as increasing the risk of mortality in girls in a neonatal supplementation trial in Guinea-Bissau [78], decreasing the rate of recovery from pneumonia [79] or possibly increasing the risk vertical transmission of HIV from mother to infant [80]. Such results suggest consideration of two factors when considering the use of high-dose vitamin A supplements. (1) Are the recipients of supplements actually at risk of deficiency, since supplements may have unintended effects in non-deficient individuals? (2) Should supplements be given during an acute illness, when inflammation may be altering vitamin A metabolism (e.g., reducing plasma retinol concentrations) for an unknown, and possibly beneficial, reason. These considerations are appropriate for other nutrients as well.

## Vitamin D

The active metabolite of vitamin D, calcitriol, can be produced by macrophages (and other cells of the innate immune system) following TLR2 activation by microbial pathogens such as *M. tuberculosis*. This stimulation induces expression of the 1-α-hydroxylase gene to produce calcitriol from 25-hydroxy vitamin D [81], the form of vitamin D that circulates in the blood but is not biologically active. Calcitriol produced by macrophages can then act in an autocrine or paracrine fashion to increase expression of the antimicrobial peptides cathelicidin and β2 defensin which mediate bacterial killing by macrophages. This activity may be a factor in host defense against tuberculosis [82]. Recent work has shown that poor vitamin D status is associated with a diagnosis of tuberculosis [83], but whether this is cause or effect is uncertain. Randomized, controlled intervention trials have been conducted using vitamin D as an adjunct therapy for treating tuberculosis. A recent meta-analysis of such trials shows that vitamin D may increase the percent of subjects responding to standard antibiotic therapy (which continues for several months) by becoming "sputum negative" for the detection of *M. tuberculosis* [84]. However, vitamin D treatment did not shorten the duration of antibiotic therapy needed to become negative, which would be an important benefit for patients and prevention programs [85]. This meta-analysis was the first to show such potential benefit though a more recently published trial in a deficient population showed no similar benefit [86], raising the question of whether there is sufficient benefit to recommend vitamin D as an adjunct therapy to tuberculosis. More encouragingly, vitamin D supplementation does appear to decrease the risk of developing acute respiratory infections (which would not include tuberculosis) in preventive studies [87]. The mechanism underlying this benefit may be, as discussed above, the role of vitamin D in the initial response of the innate immune system to infection [88]. Vitamin D supplementation has also been shown to decrease the risk of exacerbation of symptoms in adult asthma patients [89], an effect which could be due to an effect on the risk of respiratory infections, which can cause exacerbations, or to an underlying effect on asthma itself. Vitamin D can enhance the development and function of Treg cells (as well as have other effects on adaptive immunity); thus it is possible that vitamin D treatment could directly dampen inflammation in asthma or other chronic inflammatory diseases, including the autoimmune disease multiple sclerosis [90], as discussed in a recent review of the effects of vitamin D on the immune system [91].

## Vitamin E

Vitamin E is a fat-soluble antioxidant which can protect cells of the immune system against oxidative damage, which may account for some of its reported effects related to dampening inflammation in the innate immune system and supporting the proliferation of T cells [92]. Human studies on the effect of vitamin E are relatively rare, but vitamin E has been shown to promote Th1 responses in naïve CD4+ T cells [93]. In purified CD4+ T cells from young and old mice, vitamin E enhanced the formation of immune synapses between the TCRs and APCs [94]. Many of the human studies with vitamin E have been performed in elderly adults, and these data suggest that vitamin E supplementation may be important for improving the declining immune response in the aged and decreasing the risk of some infections [95].

## *Water-Soluble Vitamins*

### Vitamins $B_6$, $B_{12}$, Folate

Vitamins $B_6$, $B_{12}$, and folate play critical roles in one-carbon metabolism and are essential for the synthesis of nucleic acids and proteins [63, 96]. Therefore, deficiency impairs both T-cell and B-cell function. Impairment of proliferative responses, decreased antibody synthesis, and reduced cytokine production have been observed in humans deficient for any of these nutrients. A recent study in pregnant women at risk of deficiency showed that supplementation with vitamin $B_{12}$ enhanced the antibody response to influenza vaccination [97], suggesting that impaired immune function may be examined further as a consequence of B vitamin deficiencies.

### Vitamin C

Vitamin C is an important, water-soluble antioxidant that plays a key role in protecting immune cells against oxidative stress during immune responses [98]. Neutrophils in particular have a high cytoplasmic concentration of vitamin C and also rapidly regenerate ascorbate following activation [99], presumably to protect the neutrophil against the oxidative stress associated with bacterial killing. Human subjects fed a vitamin C-deficient diet had decreased delayed-type hypersensitivity (DTH) skin responses which are mediated by the Th1 cytokine IFN-γ [100], indicating defects in adaptive as well as innate immunity. Supplementation of these subjects with vitamin C normalized the DTH response, indicating that vitamin C is involved in the maintenance of Th1 function. In elderly subjects, vitamin C supplementation for 1 month increased the ex vivo proliferative responses of T cells to mitogen [101]. Studies in a mouse model for asthma showed high-dose supplementation with vitamin C increased the ratio of IFN-γ to IL-5 in bronchoalveolar fluid, again indicating that vitamin C supports Th1 function [102].

## *Minerals*

### Selenium

Selenium presumably exerts its activity in immune cells via its incorporation into selenoproteins [103]. Selenium is an essential component of the antioxidant enzymes glutathione peroxidase and thioredoxin reductase, both of which reduce the level of damaging reactive oxygen species generated during cellular processes. Thioredoxin reductase also regulates the redox potential of key cellular enzymes and transcription factors involved in immune responsiveness [96]. Selenoprotein knockout mice showed severe decreases in T-cell populations in the thymus, spleen, and lymph nodes [104], and T-cell proliferation, production of IL-2 after TCR activation, and antibody synthesis were defective in these mice compared to wild-type control animals. Selenium deficiency (as well as vitamin E deficiency) in mouse models of viral infection is associated with an increased occurrence of virulent virus strains that may result from an increased rate of mutation of the viral genome or perhaps from increased virus replication and opportunity for mutation [105]. Selenoproteins may also play a prominent role in redox-mediated signaling from cell-surface receptors [106], a mechanism which could be particularly important in the activation of cells of the immune system.

### Zinc

Zinc deficiency can impair key aspects of both innate and adaptive immunity, as recently reviewed [63, 84]. The function of phagocytic cells of the innate immune system, and of NK cells, is impaired by zinc deficiency [84]. Studies with humans have shown that deficiency of dietary zinc resulted in thymic atrophy, decreased numbers of peripheral T cells, and reduced IL-2 and IFN-γ production by T cells [107, 108]. Zinc-deficient individuals have a decreased DTH response due to the reduction in IFN-γ production. Zinc supplementation of children at risk of zinc deficiency in lower-income countries has decreased the risk of infectious disease, particularly diarrhea but also other infections [109]. This beneficial effect of zinc on diarrhea prevention has recently been confirmed in a meta-analysis of intervention trials [110].

### Copper and Iron

Copper and iron are components of the antioxidant enzymes superoxide dismutase and catalase, respectively. These metals along with selenium and zinc (also a component of superoxide dismutase) regulate the redox state and proliferative responses of T and B cells. T-cell proliferation is reduced in copper-deficient rats and humans [111]. Iron is actively transported by the transferrin receptor that is upregulated in activated T cells. Th1 cells are more sensitive to iron deficiency which results in a reduction in IFN-γ production and decreased proliferation. Reduction of IFN-γ production leads to decreased CTL activation and DTH responsiveness. Iron is required for the growth of microorganisms, and pathogens are specifically adapted to acquire iron in the relatively iron-poor environment of the human host [112, 113]. This need for iron by pathogens suggests that the decrease in serum iron seen during the acute phase may be an attempt by the host to restrict iron availability to pathogens. This may explain the association of hemochromatosis (which results in increased tissue iron levels) with increased severity of invasive bacterial infections [114] and the increased risk of infectious diarrhea with the use of iron supplements [115].

## Omega-3 Polyunsaturated Fatty Acids (PUFA)

Fatty acids are a major component of the phospholipid component of cell membranes. With regard to molecular structure, fatty acids have a carboxylic acid moiety at one end and a methyl group at the other. Fatty acids differ in chain length (from a few carbons to over 20), differ in the number of carbon-carbon double bonds they contain (saturated fatty acids contain none, monounsaturated fatty acids contain one, and PUFA contain two or more), and differ in the location of their double bonds (should they have any). The omega-3 (or n-3) designation indicates that there is a double bond three carbons from the methyl end of the fatty acid (omega-6 indicates six carbons and so on). Humans require omega-3 and omega-6 fatty acids in their diets because they cannot produce fatty acids with a double bond in these positions.

Omega-3 fatty acids of marine origin, particularly eicosapentaenoic acid (EPA) and docosahexaenoic acid (DHA), have well-characterized anti-inflammatory activities and are useful in treating symptoms of some chronic inflammatory diseases, including rheumatoid arthritis and perhaps asthma [116]. EPA is effective because it is so similar to arachidonic acid (AA). They are both 20 carbons long and have four double bonds, but AA, an abundant component of human cell membranes, is an omega-6 PUFA. This similarity is important because AA is a precursor for mediators of inflammation produced by monocytes, granulocytes, and, at times, lymphocytes, including prostaglandin E2 (PGE2) [117] and leukotriene B4 (LTB4) [118], to name just two. Leukotrienes mediate inflammation by enhancing leukocyte chemotaxis, phagocytosis and killing of bacteria by neutrophils and macrophages, and enhancing transcription of pro-inflammatory genes [119]. PGE2 has different effects, including enhancement of Th2 cytokines, promoting IgG1 and IgE production and diminishing synthesis of pro-inflammatory cytokines [117]. Because EPA is so similar to AA, it is also a substrate for the enzymes producing prostaglandins and leukotrienes, but the resulting omega-3-derived mediators generally have lower levels of activity. People with diets low in cold-water fish have cellular membranes with very low in EPA content, but the use of supplements or consumption of EPA-rich marine foods increases the EPA/AA ratio in the membranes of monocytes and granulocytes, resulting in relatively greater production EPA-derived eicosanoids and changes in immune function [120]. Thus increased EPA intake has anti-inflammatory effects in diseases such as rheumatoid arthritis [121] because EPA-derived eicosanoids are less inflammatory than AA-derived eicosanoids. For example, the EPA-derived leukotriene LTB5 has lower activity than LTB4 to stimulate granulocyte chemotaxis [122], which could alleviate symptoms of arthritis. EPA can also be converted to another type of lipid mediator, resolvin E1, which has direct anti-inflammatory activity including increasing production of the anti-inflammatory cytokine IL-10 as well as decreasing pro-inflammatory cytokine production by macrophages [116, 123]. Anti-inflammatory immune processes are covered in the context of helminth infections and nutrition in Chap. 12 [20].

DHA is typically found in cellular membranes at higher levels than EPA. While both EPA and DHA can be produced by chain elongation from the more commonly consumed 18-carbon, omega-3 PUFA α-linolenic acid, DHA is retained in membranes to a greater degree than EPA, presumably because it has a variety of important biological activities [116]. Consumption of DHA from supplements or fish will increase DHA levels further in the membranes of immune cells and can increase EPA levels as well because the 22-carbon DHA can be shortened by 2 carbons to form EPA. DHA intake can thus recapitulate some of the anti-inflammatory activities of EPA, described above, but also has additional activities. In particular, DHA is itself a substrate for the production of a class of anti-inflammatory mediators known as maresins, which limit recruitment of inflammatory cells, enhance apoptosis of damaged cells, and may have other activities to help dampen inflammation and resolve localized tissue damage caused by inflammation [116, 123]. In addition, DHA has anti-inflammatory activity because it can block TLR4-mediated signaling initiated by bacterial LPS [124]. This effect may be mediated by the disruption of lipid rafts in cellular membranes, which are important for signaling from cell-surface receptors such as TLR4, which is activated by LPS. Similarly, DHA may diminish the activation of T cells via the TCR and may thus dampen T-cell-mediated immune activation [125].

Thus DHA and EPA have somewhat different, but overlapping, biological effects that primarily act to dampen inflammation and immune activation. Interventions in low- and middle-income countries with fish oil or purified EPA and DHA have been rare, presumably because chronic inflammatory diseases are not a major concern, particularly among children. One recent study in the Gambia did evaluate fish oil as an intervention to improve growth by dampening intestinal inflammation and decrease intestinal permeability, but no benefits were seen [126].

# Conclusion

Given the complexity of nutritional intake and its measurement, metabolic processes, and microbial pathogenesis, we are only beginning to discover the myriad pathways of exacerbation or amelioration of infections via nutrition. Key discoveries of the value of zinc, vitamins A and D, iron, and other nutrients in battling infectious disease risks exist, but many more mysteries must be resolved. This chapter serves as an anchor to delve further into these complexities; nutritional status unpins all of the human health, and a better understanding of nutrition, infection, and immunity is a vital research priority.

# References

1. Fraher MH, O'Toole PW, Quigley EM. Techniques used to characterize the gut microbiota: a guide for the clinician. Nat Rev Gastroenterol Hepatol. 2012;9(6):312–22.
2. Niu SY, Yang J, McDermaid A, Zhao J, Kang Y, Ma Q. Bioinformatics tools for quantitative and functional metagenome and metatranscriptome data analysis in microbes. Brief Bioinform. 2018;19(6):1415–29.
3. Elson CO, Alexander KL. Host-microbiota interactions in the intestine. Digest Dis. 2015;33(2):131–6.
4. Watanabe K, Petri WA Jr. Environmental enteropathy: elusive but significant subclinical abnormalities in developing countries. EBioMedicine. 2016;10:25–32.
5. Mims CA, Nash A, Stephen J. Mims' pathogenesis of infectious disease. 5th ed. San Diego: Academic Press; 2001. xiii, 474 p.
6. Nestle FO, Di Meglio P, Qin JZ, Nickoloff BJ. Skin immune sentinels in health and disease. Nat Rev Immunol. 2009;9(10):679–91.
7. Grice EA, Kong HH, Conlan S, Deming CB, Davis J, Young AC, et al. Topographical and temporal diversity of the human skin microbiome. Science. 2009;324(5931):1190–2.
8. Feng Y, Chen CJ, Su LH, Hu S, Yu J, Chiu CH. Evolution and pathogenesis of Staphylococcus aureus: lessons learned from genotyping and comparative genomics. FEMS Microbiol Rev. 2008;32(1):23–37.
9. Hill DA, Artis D. Intestinal bacteria and the regulation of immune cell homeostasis. Annu Rev Immunol. 2010;28:623–67.
10. Bevins CL, Salzman NH. Paneth cells, antimicrobial peptides and maintenance of intestinal homeostasis. Nat Rev. 2011;9(5):356–68.
11. Ogra PL. Mucosal immunology. 2nd ed. San Diego: Academic Press; 1999. xliii, 1628 p.
12. Brandtzaeg P. Mucosal immunity: induction, dissemination, and effector functions. Scand J Immunol. 2009;70(6):505–15.
13. Sutherland DB, Suzuki K, Fagarasan S. Fostering of advanced mutualism with gut microbiota by immunoglobulin A. Immunol Rev. 2016;270(1):20–31.
14. Izcue A, Coombes JL, Powrie F. Regulatory lymphocytes and intestinal inflammation. Annu Rev Immunol. 2009;27:313–38.
15. Murphy K, Weaver C. Janeway's immunobiology. 9th ed. New York: Garland Science/Taylor & Francis Group, LLC; 2016. 904 p.

16. Kawai T, Akira S. Pathogen recognition with toll-like receptors. Curr Opin Immunol. 2005;17(4):338–44.
17. Martinon F, Mayor A, Tschopp J. The inflammasomes: guardians of the body. Annu Rev Immunol. 2009;27:229–65.
18. Serbina NV, Jia T, Hohl TM, Pamer EG. Monocyte-mediated defense against microbial pathogens. Annu Rev Immunol. 2008;26:421–52.
19. Varol C, Mildner A, Jung S. Macrophages: development and tissue specialization. Annu Rev Immunol. 2015;33:643–75.
20. Scott ME, Koski K. Soil-transmitted Helminths – does nutrition make a difference? In: Humphries DL, Scott ME, Vermund SH, editors. Nutrition and infectious disease: shifting the clinical paradigm. Totowa: Humana Press; 2020.
21. Kolaczkowska E, Kubes P. Neutrophil recruitment and function in health and inflammation. Nat Rev Immunol. 2013;13(3):159–75.
22. Bottazzi B, Doni A, Garlanda C, Mantovani A. An integrated view of humoral innate immunity: pentraxins as a paradigm. Annu Rev Immunol. 2009;28:157–83.
23. Kawai T, Akira S. Signaling to NF-kappaB by toll-like receptors. Trends Mol Med. 2007;13(11):460–9.
24. Yang D, Biragyn A, Hoover DM, Lubkowski J, Oppenheim JJ. Multiple roles of antimicrobial defensins, cathelicidins, and eosinophil-derived neurotoxin in host defense. Annu Rev Immunol. 2004;22:181–215.
25. Diebold S. Innate recognition of viruses. Immunol Lett. 2009;128(1):17–20.
26. Barffour MA, Humphries DL. Core principles: infectious disease risk in relation to macro and micronutrient status. In: Humphries DL, Scott ME, Vermund SH, editors. Nutrition and infectious disease: shifting the clinical paradigm. Totowa: Humana Press; 2020.
27. Hugman A. Hepcidin: an important new regulator of iron homeostasis. Clin Lab Haematol. 2006;28(2):75–83.
28. Wong P, Pamer EG. CD8 T cell responses to infectious pathogens. Annu Rev Immunol. 2003;21:29–70.
29. Russell JH, Ley TJ. Lymphocyte-mediated cytotoxicity. Annu Rev Immunol. 2002;20:323–70.
30. Chowdhury D, Lieberman J. Death by a thousand cuts: granzyme pathways of programmed cell death. Annu Rev Immunol. 2008;26:389–420.
31. Herbert DR, Douglas B, Zullo K. Group 2 innate lymphoid cells (ILC2): type 2 immunity and Helminth immunity. Int J Mol Sci. 2019;20(9):2276.
32. Annunziato F, Romagnani C, Romagnani S. The 3 major types of innate and adaptive cell-mediated effector immunity. J Allergy Clin Immunol. 2015;135(3):626–35.
33. Bystrom J, Clanchy FIL, Taher TE, Al-Bogami M, Ong VH, Abraham DJ, et al. Functional and phenotypic heterogeneity of Th17 cells in health and disease. Eur J Clin Investig. 2019;49(1):e13032.
34. Bettelli E, Korn T, Oukka M, Kuchroo VK. Induction and effector functions of T(H)17 cells. Nature. 2008;453(7198):1051–7.
35. Ueno A, Jeffery L, Kobayashi T, Hibi T, Ghosh S, Jijon H. Th17 plasticity and its relevance to inflammatory bowel disease. J Autoimmun. 2018;87:38–49.
36. Sakaguchi S, Yamaguchi T, Nomura T, Ono M. Regulatory T cells and immune tolerance. Cell. 2008;133(5):775–87.
37. Lu L, Cantor H. Generation and regulation of CD8(+) regulatory T cells. Cell Mol Immunol. 2008;5(6):401–6.
38. Joosse ME, Nederlof I, Walker LSK, Samsom JN. Tipping the balance: inhibitory checkpoints in intestinal homeostasis. Mucosal Immunol. 2019;12(1):21–35.
39. Stephensen CB. Burden of infection on growth failure. J Nutr. 1999;129(2S Suppl):534S–8S.
40. Owino V, Ahmed T, Freemark M, Kelly P, Loy A, Manary M, et al. Environmental enteric dysfunction and growth failure/stunting in global child health. Pediatrics. 2016;138(6):e20160641.
41. Sommer A, Tarwotjo I, Katz J. Increased risk of xerophthalmia following diarrhea and respiratory disease. Am J Clin Nutr. 1987;45(5):977–80.
42. Campos FA, Flores H, Underwood BA. Effect of an infection on vitamin A status of children as measured by the relative dose response (RDR). Am J Clin Nutr. 1987;46(1):91–4.
43. Herbert V. The five possible causes of all nutrient deficiency: illustrated by deficiencies of vitamin B 12. Am J Clin Nutr. 1973;26(1):77–86.
44. Stephensen CB. Vitamin A, infection, and immune function. Annu Rev Nutr. 2001;21:167–92.
45. Martorell R, Yarbrough C, Yarbrough S, Klein RE. The impact of ordinary illnesses on the dietary intakes of malnourished children. Am J Clin Nutr. 1980;33(2):345–50.
46. Rowland MG, Cole TJ, Whitehead RG. A quantitative study into the role of infection in determining nutritional status in Gambian village children. Br J Nutr. 1977;37(3):441–50.
47. Duggan MB, Alwar J, Milner RD. The nutritional cost of measles in Africa. Arch Dis Child. 1986;61(1):61–6.
48. Brown KH, Stallings RY, de Kanashiro HC, Lopez de Romana G, Black RE. Effects of common illnesses on infants' energy intakes from breast milk and other foods during longitudinal community-based studies in Huascar (Lima), Peru. Am J Clin Nutr. 1990;52(6):1005–13.
49. Zijlstra RT, Donovan SM, Odle J, Gelberg HB, Petschow BW, Gaskins HR. Protein-energy malnutrition delays small-intestinal recovery in neonatal pigs infected with rotavirus. J Nutr. 1997;127(6):1118–27.

50. Carrera E, Nesheim MC, Crompton DW. Lactose maldigestion in Ascaris-infected preschool children. Am J Clin Nutr. 1984;39(2):255–64.

51. Haque R, Ahmed T, Wahed MA, Mondal D, Rahman AS, Albert MJ. Low-dose beta-carotene supplementation and deworming improve serum vitamin A and beta-carotene concentrations in preschool children of Bangladesh. J Health Popul Nutr. 2010;28(3):230–7.

52. Sivakumar B, Reddy V. Absorption of labelled vitamin A in children during infection. Br J Nutr. 1972;27(2):299–304.

53. Sivakumar B, Reddy V. Absorption of vitamin A in children with ascariasis. J Trop Med Hyg. 1975;78(5):114–5.

54. Sarker SA, Wahed MA, Rahaman MM, Alam AN, Islam A, Jahan F. Persistent protein losing enteropathy in post measles diarrhoea. Arch Dis Child. 1986;61(8):739–43.

55. Crompton DW. The public health importance of hookworm disease. Parasitology. 2000;121(Suppl):S39–50.

56. Stephensen CB, Alvarez JO, Kohatsu J, Hardmeier R, Kennedy JI Jr, Gammon RB Jr. Vitamin A is excreted in the urine during acute infection. Am J Clin Nutr. 1994;60(3):388–92.

57. Mitra AK, Alvarez JO, Stephensen CB. Increased urinary retinol loss in children with severe infections. Lancet. 1998;351(9108):1033–4.

58. Mitra AK, Wahed MA, Chowdhury AK, Stephensen CB. Urinary retinol excretion in children with acute watery diarrhoea. J Health Popul Nutr. 2002;20(1):12–7.

59. Mittelsteadt AL, Hileman CO, Harris SR, Payne KM, Gripshover BM, McComsey GA. Effects of HIV and anti-retroviral therapy on resting energy expenditure in adult HIV-infected women-a matched, prospective, cross-sectional study. J Acad Nutr Diet. 2013;113(8):1037–43.

60. Melchior JC, Raguin G, Boulier A, Bouvet E, Rigaud D, Matheron S, et al. Resting energy expenditure in human immunodeficiency virus-infected patients: comparison between patients with and without secondary infections. Am J Clin Nutr. 1993;57(5):614–9.

61. Beisel WR, Sawyer WD, Ryll ED, Crozier D. Metabolic effects of intracellular infections in man. Ann Intern Med. 1967;67(4):744–79.

62. Samanta D, Mulye M, Clemente TM, Justis AV, Gilk SD. Manipulation of host cholesterol by obligate intracellular bacteria. Front Cell Infect Microbiol. 2017;7:165.

63. Raiten DJ, Sakr Ashour FA, Ross AC, Meydani SN, Dawson HD, Stephensen CB, et al. Inflammation and nutritional science for programs/policies and interpretation of research evidence (INSPIRE). J Nutr. 2015;145(5):1039S–108S.

64. Ganz T. Iron and infection. Int J Hematol. 2018;107(1):7–15.

65. Koethe JR, von Reyn CF. Protein-calorie malnutrition, macronutrient supplements, and tuberculosis. Int J Tuberc Lung Dis. 2016;20(7):857–63.

66. Moore SE, Prentice AM, Wagatsuma Y, Fulford AJ, Collinson AC, Raqib R, et al. Early-life nutritional and environmental determinants of thymic size in infants born in rural Bangladesh. Acta Paediatr. 2009;98(7):1168–75.

67. Moore SE, Fulford AJ, Wagatsuma Y, Persson LA, Arifeen SE, Prentice AM. Thymus development and infant and child mortality in rural Bangladesh. Int J Epidemiol. 2014;43(1):216–23.

68. Garly ML, Trautner SL, Marx C, Danebod K, Nielsen J, Ravn H, et al. Thymus size at 6 months of age and subsequent child mortality. J Pediatr. 2008;153(5):683–8, 8 e1–3.

69. Savino W, Dardenne M. Nutritional imbalances and infections affect the thymus: consequences on T-cell-mediated immune responses. Proc Nutr Soc. 2010;69(4):636–43.

70. Zhao Z, Murasko DM, Ross AC. The role of vitamin A in natural killer cell cytotoxicity, number and activation in the rat. Nat Immun. 1994;13(1):29–41.

71. Duriancik DM, Lackey DE, Hoag KA. Vitamin A as a regulator of antigen presenting cells. J Nutr. 2010;140(8):1395–9.

72. Cantorna MT, Nashold FE, Hayes CE. Vitamin A deficiency results in a priming environment conducive for Th1 cell development. Eur J Immunol. 1995;25(6):1673–9.

73. Pasatiempo AM, Kinoshita M, Taylor CE, Ross AC. Antibody production in vitamin A-depleted rats is impaired after immunization with bacterial polysaccharide or protein antigens. FASEB J. 1990;4(8):2518–27.

74. Ross AC. Vitamin A supplementation and retinoic acid treatment in the regulation of antibody responses in vivo. Vitam Horm. 2007;75:197–222.

75. Iwata M, Hirakiyama A, Eshima Y, Kagechika H, Kato C, Song SY. Retinoic acid imprints gut-homing specificity on T cells. Immunity. 2004;21(4):527–38.

76. Black RE, Allen LH, Bhutta ZA, Caulfield LE, de Onis M, Ezzati M, et al. Maternal and child undernutrition: global and regional exposures and health consequences. Lancet. 2008;371(9608):243–60.

77. West KP, Wu LS, Ali H, Klemm RDW, Edmond KM, Hurt L, et al. Early neonatal vitamin A supplementation and infant mortality: an individual participant data meta-analysis of randomised controlled trials. Arch Dis Child. 2019;104(3):217–26.

78. Benn CS, Fisker AB, Napirna BM, Roth A, Diness BR, Lausch KR, et al. Vitamin A supplementation and BCG vaccination at birth in low birthweight neonates: two by two factorial randomised controlled trial. BMJ. 2010;340:c1101.

79. Stephensen CB, Franchi LM, Hernandez H, Campos M, Gilman RH, Alvarez JO. Adverse effects of high-dose vitamin a supplements in children hospitalized with pneumonia. Pediatrics. 1998;101(5):E3.
80. Fawzi WW, Msamanga GI, Hunter D, Renjifo B, Antelman G, Bang H, et al. Randomized trial of vitamin supplements in relation to transmission of HIV-1 through breastfeeding and early child mortality. AIDS. 2002;16(14):1935–44.
81. Liu PT, Stenger S, Li H, Wenzel L, Tan BH, Krutzik SR, et al. Toll-like receptor triggering of a vitamin D-mediated human antimicrobial response. Science. 2006;311(5768):1770–3.
82. Martineau AR, Wilkinson KA, Newton SM, Floto RA, Norman AW, Skolimowska K, et al. IFN-gamma- and TNF-independent vitamin D-inducible human suppression of mycobacteria: the role of cathelicidin LL-37. J Immunol. 2007;178(11):7190–8.
83. Gou X, Pan L, Tang F, Gao H, Xiao D. The association between vitamin D status and tuberculosis in children: a meta-analysis. Medicine. 2018;97(35):e12179.
84. Wu D, Lewis ED, Pae M, Meydani SN. Nutritional modulation of immune function: analysis of evidence, mechanisms, and clinical relevance. Front Immunol. 2018;9:3160.
85. Wu HX, Xiong XF, Zhu M, Wei J, Zhuo KQ, Cheng DY. Effects of vitamin D supplementation on the outcomes of patients with pulmonary tuberculosis: a systematic review and meta-analysis. BMC Pulm Med. 2018;18(1):108.
86. Ganmaa D, Munkhzul B, Fawzi W, Spiegelman D, Willett WC, Bayasgalan P, et al. High-dose vitamin D3 during tuberculosis treatment in Mongolia. A randomized controlled trial. Am J Respir Crit Care Med. 2017;196(5):628–37.
87. Martineau AR, Jolliffe DA, Hooper RL, Greenberg L, Aloia JF, Bergman P, et al. Vitamin D supplementation to prevent acute respiratory tract infections: systematic review and meta-analysis of individual participant data. BMJ. 2017;356:i6583.
88. Zdrenghea MT, Makrinioti H, Bagacean C, Bush A, Johnston SL, Stanciu LA. Vitamin D modulation of innate immune responses to respiratory viral infections. Rev Med Virol. 2017;27(1):e1909.
89. Jolliffe DA, Greenberg L, Hooper RL, Griffiths CJ, Camargo CA Jr, Kerley CP, et al. Vitamin D supplementation to prevent asthma exacerbations: a systematic review and meta-analysis of individual participant data. Lancet Respir Med. 2017;5(11):881–90.
90. Cantorna MT. Vitamin D and multiple sclerosis: an update. Nutr Rev. 2008;66(10 Suppl 2):S135–8.
91. Sassi F, Tamone C, D'Amelio P. Vitamin D: nutrient, hormone, and immunomodulator. Nutrients. 2018;10(11):1656.
92. Lee GY, Han SN. The role of vitamin E in immunity. Nutrients. 2018;10(11):1614.
93. Meydani SN, Han SN, Wu D. Vitamin E and immune response in the aged: molecular mechanisms and clinical implications. Immunol Rev. 2005;205:269–84.
94. Marko MG, Ahmed T, Bunnell SC, Wu D, Chung H, Huber BT, et al. Age-associated decline in effective immune synapse formation of CD4(+) T cells is reversed by vitamin E supplementation. J Immunol. 2007;178(3):1443–9.
95. Meydani SN, Leka LS, Fine BC, Dallal GE, Keusch GT, Singh MF, et al. Vitamin E and respiratory tract infections in elderly nursing home residents: a randomized controlled trial. JAMA. 2004;292(7):828–36.
96. Wintergerst ES, Maggini S, Hornig DH. Contribution of selected vitamins and trace elements to immune function. Ann Nutr Metab. 2007;51(4):301–23.
97. Siddiqua TJ, Ahmad SM, Ahsan KB, Rashid M, Roy A, Rahman SM, et al. Vitamin B12 supplementation during pregnancy and postpartum improves B12 status of both mothers and infants but vaccine response in mothers only: a randomized clinical trial in Bangladesh. Eur J Nutr. 2016;55(1):281–93.
98. Carr AC, Maggini S. Vitamin C and immune function. Nutrients. 2017;9(11):1211.
99. Washko PW, Wang Y, Levine M. Ascorbic acid recycling in human neutrophils. J Biol Chem. 1993;268(21):15531–5.
100. Jacob RA, Kelley DS, Pianalto FS, Swendseid ME, Henning SM, Zhang JZ, et al. Immunocompetence and oxidant defense during ascorbate depletion of healthy men. Am J Clin Nutr. 1991;54(6 Suppl):1302S–9S.
101. Kennes B, Dumont I, Brohee D, Hubert C, Neve P. Effect of vitamin C supplements on cell-mediated immunity in old people. Gerontology. 1983;29(5):305–10.
102. Chang HH, Chen CS, Lin JY. High dose vitamin C supplementation increases the Th1/Th2 cytokine secretion ratio, but decreases eosinophilic infiltration in bronchoalveolar lavage fluid of ovalbumin-sensitized and challenged mice. J Agric Food Chem. 2009;57(21):10471–6.
103. Avery JC, Hoffmann PR. Selenium, selenoproteins, and immunity. Nutrients. 2018;10(9):1203.
104. Shrimali RK, Irons RD, Carlson BA, Sano Y, Gladyshev VN, Park JM, et al. Selenoproteins mediate T cell immunity through an antioxidant mechanism. J Biol Chem. 2008;283(29):20181–5.
105. Beck MA. Selenium and vitamin E status: impact on viral pathogenicity. J Nutr. 2007;137(5):1338–40.
106. Hawkes WC, Alkan Z. Regulation of redox signaling by selenoproteins. Biol Trace Elem Res. 2010;134(3):235–51.
107. Prasad AS. Zinc: role in immunit, oxidative stress and chronic inflammation. Curr Opin Clin Nutr Metab Care. 2009;12(6):646–52.
108. Overbeck S, Rink L, Haase H. Modulating the immune response by oral zinc supplementation: a single approach for multiple diseases. Arch Immunol Ther Exp. 2008;56(1):15–30.
109. Fischer Walker C, Black RE. Zinc and the risk for infectious disease. Annu Rev Nutr. 2004;24:255–75.

110. Florez ID, Veroniki AA, Al Khalifah R, Yepes-Nunez JJ, Sierra JM, Vernooij RWM, et al. Comparative effectiveness and safety of interventions for acute diarrhea and gastroenteritis in children: a systematic review and network meta-analysis. PLoS ONE. 2018;13(12):e0207701.

111. Munoz C, Rios E, Olivos J, Brunser O, Olivares M. Iron, copper and immunocompetence. Br J Nutr. 2007;98(Suppl 1):S24–8.

112. Bullen JJ, Rogers HJ, Spalding PB, Ward CG. Natural resistance, iron and infection: a challenge for clinical medicine. J Med Microbiol. 2006;55(Pt 3):251–8.

113. Cassat JE, Skaar EP. Iron in infection and immunit. Cell Host Microbe. 2013;13(5):509–19.

114. Khan FA, Fisher MA, Khakoo RA. Association of hemochromatosis with infectious diseases: expanding spectrum. Int J Infect Dis. 2007;11(6):482–7.

115. Gera T, Sachdev HP. Effect of iron supplementation on incidence of infectious illness in children: systematic review. BMJ. 2002;325(7373):1142.

116. Calder PC. Marine omega-3 fatty acids and inflammatory processes: effects, mechanisms and clinical relevance. Biochim Biophys Acta. 2015;1851(4):469–84.

117. Harris SG, Padilla J, Koumas L, Ray D, Phipps RP. Prostaglandins as modulators of immunity. Trends Immunol. 2002;23(3):144–50.

118. Radmark O, Werz O, Steinhilber D, Samuelsson B. 5-lipoxygenase: regulation of expression and enzyme activity. Trends Biochem Sci. 2007;32(7):332–41.

119. Peters-Golden M, Canetti C, Mancuso P, Coffey MJ. Leukotrienes: underappreciated mediators of innate immune responses. J Immunol. 2005;174(2):589–94.

120. Adkins Y, Kelley DS. Mechanisms underlying the cardioprotective effects of omega-3 polyunsaturated fatty acids. J Nutr Biochem. 2010;21(9):781–92.

121. Fritsche K. Fatty acids as modulators of the immune response. Annu Rev Nutr. 2006;26:45–73.

122. Moreno JJ. Differential effects of arachidonic and eicosapentaenoic acid-derived eicosanoids on polymorphonuclear transmigration across endothelial cell cultures. J Pharmacol Exp Ther. 2009;331(3):1111–7.

123. Dalli J, Serhan CN. Pro-resolving mediators in regulating and conferring macrophage function. Front Immunol. 2017;8:1400.

124. Hwang DH, Kim JA, Lee JY. Mechanisms for the activation of toll-like receptor 2/4 by saturated fatty acids and inhibition by docosahexaenoic acid. Eur J Pharmacol. 2016;785:24–35.

125. Hou TY, McMurray DN, Chapkin RS. Omega-3 fatty acids, lipid rafts, and T cell signaling. Eur J Pharmacol. 2016;785:2–9.

126. van der Merwe LF, Moore SE, Fulford AJ, Halliday KE, Drammeh S, Young S, et al. Long-chain PUFA supplementation in rural African infants: a randomized controlled trial of effects on gut integrity, growth, and cognitive development. Am J Clin Nutr. 2013;97(1):45–57.

# Chapter 4
# Bacterial Infections and Nutrition: A Primer

James A. Berkley

## Abbreviations

| | |
|---|---|
| AMR | Antimicrobial resistance |
| ATP | Adenosine triphosphate |
| BCG | Bacillus Calmette-Guérin vaccine |
| EED | Environmental enteric dysfunction |
| HIV | Human immunodeficiency virus |
| ICU | Intensive care unit |
| Ig | Immunoglobulin |
| IGF | Insulin-like growth factor |
| IL | Interleukin |
| LPS | Lipopolysaccharide |
| NET | Neutrophil extracellular trap |
| NK | Natural killer |
| RA | Retinoic acid |
| RUTF | Ready-to-use therapeutic food |
| SCFA | Small intestinal bacterial overgrowth |
| SIBO | Short-chain fatty acids |
| TB | Tuberculosis |
| Th | T helper |
| TLR | Toll-like receptor |
| VDR | Vitamin D receptor |

J. A. Berkley (✉)
Centre for Tropical Medicine and Global Health, Nuffield Department of Clinical Medicine, University of Oxford, Oxford, UK

Kenya Medical Research Institute/Wellcome Trust Research Programme, Kilifi, Kenya

Childhood Acute Illness & Nutrition (CHAIN) Network, Nairobi, Kenya
e-mail: jberkley@kemri-wellcome.org

© Springer Nature Switzerland AG 2021
D. L. Humphries et al. (eds.), *Nutrition and Infectious Diseases*, Nutrition and Health,
https://doi.org/10.1007/978-3-030-56913-6_4

# Overview

This chapter will focus on our relationships with commensal, symbiotic, and pathogenic bacteria that are present in the human microbiome, as well as concepts that link the presence of bacteria to focal or invasive diseases and clinical infections. The chapter will include a discussion of the influence of nutritional status and specific nutrients on colonization, invasion, severity, and mortality of bacterial infections. The effects of undernutrition on responses to vaccines against bacterial pathogens and the effects of antimicrobials on growth will be addressed. Examples will mostly be drawn from malnutrition in children, who globally bear the greatest burden of both undernutrition and serious morbidity from bacterial infections, and from disruptions in the commensal bacterial populations in the gastrointestinal tract that affect normal growth and development. Overnutrition and metabolic diseases also affect risks of infectious diseases, potentially through mechanisms that overlap with those observed in undernourished individuals [1]. However, these will not be the focus of this chapter. Where clinical trials are discussed, the focus will be on whether they demonstrate differences in bacterial disease incidence or mortality.

# Bacteria of Importance to Humans

Bacteria are single-cell organisms without a membrane-bound nucleus that live in almost every environment on Earth. The community of bacteria and other microbes that live together, for example, in the intestine, is referred to as the microbiome. Historically, bacterial species have been classified by their appearance under a light microscope, including their shapes (e.g., spheres, rods, spirals) and ability to take up pigment stains (e.g., the Gram stain) which characterize properties of the bacterial cell wall. When bacteria are cultured, their nutrient requirements and biochemical metabolic characteristics provide further means of identification. Although genotypic classification, including by 16s ribosomal RNA sequencing and whole-genome sequencing, is allowing us to more precisely group related species, identify separate species and sub-species, and in some cases revise the classification of the genera, nomenclature based on pigment staining characteristics remains useful in clinical practice. The effectiveness of many common antibiotics, including penicillin, often depends on their ability to penetrate bacterial cell walls where they target the synthesis of components of the bacterial cell wall.

## *Gram-Positive Bacteria*

Gram-positive bacteria have a cell wall containing peptidoglycan and take up the Gram stain. Common Gram-positive species include staphylococci, typically resident in the skin and nose, causing soft tissue and bone infections or disseminated sepsis; streptococci, in the oropharynx and skin, causing skin, throat, or cardiac infections; and pneumococci, resident in the nasopharynx, causing pneumonia, sepsis, and meningitis. Other Gram-positive bacteria may be resident in the gut, including enterococci. Gram-positive bacteria can form toxins causing food poisoning or localized tissue destruction. Lactobacilli are Gram-positive and are a major component of the gut and vaginal microbiome, acting to prevent other invasive species; they are also used in food production to ferment wine, cheese, and yoghurt. Bifidobacteria are Gram-positive anaerobes, another major component of the gut microbiome, able to ferment carbohydrates, including milk oligosaccharides in children. Lactobacilli and bifidobacteria are commonly used as probiotics, although benefits tend to be target and strain-specific. *Firmicutes*, including clostridia and bacilli, are one of the two phyla comprising more than 90% of the human microbiota.

## Gram-Negative Bacteria

Gram-negative bacteria have an additional cytoplasmic membrane in their wall and do not take up the Gram stain. Many Gram-negative bacteria express endotoxin, a lipopolysaccharide (LPS), on their cell wall which is essential for bacterial survival and a major target of human immune and inflammatory responses. One component of endotoxin, lipid A, can cause an overwhelming inflammatory response known as sepsis, with high mortality. Gram-negative bacteria include the *Enterobacteriaceae* (*Escherichia coli*, *Klebsiella*, *Salmonella*, *Shigella*, and others) resident in the gut of humans and animals and *Pseudomonas*, *Vibrio*, and *Campylobacter* species resident in the gut, water, soil, and the environment. Other Gram-negative bacteria are resident in the nasopharynx and cause pneumonia, sepsis, and meningitis, including *Neisseria* and *Haemophilus* species. However, most Gram-negative bacteria are harmless or beneficial, such as the phylum *Bacteroidetes* that are resident in soil and most notably in the human and animal intestine where they form a major component of the resident microbiota.

## Other Bacteria

*Helicobacter* (e.g., *H. pylori*), *Treponema* (e.g. *T. pallidum* causing syphilis), *Borrelia*, *Mycoplasma*, and *Rickettsia* are not classified using the Gram stain system as they have unique characteristics of shape and culture requirements or cannot be cultured.

## Mycobacteria

Mycobacteria, including *Mycobacterium tuberculosis* and nontuberculous mycobacteria, are the most common bacterial cause of death worldwide, estimated to cause 10 million cases and 1.5 million deaths each year. They do not take up the Gram stain and were originally classified by their ability to take up the Ziel-Neilson (acid-fast) stain. Mycobacteria may cause acute infection in an individual without pre-existing immunity such as young children. However, mycobacteria normally have a much slower replication cycle than other bacteria; hence they require treatment over a period of months rather than days as antibiotic treatment is only active during cell division. Mycobacteria most commonly enter a dormant phase of latent infection after exposure, usually in childhood, effectively a stalemate between the slowly replicating bacteria, the host immune response, and the "walling off" of tuberculous granuloma by fibrous tissue as a result of local inflammation. Latent infection with *M. tuberculosis* affects 25% of the world population. Latent infection may be reactivated when the stalemate is broken by a decline in host immunity due to older age, immunosuppressive drugs, or conditions such as HIV, alcoholism, or malnutrition.

## Pathogenic and Nonpathogenic Bacteria

We commonly regard bacterial species as pathogenic or nonpathogenic; however, this is an oversimplification. Within species, bacteria can be characterized by the presence of identifiable surface antigens (serotypes) and by the presence of genes conferring virulence characteristics such as invasiveness or production of a toxin. Thus, within a species, only some serotypes or genotypes may cause significant disease. Furthermore, because infection is a result of interaction with the host, a species of a particular genotype may only cause serious infection where normal barriers to infection are breached or when there is immune function compromise. Such species are known as facultatively pathogenic. For example, *Staphylococcus epidermidis* is a ubiquitous skin commensal organism and does not generally cause disease in healthy individuals. However, in an intensive care unit, among individuals with long intravenous cannulae to deliver drugs or parenteral nutrition directly to the large vessels of the central circulation, *S. epidermidis* is a common cause of sepsis, especially among preterm infants. *S. epidermidis* and other pathogens may colonize the tips of plastic cannulae and thus be introduced into the host without crossing the usual barriers to infection. There they evade immune responses and antibiotic drugs by forming biofilms to wall off and protect bacterial colonies.

## *Antimicrobial Resistance*

We live in an era when evolving bacterial antimicrobial resistance (AMR) is outstripping the rates of discovery, evaluation, and implementation of new antibiotic classes and agents. It is estimated that there are ~700,000 deaths (including ~230,000 to multidrug-resistant tuberculosis) worldwide each year, and at the current trajectory, this may rise to ~10 million deaths per year by 2050 [2]. Antibiotic resistance genes are frequently encoded in plasmids, genetic units independent of the main bacterial chromosome that are transferrable between bacteria of the same and different species. Plasmids allow rapid spread of resistance to the main classes of antibiotics in use today, including penicillins, cephalosporins, and carbapenems. The development of new classes of antibiotics is generally very expensive. Furthermore, facilities for accurate diagnosis and classification of AMR are most lacking in regions of poverty.

Malnourished individuals are at increased risk from AMR because of more frequent and more severe infections and generally longer stay as inpatients in healthcare facilities, thus increasing exposure to hospital-acquired infections. In Kenya, hospital-acquired bloodstream infection was 2.5 times more common in severely malnourished children [3]. Thus, the problem of AMR disproportionately affects individuals and communities of low economic status that are at the highest risk of bacterial infection and those with an inadequate diet or malnutrition.

## The Human-Bacterial Interface

### *Symbiotic Relationships*

The sections above may give an impression of a battleground where, at best, a stalemate is achieved between the human host and bacterial aggressors. However, the predominant features of the human host-bacteria relationship are beneficial in terms of control of more pathogenic bacterial species, immune signaling, and nutrient processing within the intestinal microbiome.

### *The Intestinal Microbiome*

Humans are exposed to bacteria from the moment of birth to the time of death. At birth, after living in a usually sterile environment in utero, a complex community that is primarily bacterial but also includes other prokaryotes (Archaea) as well as eukaryotes (Eukarya) is acquired predominantly from the birth canal and first colonizes the infant intestinal tract, oropharynx, and other spaces. This community of organisms is collectively known as the microbiota, and the overall composition of genes that are present is known as the microbiome, although microbiome and microbiota are often used as synonyms.

The infant normally acquires its first intestinal microbiome from the mother's intestinal and vaginal tracts. Not surprisingly, the intestinal microbiome of babies born by cesarean section differs from those born by vaginal delivery. The intestinal microbiome undergoes a relatively predictable process of maturation through childhood, with dramatic changes at the time of weaning and subsequent stabilization (see Fig. 4.1) [4]. Under favorable circumstances, this occurs by the age of about 3 years. In the adult body, an estimated 100 trillion microbes from 4 major phyla, *Firmicutes*, *Bacteroidetes*, *Actinobacteria*, and *Proteobacteria*, exceed the number of human cells. The intestinal microbiome has been nicely described as an "ecosystem on a leash" [5].

Major metabolic roles of the intestinal microbiome include anaerobic fermentation of dietary fiber (e.g., *Bacteroidetes* and *Bifidobacterium*) producing short-chain fatty acids including acetate, propionate, and butyrate; resistance of colonization and invasion by potentially harmful organisms; regulation and facilitation of immune development; and synthesis of vitamins and essential amino acids. Short-chain fatty acids (SCFA) provide a source of energy and also have a broad range of physiological and

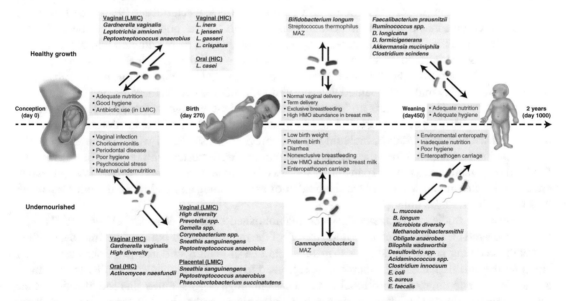

**Fig. 4.1** Key bacterial taxa at different stages of 1000 days that contribute to healthy versus undernourished growth. Current evidence suggests that a number of bacterial signatures are associated with either undernutrition or healthy growth during the first 1000 days. During pregnancy, a vaginal microbiota with low diversity and rich in *Lactobacillus* is associated with term birth and normal birth weight in high-income settings. Conversely, a more diverse vaginal microbiota, rich in *Prevotella* spp., *Gemella* spp., and *Corynebacterium*, is associated with reduced newborn LAZ. Healthy growth is associated with greater *Bifidobacterium longum* and *Streptococcus thermophilus* in the first 6 months of life, which are less prevalent in early-life undernutrition. Breastfeeding during this period is associated with greater *Bacteroides* and *Bifidobacterium*. In later childhood, higher *Akkermansia muciniphila*, *Methanobrevibacter smithii*, *Faecalibacterium prausnitzii*, *Lactobacillus*, and obligate anaerobes are associated with healthy growth, while *Escherichia coli*, *Staphylococcus aureus*, and other species are associated with severe acute malnutrition. A two-way interaction exists between an immature microbiome and the risk factors contributing to undernutrition, whereby diarrhea, nutrition, birth weight, and other factors both influence and are influenced by the "undernourished" microbiome. Image adapted from Servier Medical Art under a CC-BY license. *HICs* high-income countries, *LMICs* low- and middle-income countries, *HMO* human milk oligosaccharide, *MAZ* microbiota-for-age Z-score, *E. coli Escherichia coli*, *S. aureus Staphylococcus aureus*, *D. longicatna Dorea longicatna*. (Reprinted under a Creative Commons CC-BY License from: Robertson et al. [4])

metabolic effects. SCFAs regulate appetite, modulate immune responses, and are also involved in maintaining intestinal epithelial integrity and thus protection against bacterial invasion [6]. Other species, such as lactobacilli, produce hydrogen peroxide and other mediators that inhibit invasive bacteria and fungi. Some metabolites of the microbiome, including trimethylamine, secondary bile acids, and hydrogen sulfide, are linked to an increased risk of noncommunicable diseases [7].

The intestinal microbiome is influenced by diet, specifically by naturally occurring prebiotic compounds (favoring bacterial growth, such as oligosaccharides), by antibacterial compounds (such as antibodies and lysozyme) present in breastmilk and artificially added to commercial infant formulas along with antibiotics, and by ingestion of bacterial components (probiotics) and potentially pathogenic bacteria. During infancy and childhood, the switch from breastfeeding to non-breastmilk dietary carbohydrate components is known to have a major influence on the composition of the microbial community, and species diversity increases with age [8].

## Malnutrition and Dysbiosis

In malnourished children, the intestinal microbiome is "less mature," for the child's age, with lower diversity and a greater proportion of potentially pathogenic Enterobacteriaceae [9]. There is evidence that the microbiome may contribute to malnutrition, although "cause" and "effect" may be difficult to disentangle. When the fecal microbiomes of young Malawian twin pairs with and without kwashiorkor (edematous malnutrition) were transferred to germ-free mice fed on a typical Malawian diet, mice with the microbiome from the twin with kwashiorkor had greater weight loss during the subsequent 3 weeks compared to mice transplanted with the non-kwashiorkor twin's microbiome [10]. However, when fed a normal rodent diet, no such differential weight change occurred. Members of the Clostridiales order were overrepresented in the microbiota of children with kwashiorkor compared to their twins without kwashiorkor, including species previously associated with inflammatory bowel disease and inflammation. When the malnourished children were treated with ready to use therapeutic food (RUTF), there was a rapid expansion of species of *Bifidobacterium* and *Lactobacillus* (known to stimulate innate immunity and reduce the burden of enteropathogens) and anti-inflammatory members of the Clostridiales order [10].

However, in studies in Bangladesh, when malnourished children were fed either a RUTF or a locally prepared therapeutic diet, the "immaturity" of the microbiome of both groups improved within 1 month becoming not significantly less mature than that of healthy children [9]. Four months after stopping therapeutic feeds, their microbiome regressed to a level of immaturity similar to that found at baseline despite improved nutritional status. These findings suggest either that modification of the microbiome was due to the diet rather than nutritional recovery or that the endogenous intestinal environment (mucosal immunity and competing bacterial species) or exogenous environmental exposures had not changed. More recent trials have focused on longer-term dietary modification, for example, using microbiota-directed complementary foods, with early evidence of the types of foods that are associated with microbiota repair and that bring plasma biomarkers closer to those found in healthy children [11].

Regarding micronutrients, there is generally limited evidence of the effects of deficiency or treatment on the intestinal microbiota. An exception is iron, which is commonly given in an inorganic form to prevent or treat anemia in childhood. Iron has been associated with reductions in abundance of *Bifidobacterium* and *Lactobacillus* and increased abundances of Clostridiales in children in Kenya and in Cote d'Ivoire [12, 13]. In Kenya, those treated with iron also had an increase in bacterial virulence and toxin genes, increased intestinal fatty acid-binding protein suggesting intestinal mucosal damage, increased fecal calprotectin (a biomarker of neutrophil activity and inflammation), and increased abundance of pathogenic *E. coli* strains [12, 13]. Thus, although inorganic iron is effective in treating iron deficiency anemia, it may potentially result in significant dysbiosis and intestinal pathology. Ongoing research is investigating other forms of delivery of iron to overcome these risks and other potential infectious risks [14].

## *Environmental Enteric Dysfunction*

Environmental enteric dysfunction (EED) is a condition of chronic intestinal inflammation, increased permeability, and reduced nutrient absorptive surface affecting the majority of people living in circumstances of poverty, food insecurity, crowding, poor water and sanitation, and poor access to healthcare. EED is associated with both wasting and stunting in children and may underlie much of what is measured as malnutrition. It was first recognized in the 1960s among volunteers to poor areas in Asia from high-resource settings. Gut absorptive function recovered within 2 years of returning to a high-income environment. Blunted villi, crypt atrophy, and villous hyperplasia in the small intestine during EED reduce the area available for nutrient absorption and are accompanied by reduced lymphocyte counts in Peyer's patches (the lymphatic tissue providing surveillance and protection throughout the small intestine) and reduced mucosal immunoglobulin (Ig) A secretion. Similar histological abnormalities were demonstrated in Zambian adults and Gambian children and were associated with linear growth faltering [15–18]. Recently, the multicenter MAL-ED study in Bangladesh, Brazil, India, Nepal, Pakistan, Peru, South Africa, and Tanzania identified biomarkers of EED as being associated with increased risks of low ferritin, low retinol, and anemia in children [19].

The specific causes of EED remain unclear. The apparent correlation of inflammation and intestinal absorption with rainfall, poverty, and migration have suggested dietary and environmental factors [15, 20]. Chronic fecal-oral contamination and exposure to intestinal protozoans *Cryptosporidium* and *Giardia*, in the context of micronutrient deficiencies, are highly likely to be involved but as a relatively silent process, without overt episodes of diarrhea. Specific bacteria and small intestinal bacterial overgrowth (SIBO) may be involved, and enterotoxigenic *E. coli*, *Citrobacter rodentium*, and *H. pylori* have been implicated [15, 21–23]. In the multicenter MAL-ED study, impaired linear growth was associated with subclinical infections with the protozoan pathogen, *Giardia*, and bacteria such as *Shigella* species, enteroaggregative *E. coli*, and *Campylobacter* [24]. However, it is less clear that biomarkers of intestinal inflammation are reliable markers of the severity of EED.

Malnourished children typically have severe enteropathy, which is similar to and/or may be the same as EED [25–27]. There is concern that chronic inflammation and exposure to bacterial LPS may have consequences for the regulation and efficiency of immune responses and potentially metabolic syndromes and adult noncommunicable diseases. Besides effects on growth, EED (or perhaps the specific enteric species associated with EED) has been correlated with impaired responses to oral vaccines and impaired cognitive development [28]. However, it is difficult to eliminate the effects of confounding, and these correlations may occur as a result of similar exposures in parallel with EED, rather than being caused by EED.

## Colonization as a Precursor to Infection in the Respiratory Tract

Asymptomatic mucosal colonization is a precursor to many common bacterial infections and also facilitates transmission. The transition to invasive disease is not fully understood, and once colonized, invasive or focal bacterial infection is not necessarily associated with abundance or relative density of bacterial pathogens which have a wide natural variation in healthy children [29]. This may be partially explained by differences in the prevalence of virulent serotypes and function between colonizing and invasive strains within the same bacterial species [30, 31]. Thus, composition and virulence are likely to be more important than the numbers of bacteria. Symptomatic infection may involve colonization by new species or by new (more pathogenic) strains or serotypes, including acquisition of virulence genes or selection pressure from other resident organisms [32], or alterations in host factors including mucosal immunity (both antibody-mediated protection, such as immunoglobulin (Ig)A and cellular immunity) or in physiological factors such as disruption of tight junctions between mucosal cells that facilitates translocation of bacteria. Colonization by bacterial pathogens in the respiratory tract may be modified by concurrent viral infections [33] or by vaccination against respiratory bacterial pathogens such as *Streptococcus pneumoniae* that alters bacterial species other than the pathogens vaccinated against [29]. Viral species are also long-term residents of the respiratory and gastrointestinal tracts and can alter bacterial invasiveness by disruption of the epithelial barrier or direct effects on coresident bacteria [32].

Published studies on the influences of malnutrition on respiratory infections are relatively limited. However, malnutrition was associated with nasopharyngeal colonization with *S. pneumoniae* in studies in Ethiopia and Venezuela [34, 35], and in the latter study, colonization with *S. pneumoniae* was associated with symptomatic respiratory tract infection.

## Effect of Nutritional Status and Diet on Risks of Bacterial Infection

Multiple epidemiological observations of the increased susceptibility, severity, and duration of bacterial infections that occur in both over- and undernourished individuals suggest a secondary immune deficit [36–45]. Such deficits are of particular concern in children who are malnourished, where malnutrition has cascading physiological effects that are associated with increased risk of infection (see Fig. 4.2) [46]. The type of infection may also be determined by nutritional status. For example, diarrhea

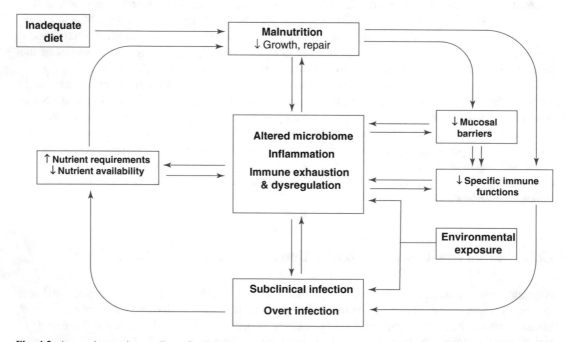

**Fig. 4.2** A growing understanding of a "vicious cycle": interactions between malnutrition, infection, and intestinal dysfunction. (Reprinted with permission from Wolters Kluwer Health: Walson and Berkley [46])

in malnourished children is more likely to be caused by bacterial pathogen rather than a viral pathogen [47]. Various immunological abnormalities have been reported among individuals with malnutrition; however investigators have not always distinguished the effects of malnutrition from those of acute concurrent infections or comorbidities. Comprehensive reviews of nutrition and immunity have been undertaken by Rytter et al. [48] and Ibrahim et al. [49] as well as Stephensen (see Chap. 3) [50].

## Barriers to Infection

Although careful studies using modern techniques are generally lacking, loss of skin and mucosal barrier function are likely to be major contributors to infection since this is the case in other conditions where such barriers are breached. The skin and wound healing are affected by malnutrition, and in addition to depigmentation or hyperpigmentation, malnourished children may have skin cracking, bullae (blistering), and skin erosion, providing a portal for bacterial infection [51]. Immune responses within the intact skin may also be affected. Other protective mechanisms, including the production of saliva containing salivary IgA, tears, and mucus, are reported to be reduced [48].

Gastric acidity is reduced in undernutrition, likely contributing to small intestinal bacterial overgrowth [52, 53]. The intestinal mucosa has a high rate of cell turnover and cell replication; thus the amino acids, folate, zinc, vitamin A, and other nutrients that are required for the transcription of new proteins from DNA may be limited. Reduced mucosal integrity and mucosal immune abnormalities [54–56], as in EED, as described above, lead to an increased translocation of bacterial products including LPS, leading to chronic inflammation and immune dysfunction [49]. Of note, translocation of bacteria from the gut to the bloodstream has been clearly documented by bacterial genotyping among severely malnourished children [57].

## Systemic Immunity, Malnutrition, and Bacterial Infections

Functions of the systemic immune system are broadly classified as "innate" and "adaptive." Innate and adaptive functions are closely interlinked, providing multiple "layers" of defense which are carefully regulated to avoid targeting the individual themselves causing bystander damage from inflammatory and pathogen-killing responses (see Chap. 3) [50].

Innate immunity is a process of recognizing molecular patterns of bacteria, other pathogens, and nucleic acids. This occurs through a set of specialized cell surface receptors, the toll-like receptors (TLRs), that induce signaling cascades within cells to release molecules that recruit, activate, and destroy pathogens and foreign materials during the first exposure. Cells including macrophages and neutrophils engulf bacteria, foreign material, and cellular debris (phagocytosis) and signal to recruit other cells through cytokines and chemokines. Neutrophils, which are the main line of cellular defense against established bacterial infections, also release granules containing superoxide free radicals that are toxic to bacteria and fungi in an intensive burst requiring energy from adenosine triphosphate (ATP). Neutrophils may also trap and kill bacteria outside the cell by forming neutrophil extracellular traps (NETs) comprising DNA, chromatin, and granule proteins. In addition, chemical cascades, such as the complement system, provide a way of marking foreign material for phagocytosis (opsonization), attracting cells, especially macrophages, to the site of infection (chemotaxis), punching holes in cell walls (lysis), and binding of pathogens together (agglutination).

Besides the impaired barrier function, it seems highly likely from the evidence of increased risks of bacterial infection and delayed recovery from susceptibility to infection compared to anthropometric recovery [58] that innate immune function is impaired. Several studies have examined circulating

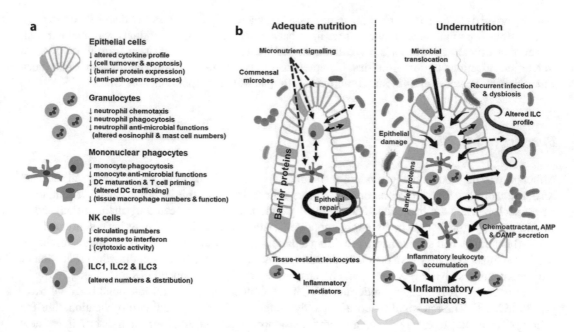

**Fig. 4.3** Summary of innate immune cell dysfunction during undernutrition. (**a**) Cellular functions where there is evidence of dysfunction from human cohort studies and animal models of undernutrition. Functions in brackets only have evidence from animal models. (**b**) Innate immune characteristics of the adequately nourished (left) vs. undernourished (right) gut. Solid arrows indicate secreted proteins and cell behavior. Dashed arrows indicate signaling pathways. Differences in the size of arrows and text indicate quantitative differences in the response between the adequately nourished and undernourished state. *AMP* antimicrobial peptides, *DAMP* damage-associated molecular patterns. (Reprinted under a free PMC article with a CC-BY license from Bourke et al. [27])

biomarkers and identified elevated pro-inflammatory markers and cytokines suggestive of innate immune activation in malnourished children (see Fig. 4.3) [26, 27, 59], but the possibility of concurrent infections, which may be subclinical, makes interpretation of these studies difficult. Few human studies have directly examined innate immune cell function in relation to malnutrition. Natural killer (NK) lymphocytes function independently as innate actors, and studies have suggested that NK cell numbers may be reduced in severe malnutrition [48]. The neutrophil functions of chemotaxis and bacterial killing capacity have been found to be impaired in some, but not all studies [48, 60–63]. Animal studies suggest that micronutrients including vitamin A, vitamin C, folate, iron, and zinc may be important in neutrophil activation, chemotaxis, adherence to other cells, and bactericidal oxidative burst, but definitive studies and clinical trials with infectious disease endpoints and other clinical endpoints are awaited [49]. Thus, we currently lack critical mechanistic information that could help better understand relationships with bacterial infections. Of particular interest is the role of micronutrients, for example, niacin/nicotinamide and vitamin A-derived retinoic acid, which are required to create neutrophil superoxides among many other cellular processes.

In contrast, adaptive immunity is built through exposure to specific antigenic molecules of pathogens (proteins, peptides, or polysaccharides) that bind to antibodies which are either free in the circulation, released at mucosal surfaces or bound to cell membranes and trigger the proliferation and activity of T and B lymphocytes. Exposure to antigens, typically delivered by specialist antigen-presenting cells such as dendritic cells, results in antibody production by B cells as well as generation of memory B cells that enable rapid and efficient future production of pathogen-specific antibodies when exposed to the pathogen again. Likewise, antigen-specific adaptive responses include cytotoxic T cells that kill cells infected by viruses or intracellular bacteria and cancer cells without harming healthy host cells, as well as memory T cells. This process of pathogen recognition through adaptive immune responses is the basis of vaccination.

There are more studies on adaptive immunity in relation to nutritional status than there are for innate immunity. Firstly, there is some evidence that both numbers and signaling functions of dendritic cells are affected by malnutrition [64, 65]. Dendritic cells are early detectors of antigens, processing and presenting them in a recognizable format to T cells, and acting as a main line of cytokine signaling between the innate and adaptive arms of the immune system. Several studies report malnutrition to be associated with atrophy of the thymus, where T lymphocytes originate, with depletion in thymic cell numbers associated with deficiencies in protein, phosphorous, and zinc [45, 49, 66]. Thymus size is seen to recover with nutritional rehabilitation. Several studies report reduced T-cell numbers [67–70], but not a specific deficit of CD4 T cells unless there is concurrent HIV [71]. There is evidence of impaired in vivo and in vitro tests of T cell function, including those involved in skin tests against tuberculin and candida antigens (delayed-type hypersensitivity) [70, 72–75]. However, studies have not always been consistent, and, as mentioned above, the effects of concurrent illness have not always been accounted for. Despite there being more studies of adaptive immunity, our picture remains incomplete. New "omic" technologies and the ability to study single-cell metabolism and responses are likely to improve knowledge in this area.

## Specific Micronutrients and Bacterial Infections

Vitamin A supplementation reduces all-cause child mortality by an estimated 12%, largely due to effects on diarrhea, but without demonstrable effect on respiratory infections [76]. Vitamin A from the diet or supplementation is converted to its active form retinoic acid (RA) which plays multiple roles in innate and adaptive systemic immunity through regulation of gene transcription (see Chap. 2) [77]. In the innate system, RA is the primary antibacterial defense mechanism, and it regulates monocyte, macrophage and neutrophil proliferation, maturation, and cytokine responses. RA is key to maintaining respiratory, gut, and urogenital epithelial integrity and production of secretory IgA [78]. In adaptive immunity, RA helps induce regulatory T cells and induces a gut-homing phenotype in T cells. These functions of RA influence tolerance and regulation of intestinal dysbiosis [79].

Vitamin D in the forms of sunlight and cod liver oil was used as an adjuvant treatment for tuberculosis (TB) (see Chap. 9) [80]. In recent years, a close relationship between vitamin D and the immune system has been established, with both antibiotic and anti-inflammatory mechanisms. Vitamin D receptors (VDR) are found on the surface of most cells of the immune system. Activation of TLRs by pathogens causes upregulation of VDRs on the surface of macrophages, inducing an antimicrobial peptide, cathelicidin, which directly kills intracellular *M. tuberculosis* [81]. Cathelicidins also have direct antibacterial effects on other bacterial species. Concurrently, vitamin D modulates T-cell proliferation and cytokine production, pushing responses away from pro-inflammatory T helper (Th)1 responses towards an anti-inflammatory Th2 response and immune regulation [82]. Thus, vitamin D is responsible for targeted, but measured, immune responses. A systematic review of vitamin D supplementation in TB patients reported an increase in the proportion of patients in whom sputum samples converted from positive for *M. tuberculosis* on microscopy and on culture and improvements in X-ray findings, but no effect on mortality [83]. There is also evidence that vitamin D supplementation reduces the incidence of acute respiratory infections in adults and children [84].

Zinc deficiency is common in low- and middle-income countries, partly due to the lowering of bioavailability by antinutrients such as phytates in many plant-based diets. Zinc is involved in multiple areas of the innate and adaptive immune system that control bacterial infections, in DNA and RNA synthesis, and in the maintenance of human cell structures (see Chap. 2) [77, 85]. Zinc deficiency is associated with thymic atrophy, reduced differentiation of immature T cells and subsequent maturation and proliferation of T cells, impaired neutrophil and macrophage chemotaxis, phagocytosis, release of superoxides, and formation of extracellular NETs, as well as impaired regulation of pro-inflammatory and anti-inflammatory cytokines and of oxidative stress [85]. Zinc supplementation is associated with a reduction in diarrhea morbidity and X-ray-confirmed pneumonia (which is more likely to be bacterial than pneumonia defined by clinical signs) incidence in children [86]. Measured blood zinc concentrations are observed to be decreased in patients with sepsis, possibly due to redistribution to decrease zinc availability of zinc as a nutrient for replicating bacteria and, in a crisis, to shift immune responses towards innate responses rather than slower adaptive responses to potentially overwhelming bacterial infection [87].

Iron deficiency anemia remains widespread in preschool and school-aged children and pregnant women. Iron supplementation is commonly given in these groups. However, iron is also an essential micronutrient for the replication of most bacterial species. Many bacteria, including those within the gut microbiota, pathogenic *Enterobacteriaceae* (including *E. coli*, *Salmonella*, *Vibrio*, and *Klebsiella* species), and *Listeria* species produce siderophores, which scavenge free iron and form complexes that are transported into bacterial cells by membrane receptors. Thus, iron is involved in a "tug of war" between bacteria and humans (and other mammals) [88]. Consequently, iron absorption and circulating concentration are normally tightly regulated by the hormone, hepcidin, and iron-binding proteins, ferritin and transferrin (see Chap. 2) [77]. When required, such as during inflammation or infection, raised serum hepcidin causes iron to be redistributed and sequestered within macrophages and the liver. Some bacterial pathogens have evolved strategies to scavenge iron, such as *Neisseria meningitides* that obtains iron from iron-binding proteins and *E. coli* that obtains iron from hemoglobin [89]. There is also data from animal studies indicating that iron and mechanisms involving siderophores contribute to bacterial virulence and tissue damage during infection [90]. Free iron overload may occur in individuals with conditions that are dependent on regular blood transfusion or with familial hemochromatosis and is associated with serious infections with the iron-scavenging bacteria mentioned above.

Oral iron supplementation is associated with intestinal inflammation and dysbiosis and an increased risk of diarrhea. Among children with low hemoglobin concentrations, iron supplementation is associated with improved motor and mental development [91]. However, it is unclear where the upper limit of beneficial hemoglobin lies and whether there is harm in iron-replete children. However, despite these findings, and ongoing concerns in settings where malaria-surveillance and treatment services are unavailable (see Chap. 11) [92], an increased risk of serious bacterial infections has not been attributed to iron supplementation.

## Antibacterial Vaccine Responses

The major bacterial species that children (and sometimes adults) are vaccinated against include *Mycobacterium tuberculosis* causing TB; *Bordetella pertussis* causing whooping cough; *Corynebacterium diphtheria* causing diphtheria; *Haemophilus influenzae* causing pneumonia and meningitis; *Streptococcus pneumoniae* causing pneumonia, sepsis, and meningitis; *Neisseria meningitidis* causing sepsis and meningitis; *Pasteurella pestis* causing plague; *Salmonella typhi* causing typhoid fever; and *Vibrio cholera* causing cholera.

Several types of vaccines exist. Live vaccines are attenuated, but viable bacterial organisms induce a protective response (typically a T-cell and B-cell response, as in a natural infection) and include the bacillus Calmette-Guérin (BCG) vaccine against TB and oral typhoid vaccine. Live vaccines against viruses, such as measles vaccine, may also protect against secondary bacterial infections. Inactivated (non-live) vaccines come in several forms and typically require several doses. Whole bacterial cell inactivated vaccines are used against pertussis, typhoid, cholera, and plague. Protein vaccines comprise purified or recombinant protein antigens from a pathogen, such as the diphtheria toxoid vaccine.

Polysaccharide vaccines comprise long-chain sugars from the surface capsule of bacteria and may include several serotypes of a bacterial species; they are used against *S. pneumoniae, H. influenzae, N. meningitidis*, and *S. typhi* infections. Polysaccharide conjugate vaccines elicit B-cell responses (hence antibody production) without the need for accompanying T-cell support and therefore are effective in infancy. Plain polysaccharide vaccines without a protein conjugate are not reliably effective in children under 2 years of age but are used in older children and adults, such as the 23-valent *S. pneumoniae* polysaccharide vaccine.

In determining the effectiveness of vaccines, the gold standard is a clinical trial with a specific disease incidence endpoint. However, these are large and expensive and may not be feasible for rare diseases. Antibody concentrations (titer) can be measured in the blood. However, not all antibodies are equally important in controlling infection and other assays that assess the affinity of the antibody for a pathogen or the ability of the antibody to neutralize a pathogen are more specific. Where a vaccine (or natural exposure) induces a T cell response, the resulting T cell cytokine response to pathogen antigens may be measured in a blood sample.

Polysaccharide-protein conjugate vaccines are key to efforts to reduce child mortality, as they target pneumonia, sepsis, and meningitis. In South Africa, the 13-valent pneumococcal conjugate vaccine was similarly protective against invasive pneumococcal disease in malnourished infants and children as in well-nourished children [93]. Other studies have generally examined antibody responses only. In Gambian children, plain polysaccharide vaccine responses in children aged above 5 years were unrelated to anthropometry or measured micronutrient status [94].

While there is no recent epidemiological evidence of an increased burden of diphtheria associated with undernutrition in children, studies of antibody titers following diphtheria protein vaccines suggest there may be variation by season of birth, stunting, and underweight in some studies but not others, although titers are likely still to be within a protective range [95, 96]. For killed typhoid vaccine, South African children with severe malnutrition have been shown to have similar responses to well-nourished children [95].

Generally, BCG has lower efficacy against pulmonary TB in low-income countries than in more wealthy nations, whereas protection against disseminated TB and TB meningitis appear preserved in all settings. Responses to live BCG vaccine have been examined in older studies (25–50 years ago) by skin tests of response to a purified protein derivative of *M. tuberculosis*, tuberculin (TST), indicating delayed-type hypersensitivity mediated by T cells, reporting reduced responses in malnutrition [70, 72–75]. More recent studies show that Gambian children who were undernourished (at the time of assessment rather than at the time of vaccination) had similar TST responses to well-nourished children, with similar rates of latent and active TB [97]. In an animal model, malnutrition did not alter the T-cell number, but it did impair T-cell cytokine responses during TB infection in BCG-vaccinated mice, which was reversible on refeeding [98].

Overall, the limited data suggest that, as far as they have been measured, there is limited if any clinically meaningful impact of undernutrition on the efficacy of currently used antibacterial (?) vaccines. However, only rarely have actual disease endpoints been examined, and reviews have identified questionable quality of studies and heterogeneity of study designs as problems in this area [95].

## Nutrients in Treatment of Serious Bacterial Infection

There is growing interest in immunometabolism (the metabolism and substrate requirements of immune cells), as well as immunonutrition (the requirements of individuals to maintain or restore for normal immune function), with most research taking place in relation to surgery, oncology, and sepsis. Although outcomes of serious infection are known to be worse in undernourished individuals, there is evidence from the well-conducted PEPaNIC trial that, in bacterial sepsis, initiating parenteral or enteral feeding in the first 24 h, rather than a week later, is harmful [99]. This effect was most closely related to amino acid doses, which were associated with an increase in new infections and greater dependency on the intensive care unit (ICU) care [100]. In contrast to amino acid doses, early glucose and lipid administration was associated with fewer infections and earlier ICU discharge. Specific amino acids, including arginine and glutamine, and other nutrients, including omega-3 fatty acids, have been investigated as immune adjuvants in sepsis, but as yet there is no clear evidence of reduced mortality [101]. Deficiencies of vitamin A, vitamin D, or zinc are common in patients with sepsis [102–104]. However, several trials have examined vitamin A, vitamin D, or zinc as adjuvants to pneumonia treatment without generating any clear evidence of benefit in terms of mortality or treatment failure rates [105–107]. The results of larger trials are awaited, and other therapeutic targets such as mitochondrial function are being targeted [108].

## Effects of Bacterial Infection on Host Nutritional Status

Diarrhea is associated with malabsorption and marked losses of protein, vitamin A, zinc, and other micronutrients (see Chap. 8) [109–111]. Bacteria require nutrients for their proliferation and metabolism. However, the predominant effects on human nutrition are from physiological and immunological host responses [112–115]. Besides anorexia due to illness, infections are associated with net protein and energy loss. Amino acids and micronutrients are diverted to meet the requirements of generating acute-phase proteins for the host response [116–119]. Increased body temperature has evolved to inhibit bacterial replication, but this comes at a cost of increased metabolic work and depends on the availability of energy (ATP) and enzymes that catalyze these reactions. A one-degree centigrade increase above normal body temperature is estimated to cost an additional 7–13% over resting energy expenditure [120–122].

Interleukin (IL) 6 and other mediators involved in the activation of inflammatory cascades cause reduced appetite and loss of lean tissue and fat [17, 114, 123]. These inflammatory pathways also act directly on insulin-like growth factor (IGF)1 that is responsible for linear growth in children; thus inflammation contributes to stunting. Severely malnourished children may expend less energy and protein because of a temporary reduction in less essential physiological processes through reductive adaptation in response to malnutrition [117], but nutritional costs of infection may impair catch-up growth [17, 124].

## Conclusions

Bacterial infections remain a major cause of adult and pediatric morbidity and mortality. Current evidence suggests that their impact is likely to dramatically increase with the continued spread of transferrable bacterial genes conferring resistance to most of the currently available antibiotics. There is strong evidence that bacterial infections are more common, severe, and fatal in malnourished individuals. However, evidence from trials of nutritional interventions for either prevention or treatment of bacterial infections is weak. It is notable that, when systematically reviewed, these trials have often been observed to be small and of low quality. New tools and techniques are providing opportunities for improving our understanding of pathogen biology, of the relationships between metabolism and nutrients and the immune system, and of the microbiome and its potential for manipulation. This understanding, combined with rigorous trials, is anticipated to lead to targeted and effective nutritional strategies for the prevention and treatment of bacterial infections. Prevention of infections through vaccination and improved water, sanitation, and living conditions is also likely to reduce the burden of endemic malnutrition in low- and middle-income countries.

# References

1. Bourke CD, Berkley JA, Prendergast AJ. Immune dysfunction as a cause and consequence of malnutrition. Trends Immunol. 2016;37(6):386–98.
2. Report to the Secretary-General of the United Nations. No time to wait: securing the future from drug-resistant infections. 2019. Available from: https://www.who.int/antimicrobial-resistance/interagency-coordination-group/IACG_final_report_EN.pdf.
3. Aiken AM, Mturi N, Njuguna P, Mohammed S, Berkley JA, Mwangi I, et al. Risk and causes of paediatric hospital-acquired bacteraemia in Kilifi District Hospital, Kenya: a prospective cohort study. Lancet. 2011;378(9808):2021–7.
4. Robertson RC, Manges AR, Finlay BB, Prendergast AJ. The human microbiome and child growth—first 1000 days and beyond. Trends Microbiol. 2019;27(2):131–47.
5. Foster KR, Schluter J, Coyte KZ, Rakoff-Nahoum S. The evolution of the host microbiome as an ecosystem on a leash. Nature. 2017;548(7665):43–51.
6. Mohajeri MH, Brummer RJM, Rastall RA, Weersma RK, Harmsen HJM, Faas M, et al. The role of the microbiome for human health: from basic science to clinical applications. Eur J Nutr. 2018;57(Suppl 1):1–14.
7. Rath S, Rud T, Karch A, Pieper DH, Vital M. Pathogenic functions of host microbiota. Microbiome. 2018;6(1):174.
8. Singh RK, Chang HW, Yan D, Lee KM, Ucmak D, Wong K, et al. Influence of diet on the gut microbiome and implications for human health. J Transl Med. 2017;15(1):73.
9. Subramanian S, Huq S, Yatsunenko T, Haque R, Mahfuz M, Alam MA, et al. Persistent gut microbiota immaturity in malnourished Bangladeshi children. Nature. 2014;510(7505):417–21.
10. Smith MI, Yatsunenko T, Manary MJ, Trehan I, Mkakosya R, Cheng J, et al. Gut microbiomes of Malawian twin pairs discordant for kwashiorkor. Science. 2013;339(6119):548–54.
11. Gehrig JL, Venkatesh S, Chang HW, Hibberd MC, Kung VL, Cheng J, et al. Effects of microbiota-directed foods in gnotobiotic animals and undernourished children. Science. 2019;365(6449):eaau4732.
12. Zimmermann MB, Chassard C, Rohner F, N'Goran EK, Nindjin C, Dostal A, et al. The effects of iron fortification on the gut microbiota in African children: a randomized controlled trial in Cote d'Ivoire. Am J Clin Nutr. 2010;92(6):1406–15.
13. Paganini D, Uyoga MA, Kortman GAM, Cercamondi CI, Moretti D, Barth-Jaeggi T, et al. Prebiotic galacto-oligosaccharides mitigate the adverse effects of iron fortification on the gut microbiome: a randomised controlled study in Kenyan infants. Gut. 2017;66(11):1956–67.
14. Prentice AM, Mendoza YA, Pereira D, Cerami C, Wegmuller R, Constable A, et al. Dietary strategies for improving iron status: balancing safety and efficacy. Nutr Rev. 2017;75(1):49–60.
15. Kelly P, Menzies I, Crane R, Zulu I, Nickols C, Feakins R, et al. Responses of small intestinal architecture and function over time to environmental factors in a tropical population. Am J Trop Med Hyg. 2004;70(4):412–9.
16. Lunn PG, Northrop-Clewes CA, Downes RM. Intestinal permeability, mucosal injury, and growth faltering in Gambian infants. Lancet. 1991;338(8772):907–10.
17. Campbell DI, Elia M, Lunn PG. Growth faltering in rural Gambian infants is associated with impaired small intestinal barrier function, leading to endotoxemia and systemic inflammation. J Nutr. 2003;133(5):1332–8.
18. Campbell DI, McPhail G, Lunn PG, Elia M, Jeffries DJ. Intestinal inflammation measured by fecal neopterin in Gambian children with enteropathy: association with growth failure, Giardia lamblia, and intestinal permeability. J Pediatr Gastroenterol Nutr. 2004;39(2):153–7.
19. Richard SA, McCormick BJJ, Murray-Kolb LE, Lee GO, Seidman JC, Mahfuz M, et al. Enteric dysfunction and other factors associated with attained size at 5 years: MAL-ED birth cohort study findings. Am J Clin Nutr. 2019;110(1):131–8.
20. Menzies IS, Zuckerman MJ, Nukajam WS, Somasundaram SG, Murphy B, Jenkins AP, et al. Geography of intestinal permeability and absorption. Gut. 1999;44(4):483–9.
21. Sullivan PB, Thomas JE, Wight DG, Neale G, Eastham EJ, Corrah T, et al. Helicobacter pylori in Gambian children with chronic diarrhoea and malnutrition. Arch Dis Child. 1990;65(2):189–91.
22. Dale A, Thomas JE, Darboe MK, Coward WA, Harding M, Weaver LT. Helicobacter pylori infection, gastric acid secretion, and infant growth. J Pediatr Gastroenterol Nutr. 1998;26(4):393–7.
23. Thomas JE, Dale A, Bunn JE, Harding M, Coward WA, Cole TJ, et al. Early Helicobacter pylori colonisation: the association with growth faltering in The Gambia. Arch Dis Child. 2004;89(12):1149–54.
24. Rogawski ET, Liu J, Platts-Mills JA, Kabir F, Lertsethtakarn P, Siguas M, et al. Use of quantitative molecular diagnostic methods to investigate the effect of enteropathogen infections on linear growth in children in low-resource settings: longitudinal analysis of results from the MAL-ED cohort study. Lancet Glob Health. 2018;6(12):e1319–e28.
25. Louis-Auguste J, Kelly P. Tropical enteropathies. Curr Gastroenterol Rep. 2017;19(7):29.

26. Attia S, Versloot CJ, Voskuijl W, van Vliet SJ, Di Giovanni V, Zhang L, et al. Mortality in children with complicated severe acute malnutrition is related to intestinal and systemic inflammation: an observational cohort study. Am J Clin Nutr. 2016;104(5):1441–9.

27. Bourke CD, Jones KDJ, Prendergast AJ. Current understanding of innate immune cell dysfunction in childhood undernutrition. Front Immunol. 2019;10:1728. https://doi.org/10.3389/fimmu.2019.01728. eCollection 2019. PMID: 31417545. PMID: 31417545.

28. Bartelt LA, Bolick DT, Guerrant RL. Disentangling microbial mediators of malnutrition: modeling environmental enteric dysfunction. Cell Mol Gastroenterol Hepatol. 2019;7(3):692–707.

29. Boelsen LK, Dunne EM, Mika M, Eggers S, Nguyen CD, Ratu FT, et al. The association between pneumococcal vaccination, ethnicity, and the nasopharyngeal microbiota of children in Fiji. Microbiome. 2019;7(1):106.

30. Seale AC, Koech AC, Sheppard AE, Barsosio HC, Langat J, Anyango E, et al. Maternal colonization with Streptococcus agalactiae and associated stillbirth and neonatal disease in coastal Kenya. Nat Microbiol. 2016;1(7):16067.

31. Bittaye M, Cash P, Forbes K. Proteomic variation and diversity in clinical Streptococcus pneumoniae isolates from invasive and non-invasive sites. PLoS ONE. 2017;12(6):e0179075.

32. Bosch AA, Biesbroek G, Trzcinski K, Sanders EA, Bogaert D. Viral and bacterial interactions in the upper respiratory tract. PLoS Pathog. 2013;9(1):e1003057.

33. Morpeth SC, Munywoki P, Hammitt LL, Bett A, Bottomley C, Onyango CO, et al. Impact of viral upper respiratory tract infection on the concentration of nasopharyngeal pneumococcal carriage among Kenyan children. Sci Rep. 2018;8(1):11030.

34. Verhagen LM, Gomez-Castellano K, Snelders E, Rivera-Olivero I, Pocaterra L, Melchers WJ, et al. Respiratory infections in Enepa Amerindians are related to malnutrition and Streptococcus pneumoniae carriage. J Infect. 2013;67(4):273–81.

35. Gebre T, Tadesse M, Aragaw D, Feye D, Beyene HB, Seyoum D, et al. Nasopharyngeal carriage and antimicrobial susceptibility patterns of Streptococcus pneumoniae among children under five in Southwest Ethiopia. Children. 2017;4(4):27.

36. Zaman K, Baqui AH, Yunus M, Sack RB, Bateman OM, Chowdhury HR, et al. Association between nutritional status, cell-mediated immune status and acute lower respiratory infections in Bangladeshi children. Eur J Clin Nutr. 1996;50(5):309–14.

37. Zaman K, Baqui AH, Yunus M, Sack RB, Chowdhury HR, Black RE. Malnutrition, cell-mediated immune deficiency and acute upper respiratory infections in rural Bangladeshi children. Acta Paediatr. 1997;86(9):923–7.

38. Lindtjørn B, Alemu T, Bjorvatn B. Nutritional status and risk of infection among Ethiopian children. J Trop Pediatr. 1993;39(2):76–82.

39. Caulfield LE, de Onis M, Blossner M, Black RE. Undernutrition as an underlying cause of child deaths associated with diarrhea, pneumonia, malaria, and measles. Am J Clin Nutr. 2004;80(1):193–8.

40. Pickering H, Hayes RJ, Tomkins AM, Carson D, Dunn DT. Alternative measures of diarrhoeal morbidity and their association with social and environmental factors in urban children in The Gambia. Trans R Soc Trop Med Hyg. 1987;81(5):853–9.

41. Waterlow JC, Tomkins AM, Grantham-McGregor SM. Protein energy malnutrition. London: Edward Arnold; 1992.

42. Hughes WT, Price RA, Sisko F, Havron WS, Kafatos AG, Schonland M, et al. Protein-calorie malnutrition. A host determinant for Pneumocystis carinii infection. Am J Dis Child. 1974;128(1):44–52.

43. Russian DA, Levine SJ. Pneumocystis carinii pneumonia in patients without HIV infection. Am J Med Sci. 2001;321(1):56–65.

44. Tomashefski JF Jr, Butler T, Islam M. Histopathology and etiology of childhood pneumonia: an autopsy study of 93 patients in Bangladesh. Pathology. 1989;21(2):71–8.

45. Purtilo DT, Connor DH. Fatal infections in protein-calorie malnourished children with thymolymphatic atrophy. Arch Dis Child. 1975;50(2):149–52.

46. Walson JL, Berkley JA. The impact of malnutrition on childhood infections. Curr Opin Infect Dis. 2018;31(3):231–6.

47. Tickell KD, Pavlinac PB, John-Stewart GC, Denno DM, Richardson BA, Naulikha JM, et al. Impact of childhood nutritional status on pathogen prevalence and severity of acute diarrhea. Am J Trop Med Hyg. 2017;97(5):1337–44.

48. Rytter MJ, Kolte L, Briend A, Friis H, Christensen VB. The immune system in children with malnutrition—a systematic review. PLoS ONE. 2014;9(8):e105017.

49. Ibrahim MK, Zambruni M, Melby CL, Melby PC. Impact of childhood malnutrition on host defense and infection. Clin Microbiol Rev. 2017;30(4):919–71.

50. Stephensen CB. Primer on immune response and interface with malnutrition. In: Humphries DL, Scott ME, Vermund SH, editors. Nutrition and infectious disease: shifting the clinical paradigm. Totowa: Humana Press; 2020.

51. Heilskov S, Vestergaard C, Babirekere E, Ritz C, Namusoke H, Rytter M, et al. Characterization and scoring of skin changes in severe acute malnutrition in children between 6 months and 5 years of age. J Eur Acad Dermatol Venereol. 2015;29(12):2463–9.

52. Gilman RH, Partanen R, Brown KH, Spira WM, Khanam S, Greenberg B, et al. Decreased gastric acid secretion and bacterial colonization of the stomach in severely malnourished Bangladeshi children. Gastroenterology. 1988;94(6):1308–14.

53. Martinsen TC, Bergh K, Waldum HL. Gastric juice: a barrier against infectious diseases. Basic Clin Pharmacol Toxicol. 2005;96(2):94–102.

54. Chandra RK, Wadhwa M. Nutritional modulation of intestinal mucosal immunity. Immunol Investig. 1989;18(1–4):119–26.

55. Sirisinha S, Suskind R, Edelman R, Asvapaka C, Olson RE. Secretory and serum IgA in children with protein-calorie malnutrition. Pediatrics. 1975;55(2):166–70.

56. Reddy V, Raghuramulu N, Bhaskaram C. Secretory IgA in protein-calorie malnutrition. Arch Dis Child. 1976;51(11):871–4.

57. Youssef M, Al Shurman A, Chachaty E, Bsoul AR, Andremont A. Use of molecular typing to investigate bacterial translocation from the intestinal tract in malnourished children with Gram-negative bacteremia. Clin Microbiol Infect. 1998;4(2):70–4.

58. Ngari MM, Mwalekwa L, Timbwa M, Hamid F, Ali R, Iversen PO, et al. Changes in susceptibility to life-threatening infections after treatment for complicated severe malnutrition in Kenya. Am J Clin Nutr. 2018;107(4):626–34.

59. Njunge JM, Gwela A, Kibinge NK, Ngari M, Nyamako L, Nyatichi E, et al. Biomarkers of post-discharge mortality among children with complicated severe acute malnutrition. Sci Rep. 2019;9(1):5981.

60. Ortiz R, Campos C, Gomez JL, Espinoza M, Ramos-Motilla M, Betancourt M. Effect of renutrition on the proliferation kinetics of PHA stimulated lymphocytes from malnourished children. Mutat Res. 1995;334(2):235–41.

61. Hughes S, Kelly P. Interactions of malnutrition and immune impairment, with specific reference to immunity against parasites. Parasite Immunol. 2006;28(11):577–88.

62. Gotch FM, Spry CJ, Mowat AG, Beeson PB, Maclennan IC. Reversible granulocyte killing defect in anorexia nervosa. Clin Exp Immunol. 1975;21(2):244–9.

63. Jose DG, Shelton M, Tauro GP, Belbin R, Hosking CS. Deficiency of immunological and phagocytic function in aboriginal children with protein-calorie malnutrition. Med J Aust. 1975;2(18):699–705.

64. Abe M, Akbar F, Matsuura B, Horiike N, Onji M. Defective antigen-presenting capacity of murine dendritic cells during starvation. Nutrition. 2003;19(3):265–9.

65. Hughes SM, Amadi B, Mwiya M, Nkamba H, Tomkins A, Goldblatt D. Dendritic cell anergy results from endotoxemia in severe malnutrition. J Immunol. 2009;183(4):2818–26.

66. Rytter MJ, Namusoke H, Ritz C, Michaelsen KF, Briend A, Friis H, et al. Correlates of thymus size and changes during treatment of children with severe acute malnutrition: a cohort study. BMC Pediatr. 2017;17(1):70.

67. Chevalier P, Sevilla R, Sejas E, Zalles L, Belmonte G, Parent G. Immune recovery of malnourished children takes longer than nutritional recovery: implications for treatment and discharge. J Trop Pediatr. 1998;44(5):304–7.

68. Parent G, Chevalier P, Zalles L, Sevilla R, Bustos M, Dhenin JM, et al. In vitro lymphocyte-differentiating effects of thymulin (Zn-FTS) on lymphocyte subpopulations of severely malnourished children. Am J Clin Nutr. 1994;60(2):274–8.

69. Smythe PM, Brereton-Stiles GG, Grace HJ, Mafoyane A, Schonland M, Coovadia HM, et al. Thymolymphatic deficiency and depression of cell-mediated immunity in protein-calorie malnutrition. Lancet. 1971;2(7731): 939–43.

70. Najera O, Gonzalez C, Toledo G, Lopez L, Ortiz R. Flow cytometry study of lymphocyte subsets in malnourished and well-nourished children with bacterial infections. Clin Diagn Lab Immunol. 2004;11(3):577–80.

71. Hughes SM, Amadi B, Mwiya M, Nkamba H, Mulundu G, Tomkins A, et al. CD4 counts decline despite nutritional recovery in HIV-infected Zambian children with severe malnutrition. Pediatrics. 2009;123(2):e347–51.

72. Najera O, Gonzalez C, Toledo G, Lopez L, Cortes E, Betancourt M, et al. CD45RA and CD45RO isoforms in infected malnourished and infected well-nourished children. Clin Exp Immunol. 2001;126(3):461–5.

73. Allende LM, Corell A, Manzanares J, Madruga D, Marcos A, Madrono A, et al. Immunodeficiency associated with anorexia nervosa is secondary and improves after refeeding. Immunology. 1998;94(4):543–51.

74. Fakhir S, Ahmad P, Faridi MA, Rattan A. Cell-mediated immune responses in malnourished host. J Trop Pediatr. 1989;35(4):175–8.

75. Rodriguez L, Graniel J, Ortiz R. Effect of leptin on activation and cytokine synthesis in peripheral blood lymphocytes of malnourished infected children. Clin Exp Immunol. 2007;148:478–85.

76. Imdad A, Mayo-Wilson E, Herzer K, Bhutta ZA. Vitamin A supplementation for preventing morbidity and mortality in children from six months to five years of age. Cochrane Database Syst Rev. 2017;3:CD008524.

77. Barffour MA, Humphries DL. Core principles: infectious disease risk in relation to macro and micronutrient status. In: Humphries DL, Scott ME, Vermund SH, editors. Nutrition and infectious disease: shifting the clinical paradigm. Totowa: Humana Press; 2020.

78. Villamor E, Fawzi WW. Effects of vitamin a supplementation on immune responses and correlation with clinical outcomes. Clin Microbiol Rev. 2005;18(3):446–64.

79. Oliveira LM, Teixeira FME, Sato MN. Impact of retinoic acid on immune cells and inflammatory diseases. Mediat Inflamm. 2018;2018:3067126.

80. Wanke C, Baum M. [To be determined]. In: Humphries DL, Scott ME, Vermund SH, editors. Nutrition and infectious disease: shifting the clinical paradigm. New York: Springer; 2020.

81. Liu PT, Stenger S, Li H, Wenzel L, Tan BH, Krutzik SR, et al. Toll-like receptor triggering of a vitamin D-mediated human antimicrobial response. Science. 2006;311(5768):1770–3.

82. Gombart AF. The vitamin D-antimicrobial peptide pathway and its role in protection against infection. Future Microbiol. 2009;4(9):1151–65.

83. Wu HX, Xiong XF, Zhu M, Wei J, Zhuo KQ, Cheng DY. Effects of vitamin D supplementation on the outcomes of patients with pulmonary tuberculosis: a systematic review and meta-analysis. BMC Pulm Med. 2018;18(1):108.

84. Yakoob MY, Salam RA, Khan FR, Bhutta ZA. Vitamin D supplementation for preventing infections in children under five years of age. Cochrane Database Syst Rev. 2016;11:CD008824.

85. Gammoh NZ, Rink L. Zinc in infection and inflammation. Nutrients. 2017;9(6):624.

86. Lassi ZS, Moin A, Bhutta ZA. Zinc supplementation for the prevention of pneumonia in children aged 2 months to 59 months. Cochrane Database Syst Rev. 2016;12:CD005978.

87. Alker W, Haase H. Zinc and Sepsis. Nutrients. 2018;10(8):976.

88. Golonka R, Yeoh BS, Vijay-Kumar M. The iron tug-of-war between bacterial siderophores and innate immunity. J Innate Immun. 2019;11(3):249–62.

89. Parrow NL, Fleming RE, Minnick MF. Sequestration and scavenging of iron in infection. Infect Immun. 2013;81(10):3503–14.

90. Holden VI, Breen P, Houle S, Dozois CM, Bachman MA. Klebsiella pneumoniae Siderophores induce inflammation, bacterial dissemination, and HIF-1alpha stabilization during pneumonia. MBio. 2016;7(5):e01397–16.

91. Larson LM, Kubes JN, Ramirez-Luzuriaga MJ, Khishen S, A HS, Prado EL. Effects of increased hemoglobin on child growth, development, and disease: a systematic review and meta-analysis. Ann N Y Acad Sci. 2019;1450:83–104.

92. Kim HH, Bei AK. Nutritional frameworks in malaria. In: Humphries DL, Scott ME, Vermund SH, editors. Nutrition and infectious disease: shifting the clinical paradigm. Totowa: Humana Press; 2020.

93. Cohen C, von Mollendorf C, de Gouveia L, Lengana S, Meiring S, Quan V, et al. Effectiveness of the 13-valent pneumococcal conjugate vaccine against invasive pneumococcal disease in South African children: a case-control study. Lancet Glob Health. 2017;5(3):e359–e69.

94. Moore SE, Goldblatt D, Bates CJ, Prentice AM. Impact of nutritional status on antibody responses to different vaccines in undernourished Gambian children. Acta Paediatr. 2003;92(2):170–6.

95. Prendergast AJ. Malnutrition and vaccination in developing countries. Philos Trans R Soc Lond Ser B Biol Sci. 2015;370(1671):20140141.

96. Savy M, Edmond K, Fine PE, Hall A, Hennig BJ, Moore SE, et al. Landscape analysis of interactions between nutrition and vaccine responses in children. J Nutr. 2009;139(11):2154S–218S.

97. Adetifa IM, Muhammad AK, Jeffries D, Donkor S, Borgdorff MW, Corrah T, et al. A tuberculin skin test survey and the annual risk of Mycobacterium tuberculosis infection in Gambian school children. PLoS ONE. 2015;10(10):e0139354.

98. Hoang T, Agger EM, Cassidy JP, Christensen JP, Andersen P. Protein energy malnutrition during vaccination has limited influence on vaccine efficacy but abolishes immunity if administered during Mycobacterium tuberculosis infection. Infect Immun. 2015;83(5):2118–26.

99. van Puffelen E, Hulst JM, Vanhorebeek I, Dulfer K, Van den Berghe G, Verbruggen S, et al. Outcomes of delaying parenteral nutrition for 1 week vs initiation within 24 hours among undernourished children in pediatric intensive care: a subanalysis of the PEPaNIC randomized clinical trial. JAMA Netw Open. 2018;1(5):e182668.

100. Vanhorebeek I, Verbruggen S, Casaer MP, Gunst J, Wouters PJ, Hanot J, et al. Effect of early supplemental parenteral nutrition in the paediatric ICU: a preplanned observational study of post-randomisation treatments in the PEPaNIC trial. Lancet Respir Med. 2017;5(6):475–83.

101. Tao W, Li PS, Shen Z, Shu YS, Liu S. Effects of omega-3 fatty acid nutrition on mortality in septic patients: a meta-analysis of randomized controlled trials. BMC Anesthesiol. 2016;16(1):39.

102. Zhang X, Yang K, Chen L, Liao X, Deng L, Chen S, et al. Vitamin A deficiency in critically ill children with sepsis. Crit Care. 2019;23(1):267.

103. Ponnarmeni S, Kumar Angurana S, Singhi S, Bansal A, Dayal D, Kaur R, et al. Vitamin D deficiency in critically ill children with sepsis. Paediatr Int Child H. 2016;36(1):15–21.

104. Saleh NY, Abo El Fotoh WMM. Low serum zinc level: the relationship with severe pneumonia and survival in critically ill children. Int J Clin Pract. 2018;72(6):e13211.

105. Tie HT, Tan Q, Luo MZ, Li Q, Yu JL, Wu QC. Zinc as an adjunct to antibiotics for the treatment of severe pneumonia in children <5 years: a meta-analysis of randomised-controlled trials. Br J Nutr. 2016;115(5):807–16.

106. Das RR, Singh M, Naik SS. Vitamin D as an adjunct to antibiotics for the treatment of acute childhood pneumonia. Cochrane Database Syst Rev. 2018;7:CD011597.
107. Thorne-Lyman A, Fawzi WW. Vitamin A supplementation, infectious disease and child mortality: a summary of the evidence. Nestle Nutr Inst Workshop Ser. 2012;70:79–90.
108. Leite HP, de Lima LF. Metabolic resuscitation in sepsis: a necessary step beyond the hemodynamic? J Thorac Dis. 2016;8(7):E552–7.
109. Castillo-Duran C, Vial P, Uauy R. Oral copper supplementation: effect on copper and zinc balance during acute gastroenteritis in infants. Am J Clin Nutr. 1990;51(6):1088–92.
110. Mitra AK, Wahed MA, Chowdhury AK, Stephensen CB. Urinary retinol excretion in children with acute watery diarrhoea. J Health Popul Nutr. 2002;20(1):12–7.
111. Siddiqui F, Belayneh G, Bhutta ZA. Nutrition and diarrheal disease and enteric pathogens. In: Humphries DL, Scott ME, Vermund SH, editors. Nutrition and infectious disease: shifting the clinical paradigm. Totowa: Humana Press; 2020.
112. Pelletier DL, Frongillo EA Jr, Habicht JP. Epidemiologic evidence for a potentiating effect of malnutrition on child mortality. Am J Public Health. 1993;83(8):1130–3.
113. Scrimshaw NS, Taylor CE, Gordon JE. Interactions of nutrition and infection. Monogr Ser World Health Organ. 1968;57:3–329.
114. Bhutta ZA. Effect of infections and environmental factors on growth and nutritional status in developing countries. J Pediatr Gastroenterol Nutr. 2006;43(Suppl 3):S13–21.
115. Black RE. Would control of childhood infectious diseases reduce malnutrition? Acta Paediatr Scand Suppl. 1991;374:133–40.
116. Manary MJ, Broadhead RL, Yarasheski KE. Whole-body protein kinetics in marasmus and kwashiorkor during acute infection. Am J Clin Nutr. 1998;67(6):1205–9.
117. Manary MJ, Yarasheski KE, Berger R, Abrams ET, Hart CA, Broadhead RL. Whole-body leucine kinetics and the acute phase response during acute infection in marasmic Malawian children. Pediatr Res. 2004;55(6):940–6.
118. Tomkins AM, Garlick PJ, Schofield WN, Waterlow JC. The combined effects of infection and malnutrition on protein metabolism in children. Clin Sci (Lond). 1983;65(3):313–24.
119. Waterlow JC, Golden J, Picou D. The measurements of rates of protein turnover, synthesis, and breakdown in man and the effects of nutritional status and surgical injury. Am J Clin Nutr. 1977;30(8):1333–9.
120. Benhariz M, Goulet O, Salas J, Colomb V, Ricour C. Energy cost of fever in children on total parenteral nutrition. Clin Nutr. 1997;16(5):251–5.
121. Du Bois EF. The basal metabolism of fever. JAMA. 1921;77:352–5.
122. Stettler N, Schutz Y, Whitehead R, Jequier E. Effect of malaria and fever on energy metabolism in Gambian children. Pediatr Res. 1992;31(2):102–6.
123. Saez-Llorens X, Lagrutta F. The acute phase host reaction during bacterial infection and its clinical impact in children. Pediatr Infect Dis J. 1993;12(1):83–7.
124. Stephensen CB. Burden of infection on growth failure. J Nutr. 1999;129(2S Suppl):534S–8S.

# Chapter 5
# Viral Infections and Nutrition: Influenza Virus as a Case Study

**William David Green, Erik A. Karlsson, and Melinda A. Beck**

## Abbreviations

| | |
|---|---|
| AIDS | Acquired immunodeficiency syndrome |
| aOR | Adjusted odds ratio |
| BMI | Body mass index |
| cccDNA | Covalently closed circular DNA |
| CCR5 | C-C chemokine receptor 5 |
| CXCR4 | C-X-C chemokine receptor 4 |
| DAA | Direct-acting antiviral |
| DNA | Deoxyribonucleic acid |
| dsDNA | Double-stranded DNA |
| GPx | Glutathione peroxidase |
| H1N1 | Hemagglutinin 1 neuraminidase 1 |
| HA | Hemagglutinin |
| HBV | Hepatitis B virus |
| HCV | Hepatitis C virus |
| HIV | Human immunodeficiency virus |
| HRV | Human rhinovirus |
| HSV | Herpes simplex virus |
| ICAM-1 | Intercellular adhesion molecule 1 |
| ICTV | International Committee on Taxonomy of Viruses |
| IFN | Interferon |
| Ig | Immunoglobulin |
| LAT | Latency-associated transcripts |
| mRNA | Messenger RNA |
| NA | Neuraminidase |
| NK cells | Natural killer cells |

W. D. Green · M. A. Beck (✉)
Department of Nutrition, Gilling's School of Global Public Health, University of North Carolina, Chapel Hill, NC, USA
e-mail: melinda_beck@med.unc.edu

E. A. Karlsson
Virology Unit, Institut Pasteur du Cambodge, Phnom Penh, Cambodia

© Springer Nature Switzerland AG 2021
D. L. Humphries et al. (eds.), *Nutrition and Infectious Diseases*, Nutrition and Health,
https://doi.org/10.1007/978-3-030-56913-6_5

| rcDNA | Relaxed circle DNA |
| RNA | Ribonucleic acid |
| ROS | Reactive oxygen species |
| ssDNA | Single-stranded DNA |
| ssRNA | Single-stranded RNA |
| TGF | Transforming growth factor |
| TNF | Tumor necrosis factor |
| UVB | Ultraviolet B |
| VDR | Vitamin D receptor |
| VKA | Vitamin K antagonist |
| WHO | World Health Organization |

**Key Points**
- Adequate nutrition is essential for innate and adaptive immune protection from viral infections.
- Malnutrition, including obesity and micronutrient deficiencies, increases risk for influenza infection in adults and children.
- Rising trends in global malnutrition burden are a serious public health risk for influenza epidemics and pandemics despite vaccination efforts.

## Brief Overview of Viruses

The International Committee on Taxonomy of Viruses (ICTV) is responsible for the taxonomic and nomenclature for all viruses. In general, viruses are classified by a variety of features: nucleic acid (DNA vs RNA), number of nucleic acid strands, conformation of the strands (linear, circular), sense (+ or − or antisense), presence or absence of 5′ terminal caps, terminal proteins or poly (A) tracts, morphology, physiochemical properties (e.g., stability to heat, pH), content and nature of proteins, lipids and carbohydrates, genomic organization and replication, antigenic properties, and biological properties (e.g., host range, mode of transmission, cell and tissue tropisms). Viruses have also been classified based on their nucleic acid alone, with dsDNA versus ssDNA viruses, and ssRNA further divided into − sense or + sense. Some viruses are enveloped, that is, they contain portions of the host cell membrane that cover the viral protein capsid. Because the viral envelope contains the lipid bilayer of the host cell, enveloped viruses are easier to neutralize with heat and detergents and have limited ability to survive for long periods of time outside of the host cell due their sensitivity to desiccation.

The complete viral taxonomy can be downloaded from the ICTV website (https://talk.ictvonline.org/taxonomy/). As of this writing, there is 1 phylum, 2 subphyla, 6 classes, 14 orders, 5 suborders, 143 subfamilies, 846 genera, and 4958 species of known viruses [1].

### Viral Structure and Replication

Viral structure and replication varies widely among viruses. In general, viruses use host cells for replication, as they are unable to reproduce without a host. Viruses outside of the host, referred to as virions, must enter a host cell in order to use the host's machinery for DNA and protein synthesis. Once inside, viruses reproduce by the lytic or lysogenic cycles. The lytic cycle refers to the immediate replication and spread of the virus, causing lysis of the host cell. In contrast, lysogenic replication involves incorporation of viral nucleic acid into the host cell's genome, allowing routine replication along with the host cell genome until conditions are more favorable and a lytic cycle can be triggered. A few examples of viruses important to human health are reviewed below as examples of the complexity of differences among viral species.

## Rotavirus (Reoviridae)

Rotaviruses are responsible for 34–50% of hospitalizations of young children and infants due to their ability to cause severe diarrhea. These viruses have a distinct morphology, similar to a wheel, made up of a well-defined rim with short spikes resembling wheel spokes (hence the name derived from the Latin word "rota," meaning wheel). Rotaviruses do not contain a viral envelope. Rotaviruses replicate in the enterocytes of the gastrointestinal tract, and their viral protein capsid makes them resistant to stomach acid. Entering the cell via endocytosis, the segmented dsRNA is used as mRNA for production of viral proteins and gene replication. Following assembly of the virus within the cell cytoplasm, the virus exits the cell by budding from the host membrane. Diarrhea results from loss of the infected enterocytes resulting in malabsorption. Rotaviruses generally spread through the fecal-oral route via direct (person to person) or indirect (through contaminated food and water) transmission [2].

## *Measles (Paramyxoviridae)*

Measles is a highly contagious non-segmented negative-sense RNA virus. The virus itself contains six structural proteins and two non-structural proteins. A transmembrane hemagglutinin protein is present on the surface of the virus, which binds to host cellular receptors found on a number of immune cells, including lymphocytes, monocytes, macrophages, and dendritic cells. The measles virus is also able to recognize and bind to an epithelial cell receptor present on a broad range of cell types, allowing infection of many cells and tissues. Measles virus is spread through respiratory droplets and initially infects immune cells of the respiratory tract. These infected immune cells then travel throughout the body, spreading the virus to almost all organ systems. In exiting the host cell, the virus picks up a lipid-containing envelope from the host cell membrane. Measles infection initially results in fever and cough, coryza (nasal inflammation), and conjunctivitis. The characteristic measles rash consisting of perivascular, lymphocytic infiltrates generally occurs 3–4 days after fever onset. In cases with complications, measles recovery usually occurs within 1 week of the appearance of the rash, due to control by the host immune response. Immunocompromised patients or undernourished children, particularly those with vitamin A deficiency, pregnant women, and young infants are at risk for measles complications. Complications can include pneumonia, diarrhea, and blindness and for pregnant women a risk of low birthrate, spontaneous abortion, and fetal and maternal death [3].

## *Herpes Simplex Virus* (Herpesviridae)

Herpes simplex viruses (HSV) 1 and 2 are large, double-stranded DNA viruses with an icosahedral capsid. There are at least 84 viral genes coded by both HSV-1 and HSV-2, which share about 83% of their aligned nucleotides. The host-derived lipid envelope contains 11 virally encoded glycoproteins. HSV enters host cells by binding to three different cellular receptors and fusing the viral envelope with the host membrane. Viral DNA then enters the nucleus where viral transcription, viral DNA replication, and assembly of new capsids occur. These viruses are able to establish latency, in which the virus fuses with the axon of nerves and travels along sensory fibers in a retrograde fashion to the ganglion of the trigeminal and sacral nuclei. The viral genome becomes circular during latency and produces latency-associated transcripts (LAT) that protect the neuron from apoptosis, ensuring survival of the latent virus. Physical or emotional stress or other stressors such as fever, trauma, or hormonal imbalances can trigger reactivation of the virus, whereby the virus travels back down the sensory nerves to cutaneous nerve endings resulting in a viral eruption in the skin. Viral transmission occurs through close physical contact, and because these viruses can become latent, individuals can have recurrent infections due to reactivation of the latent virus [4].

## *Ebola Virus* (Filoviridae)

Ebola virus is one of the deadliest of epidemic viral diseases, with a case mortality rate for Ebola Zaire strain of 88% and Ebola Sudan strain of 60%. However, with effective supportive care, the mortality rate can fall into the 40% range. Ebola virus is a non-segmented negative-strand RNA virus, which codes for seven viral proteins. The virus infects cells by attaching to a number of cellular molecules and enters cells mainly by micropinocytosis. Ebola outbreaks have occurred across the entire equatorial belt of Africa, frequently in areas where it had not been seen previously. The animal reservoir for Ebola has not been definitely identified, although migratory bats have been implicated. Human-to-human spread occurs via exposure of mucous membranes or nonintact skin to infectious body fluids or tissues. Ebola targets cells of the monocyte/macrophage lineage, including dendritic cells. These virus-infected cells then disseminate the virus throughout the bloodstream resulting in immune suppression and immune overactivation, disordered coagulation, tissue damage, hemorrhage, organ failure, and death within 10 days of symptom onset without adequate supportive care [5].

## *HIV* (Retroviridae)

Human immunodeficiency virus (HIV) has been pandemic for over 30 years, and advanced HIV disease was originally termed acquired immune deficiency syndrome (AIDS). Nearly all HIV infections are with type 1 (HIV-1). HIV-2 is less common and overall less virulent. A distinguishing feature of HIV is the reverse transcription of an RNA viral genome into a DNA copy, which is then subsequently integrated into the host genome. The HIV particle consists of a viral envelope surrounding a capsid core containing two copies of ssRNA and the viral enzymes reverse transcriptase, integrase, and protease. HIV attaches to the CD4 T cell receptor and the chemokine co-receptors CCR5 and CXCR5. This leads to fusion of the viral envelope with the host cell membrane, releasing the viral contents into the cytoplasm of the infected cell. Viral reverse transcriptase will then reverse transcribe the viral RNA into double-stranded DNA. This dsDNA will move into the host cell nucleus and will be incorporated into the host DNA by the viral integrase protein. This integrated viral DNA will be transcribed and translated into viral polyprotein using host cell machinery. Infection of CD4 T cells results in their destruction, making individuals infected with HIV highly susceptible to opportunistic infections and the development of tumors (see Chap. 3) [6]. Recent improvements in anti-retroviral drug treatments for HIV have resulted in infected persons living nearly as long as non-infected individuals, without developing the classical presentation of classic HIV-related disease (e.g., candidiasis, cryptococcosis, Kaposi sarcoma) (see Chap. 9) [7].

## *Hepatitis B* (Hepadnaviridae)

Rather than causing an acute, short-lived infection, infection with hepatitis B virus (HBV) can result in a chronic infection. It currently infects over 250 million people worldwide, and the resulting chronic inflammation causes 800,000 deaths annually due to liver cirrhosis and hepatocellular carcinoma. HBV, one of the smallest DNA viruses, is an enveloped virus with a nucleocapsid core enclosing a partially double-stranded DNA in a relaxed circle (rcDNA) along with a viral polymerase protein. The viral receptor is a bile acid transporter expressed on hepatocytes. Once bound to the receptor, the virus is internalized through clathrin-mediated endocytosis. The rcDNA is delivered to the nucleus where the rcDNA is converted into the covalently closed circular DNA (cccDNA) form, which constitutes the template for the viral transcription. The transcripts then move to the cytoplasm for translation into viral proteins. Once assembled, the viruses leave the infected cell by budding. The virus is not directly cytopathic, and the pathology observed in the liver is due to activation of cytotoxic T cells. Chronic infection with HBV is maintained by the presence of the cccDNA, which persists throughout the lifespan of the infected hepatocyte. Acute infections can be symptomatic with jaundice, fatigue, nausea, vomiting, and abdominal pain. Chronic HBV infection is broken down into three phases: the immune-tolerant phase with minimal liver inflammation, the immune-active phase associated with active liver inflammation, and the inactive hepatitis B phase, characterized by the presence of HBV antigen with mild or inactive liver disease. The inactive phase can last for decades, and about 20% of chronically infected patients develop cirrhosis, with a risk of hepatocellular carcinoma 100 times that of healthy controls. HBV is spread via sex with an infected partner, sharing of needles, from an infected mother to child, and by accidental needle sticks [8].

## *Hepatitis C* (Flaviviridae)

Similar to hepatitis B, hepatitis C (HCV) causes chronic liver infection. This spherical, enveloped, positive-strand RNA virus causes acute liver infection leading to viral peaks within the first 8–12 weeks [9]. The initial lytic phase is followed by a dormant and chronic infection phase similar to HBV. Unlike hepatitis B virus, there is currently no effective vaccine [10]. Thus, approximately 50–85% of infected individuals develop long-term hepatic infection often leading to fibrosis, cirrhosis, and hepatocellular carcinoma [10, 11]. HCV affects 3–5 million Americans with a global burden of 63–107 million [12]. Since identification in 1989, improved blood screening has reduced US incidence rates [13], with the highest at-risk populations remaining males born between 1945 and 1965 [11]. However, since 2006, resurgence in HCV incidence has occurred alongside growing rates of intravenous drug use in younger adults [14]. Recent advancements in direct-acting antiviral (DAA) therapy have allowed for nearly 100% curative rates of HCV by targeting the RNA polymerase, NS3/NS4 protease, and NS5A proteins of HCV [15, 16]. Nonetheless, due to lack of screening and high cost of DAA treatment, the public health burden of HCV remains high.

## *Rhinovirus* (Picornaviridae)

There are about 150 human rhinovirus (HRV) serotypes that are responsible for more than 50% of upper respiratory tract infections. The main site for HRV infections is the nasal mucosa. HRV are non-enveloped, ssRNA genome within an icosahedral protein capsid. The major group of HRVs binds the

ICAM-1 molecule on the surface of ciliated epithelial cells of the upper respiratory tract. Upon entering the cells through receptor-mediated endocytosis, the RNA is released into the cytoplasm whereupon the viral RNA is translated into a polyprotein, which is then cleaved into individual viral proteins. The viral progeny are released from the cells through a non-lytic mechanism. Although HRVs are mainly found in the upper respiratory tract, they can be found in ciliated epithelial cells of the lower respiratory tract as well. HRVs are transmitted person to person via contact (direct or through fomites) or by aerosol. HRV infection is generally self-limiting, causing what is typically known as the "common cold" ranging from asymptomatic infection to symptoms such as rhinorrhea, nasal congestion, sore throat, headache, and malaise. Despite the mildness of the illness, infections with HRV are responsible for a considerable economic burden estimated to be close to $40 billion annually in costs [17].

## *Coronaviruses* (**Coronaviridae**)

Coronaviruses comprise a family of enveloped positive-strand RNA viruses. The characteristic "corona" or crown-like morphology was first observed by electron microscopy in the late 1960s [18], giving rise to the family name. Coronaviruses infect numerous animal species including humans and can be divided into four main groups or genera: α, β, γ, and δ [19]. Generally, coronaviruses cause acute and chronic respiratory, enteric, and central nervous system (CNS) diseases. Predominant human coronaviruses, NL-63, OC43, and 229E, cause mild respiratory infections often referred to as the common cold [20]. In 2002 in Guangdong, China, emergence of a Severe Acute Respiratory Syndrome Coronavirus (SARS-CoV) marked the first accounted outbreak of severe coronavirus disease in humans. Two other severe coronaviruses have recently emerged in humans: the Middle Eastern Respiratory Coronavirus (MERS-CoV), which surfaced in 2012 in Saudi Arabia, and the Severe Acute Respiratory Coronavirus-2 (SARS-CoV-2), in 2019 from Wuhan, China [21]. This most recent novel β-coronavirus outbreak has sparked the Coronavirus Disease 2019 (COVID-19) pandemic, which has caused over 28 million confirmed global cases and 922,252 deaths as of September 14, 2020 [22].

   Coronaviruses consist of structural spike (S), membrane (M), envelope (E), and nucleocapsid (N) proteins. Importantly, SARS-CoV-2 infects humans primarily through the respiratory system, where the viral S protein binds the angiotensin converting enzyme 2 receptor (ACE2) of the host, allowing viral entry with the help of the viral transmembrane protease serine 2 (TMPRSS2) [19]. However, given the widespread expression of ACE2 in the heart, kidney, ileum, and bladder, SARS-CoV-2 can infect numerous tissues and has thus been considered an endothelial disease [23]. Individuals at high risk of severe COVID-19 include the elderly (>65 years of age), immunocompromised, pregnant women, children under 5 years, and individuals with comorbidities including chronic kidney disease, heart disease, hypertension, type 2 diabetes, and chronic obstructive pulmonary disease [24, 25]. A recent meta-analysis by Popkin et al. identified obesity as a significant driver of COVID-19 incidence, hospitalization, severity, and mortality [26]. Of particular worry, similar to individuals with obesity and influenza infection [27, 28], SARS-CoV-2 infection and/or vaccination may lead to a decreased memory immune response, which could increase the vulnerability of populations with obesity to reinfection. Morbidity and mortality from COVID-19 primarily result from the development of acute respiratory distress syndrome (ARDS) caused by the immune-generated cytokine storm [29–31]. Among 60 COVID-19 patients with clinical status varying from mild to critical and studied a median of 10 days post disease onset, more severe disease correlated with greater lymphopenia, activation of both innate and inflammatory pathways (e.g., excessive NF-kB-driven inflammatory response with higher IL-6 and TNF-α), and higher SARS-CoV-2 viral loads [32]. While both interferon (IFN) and TNF-α responses increased in

milder cases, they were diminished in more critical cases. The severe decline in type I IFN deficiency in the blood was a hallmark of critical COVID-19 disease in this case series and is now the
subject of research towards combined therapies. Early data suggests that asymptomatic infections
or coronavirus viral protection may be in part due to T-cell mediated immunity [33–35], and ongoing efforts continue to detail the immune response and pathophysiology of COVID-19 [36, 37].
Further, Zabetakis et al. summarize the influence of diet and nutritional status of key micronutrients
such as zinc, copper, vitamin D, and vitamin C on COVID-19 and speculate on how nutrient factors
may help ameliorate COVID-19 severity [38]. New information is constantly being added to
improve the understanding of SARS-CoV-2 and COVID-19.

## Influenza Virus: A Case Study

The influenza virus is a segmented, negative-strand RNA virus of the family *Orthomyxoviridae*. The
outer structure is composed of a lipid bilayer with two predominant glycoproteins, hemagglutinin
(HA) and neuraminidase (NA). These viral proteins facilitate viral entry and exit through binding of
sialic acid residues on host cells, allowing the influenza virion to infect host cells [39]. There are four
known types of influenza virus, classified as influenza A, B, C, and D. Influenza A and B cause most
human illness and have 8 RNA segments encoding 11 viral proteins. Influenza C and D both have 7
RNA segments with 9 viral proteins, with influenza C rarely occurring in humans and causing mild
illness [40] and influenza D mostly affecting cattle [41]. Influenza A viruses are further classified by
subtype depending on the HA and NA viral proteins, with HA having 18 different subtypes and NA
11. Other important proteins for influenza virus replication include the RNA-dependent RNA polymerase chain complex (PA, PB1, and PB2), the ion matrix channel protein (M), and the nucleoprotein
(NP) [42]. Current nomenclature for influenza viruses follows international standards set by the WHO
in 1979 [43], where influenza viruses are named by (1) antigenic type (A, B, or C), (2) host of origin,
(3) geographical region, (4) strain number, (5) year of isolation, and (6) the hemagglutinin or neuraminidase description (e.g., H1N1). For example, the 2009 pandemic swine flu caused by influenza A
(H1N1) virus is named "A/California/7/2009 (H1N1)."

Infection with influenza virus results in respiratory illness commonly referred to as the flu.
Symptoms include fever (over 100 °F), chills, headaches, fatigue, cough, and body aches or pains.
Unlike other respiratory viral infections, influenza has a fast onset and can last up to 14 days [44].
Transmission occurs between humans during colder winter months through airborne droplets of
infected hosts, causing significant morbidity and mortality [45, 46]. Influenza-related complications
include viral or bacterial pneumonia, dehydration, and death [47]. Due to their highly mutable
nature, influenza viruses go through continual antigenic drift as a result of minor changes in HA or
NA. This subtle adaptation allows the virus to evade the host antibody response and infect otherwise
immune-protected populations [48]. Occasionally influenza viruses can go through a major antigenic shift usually through a zoonotic transfer from swine or birds to humans, resulting in a dramatic
change in viral proteins and causing pandemic outbreak as evidenced by the 2009 swine H1N1 pandemic [49, 50].

Yearly vaccination remains the primary method of influenza prevention. In general, vaccines target
the adaptive immune system by eliciting immunological memory through a protective antibody
response and cellular or T cell response. For influenza vaccines, yearly formulations target HA proteins as they are the most abundant glycoprotein and critical for viral envelopment into the host cell
[39, 51, 52]. Antiviral therapies, however, target influenza NA proteins to prevent the spread of influenza after infection [40]. Despite these developments, each year 5–15% of the world population con-
tracts influenza virus, causing approximately half a million cases of severe illness, influenza-related

complications, and death. Importantly, young children, the elderly, and individuals with chronic diseases are particularly susceptible to influenza [53].

The remainder of this chapter will focus on what is currently known about the impact of nutritional status on influenza infection.

## Influenza and the Host-Nutrient Environment

Nutrition influences the immune response to infectious diseases in numerous ways. Figure 5.1 provides an overview of the immune response to influenza virus infection/vaccination and the points at which host nutrition impacts these responses. Micronutrients facilitate the production of enzymes, hormones, and other constituents essential for growth, development, and metabolism of innate and adaptive immune cells (see Chap. 3) [6]. Macronutrients provide the amino acid building blocks and metabolic fuels required for these cells to develop, function, and survive. On a global scale, malnutrition and infection remain the cause of over half of preventable deaths worldwide, especially in

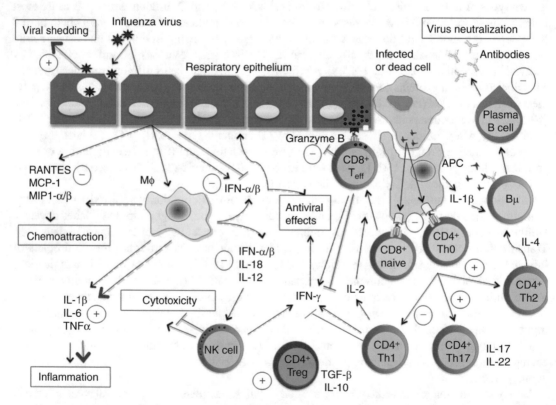

**Fig. 5.1** Immune response to influenza virus in the malnourished host. Influenza infection of the respiratory epithelium elicits a robust innate and adaptive immune response, hallmarked by production of chemoattractants, inflammatory cytokines, and neutralizing antibodies. In malnutrition (red), impairments in numerous immune response mechanisms result in greater inflammation and reduced viral clearance. These reductions in immune cell-mediated cytokine and antibody production increase risk of influenza morbidity and mortality. *IL* interleukin, *MCP* monocyte chemoattractant protein, *TNF* tumor necrosis factor, *IFN* interferon, *NK* natural killer cell, *RANTES* regulated on activation normal T cell expressed and secreted, *APC* antigen-presenting cell, *MIP* macrophage inflammatory protein, *TGF-β* transforming growth factor beta, $T_{reg}$ T regulatory cell, $T_{eff}$ T effector cell. (Reprinted with permission from Karlsson and Beck [257])

children [54]. However, recent trends in obesity rates in resource-rich and resource-poor nations demonstrate a strong link between obesity and infectious disease outcomes [55]. Lack of proper nutrition, whether it is micronutrient deficiencies, stunting or wasting from caloric malnutrition, or even obesity-related malnutrition, can lead to decreased immune function and increased susceptibility to infection [54, 56, 57]. What has become known as the "triple burden of malnutrition" is a concern for many resource-poor countries, in which stunting or wasting, micronutrient deficiencies, and obesity are all present together within the population.

Furthermore, infection can worsen malnutrition through several mechanisms such as infection-associated anorexia, altered metabolic rate, and altered dietary absorption, further complicating infection susceptibility and severity [58]. Indeed, the frequency of infectious diseases has been shown to increase the risk of poor nutrition [59]. Nutritional status of the host has also been shown to affect the invading pathogen itself. Host nutritional status, especially micronutrient status, can drive pathogen mutation and evolution [60]. Therefore, it is apparent that the interactions between nutritional status and infectious disease are not unidirectional and the degree of interplay between host, pathogen, and nutrition can become extremely complex (see Chap. 1) [61].

## Malnutrition, Obesity, and the Triple Burden

Malnutrition and infection remain a critical public health problem accounting for the largest number of preventable deaths and disabilities worldwide. Chronic undernutrition, which can lead to stunting, defined as low height for age, and/or wasting, low weight for height, is predictor of poor outcomes from infections [62]. For influenza virus, children under the age of 5 are at high risk for influenza infection, comorbidity, and death [63]. Further, malnutrition is recognized as a risk factor in this already vulnerable population. However, recent meta-analyses acknowledge the lack of information on undernutrition and influenza infection and on vaccination efficacy and effectiveness, especially for low- to middle-income countries like those in Africa [64, 65].

Recently, data from influenza-associated hospitalizations in two provinces of South Africa from 2012 to 2015 identified children under 59 months and adults over age 65 as having the greatest adjusted odds ratio (aOR) of influenza-related hospitalizations compared to individuals age 5–24, with similar findings to those seen in high-income countries. Alarmingly, malnourished children (2.4 aOR) and obese adults (21.3 aOR) had even greater risk of influenza hospitalization [66]. In mice, protein malnutrition has been shown to impair antibody production and cytotoxic CD8+ T cell function, while increasing lung inflammation and mortality following influenza infection (see Chap. 3) [6]. However, return to an adequate protein diet improved viral clearance and protective immunity upon influenza viral challenge [67].

Considered by some as a modern phenomenon, obesity has exploded within the past few decades [68]. Defined as a body mass index (BMI) or weight by height ratio of $30.0$ kg/m$^2$ or greater, obesity results from chronic excess caloric consumption beyond energy expenditure. For the first time in history in 2014, obese adults outnumber underweight adults worldwide, with 10.8% of men and 15.9% of women classified as obese [68]. In the United States alone, obesity prevalence has reached 36.5%, with another one third overweight (BMI 25.0–29.9 kg/m$^2$) [69]. Since its meteoric rise beginning in the 1960s, obesity has demonstrated a strong and causal relationship with chronic conditions like type II diabetes, kidney disease, and cardiovascular disease. This phenomenon and the various metabolic, psychological, and social factors responsible have been reviewed thoroughly elsewhere [70–72].

Obesity has also been linked to increased incidences of infectious diseases. Following the 2009 swine H1N1 influenza pandemic, obesity was recognized as an independent risk factor for greater influenza-related morbidity and mortality [73]. Obese subjects also have increased rates of hospitalization and death from both seasonal and pandemic influenza infection [74–76], with obese-related complications independent of other comorbidities [73]. Influenza vaccination of obese adults compared to lean adults results in decreased antibody response at 1-year post-vaccination [77]. Interestingly, influenza-vaccinated overweight and obese adults have decreased CD4+ and CD8+ T cell activation and function [51], with two times greater risk of influenza or influenza-like illness despite equivalent 30-day post-vaccination antibody response [78].

Unlike specific micronutrient deficiencies, obesity is a multisystem disorder and is inherently a metabolic disease characterized by alterations in systemic metabolism, including insulin resistance, elevated glucose levels, altered adipokines (e.g., increased leptin, decreased adiponectin), and lipid accumulation, contributing to the development of "metabolic syndrome." In any given year, roughly 3000–56,000 people die from influenza in the United States [79]. In pandemic years, as was the case in 2009 with the pandemic H1N1 influenza outbreak, roughly 500 million people in high-risk populations like children, the elderly, and the obese are at greater risk of influenza infection. Despite the observation of greater risk to obese individuals of influenza, the mechanistic causes of impairment against influenza immunity remain largely unknown. For insights into some potential mechanisms through which obesity may impair the immune response to influenza, refer to the work by Karlsson et al. [80].

## Vitamins and Influenza Virus

Vitamins are essential, organic nutrients that are critical for immune defenses. As organic compounds, vitamins are extremely susceptible to degradation by heat, pH, and air. Therefore, obtaining vitamins from food and other sources into the body can be difficult due to inactivation by cooking, storage, and even simple exposure to air. This instability and the fragile nature of these compounds and decreased access to a varied diet of fruits and vegetables mean that vitamin deficiencies are widespread in many developing countries. Vitamin deficiencies impair both innate and adaptive immunity and can be important immunomodulators during infection (see Chaps. 2 and 3) [6, 81]. Interactions of vitamins with the immune system and impact on influenza infection are outlined in Table 5.1.

### Respiratory Infections and Vitamin A

Vitamin A deficiency is a major nutritional concern, especially in low-income countries, and can lead to many health consequences. Xerophthalmia, the most specific vitamin A deficiency, is the leading preventable cause of blindness in children, and it is estimated that approximately 190 million preschool-aged children and 19 million pregnant women have low vitamin A status worldwide [82]. Vitamin A is vital for processes such as vision and reproduction [83]; however it is also apparent that vitamin A is important for the resistance to infection. Indeed, vitamin A deficiency is implicated as a major contributor to the high infectious disease mortality rates in young children [84, 85]. The role of vitamin A in immune function was first recognized at the beginning of the twentieth century, when it was dubbed the "anti-infective" vitamin [86, 87]. Since then, the role of vitamin A in modulating immunity and its anti-infective effects have been well studied for reducing the mortality of measles and diarrhea [85, 88], and vitamin A is integral in maintaining the respiratory and intestinal epithelium [89]. Vitamin A-deficient children have an increased risk of developing respiratory disease [90]. Interestingly, while it appears that correction of xerophthalmia can provide modest benefit in decreasing disease incidence [90, 91], studies suggest that vitamin A supplementation does not diminish severity or duration of respiratory infections and may slow recovery in individuals with normal

**Table 5.1** Vitamins and influenza response

| Vitamin | Other names | Possible functions in influenza infection and vaccination | Effects of deficiency | Effects of supplementation | Effects on vaccination | References |
|---|---|---|---|---|---|---|
| A | Retinol, retinal, retinoic acid, and several provitamin A carotenoids (e.g., β-carotene) | Epithelial barrier maintenance and function | Possible increased susceptibility to respiratory infection | No decrease in severity or duration of respiratory infections | Deficiency may result in decreased antibody response | [82, 86–99] |
| | | Antibody production | Decreased regeneration of respiratory epithelium | May slow recovery in individuals with adequate levels | Improved antibody response with supplementation | |
| | | | | Over-supplementation may exacerbate damage to respiratory tract | | |
| B | Pyridoxine, folate, $B_{12}$ | Possible immunocompromised state due to anemia | Increased burden of respiratory infections and impaired immune responses | Not yet fully studied | Deficiency associated with decreased antibody responses in vivo | [81, 100, 145–149] |
| | | Lymphocyte maturation, growth, and activity | | | Supplementation increases vaccine responses in humans | |
| | | Antibody production | | | | |
| C | Ascorbic acid | Enhanced immune function | Increased burden of respiratory infections and impaired immune responses | Possible beneficial effect of high-dose supplementation | Not yet fully studied | [81, 150–165] |
| | | Counteract free radicals and lipid peroxidation | | | | |
| D | Cholecalciferol, calcifediol, calcidiol | Inverse association between vitamin D status and respiratory tract infection prevalence | Inverse association between vitamin D status and respiratory tract infection prevalence | Supplementation may decrease incidence of viral respiratory infections—influenza-specific results inconclusive | Deficiency not conclusively linked with decreased antibody response | [106–128] |
| | | Altered expression of antiviral and inflammatory signals | | | | |
| E | Tocopherols, tocotrienols | Increases in lymphocyte proliferation, NK cell, and macrophage activity | Deficiency is extremely rare | Decreased morbidity and viral titers in vivo | Component of adjuvant vaccine therapies | [129–138] |
| | | Stabilize influenza-associated lipid peroxidation | | | | |
| | | Antibody production | | | | |
| K | Phylloquinone, menaquinone | Not yet fully studied | Not yet fully studied | Not yet fully studied | Vaccination during vitamin K agonist regimen can possibly increase anticoagulation | [139–142] |

vitamin A levels. Supplementation over dietary needs may even exacerbate damage to the respiratory tract by increasing the inflammatory response [88, 92–95].

The majority of epidemiological observations and clinical trials looking at vitamin A and respiratory infections have focused on all-cause pneumonia and respiratory syncytial virus (RSV) infections, so little is known about the specific association between influenza and vitamin A in the clinical setting. In the laboratory setting, neither vitamin A deficiency nor high-level dietary vitamin A influenced influenza morbidity or mortality or viral clearance in mice [96, 97]. Vitamin A deficiency did decrease regeneration of the normal respiratory epithelium in vitamin A-deficient mice, suggesting increased risk of secondary bacterial infections in individuals with xerophthalmia [97]. Changes in vitamin A status do appear to affect influenza A-specific immunoglobulin (Ig) levels, with deficiency decreasing the salivary IgA response and increasing serum IgG [97–99], while high-level dietary supplementation increases IgA and decreases IgG [96]. Therefore, the utility of vitamin A supplementation in treating or preventing influenza infection appears to be limited; however, in mice and humans, vitamin A supplementation has been shown to improve antibody responses to vaccination [56, 100–103], and vitamin A preparations have been successfully used as parts of adjuvant formulations [104].

## Influenza and Vitamin D

Vitamin D insufficiency and hypovitaminosis D are major global concerns, estimated to affect over one billion people worldwide [105–107]. Obtained through both diet and UV-mediated synthesis via exposure to sunlight, the classical role of vitamin D is to regulate calcium homeostasis and skeletal health, and deficiency is associated with rickets and osteoporosis (see Chap. 2) [81, 107]. However, the prevalence of the vitamin D receptor (VDR) throughout the body indicates vitamin D is important for more than skeletal health [108, 109]. The discovery that cells of the immune system express the VDR and can metabolize the active form of vitamin D (calcitriol; 1,25-dihydroxyvitamin D) suggests vitamin D is important for immune responses, especially expression of antiviral and inflammatory signals to combat infectious disease. Undeniably, vitamin D has since been shown to be important for the response to both bacterial and viral pathogens. The specific effects of vitamin D on the immune and adaptive response to infection have been reviewed previously [110–114].

Numerous in vitro studies demonstrate how changes in the immune system lead to increased risk of respiratory infections [115], and early studies in mice suggested a link between low vitamin D status and greater influenza infection [116]. In humans, an inverse association between serum vitamin D levels and incidence of respiratory infection has been observed in both adults and children [117]. Interestingly, it has been hypothesized that there may be a seasonal association between vitamin D status and influenza infection. While vitamin D can be obtained from dietary intake, very few foods naturally contain significant amounts of vitamin D. Therefore the most important source of vitamin D is through UV-B exposure from sunlight on the skin. Increased incidence of influenza (and other respiratory infections) occurs in the winter months during times of decreased sunlight and vitamin D levels; however, the seasonal fluctuations in vitamin D levels do not consistently match seasonal patterns in influenza, suggesting vitamin D is unlikely to be a significant factor in the seasonality of influenza [118]. In terms of vitamin D supplementation to prevent respiratory illness, UV radiation exposure and cod liver oil supplementation have both been found to decrease incidence of viral respiratory infections [119]; however, influenza-specific results have been inconclusive. Some studies have shown a modest protective effect, while others show no differences between supplemented and unsupplemented groups [120–123]. In the case of influenza vaccination, vitamin D deficiency has not been associated with decreased vaccine response [124, 125]. Meanwhile, data on vitamin D supplementation show some modest increases in vaccine response observed in vivo [102], but no conclusive evidence has been observed in human trials [126, 127].

## Influenza and Vitamin E

In humans, vitamin E deficiency is extremely rare. However, vitamin E deficiency does occur in infants and as a result of genetic abnormalities in fat absorption [128]. As a fat-soluble vitamin, Vitamin E functions as an antioxidant mainly by preventing the oxidation of polyunsaturated fatty acids in membranes [129]. Vitamin E is comprised of a family of tocopherols and tocotrienols. Alpha-tocopherol is the form preferentially secreted by the liver into the plasma for uptake by tissues. Vitamin E supplementation has also been shown to support the immune response and is associated with increases in lymphocyte proliferation in response to mitogen stimulation as well as NK cell and macrophage activity (see Chap. 2) [81]. In addition, vitamin E supplementation has been associated with increased resistance to infection, especially in the elderly [129].

Vitamin E supplementation has been found to significantly improve the response to influenza both in vivo and in human trials. Mice given vitamin E-supplemented diets display significantly decreased morbidity and lung viral titers following influenza infection compared to controls [130, 131]. Vitamin E supplementation was also shown to stabilize influenza-associated lipid peroxidation [132, 133]. In addition, when vitamin E supplementation was compared with other forms of antioxidants, vitamin E was the only effective agent at reducing both morbidity and viral titer following an influenza challenge, indicating that other mechanisms may be associated with vitamin E intake aside from its anti-oxidant properties [134]. Vitamin E supplementation has also been shown to alleviate secondary bacterial infection following an influenza challenge in a mouse model [135]. Vitamin E has also been found to be a potent component of adjuvant preparations, and α-tocopherol is a critical component of a new generation of squalene-containing oil-in-water emulsion adjuvants licensed for use in influenza vaccines [136, 137].

## Influenza Vaccination and Vitamin K

The role of vitamin K in coagulation and in skeletal health has been well established; however, vitamin K is one of the least studied vitamins in terms of its impact on immune function [138]. Vitamin K deficiency is rare in healthy adults, but newborn infants are particularly susceptible, and prophylactic vitamin K supplementation is common practice [139]. While the role of vitamin K in influenza infection has not been studied, there have been some reports that influenza vaccination can have negative interactions with vitamin K antagonist (VKA) therapies. Observational studies suggest that influenza vaccination during a VKA regimen could increase the anticoagulation function of these drugs. However, to date, this theory has not been proven, and clinical trials have indicated that influenza vaccination is safe in individuals receiving VKAs [140, 141].

## Vitamin B Complex and Influenza Vaccine Response

The B vitamin group consists of 8+ chemically distinct compounds that are vital for cell metabolism. The better understood B vitamins involved in immune function include $B_6$ (pyridoxine), $B_9$ (folate), and $B_{12}$ (cobalamin), which are implicated in cell proliferation and erythrocyte production as well as protein biosynthesis (see Chap. 2) [81]. Deficiencies in these nutrients result in anemia, making it difficult to determine whether the immunocompromised state is due to vitamin deficiency or from the more general state of anemia. Vitamin $B_6$ is essential for nucleic acid and protein biosynthesis and, therefore, is vital for antibody and cytokine production. Human $B_6$ deficiency and marginal $B_6$

deficiency result in decreased lymphocyte maturation, growth, and activity, as well as decreased antibody production, and supplementation can reverse these effects [142–144]. Vitamin $B_{12}$ is involved in one-carbon metabolism, and vitamin $B_{12}$-deficient patients have been shown to have altered lymphocyte populations and decreased NK cell activity [145]. In addition, $B_{12}$ deficiency has also been associated with decreased antibody response to vaccination [146]. Due to the difference in each of the B complex vitamins, it is difficult to determine the exact impact on influenza infection; however, deficits in vitamin $B_6$ and $B_{12}$ have been associated with a higher burden of respiratory infections and impaired immune responses in elderly individuals [147]. In addition, vitamin B deficiency has been associated with decreased antibody responses to influenza vaccination in mice [148], and $B_{12}$ supplementation has been shown to increase vaccine response in pregnant women [149].

## Influenza Infection and Vitamin C (Ascorbic Acid)

While severe vitamin C deficiency, also known as scurvy, is relatively rare in developed countries, almost 10–14% of the population is thought to be below the recommended dietary levels of vitamin C intake, mainly in low-income groups [150, 151]. Vitamin C is essential for mammalian health and is important in many vital processes throughout the body [152]. Interestingly, while vitamin C is synthesized from glucose in the liver of most mammalian species, humans, nonhuman primates, guinea pigs, and some fruit bats have evolved to lack the key enzyme to endogenously synthesize vitamin C [153]. Therefore, it is vital that humans have adequate vitamin C in their diets. As an antioxidant vitamin, the effects of vitamin C on the immune system have been well studied. Antioxidants, such as vitamin C, are particularly important for cells of the immune system that are exposed to high concentrations of reactive oxygen species (ROS) as a result of immune activation (see Chap. 2) [81]. While ROS play essential roles in killing invading pathogens, free radicals and lipid peroxidation are immunosuppressive, and antioxidants serve to counteract their effects [59, 142, 154]. Ascorbic acid markedly enhances immune functions, is found in high concentrations in leukocytes, and can be readily utilized during an infectious event. In addition, animals deficient in vitamin C have impaired immune function, and high levels of vitamin C can increase the immune response [138, 155, 156]. While the exact mechanism by which vitamin C enhances immune response has not been fully studied, it is generally accepted that vitamin C can "boost" immune function. Indeed, high daily intake of vitamin C has been considered to be preventive of many infections [157–159].

There has been considerable interest in vitamin C supplementation during influenza infection, spurred, perhaps, by Linus Pauling's famous claim that ascorbic acid has a physiologic effect on the common cold [160]. Since then, a number of studies have been conducted to observe the effects of ascorbic acid on respiratory infections both in vivo and in vitro. Based on reviews of these studies, vitamin C has been hypothesized as a potential preventative for the next influenza pandemic [161, 162]. Similar to the B complex vitamins, vitamin C deficiency has been associated with higher burden of respiratory infections and impaired immune responses [147]. In laboratory mice lacking the enzyme necessary to form endogenous vitamin C, ascorbic acid deficiency increased influenza-associated lung pathology but not viral titers [163]. In addition, vitamin C has been shown to be associated with the generation of antiviral cytokines critical for early protection against influenza infection [164]. While there appears to be some contention in the literature, clinical trials have shown a positive correlation between high-dose vitamin C supplementation and prevention of cold and flu symptoms; however, only a few trials have observed effects on clinically confirmed influenza. Supplementation of vitamin C to hospitalized influenza-infected patients appears to reduce the severity of influenza-related complications and duration of stay [165]. In addition to the immune effects, vitamin C has also been shown to have influenza-specific antiviral effects, significantly reducing influenza virus proliferation (Reviewed in [161, 162]). To date, no significant information is available on vitamin C status and response to influenza vaccination itself.

# Minerals and Influenza Virus

There has been a significant amount of research in the last part of the twentieth century and early twenty-first century establishing the importance of trace element nutrition in protection against infection. Generally, trace elements have been found to be extremely important for number and function of immune cells, and correction of deficiency can generally restore immune functionality [166]. Macrominerals include magnesium, calcium, phosphorous, and potassium. A large number of trace minerals have been found in human tissues, but only a few of these have been found to be essential for survival. These elements include cobalt, copper, iodine, iron, manganese, molybdenum, selenium, and zinc. There is a lack of consensus on the essentiality of arsenic, boron, nickel, and vanadium for human health; however, they are considered to be essential for some species. In addition, fluoride and chromium have also been implicated in human health. Deficiencies in essential trace elements can arise through inadequate intake from poor diet or from a number of secondary pathways including genetic factors, nutritional interactions, physiological stressors, and exposure to drugs or other chemicals or toxicants. Prolonged deficiency in an essential mineral can ultimately result in death of an individual. In addition to deficiency, host needs of these nutrients must be balanced since acute high-level or chronic low-level exposure can result in toxicity that can also have deleterious effects. While much remains to be learned about the interactions of these elements and resistance to influenza infection, several elements have been studied for their roles in the response to influenza. Interactions of essential trace elements with the immune system and impact on influenza infection are outlined in Table 5.2.

## *Calcium (Ca) and Influenza Viral Replication*

Calcium is required for bone formation, repair, and supporting skeletal growth. Due to the lack of biochemical indicators of Ca status, the global prevalence of calcium deficiency is unknown; however, it can be estimated by dietary intake. Ca intakes are the highest in North America and Europe, and the lowest intakes are found in developing countries, especially in Asia. The association between hypo- or hypercalcemia and influenza infection has not been well studied. However, Ca is also a critical cellular signal involved in numerous processes throughout the cell (see Chap. 2). Strong evidence supports the role of Ca in influenza A virus entry into the cell through Ca-binding domains on neuraminidase as well as Ca-dependent signaling involved in clathrin-mediated and clathrin-independent endocytosis of influenza A virus [167]. Several antiviral medications for influenza target Ca-mediated signaling in order to reduce symptoms and disease burden. For example, the Ca channel blocking drugs, verapamil and chlorpromazine, limit influenza viral replication by inhibiting calmodulin-dependent signaling and viral assembly [168].

## *Magnesium (Mg) and Influenza Inflammation*

Of the macrominerals, magnesium has been the most studied in connection to the immune response. While Mg deficiency is rare in humans, low serum Mg (hypomagnesemia) is quite common. It has been estimated that most population groups do not ingest the recommended daily allowance of Mg, most likely due to the increased consumption of refined and processed foods that are generally low in Mg. Indeed, only 48% of individuals in the United States are estimated to intake the recommended levels of Mg [169, 170]. Mg is involved in a

**Table 5.2** Minerals and influenza

| Macro/micro | Mineral | Chemical symbol | Possible functions in influenza infection and vaccination | Effects of deficiency | Effects of supplementation | Effects on vaccination | References |
|---|---|---|---|---|---|---|---|
| Macro | Calcium | Ca | Viral entry through Ca-mediated neuraminidase activity<br>Ca signaling targeted by antiviral medications | Not yet fully studied | Not yet fully studied | Not yet fully studied | [167, 168] |
| | Magnesium | Mg | Metabolic processes involved in immune cell function<br>Important for lung cell function | Thymic atrophy/decreased cellular and humoral responses<br>Low serum magnesium associated with hospitalization for acute respiratory infection in children | Not yet fully studied | Not yet fully studied | [53, 169–174] |
| | Phosphorous | P | Not yet fully studied | Not yet fully studied | Not yet fully studied | Not yet fully studied | [175] |
| | Potassium | K | Not yet fully studied | Not yet fully studied | Not yet fully studied | Not yet fully studied | [175, 176] |
| Micro | Copper | Cu | Essential for antioxidant properties associated with function of the immune system | Leads to impaired immune function | Can lead to immunosuppression | Not yet fully studied | [100, 177–184] |
| | Iron | Fe | Essential for function of the immune system | Decreased neutrophil function, decreased numbers and function of lymphocytes and NK cells, and decreased cytokine production<br>Increased susceptibility to infection | Can correct immunosuppression associated with iron deficiency<br>Iron overload and supplementation associated with increased susceptibility to infection | Deficiency leads to possible decreased humoral responses | [185–195] |

| | | | | | | |
|---|---|---|---|---|---|---|
| Selenium | Se | Essential for selenoproteins, notably glutathione peroxidase, involved in oxidative stress response of immune cells | Increased survival from influenza infection due to less lung inflammation. May allow more mutations in influenza viral genome | Supplementation reduced mortality in murine model | Not yet fully studied | [196–204] |
| Zinc | Zn | Essential for the functions of neutrophils, NK cells, and macrophages as well as the growth of T and B cells | Increased susceptibility to parasitic, viral, and bacterial infections | Possible decreased duration and severity of symptoms from respiratory disease. Possible decreased risk of upper respiratory tract infections and pneumonia | Supplementation can improve humoral responses. No beneficial effect observed for influenza vaccination | [81, 166, 205–215] |
| Arsenic | As | Damages lung function and potentially impairs immune protection in lungs | Not yet fully studied | Increased severity, morbidity, and mortality upon high exposure | Not yet fully studied | [216–226] |

number of metabolic processes including immune function (see Chap. 2). In experimental animal models, Mg deficiency has been associated with thymic atrophy as well as decreased cellular and humoral responses [171]. In addition, hypomagnesemia is considered to cause a pro-inflammatory state and is a potent inducer of a generalized inflammatory response in the body [172]. While very few studies have looked at hypomagnesemia or Mg deficiency in regard to influenza infection, there has been some association of low serum Mg with hospitalization for acute respiratory infection in children [173]. In addition, the inflammation associated with low Mg status has been implicated in exacerbating the development of both asthma and diabetes, known risk factors for susceptibility to severe influenza infection [53, 170, 174].

## Phosphorous (P)

Following Ca, phosphorous is the most abundant mineral in the body. While P deficiency in healthy individuals is rare, diabetes, celiac disease, starvation, and alcoholism can all decrease levels of phosphorous in the body. In addition, taking certain antacids and diuretics can also lower P levels [175]. The association between low P levels and influenza infection has not been well studied; however, low P is associated with high-risk conditions known to increase severity of influenza.

## Influenza and Potassium (K)

Potassium) is a vital nutrient in the body essential for nerve and muscle function. Hypokalemia (low K) can be a serious concern and, at its most severe, can lead to abnormal heart function. Most commonly, low K is a result of excessive loss through urination, vomiting, or the digestive tract [175]. While low K has not been associated with increasing influenza infection severity per se, influenza infection has been associated with causing low K through gastrointestinal distress associated with the clinical manifestations [176]. These deficiencies are mainly seen in high-risk groups such as the elderly and children who may develop more severe forms of disease.

## Influenza and Copper (Cu)

Copper is found in a number of foodstuffs and is required for several processes within the body. While Cu was clearly demonstrated to be an essential trace element for mammalian life in the 1920s and 1930s, Cu deficiency was not described until the 1960s. Severe Cu deficiency from food intake is rare; however, long-term, marginally acquired Cu deficiency may be underdiagnosed, as it has been estimated that 25% of people do not ingest the recommended amount of Cu. Cu deficiencies can also occur from genetic abnormalities, such as Menkes syndrome, or from secondary deficiencies associated with ingestion of other nutrients such as molybdenum [177, 178]. Similar to deficiencies in Vitamin E and selenium, Cu deficiency has been associated with increased levels of oxidative stress, and Cu is essential to the immune system in humans and animals for its antioxidant properties (see Chap. 2). Numerous studies have shown that both Cu deficiency and high intake can lead to impaired immune function [142, 179, 180] and increased severity of viral infection [181]. While humans and other mammals are generally protected from excess dietary Cu levels, Cu overload can occur via ingestion or genetic abnormalities [182]. Increased Cu intake has been shown to cause immunosuppression in mice [183]. While not much is known about Cu toxicity and influenza, severe complications from influenza infection have been associated with Wilson's disease [184].

## *Iron (Fe) and Influenza Infection*

Despite an abundance of iron on earth, Fe deficiency anemia is one of the most common nutrient deficiencies worldwide [185]. Several reviews have addressed the associations between Fe and the immune system [186–191]. Interestingly, Fe status can act as double-edged sword to the host. While Fe is necessary for proper immune function, invading pathogens also require access to Fe for replication and survival as well. Therefore, it is necessary for the host to restrict pathogen access to Fe while maintaining adequate Fe levels to mount an adequate immune response and to avoid excess Fe that could cause free radical damage. Many cells of the immune system play a part in this homeostasis, especially macrophages. The interactions between Fe and susceptibility to infection are complex. Fe is required for many aspects of the immune response, and inadequate intake of Fe can lead to decreased neutrophil function, decreased numbers and function of lymphocytes and NK cells, and decreased cytokine production (see Chap. 2) [81]. These changes can be reversed by Fe supplementation. In addition, many Fe-associated genes and proteins, such as transferrin and ferritin, are present in cells of the immune system and certain Fe-containing proteins, such as lactoferrin, have antimicrobial properties themselves [192]. Fe overload and supplementation have also been associated in vivo and in human populations with increased susceptibility to infection, especially from pulmonary tuberculosis and malaria.

Fe-containing enzymes have also been investigated for their antiviral activity against influenza. Lactoferrin has been found to inhibit influenza-associated cytopathic effects in vitro [193, 194]. While severe anemia has been associated with decreased humoral responses to influenza vaccination in the laboratory setting, it does not appear that moderate Fe deficiency severely impacts the humoral response in humans [195].

## *Selenium (Se) and Influenza*

Selenium has been shown to be particularly important for immune function (see Chap. 2) [196, 197]. Se is a naturally occurring, essential trace element, and the penultimate source of Se is from rocks and soils. Generally limestone and sandstone contain lower levels than shale. Se bioaccumulates in food chains, and dietary uptake of Se depends on concentrations in water and food sources. There are numerous places on the planet with inadequate Se in soil resulting in deficiency in humans and domestic animals fed with plants grown in Se-deficient soils [198]. Se is very important for several aspects of the immune system and susceptibility to disease. The significance of host Se status is based on properties of the amino acid selenocysteine acting as the catalytic center of several selenoenzymes such as glutathione peroxidase (GPx). Selenoproteins are involved in the activation, proliferation, and differentiation of cells that drive innate and adaptive immune responses (see Chap. 2) [81]. Dietary Se and selenoproteins are important for initiating or enhancing immunity, and they are also involved in immunoregulation, which is crucial for preventing excessive responses [197].

Yu et al. [199] demonstrated that supplementing mice with Se markedly reduced mortality from H1N1 infection. Although there were no differences in viral titers between supplemented and non-supplemented mice, decreased TNF-$\alpha$ and IFN-$\gamma$ in the non-supplemented group demonstrate that Se can enhance the immune response. A deficiency in Se has also been reported to alter epithelial cell morphology and the response to influenza infection [200]. Sheridan et al. [201] demonstrated that mice with reduced selenoproteins due to expression of a transgene carrying a mutant selenocysteine tRNA had altered chemokine levels and slower viral clearance. Interestingly, Li and Beck [202] saw an increased survival in Se-deficient mice infected with a highly pathogenic mouse strain of influenza, likely due to reduced lung inflammation as a consequence of Se deficiency. Finally, a deficiency in Se may allow increased mutations to occur in the influenza viral genome, presumably due to the reduced immune response [203, 204].

## Zinc (Zn) and Respiratory Infection

Zinc is vital for catalytic processes as well as functioning as a structural and regulatory ion. It can also act as an antioxidant, and Zn is an important element in prevention of free radical formation. The essentiality of Zn for animals and plants has been known since the mid-1800s; however, Zn deficiency was not thought to be an issue in humans until the mid-1900s when it was identified in populations in the Middle East. Today, it is estimated that Zn deficiency affects billions of individuals in the developing world, and even a small deficiency in Zn can have deleterious effects resulting in premature loss of life, most likely from increased susceptibility to infection. Approximately 12% of the US population does not consume the estimated average requirement of Zn. The interactions of Zn and the immune system have been recently reviewed, and Zn deficiency has been shown to be essential for the functions of neutrophils, NK cells, and macrophages as well as the growth of T and B cells (see Chap. 2) [81]. Zn-deficient individuals are thought to be extremely susceptible to parasitic, viral, and bacterial infections. While Zn supplementation can help to ameliorate immune defects in Zn deficiency, long-term, high-dose intake of Zn may provoke accumulation and subsequent immune deficiency [205–209].

While it does not appear that Zn intake has been directly correlated with incidence or severity of influenza infection, Zn has been found to be important for respiratory diseases. Zn supplementation has been shown to be beneficial for decreasing duration and severity of symptoms of the common cold in several studies [210]; however, others have shown no association. The differences in these trials may be due to inadequate sample sizes, dosages, or formulations to observe adequate protections. In addition, Zn supplementation has been shown to possibly decrease the risk of upper respiratory tract infections and pneumonia [166, 205]. In terms of vaccination, while Zn supplementation has been shown to increase seroconversion following an oral cholera vaccine in children [211] and can raise immune system responsiveness in immunocompromised individuals, no beneficial effect has been seen between Zn supplementation and influenza vaccination [212, 213]. Due to the high prevalence of mild Zn deficiency and the finding that Zn supplementation can improve immune response to infection, it has been suggested that Zn should be considered as a possible preventative therapy for influenza infection [214, 215].

## Arsenic (As) and Influenza

While there is a lack of consensus on the essentiality of arsenic for human health, As is a recognized toxicant and carcinogen. Hundreds of millions of people worldwide ingest excessive amounts of As through drinking water and food, and chronic exposure to As is considered a significant environmental health concern. In the United States alone, 25 million people may be exposed to As levels high above the standard for exposure through consumption of water from private wells [216–218]. Chronic As exposure is associated with a number of diseases including certain cancers, cardiovascular disease, and diabetes [216, 219–221]. As has been found to be a potent immunomodulatory agent [222].

Chronic As exposure has been associated with pulmonary effects such as cough and shortness of breath, and As has been linked with a number of pulmonary disorders such as impaired lung function, lung cancer, and chronic respiratory illness [216, 223]. Recently, As exposure has also been found to alter the immune response to influenza infection. Spurred by the ecological association between high As exposure in the Southwestern United States and Mexico and the emergence of the 2009 influenza H1N1 pandemic, it was hypothesized that chronic As exposure could exacerbate influenza infection. Mice exposed to high levels of As in their drinking water experienced significantly increased morbidity and viral titers compared to untreated controls following influenza infection, most likely due to a compromised immune response [224]. In addition, taking data from the 2009 pandemic, As exposure has also been quantitatively linked with severity of influenza infection in a dose-dependent manner [225]. Early life exposure to As can also affect the response to influenza virus infection. Mice exposed to As in utero and throughout postnatal life were infected with influenza at 1 week of age. Those exposed to As had reduced lung clearance of the virus and increased inflammation compared to mice not exposed to As. In addition, at 8 weeks post-influenza infection, As-exposed mice had increased airway hyperresponsiveness, with defects in lung mechanics [226]. While the mechanistic links between As exposure and increased risk of influenza infection are still being investigated, it does appear that chronic As exposure is associated with increased influenza severity.

## Life Stages Influence Micronutrient Needs and Influenza

### *Pregnancy/Breastfeeding*

The health and nutrition of pregnant and lactating woman has always been a major concern, and the nutritional and immune status of the mother can affect not only her own health but also the health of her child. During the gestational period, increased requirements for several nutrients can occur in varying amounts [227, 228]. The most frequent nutritional complication associated with pregnancy is anemia from Fe and/or folate deficiency [229]. In addition, pregnant women have increased requirements for other specific nutrients such as vitamin A and Zn [230, 231]. Indeed, approximately 80% of pregnant women worldwide may be Zn-deficient [232]. Aside from changes in nutritional status and their impact on immune function, the altered immune status of pregnant women required for fetal growth can also be favorable for the development of certain infections. The burden of pregnancy and influenza infection has been reviewed in depth elsewhere [233].

Lactation is even more nutritionally demanding for a woman than pregnancy and is also an extremely vulnerable time for the infant. Indeed, breastfeeding has been associated with protection from gastrointestinal and respiratory infections in infants [234]. In regard to influenza infection, maternal IgA from breast milk provides vital mucosal protection against influenza virus by directly binding sialic acid residues to the C-terminal portion of IgA, preventing neuraminidase activity [235]. This type of passive immunity, where antigen resistance is acquired from an external source like breast milk, helps provide protection for the infant while the infant's immune system develops. Additional immunological and non-immunological factors provide protective functions to infants against influenza infection. These include cytokines such as type I interferon (IFN), transforming growth factor (TGF) alpha, immune cells (B cells, macrophages, T cells, NK cells), and non-immune factors found in breast milk [236].

Aside from maternal IgA and IgM which help to protect the infant from infection, it is well known that milk also contains various non-antibody components with known antiviral activity, such as lactoferrin [192, 237]. Lactoferrin, found in the colostrum, inhibits influenza absorption while enhancing the cellular machinery in breast milk [238]. Other bioactive compounds such as glycans and lipoprotein lipases can prevent influenza infection through viral envelope inactivation and cell lysis [239, 240]. While vitamin A requirements increase only slightly during pregnancy, these requirements almost double during lactation since healthy term infants are born with very low stores of vitamin A and must obtain their stores from lactation. While many micronutrients remain adequate in breast milk despite maternal undernutrition, retinol in breast milk varies with maternal vitamin A status [241].

## Aging

In 2017, approximately 13% of the global population was aged 60 or older, and 2% were over the age of 80. These numbers are projected to triple by 2050 [242]. Aging is associated with significant undernutrition and subsequent adverse health outcomes [243]. Decreases in appetite and/or food intake result in "anorexia of aging" caused by a failure to ingest essential nutritional requirements. Coupled with physiological changes associated with aging, this anorexia can lead to significant deficiencies in a number of essential micronutrients [244]. Interestingly, in some populations, micronutrient deficiencies are directly associated with a high prevalence of overweight and obesity, suggesting high consumption of energy-dense but micronutrient-poor foods [245, 246].

Vitamin D appears to be particularly affected by aging. Several studies globally have found that the majority of free-living adults over 65 years of age have clinical vitamin D deficiency. Aside from Vitamin D, it is estimated that almost 15% of elderly individuals have low serum vitamin $B_{12}$ concentrations, and $B_{12}$ supplementation has been shown to increase innate and adaptive immunity in elderly populations [142, 247]. In addition, elderly individuals are also susceptible to Zn deficiency. It is estimated that 40% of men and 45% of women over the age of 50 consume less than the estimated requirement of Zn and that plasma Zn levels decline with age [248]. Low serum Zn was associated with increased risk of mortality, and elderly individuals with normal Zn levels had decreased incidence and duration of pneumonia [249].

It is well established that adults over the age of 65 have greater risk of influenza morbidity and mortality [63, 250]. For this reason, elderly adults represent a major population group targeted for influenza vaccination programs to help reduce influenza burden. Vaccine effectiveness in elderly adults has long been a contentious point, suggested as the primary cause for greater risk in the elderly compared to younger adults. Russell et al. [251] compared vaccine effectiveness (VE) of adults over 65 with younger adults from 2011–2012 to 2015–2016. Their analysis of 20,022 adults contained 4785 confirmed cases (24%) of influenza within the United States, finding no difference in VE between subjects 18–49 years and adults ≥65 years. Furthermore, they found no difference in VE influenza subtype (A/H1N1, A/H3N2, or B lineage) [251]. However, influenza vaccine effectiveness for elderly adults has previously been reported to be significantly lower in some vaccine seasons [252, 253], with VE low during years when A/H3N2 was the dominant circulating strain [254]. Decreases in nutritional status have been significantly associated with the decreased vaccine responsiveness of elderly individuals compared with nutritionally adequate controls [255].

## The Future of Nutrition at the Host-Influenza Interface

As seen in this chapter, the influence of nutrition on influenza is complex. Influenza provides an important case study because of the continuous threat of global pandemics from these viruses. This significant public health threat was dramatically shown with the so-called "Spanish flu" epidemic of 1918. Over 50 million persons, mostly previously healthy young adults, are thought to have died on 6 continents; perhaps the worst pandemic in world history until the HIV/AIDS epidemic was recognized in 1981 [256]. Influenza pandemics continue to occur, increasing the death rate beyond the "usual" rate of typical seasonal influenza infections. Because of the ability of segmented influenza virus genome to re-assort and our close proximity to both porcine and avian hosts, we face the risk of a human-adapted strain that might integrate genetic material from a more virulent avian- or porcine-adapted influenza strain, making a new human pathogen far more lethal. As we have shown in this chapter, the nutritional status of the host can make individuals more susceptible, both to epidemic and pandemic strains of virus.

Over- and undernutrition, as well as micronutrient deficiencies, play a significant role in increasing the risk of influenza morbidity and mortality. The global prevalence of the triple burden of malnutrition (underweight, overweight, and micronutrient deficiencies together) coupled with endemic, emerging, and re-emerging infectious diseases makes it imperative to continue to understand the nutrition-infection-immunity axis. The increase in obesity and other non-communicable diseases as well as the consumption of energy-dense and nutrient-poor foods means that micronutrient deficiencies and obesity will continue to be a problem while being coupled with other high-risk nutritional states. Interestingly, these deficiencies can occur not only in humans but also in animals that can act as vectors and reservoirs such as poultry and swine. Improving nutritional health worldwide is imperative for reducing the burden of infectious diseases, including influenza.

# References

 1. Lefkowitz EJ, Dempsey DM, Hendrickson RC, Orton RJ, Siddell SG, Smith DB. Virus taxonomy: the database of the international committee on taxonomy of viruses (ICTV). Nucleic Acids Res. 2018;46(D1):D708–17.
 2. Esona MD, Gautam R. Rotavirus. Clin Lab Med. 2015;35(2):363–91.
 3. Moss WJ. Measles. Lancet. 2017;390(10111):2490–502.
 4. Widener RW, Whitley RJ. Herpes simplex virus. Handb Clin Neurol. 2014;123:251–63.
 5. Baseler L, Chertow DS, Johnson KM, Feldmann H, Morens DM. The pathogenesis of Ebola virus disease. Annu Rev Pathol. 2017;12:387–418.
 6. Stephensen CB. Primer on immune response and interface with malnutrition. In: Humphries DL, Scott ME, Vermund SH, editors. Nutrition and infectious disease: shifting the clinical paradigm. Switerzerland: Springer Nature; 2020.
 7. Lucas S, Nelson AM. HIV and the spectrum of human disease. J Pathol. 2015;235(2):229–41.
 8. Karayiannis P. Hepatitis B virus: virology, molecular biology, life cycle and intrahepatic spread. Hepatol Int. 2017;11(6):500–8.
 9. Basit H, Tyagi I, Koirala J. Hepatitis C. [Updated 2019 May 15]. In: StatPearls [Internet]. Treasure Island FL: StatPearls Publishing; 2019. https://www.ncbi.nlm.nih.gov/books/NBK430897/. Accessed 12 Oct 2019.
10. Li H-C, Lo S-Y. Hepatitis C virus: virology, diagnosis and treatment. World J Hepatol. 2015;7(10):1377–89.
11. Mukhtar NA, Ness EM, Jhaveri M, Fix OK, Hart M, Dale C, et al. Epidemiologic features of a large hepatitis C cohort evaluated in a major health system in the western United States. Ann Hepatol. 2019;18(2):360–5.
12. Manns MP, Buti M, Gane E, Pawlotsky JM, Razavi H, Terrault N, et al. Hepatitis C virus infection. Nat Rev Dis Primers. 2017;3:17006.
13. Rosenberg ES, Hall EW, Sullivan PS, Sanchez TH, Workowski KA, Ward JW, et al. Estimation of state-level prevalence of hepatitis C virus infection, US states and District of Columbia, 2010. Clin Infect Dis. 2017;64(11):1573–81.
14. Suryaprasad AG, White JZ, Xu F, Eichler BA, Hamilton J, Patel A, et al. Emerging epidemic of hepatitis C virus infections among young nonurban persons who inject drugs in the United States, 2006–2012. Clin Infect Dis. 2014;59(10):1411–9.
15. Burstow NJ, Mohamed Z, Gomaa AI, Sonderup MW, Cook NA, Waked I, et al. Hepatitis C treatment: where are we now? Int J Gen Med. 2017;10:39–52.
16. Zeuzem S. Treatment options in hepatitis C. Dtsch Arztebl Int. 2017;114(1–02):11–21.
17. Jacobs SE, Lamson DM, St George K, Walsh TJ. Human rhinoviruses. Clin Microbiol Rev. 2013;26(1):135–62.
18. Tyrell DA. Coronaviruses. Nature, (London). 1968;220:650.
19. Yuki K, Fujiogi M, Koutsogiannaki S. COVID-19 pathophysiology: A review. Clin Immunol. 2020;215:108427.
20. Weiss SR, Navas-Martin S. Coronavirus Pathogenesis and the Emerging Pathogen Severe Acute Respiratory Syndrome Coronavirus. Microbiol Mol Biol Rev. 2005;69(4):635–64.
21. Peeri NC, Shrestha N, Rahman MS, Zaki R, Tan Z, Bibi S, et al. The SARS, MERS and novel coronavirus (COVID-19) epidemics, the newest and biggest global health threats: what lessons have we learned? Int J Epidemiol. 2020;49(3):717–26.
22. WHO coronavirus disease (COVID-19) dashboard. Geneva: World Health Organization. Available Online: https://covid19.who.int/. Last cited: 14 Sept 2020.

23. Libby P, Lüscher T. COVID-19 is, in the end, an endothelial disease. Eur Heart J. 2020;41(32):3038–44.
24. Petrilli CM, Jones SA, Yang J, Rajagopalan H, O'Donnell LF, Chernyak Y, et al. Factors associated with hospitalization and critical illness among 4,103 patients with COVID-19 disease in New York City. medRxiv. 2020:2020.04.08.20057794.
25. Richardson SHJ, Narasimhan M, Crawford JM, McGinn T, Davidson KW, Barnaby DP, Becker LB, Chelico JD, Cohen SL, Cookingham J, Coppa K, Diefenbach MA, Dominello AJ, Duer-Hefele J, Falzon L, Gitlin J, Hajizadeh N, Harvin TG, Hirschwerk DA, Kim EJ, Kozel ZM, Marrast LM, Mogavero JN, Osorio GA, Qiu M, Zanos TP, the Northwell COVID-19 Research Consortium. Presenting characteristics, comorbidities, and outcomes among 5700 patients hospitalized With COVID-19 in the New York City Area. JAMA. 2020;323(20):2052–9.
26. Popkin BM, Du S, Green WD, Beck MA, Algaith T, Herbst CH, et al. Individuals with obesity and COVID-19: A global perspective on the epidemiology and biological relationships. Obes Rev. 2020;21(11):1–17. https://doi.org/10.1111/obr.13128.
27. Paich HA, Sheridan PA, Handy J, Karlsson EA, Schultz-Cherry S, Hudgens MG, et al. Overweight and obese adult humans have a defective cellular immune response to pandemic H1N1 influenza A virus. Obes (Silver Spring). 2013;21(11):2377–86.
28. Neidich SD, Green WD, Rebeles J, Karlsson EA, Schultz-Cherry S, Noah TL, et al. Increased risk of influenza among vaccinated adults who are obese. Int J Obes (Lond). 2017;41:1324–30.
29. Moore BJB, June CH. Cytokine release syndrome in severe COVID-19. Science. 2020;368(6490):473–4.
30. Ruan Q, Yang K, Wang W, Jiang L, Song J. Clinical predictors of mortality due to COVID-19 based on an analysis of data of 150 patients from Wuhan, China. Intensive Care Med. 2020;46(5):846–8.
31. Mehta P, McAuley DF, Brown M, Sanchez E, Tattersall RS, Manson JJ. COVID-19: consider cytokine storm syndromes and immunosuppression. Lancet (London, England). 2020;395(10229):1033–4.
32. Hadjadj J, Yatim N, Barnabei L, Corneau A, Boussier J, Smith N, et al. Impaired type I interferon activity and inflammatory responses in severe COVID-19 patients. Science. 2020;369(6504):718–24.
33. Le Bert N, Tan AT, Kunasegaran K, Tham CYL, Hafezi M, Chia A, et al. SARS-CoV-2-specific T cell immunity in cases of COVID-19 and SARS, and uninfected controls. Nature. 2020;584(7821):457–62.
34. Braun J, Loyal L, Frentsch M, Wendisch D, Georg P, Kurth F, et al. Presence of SARS-CoV-2 reactive T cells in COVID-19 patients and healthy donors. medRxiv. 2020;2020.04.17.20061440.
35. Grifoni A, Weiskopf D, Ramirez SI, Mateus J, Dan JM, Moderbacher CR, et al. Targets of T cell responses to SARS-CoV-2 coronavirus in humans with COVID-19 disease and unexposed individuals. Cell. 2020;181(7):1489–501.e15.
36. Tay MZ, Poh CM, Renia L, MacAry PA, Ng LFP. The trinity of COVID-19: immunity, inflammation and intervention. Nat Rev Immunol. 2020;20(6):363–74.
37. Vabret N, Britton GJ, Gruber C, Hegde S, Kim J, Kuksin M, et al. Immunology of COVID-19: current state of the science. Immunity. 2020;52(6):910–41.
38. Zabetakis I, Lordan R, Norton C, Tsoupras A. COVID-19: the inflammation link and the role of nutrition in potential mitigation. Nutrients. 2020;12(5):1466.
39. Shi Y, Wu Y, Zhang W, Qi J, Gao GF. Enabling the 'host jump': structural determinants of receptor-binding specificity in influenza A viruses. Nat Rev Microbiol. 2014;12(12):822–31.
40. Kamps BS, Hoffmann C, Preiser W, Behrens G. Influenza report 2006: Paris: Flying Publisher; 2006. www.influenzareport.com. Accessed 12 Oct 2019.
41. Centers for Disease Control. Types of influenza viruses 2017 [updated September 15, 2016]. https://www.cdc.gov/flu/about/viruses/types.htm. Accessed 12 Oct 2019.
42. Bouvier NM, Palese P. The biology of influenza viruses. Vaccine. 2008;26(Suppl 4):D49–53.
43. WHO. A revision of the system of nomenclature for influenza viruses: a WHO memorandum. Bull World Health Organ. 1980;58(4):585–91.
44. Banning M. Influenza: incidence, symptoms and treatment. Br J Nurs. 2005;14(22):1192–7.
45. Murphy B, Webster R. Orthomyxoviruses. 3rd ed. Fields B, ed. Philadelphia: Lippincott-Raven; 1997.
46. Lowen AC, Mubareka S, Steel J, Palese P. Influenza virus transmission is dependent on relative humidity and temperature. PLoS Pathog. 2007;3(10):1470–6.
47. Advisory Committee on Immunization Practices Prevention and Control of Influenza. Recommendations of the advisory committee on immunization practices (ACIP). MMWR Recomm Rep. 2006;55(RR-10):1–42.
48. Treanor J. Influenza vaccine—outmaneuvering antigenic shift and drift. N Engl J Med. 2004;350(3):218–20.
49. Michaelis M, Doerr H, Cinatl J. An influenza A H1N1 virus revival pandemic H1N1/09 virus. Infection. 2009;37(5):381–9.
50. Cohen J, Enserink M. After delays, WHO agrees: the 2009 pandemic has begun. Science. 2009;324(5934):1496–7.
51. Paich HA, Sheridan PA, Handy J, Karlsson EA, Schultz-Cherry S, Hudgens MG, et al. Overweight and obese adult humans have a defective cellular immune response to pandemic H1N1 influenza A virus. Obesity (Silver Spring). 2013;21(11):2377–86.
52. Ito T, Couceiro JN, Kelm S, Baum LG, Krauss S, Castrucci MR, et al. Molecular basis for the generation in pigs of influenza a viruses with pandemic potential. J Virol. 1998;72(9):7367–73.

53. World Health Organization. WHO factsheet 211: influenza (seasonal). Geneva: World Health Organization; 2009. http://www.who.int/mediacentre/factsheets/fs211/en/index.htm. Accessed 7 Oct 2019.
54. Ibrahim MK, Zambruni M, Melby CL, Melby PC. Impact of childhood malnutrition on host defense and infection. Clin Microbiol Rev. 2017;30(4):919–71.
55. Huttunen R, Syrjanen J. Obesity and the risk and outcome of infection. Int J Obes. 2013;37(3):333–40.
56. Wintergerst ES, Maggini S, Hornig DH. Contribution of selected vitamins and trace elements to immune function. Ann Nutr Metab. 2007;51(4):301–23.
57. Labadarios D, Steyn NP. Nutritional disorders in Africa: the triple burden. Nutrition. 2005;21(1):2–3.
58. Thurnham DI, Northrop-Clewes CA. Effects of infection on nutritional and immune status. In: Hughes DA, Darlington LG, Bendich A, editors. Diet and human immune function. Nutrition and health. Totowa: Humana Press; 2004. p. 35–66.
59. Calder PC, Jackson AA. Undernutrition, infection and immune function. Nutr Res Rev. 2002;13:3–29.
60. Beck MA, Handy J, Levander OA. Host nutritional status: the neglected virulence factor. Trends Microbiol. 2004;12(9):417–23.
61. Humphries DL, Scott ME, Vermund SH. Pathways linking nutritional status and infectious disease. In: Humphries D, Scott ME, Vermund SH, editors. Nutrition and infectious disease: shifting the clinical paradigm. Cham: Springer Nature; 2020.
62. Caulfield LE, Richard SA, Rivera JA, Musgrove P, Black RE. Stunting, wasting, and micronutrient deficiency disorders. Disease control priorities in developing countries. 2nd ed. Washington, DC: The International Bank for Reconstruction and Development/The World Bank; 2006.
63. Zhou H, Thompson WW, Viboud CG, Ringholz CM, Cheng PY, Steiner C, et al. Hospitalizations associated with influenza and respiratory syncytial virus in the United States, 1993–2008. Clin Infect Dis. 2012;54(10):1427–36.
64. Lindsey BB, Armitage EP, Kampmann B, de Silva TI. The efficacy, effectiveness, and immunogenicity of influenza vaccines in Africa: a systematic review. Lancet Infect Dis. 2019;19(4):e110–e9.
65. Fischer WA 2nd, Gong M, Bhagwanjee S, Sevransky J. Global burden of influenza as a cause of cardiopulmonary morbidity and mortality. Glob Heart. 2014;9(3):325–36.
66. Tempia S, Walaza S, Moyes J, Cohen AL, von Mollendorf C, Treurnicht FK, et al. Risk factors for influenza-associated severe acute respiratory illness hospitalization in South Africa, 2012–2015. Open Forum Infect Dis. 2017;4(1):ofw262.
67. Taylor AK, Cao W, Vora KP, De La Cruz J, Shieh WJ, Zaki SR, et al. Protein energy malnutrition decreases immunity and increases susceptibility to influenza infection in mice. J Infect Dis. 2013;207(3):501–10.
68. Collaboration NRF. Trends in adult body-mass index in 200 countries from 1975 to 2014: a pooled analysis of 1698 population-based measurement studies with 19.2 million participants. Lancet. 2016;387:1377–96.
69. Ogden CL, Carroll MD, Fryar CD, Flegal KM. Prevalence of obesity among adults and youth- United States, 2011–2014. NCHS data brief. 2015;no 219.
70. Mitchell NS, Catenacci VA, Wyatt HR, Hill JO. Obesity: overview of an epidemic. Psychiatr Clin North Am. 2011;34(4):717–32.
71. Roth J, Sahota N, Patel P, Mehdi SF, Wiese MM, Mahboob HB, et al. Obesity paradox, obesity orthodox, and the metabolic syndrome: an approach to unity. Mol Med. 2016;22:873–85.
72. Jung UJ, Choi M-S. Obesity and its metabolic complications: the role of Adipokines and the relationship between obesity, inflammation, insulin resistance, dyslipidemia and nonalcoholic fatty liver disease. Int J Mol Sci. 2014;15(4):6184–223.
73. Louie JK, Acosta M, Samuel MC, Schechter R, Vugia DJ, Harriman K, et al. A novel risk factor for a novel virus: obesity and 2009 pandemic influenza A (H1N1). Clin Infect Dis. 2011;52(3):301–12.
74. Kwong JC, Campitelli MA, Rosella LC. Obesity and respiratory hospitalizations during influenza seasons in Ontario, Canada: a cohort study. Clin Infect Dis. 2011;53(5):413–21.
75. Yu H, Feng Z, Uyeki TM, Liao Q, Zhou L, Feng L, et al. Risk factors for severe illness with 2009 pandemic influenza A (H1N1) virus infection in China. Clin Infect Dis. 2011;52(4):457–65.
76. Morgan OW, Bramley A, Fowlkes A, Freedman DS, Taylor TH, Gargiullo P, et al. Morbid obesity as a risk factor for hospitalization and death due to 2009 pandemic influenza A (H1N1) disease. PLoS ONE. 2010;5(3):e9694.
77. Sheridan PA, Paich HA, Handy J, Karlsson EA, Schultz-Cherry S, Hudgens M, et al. The antibody response to influenza vaccination is not impaired in type 2 diabetics. Vaccine. 2015;33(29):3306–13.
78. Neidich SD, Green WD, Rebeles J, Karlsson EA, Schultz-Cherry S, Noah TL, et al. Increased risk of influenza among vaccinated adults who are obese. Int J Obes. 2017;41:1324–30.
79. Centers for Disease Control and Prevention (CDC). Estimates of deaths associated with seasonal influenza—United States, 1976–2007. Morb Mortal Wkly Rep. 2010;59(33):1057–89.
80. Karlsson EA, Milner JJ, Green WD, Rebeles J, Schultz-Cherry S, Beck MA. Chapter 10—influence of obesity on the response to influenza infection and vaccination. In: Johnston RA, Suratt BT, editors. Mechanisms and manifestations of obesity in lung disease. Cambridge, MA: Academic Press; 2019. p. 227–59.
81. Barffour MA, Humphries DL. Core principles: infectious disease risk in relation to macro and micronutrient status. In: Humphries DL, Scott ME, Vermund SH, editors. Nutrition and infectious disease: shifting the clinical paradigm. Cham: Springer Nature; 2020.

82. World Health Organization. Global prevalence of vitamin A deficiency in populations at risk 1995–2005. WHO global database on vitamin A deficiency. Geneva: World Health Organization; 2009.

83. Rucker R. Vitamins: overview and metabolic functions. In: Gershwin ME, German JB, Keen CL, editors. Nutrition and immunology: principles and practice. Totowa: Humana Press; 2000.

84. Sommer A, Davidson FR, Annecy A. Assessment and control of vitamin A deficiency: the Annecy accords. J Nutr. 2002;132(9 Suppl):2845S–50S.

85. Glasziou PP, Mackerras DE. Vitamin A supplementation in infectious diseases: a meta-analysis. BMJ. 1993;306(6874):366–70.

86. Greene HN, Mellanby E. Vitamin A as an anti-infectve agent. BMJ. 1928;2:691–6.

87. Semba RD. Vitamin A as "anti-infective" therapy. J Nutr. 1999;129:783–91.

88. Stephenson CB. Vitamin A, infection, and immune function. Annu Rev Nutr. 2001;21:167–92.

89. Maggini S, Wintergerst ES, Beveridge S, Hornig DH. Selected vitamins and trace elements support immune function by strengthening epithelial barriers and cellular and humoral immune responses. Br J Nutr. 2007;98(S1):S29–35.

90. Sommer A, Katz J, Tarwotjo I. Increased risk of respiratory disease and diarrhea in children with preexisting mild vitamin A deficiency. Am J Clin Nutr. 1984;40(5):1090–5.

91. Bloem MW, Hye A, Wijnroks M, Ralte A, West KP Jr, Sommer A. The role of universal distribution of vitamin A capsules in combatting vitamin A deficiency in Bangladesh. Am J Epidemiol. 1995;142(8):843–55.

92. Abdeljaber MH, Monto AS, Tilden RL, Schork MA, Tarwotjo I. The impact of vitamin A supplementation on morbidity: a randomized community intervention trial. Am J Public Health. 1991;81(12):1654–6.

93. Bresee JS, Fischer M, Dowell SF, Johnston BD, Biggs VM, Levine RS, et al. Vitamin A therapy for children with respiratory syncytial virus infection: a multicenter trial in the United States. Pediatr Infect Dis J. 1996;15(9):777–82.

94. Dibley MJ, Sadjimin T, Kjolhede CL, Moulton LH. Vitamin A supplementation fails to reduce incidence of acute respiratory illness and diarrhea in preschool-age Indonesian children. J Nutr. 1996;126(2):434–42.

95. Stephenson CB, Franchi LM, Hernandez H, Campos M, Gilman RH, Alvarez JO. Adverse effects of high-dose vitamin A supplements in children hospitalized with pneumonia. Pediatrics. 1998;101:e3.

96. Cui D, Moldoveanu Z, Stephensen CB. High-level dietary vitamin A enhances T-helper type 2 cytokine production and secretory immunoglobulin A response to influenza A virus infection in BALB/c mice. J Nutr. 2000;130(5):1132–9.

97. Stephensen CB, Blount SR, Schoeb TR, Park JY. Vitamin A deficiency impairs some aspects of the host response to influenza A virus infection in BALB/c mice. J Nutr. 1993;123(5):823–33.

98. Gangopadhyay NN, Moldoveanu Z, Stephensen CB. Vitamin A deficiency has different effects on immunoglobulin A production and transport during influenza A infection in BALB/c mice. J Nutr. 1996;126(12):2960–7.

99. Stephensen CB, Moldoveanu Z, Gangopadhyay NN. Vitamin A deficiency diminishes the salivary immunoglobulin A response and enhances the serum immunoglobulin G response to influenza A virus infection in BALB/c mice. J Nutr. 1996;126(1):94–102.

100. Surman SL, Rudraraju R, Sealy R, Jones B, Hurwitz JL. Vitamin A deficiency disrupts vaccine-induced antibody-forming cells and the balance of IgA/IgG isotypes in the upper and lower respiratory tract. Viral Immunol. 2012;25(4):341–4.

101. Hanekom WA, Yogev R, Heald LM, Edwards KM, Hussey GD, Chadwick EG. Effect of vitamin A therapy on serologic responses and viral load changes after influenza vaccination in children infected with the human immunodeficiency virus. J Pediatr. 2000;136(4):550–2.

102. Surman SL, Penkert RR, Jones BG, Sealy RE, Hurwitz JL. Vitamin supplementation at the time of immunization with a cold-adapted influenza virus vaccine corrects poor mucosal antibody responses in mice deficient for vitamins A and D. Clin Vaccine Immunol. 2016;23(3):219–27.

103. Jones BG, Oshansky CM, Bajracharya R, Tang L, Sun Y, Wong SS, et al. Retinol binding protein and vitamin D associations with serum antibody isotypes, serum influenza virus-specific neutralizing activities and airway cytokine profiles. Clin Exp Immunol. 2016;183(2):239–47.

104. Patel S, Faraj Y, Duso KD, Reiley WW, Karlsson AE, Schultz-Cherry S, et al. Comparative safety and efficacy profile of a novel oil in water vaccine adjuvant comprising vitamins A and E and a Catechin in protective anti-influenza immunity. Nutrients. 2017;9(5):516.

105. Mithal A, Wahl DA, Bonjour JP, Burckhardt P, Dawson-Hughes B, Eisman JA, et al. Global vitamin D status and determinants of hypovitaminosis D. Osteoporos Int. 2009;20(11):1807–20.

106. Hagenau T, Vest R, Gissel TN, Poulsen CS, Erlandsen M, Mosekilde L, et al. Global vitamin D levels in relation to age, gender, skin pigmentation and latitude: an ecologic meta-regression analysis. Osteoporos Int. 2009;20(1):133–40.

107. Holick MF. Vitamin D deficiency. N Engl J Med. 2007;357:266–81.

108. DeLuca HF. Overview of general physiologic features and functions of vitamin D. Am J Clin Nutr. 2004;80:1689S–96S.

109. Maalouf NM. The noncalcitropic actions of vitamin D: recent clinical developments. Curr Opin Nephrol Hypertens. 2008;17:408–15.

110. Baeke F, Gysemans C, Korf H, Mathieu C. Vitamin D insufficiency: implications for the immune system. Pediatr Nephrol. 2010;25(9):1597–606.
111. Baeke F, Takiishi T, Korf H, Gysemans C, Mathieu C. Vitamin D: modulator of the immune system. Curr Opin Pharmacol. 2010;10(4):482–96.
112. Bikle DD. Vitamin D and the immune system: role in protection against bacterial infection. Curr Opin Nephrol Hypertens. 2008;17(4):348–52.
113. Beard JA, Bearden A, Striker R. Vitamin D and the anti-viral state. J Clin Virol. 2011;50(3):194–200.
114. Greiller C, Martineau A. Modulation of the immune response to respiratory viruses by vitamin D. Nutrients. 2015;7(6):4240.
115. Lacoma A, Mateo L, Blanco I, Mendez MJ, Rodrigo C, Latorre I, et al. Impact of host genetics and biological response modifiers on respiratory tract infections. Front Immunol. 2019;10:1013.
116. Young GA, Underhal NR, Carpenter LE. Vitamin-D intake and susceptibility of mice to experimental swine influenza virus infection. Proc Soc Exp Biol Med. 1949;72:695–7.
117. Ginde AA, Mansbach JM, Camargo CA Jr. Association between serum 25-hydroxyvitamin d level and upper respiratory tract infection in the third national health and nutrition examination survey. Arch Intern Med. 2009;169(4):384–90.
118. Shaman J, Jeon CY, Giovannucci E, Lipsitch M. Shortcomings of vitamin D-based model simulations of seasonal influenza. PLoS ONE. 2011;6(6):e20743.
119. Cannell JJ, Veith R, Umhau JC, Holick MF, Grant WB, Mandronich S, et al. Epidemic influenza and vitamin D. Epidemiol Infect. 2006;134:1129–40.
120. Khoo AL, Chai L, Koenen H, Joosten I, Netea M, van der Ven A. Translating the role of vitamin D3 in infectious diseases. Crit Rev Microbiol. 2012;38(2):122–35.
121. Taylor CE, Camargo CA. Impact of micronutrients on respiratory infections. Nutr Rev. 2012;69(5):259–69.
122. Sundaram ME, Coleman LA. Vitamin D and influenza. Adv Nutr. 2012;3(4):517–25.
123. Nanri A, Nakamoto K, Sakamoto N, Imai T, Akter S, Nonaka D, et al. Association of serum 25-hydroxyvitamin D with influenza in case-control study nested in a cohort of Japanese employees. Clin Nutr. 2017;36(5):1288–93.
124. Crum-Cianflone NF, Won S, Lee R, Lalani T, Ganesan A, Burgess T, et al. Vitamin D levels and influenza vaccine immunogenicity among HIV-infected and HIV-uninfected adults. Vaccine. 2016;34(41):5040–6.
125. Sundaram ME, Talbot HK, Zhu Y, Griffin MR, Spencer S, Shay DK, et al. Vitamin D is not associated with serologic response to influenza vaccine in adults over 50 years old. Vaccine. 2013;31(16):2057–61.
126. Principi N, Marchisio P, Terranova L, Zampiero A, Baggi E, Daleno C, et al. Impact of vitamin D administration on immunogenicity of trivalent inactivated influenza vaccine in previously unvaccinated children. Hum Vaccin Immunother. 2013;9(5):969–74.
127. Principi N, Esposito S. Vitamin D and influenza vaccination. Hum Vaccin Immunother. 2013;9(5):976.
128. Brigelius-Flohe R, Traber MG. Vitamin E: function and metabolism. FASEB J. 1999;13(10):1145–55.
129. Meydani SN, Han SN, Wu D. Vitamin E and immune response in the aged: molecular mechanism and clinical implications. Immunol Rev. 2005;205:269–84.
130. Han SN, Wu D, Ha WK, Beharka A, Smith DE, Bender BS, et al. Vitamin E supplementation increases T helper 1 cytokine production in old mice infected with influenza virus. Immunology. 2000;100(4):487–93.
131. Hayek MG, Taylor SF, Bender BS, Han SN, Meydani M, Smith DE, et al. Vitamin E supplementation decreases lung virus titers in mice infected with influenza. J Infect Dis. 1997;176(1):273–6.
132. Mileva M, Bakalova R, Tancheva L, Galabov A, Ribarov S. Effect of vitamin E supplementation on lipid peroxidation in blood and lung of influenza virus infected mice. Comp Immunol Microbiol Infect Dis. 2002;25(1):1–11.
133. Mileva M, Tancheva L, Bakalova R, Galabov A, Savov V, Ribarov S. Effect of vitamin E on lipid peroxidation and liver monooxigenase activity in experimental influenza virus infection. Toxicol Lett. 2000;114(1–3):39–45.
134. Han SN, Meydani M, Wu D, Bender BS, Smith DE, Vina J, et al. Effect of long-term dietary antioxidant supplementation on influenza virus infection. J Gerontol A Biol Sci Med Sci. 2000;55(10):B496–503.
135. Gay R, Han SN, Marko M, Belisle S, Bronson R, Meydani SN. The effect of vitamin E on secondary bacterial infection after influenza infection in young and old mice. Ann N Y Acad Sci. 2004;1031:418–21.
136. Quintilio W, de Freitas FA, Rodriguez D, Kubrusly FS, Yourtov D, Miyaki C, et al. Vitamins as influenza vaccine adjuvant components. Arch Virol. 2016;161(10):2787–95.
137. Tegenge MA, Mitkus RJ. A first-generation physiologically based pharmacokinetic (PBPK) model of alpha-tocopherol in human influenza vaccine adjuvant. Regul Toxicol Pharmacol. 2015;71(3):353–64.
138. Ramakrishnan U, Webb AL, Ologoudou K. Infection, immunity, and vitamins. In: Gershwin ME, Nestel P, Keen CL, editors. Handbook of nutrition and immunity. Totowa: Humana Press; 2004. p. 93–115.
139. Leaf AA. Vitamins for babies and young children. Arch Dis Child. 2007;92(2):160–4.
140. Carroll DN, Carroll DG. Fatal intracranial bleed potentially due to a warfarin and influenza vaccine interaction. Ann Pharmacother. 2009;43(4):754–60.
141. Iorio A, Basileo M, Marcucci M, Guercini F, Camilloni B, Paccamiccio E, et al. Influenza vaccination and vitamin K antagonist treatment: a placebo-controlled, randomized, double-blind crossover study. Arch Intern Med. 2010;170(7):609–16.

142. Maggini S, Wintergerst ES, Beveridge S, Horning DH. Selected vitamins and trace elements support immune function by strengthening epithelial barriers and cellular and humoral immune responses. Br J Nutr. 2007;98(Suppl 1):S29–35.

143. Rall LC, Meydani SN. Vitamin B6 and immune competence. Nutr Rev. 1993;51(8):217–25.

144. Trakatellis A, Dimitriadou A, Trakatelli M. Pyridoxine deficiency: new approaches in immunosuppression and chemotherapy. Postgrad Med J. 1997;73(864):617–22.

145. Fata FT, Herzlich BC, Schiffman G, Ast AL. Impaired antibody responses to pneumococcal polysaccharide in elderly patients with low serum vitamin B12 levels. Ann Intern Med. 1996;124(3):299–304.

146. Tamura J, Kubota K, Murakami H, Sawamura M, Matsushima T, Tamura T, et al. Immunomodulation by vitamin B12: augmentation of CD8+ T lymphocytes and natural killer (NK) cell activity in vitamin B12-deficient patients by methyl-B12 treatment. Clin Exp Immunol. 1999;116(1):28–32.

147. Hamer DH, Sempértegui F, Estrella B, Tucker KL, Rodríguez A, Egas J, et al. Micronutrient deficiencies are associated with impaired immune response and higher burden of respiratory infections in elderly Ecuadorians. J Nutr. 2009;139(1):113–9.

148. Axelrod AE, Hopper S. Effects of pantothenic acid, pyridoxine and thiamine deficiencies upon antibody formation to influenza virus PR-8 in rats. J Nutr. 1960;72(3):325–30.

149. Siddiqua TJ, Ahmad SM, Ahsan KB, Rashid M, Roy A, Rahman SM, et al. Vitamin B12 supplementation during pregnancy and postpartum improves B12 status of both mothers and infants but vaccine response in mothers only: a randomized clinical trial in Bangladesh. Eur J Nutr. 2016;55(1):281–93.

150. Schleicher RL, Carroll MD, Ford ES, Lacher DA. Serum vitamin C and the prevalence of vitamin C deficiency in the United States: 2003–2004 National Health and Nutrition Examination Survey (NHANES). Am J Clin Nutr. 2009;90(5):1252–63.

151. Velandia B, Centor R, McConnell V, Shah M. Scurvy is still present in developed countries. J Gen Intern Med. 2008;23(8):1281–4.

152. Chatterjee IB, Majumder AK, Nandi BK, Subramanian N. Synthesis and some major functions of vitamin C in animals. Ann N Y Acad Sci. 1975;258:24–47.

153. Nishikimi M, Yagi K. Biochemistry and molecuar biology of ascorbic acid biosynthesis. Subcell Biochem. 1996;25:17–39.

154. Hughes DA. Antioxidant vitamins and immune function. In: Calder PC, Field CJ, Gill HS, editors. Nutrition and immune function. Wallingford: CAB International; 2000. p. 171–91.

155. Long KZ, Santos JI. Vitamins and the regulation of the immune response. Pediatr Infect Dis J. 1999;18:283–90.

156. Wintergerst ES, Maggini S, Hornig DH. Immune enhancing role of vitamin C and zinc and effect on clinical conditions. Ann Nutr Metab. 2006;50:85–94.

157. Klenner FR. Massive doses of vitamin C and the virus diseases. South Med Surg. 1951;113(4):101–7.

158. Klenner FR. The treatment of poliomyelitis and other virus diseases with vitamin C. South Med Surg. 1949;111(7):209–14.

159. Klenner FR. Virus pneumonia and its treatment with vitamin C. South Med Surg. 1948;110(2):36–8.

160. Pauling LJ. How to live longer and feel better. New York: Avon Books; 1987.

161. Banerjee D, Kaul D. Combined inhalational and oral supplementation of ascorbic acid may prevent influenza pandemic emergency: a hypothesis. Nutrition. 2010;26:128–32.

162. Ely JTA. Ascorbic acid role in containment of the world avian flu pandemic. Exp Biol Med. 2007;232:847–51.

163. Li W, Maeda N, Beck MA. Vitamin C deficiency increases the lung pathology of influenza virus-infected gulo-/-mice. J Nutr. 2006;136(10):2611–6.

164. Kim Y, Kim H, Bae S, Choi J, Lim SY, Lee N, et al. Vitamin C is an essential factor on the anti-viral immune responses through the production of interferon-α/β at the initial stage of influenza A virus (H3N2) infection. Immune Netw. 2013;13(2):70–4.

165. Hemilä H. Vitamin C and infections. Nutrients. 2017;9(4):339.

166. Failla ML. Trace elements and host defense: recent advances and continuing challenges. J Nutr. 2003;133(Suppl):1443S–7S.

167. Lawrenz M, Wereszczynski J, Amaro R, Walker R, Roitberg A, McCammon JA. Impact of calcium on N1 influenza neuraminidase dynamics and binding free energy. Proteins. 2010;78(11):2523–32.

168. Nugent KM, Shanley JD. Verapamil inhibits influenza A virus replication. Arch Virol. 1984;81(1–2):163–70.

169. United States Department of Agriculture. Community nutrition mapping project 2009. Available from: http://www.ars.usda.gov/Services/docs.htm?docid=15656. Accessed 7 Oct 2019.

170. Rosanoff A, Weaver CM, Rude RK. Suboptimal magnesium status in the United States: are the health consequences underestimated? Nutr Rev. 2012;70(3):153–64.

171. Malpuech-Brugère C, Nowacki W, Gueux E, Kuryszko J, Rock E, Rayssiguier Y, et al. Accelerated thymus involution in magnesium-deficient rats is related to enhanced apoptosis and sensitivity to oxidative stress. Br J Nutr. 1999;81(5):405–11.

172. Weglicki WB. Hypomagnesemia and inflammation: clinical and basic aspects. Annu Rev Nutr. 2012;32:55–71.
173. Floriańczyk B, Karska M, Bednarek A. The level of magnesium in the serum of children hospitalized for severe respiratory infections. Ann Univ Mariae Curie Sklodowska Med. 2001;56:243–7.
174. Centers for Disease Control. Flu and people with diabetes Atlanta: Centers for Disease Control; 2013. Available from: http://www.cdc.gov/flu/diabetes/. Accessed 7 Oct 2019.
175. Moe SM. Disorders involving calcium, phosphorus, and magnesium. Prim Care. 2008;35(2):215–vi.
176. Blair JR, Meriwether TW. Hypokalemic periodic paralysis and influenza. JAMA. 1972;220(12):1617.
177. Stern BR. Essentiality and toxicity in copper health rish assessment: overview, update and regulatory considerations. J Toxicol Environ Health. 2010;73:114–27.
178. Beshgetoor D, Hambidge M. Clinical conditions altering copper metabolism in humans. Am J Clin Nutr. 1998;67(Suppl):1017S–21S.
179. Keen CL, Uriu-Adams JY, Ensunsa JL, Gershwin ME. Trace elements/minerals and immunity. In: Gershwin ME, Nestel P, Keen CL, editors. Handbook of nutrition and immunity. Totowa: Humana Press; 2004. p. 117–40.
180. Bonham M, O'Connor JM, Hannigan BM, Strain JJ. The immune system as a physiological indicator of marginal copper status? Br J Nutr. 2002;87(5):393–403.
181. Smith AD, Botero S, Levander OA. Copper deficiency increases the virulence of amyocarditic and myocarditic strains of coxsackievirus B3 in mice. J Nutr. 2008;138:849–55.
182. Scheiber I, Dringen R, Mercer JF. Copper: effects of deficiency and overload. In: Sigel A, Sigel H, Sigel R, editors. Interrelations between essential metal ions and human diseases. Metal ions in life sciences, vol. 13. Dordrecht: Springer; 2013.
183. Mitra S, Keswani T, Ghosh N, Goswami S, Datta A, Das S, et al. Copper induced immunotoxicity promote differential apoptotic pathways in spleen and thymus. Toxicology. 2013;306:74–84.
184. Sultan Tosun M, Tuna V, Ertekin V, Orbak Z. Swine-origin influenza a (H1N1) infection with acute respiratory distress syndrome in a child with Wilson disease. Minerva Anestesiol. 2010;76(7):559–60.
185. Miller JL. Iron deficiency Anemia: a common and curable disease. Cold Spring Harb Perspect Med. 2013;3(7):a011866.
186. Schaible UE, Kaufmann SHE. Iron and microbial infection. Nat Rev Microbiol. 2004;2:946–53.
187. Weiss G. Iron and immunity: a double-edged sword. J Clin Invest. 2002;32(Suppl 1):70–8.
188. Oppenheimer SJ. Iron and its relation to immunity and infectious disease. J Nutr. 2001;131:616S–35S.
189. Cherayil BJ. Iron and immunity: immunological consequences of iron deficiency and overload. Arch Immunol Ther Exp. 2010;58(6):407–15.
190. Ward RJ, Crichton RR, Taylor DL, Corte LD, Srai SK, Dexter DT. Iron and the immune system. J Neural Transm. 2011;118:315–28.
191. Johnson EE, Wessling-Resnick M. Iron metabolism and the innate immune response to infection. Microbes Infect. 2012;14:207–16.
192. Valenti P, Antonini G. Lactoferrin: an important host defence against microbial and viral attack. Cell Mol Life Sci. 2005;62:2576–87.
193. Pietrantoni A, Ammendolia MG, Superti F. Bovine lactoferrin: involvement of metal saturation and carbohydrates in the inhibition of influenza virus infection. Biochem Cell Biol. 2012;90(3):442–8.
194. Pietrantoni A, Dofrelli E, Tinari A, Ammendolia MG, Puzelli S, Fabiani C, et al. Bovine lactoferrin inhibits influenza A virus induced programmed cell death in vitro. Biometals. 2010;23(3):465–75.
195. Dhur A, Galan P, Hannoun C, Huot K, Hercberg S. Effects of iron deficiency upon the antibody response to influenza virus in rats. J Nutr Biochem. 1990;1(12):629–34.
196. Hoffmann PR, Berry MJ. The influence of selenium on immune responses. Mol Nutr Food Res. 2008;52(11):1273–80.
197. Avery JC, Hoffmann PR. Selenium, selenoproteins, and immunity. Nutrients. 2018;10(9):1203.
198. Oldfield JE. Selenium world atlas. Grimbergen: Selenium-tellurium Development Association; 2002.
199. Yu L, Sun L, Nan Y, Zhu LY. Protection from H1N1 influenza virus infections in mice by supplementation with selenium: a comparison with selenium-deficient mice. Biol Trace Elem Res. 2011;141(1–3):254–61.
200. Jaspers I, Zhang W, Brighton LE, Carson JL, Styblo M, Beck MA. Selenium deficiency alters epithelial cell morphology and responses to influenza. Free Radic Biol Med. 2007;42(12):1826–37.
201. Sheridan PA, Zhong N, Carlson BA, Perella CM, Hatfield DL, Beck MA. Decreased selenoprotein expression alters the immune response during influenza virus infection in mice. J Nutr. 2007;137(6):1466–71.
202. Li W, Beck MA. Selenium deficiency induced an altered immune response and increased survival following influenza A/Puerto Rico/8/34 infection. Exp Biol Med (Maywood). 2007;232(3):412–9.
203. Nelson HK, Shi Q, Van Dael P, Schiffrin EJ, Blum S, Barclay D, et al. Host nutritional selenium status as a driving force for influenza virus mutations. FASEB J. 2001;15(10):1846–8.
204. Harthill M. Review: micronutrient selenium deficiency influences evolution of some viral infectious diseases. Biol Trace Elem Res. 2011;143(3):1325–36.
205. Prasad AS. Impact of the discovery of human zinc deficiency on health. J Am Coll Nutr. 2009;28(3):257–65.

206. Chasapis CT, Loutsidou AC, Spiliopoulou CA, Stefanidou ME. Zinc and human health: an update. Arch Toxicol. 2012;86:521–36.
207. Wong CP, Ho E. Zinc and its role in age-related inflammation and immune dysfunction. Mol Nutr Food Res. 2012;56:77–87.
208. Stefanidou M, Maravelias C, Dona A, Spiliopoulou C. Zinc: a multipurpose trace element. Arch Toxicol. 2006;80:1–9.
209. Prasad AS. Zinc in human health: effect of zinc on immune cells. Mol Med. 2008;14(5–6):353–7.
210. Rao G, Rowland K. PURLs: zinc for the common cold—not if, but when. J Fam Pract. 2011;60(11):669–71.
211. Overbeck S, Rink L, Haase H. Modulating the immne response by oral zinc supplementation: a single approach for multiple diseases. Arch Immunol Ther Exp. 2008;56:15–30.
212. Provinciali M, Montenovo A, Di Stefano G, Colombo M, Daghetta L, Cairati M, et al. Effect of zinc or zinc plus arginine supplementation on antibody titre and lymphocyte subsets after influenza vaccination in elderly subjects: a randomized controlled trial. Age Ageing. 1998;27(6):715–22.
213. Turk S, Bozfakiglu S, Ecder ST, Kahraman T, Gurel N, Erkoc R, et al. Effects of zinc supplementation on the immune system and on antibody response to mulivalent influenza vaccine in hemodialysis patients. Int J Artif Organs. 1998;21(5):274–8.
214. Sandstead HH, Prasad AS. Zinc intake and resistance to H1N1 influenza. Am J Public Health. 2010;100(6):970–1.
215. Zinc for colds: not much benefit…but there is a way to prevent flu. Child Health Alert. 2007;25:2–3.
216. Rahman MM, Ng JC, Naidu R. Chronic exposure of arsenic via drinking water and its adverse health impacts on humans. Environ Geochem Health. 2009;31(Suppl 1):189–200.
217. National Research Council (US) subcommittee to update the 1999 arsenic in drinking water report. Arsenic in drinking water: 2001 Update. 2001.
218. Shankar S, Shanker U. Shikha. Arsenic contamination of groundwater: a review of sources, prevalence, health risks, and strategies for mitigation. Sci World J. 2014;2014:304524.
219. Abernathy CO, Liu YP, Longfellow D, Aposhian HV, Beck B, Fowler B, et al. Arsenic: health effects, mechanisms of actions, and research issues. Environ Health Perspect. 1999;107(7):593–7.
220. Huang CF, Chen YW, Yang CY, Tsai KS, Yang RS, Liu SH. Arsenic and diabetes: current perspectives. Kaohsiung J Med Sci. 2011;27(9):402–10.
221. Tapio S, Grosche B. Arsenic in the aetiology of cancer. Mutation Res. 2006;612(3):215–46.
222. Dangleben NL, Skibola CF, Smith MT. Arsenic immunotoxicity: a review. Environ Health. 2013;12(1):73.
223. Soto-Martinez M, Sly PD. Relationship between environmental exposures in children and adult lung disease: the case for outdoor exposures. Chron Respir Dis. 2010;7(3):173–86.
224. Kozul CD, Ely KH, Enelow RI, Hamilton JH. Low-dose arsenic comprmises the immune response to influenza A infection in vivo. Environ Health Perspect. 2009;117(9):1441–7.
225. Liao CM, Chio CP, Cheng YH, Hsieh NH, Chen WY, Chen SC. Quantitative links between arsenic exposure and influenza A (H1N1) infection-associated lung function exacerbations risk. Risk Anal. 2011;31(8):1281–94.
226. Ramsey KA, Foong RE, Sly PD, Larcombe AN, Zosky GR. Early life arsenic exposure and acute and long-term responses to influenza A infection in mice. Environ Health Perspect. 2013;121(10):1187–93.
227. Costello AM, Osrin D. Micronutrient status during pregnancy and outcomes for newborn infants in developing countries. J Nutr. 2003;133(5 Suppl 2):1757S–64S.
228. Konje JC, Ladipo OA. Nutrition and obstructed labor. Am J Clin Nutr. 2000;72(1 Suppl):291S–7S.
229. Stoltzfus RJ. Iron-deficiency anemia: reexamining the nature and magnitude of the public health problem. Summary: implications for research and programs. J Nutr. 2001;131(2S–2):697S–700S; discussion S–1S.
230. Chaffee BW, King JC. Effect of zinc supplementation on pregnancy and infant outcomes: a systematic review. Paediatr Perinat Epidemiol. 2012;26(Suppl 1):118–37.
231. Strobel M, Tinz J, Biesalski HK. The importance of beta-carotene as a source of vitamin A with special regard to pregnant and breastfeeding women. Eur J Nutr. 2007;46(Suppl 1):I1–20.
232. Caulfield LE, Zavaleta N, Shankar AH, Merialdi M. Potential contribution of maternal zinc supplementation during pregnancy to maternal and child survival. Am J Clin Nutr. 1998;68(2 Suppl):499S–508S.
233. Karlsson EA, Marcelin G, Webby RJ, Schultz-Cherry S. Review on the impact of pregnancy and obesity on influenza virus infection. Influenza Other Respir Viruses. 2012;6(6):449–60.
234. Ip S, Chung M, Raman G, Chew P, Magula N, DeVine D, et al. Breastfeeding and maternal and infant health outcomes in developed countries. Evid Rep Technol Assess (Full Rep). 2007;153:1–186.
235. Maurer MA, Meyer L, Bianchi M, Turner HL, Le NPL, Steck M, et al. Glycosylation of human IgA directly inhibits influenza A and other sialic-acid-binding viruses. Cell Rep. 2018;23(1):90–9.
236. Prameela KK. Breastfeeding—anti-viral potential and relevance to the influenza virus pandemic. Med J Malaysia. 2011;66(2):166–9; quiz 70.
237. May JT. Microbial contaminants and antimicrobial properties of human milk. Microbiol Sci. 1988;5:42–6.

238. Ward PP, Paz E, Conneely OM. Multifunctional roles of lactoferrin: a critical overview. Cell Mol Life Sci. 2005;62(22):2540–8.
239. Morrow AL, Ruiz-Palacios GM, Jiang X, Newburg DS. Human-milk glycans that inhibit pathogen binding protect breast-feeding infants against infectious diarrhea. J Nutr. 2005;135(5):1304–7.
240. Thormar H, Isaacs CE, Brown HR, Barshatzky MR, Pessolano T. Inactivation of enveloped viruses and killing of cells by fatty acids and monoglycerides. Antimicrob Agents Chemother. 1987;31(1):27–31.
241. Miller M, Humphrey J, Johnson E, Marinda E, Brookmeyer R, Katz J. Why do children become vitamin A deficient? J Nutr. 2002;132(9 Suppl):2867S–80S.
242. United Nations Department of Economic and Social Affairs Population Division. World population prospects: the 2017 revision, key findings and advance tables. 2017.
243. Crogan NL. Nutritional problems affecting older adults. Nurs Clin North Am. 2017;52(3):433–45.
244. Landi F, Calvani R, Tosato M, Martone AM, Ortolani E, Savera G, et al. Anorexia of aging: risk factors, consequences, and potential treatments. Nutrients. 2016;8(2):69.
245. Via M. The malnutrition of obesity: micronutrient deficiencies that promote diabetes. ISRN Endocrinol. 2012;2012:103472.
246. Perez-Escamilla R, Bermudez O, Buccini GS, Kumanyika S, Lutter CK, Monsivais P, et al. Nutrition disparities and the global burden of malnutrition. BMJ. 2018;361:k2252.
247. Stabler SP, Lindenbaum J, Allen RH. Vitamin B-12 deficiency in the elderly: current dilemmas. Am J Clin Nutr. 1997;66(4):741–9.
248. Ervin RB, Kennedy-Stephenson J. Mineral intakes of elderly adult supplement and non-supplement users in the third national health and nutrition examination survey. J Nutr. 2002;132(11):3422–7.
249. Meydani SN, Barnett JB, Dallal GE, Fine BC, Jaques PF, Leka LS, et al. Serum zinc and pneumonia in nursing home elderly. Am J Clin Nutr. 2007;86:1167–73.
250. Thompson WW, Shay DK, Weintraub E, Brammer L, Cox N, Anderson LJ, et al. Mortality associated with influenza and respiratory syncytial virus in the United States. JAMA. 2003;289(2):179–86.
251. Russell K, Chung JR, Monto AS, Martin ET, Belongia EA, McLean HQ, et al. Influenza vaccine effectiveness in older adults compared with younger adults over five seasons. Vaccine. 2018;36(10):1272–8.
252. Ohmit SE, Thompson MG, Petrie JG, Thaker SN, Jackson ML, Belongia EA, et al. Influenza vaccine effectiveness in the 2011–2012 season: protection against each circulating virus and the effect of prior vaccination on estimates. Clin Infect Dis. 2014;58(3):319–27.
253. McLean HQ, Thompson MG, Sundaram ME, Kieke BA, Gaglani M, Murthy K, et al. Influenza vaccine effectiveness in the United States during 2012–2013: variable protection by age and virus type. J Infect Dis. 2015;211(10):1529–40.
254. Osterholm MT, Kelley NS, Sommer A, Belongia EA. Efficacy and effectiveness of influenza vaccines: a systematic review and meta-analysis. Lancet Infect Dis. 2012;12(1):36–44.
255. Fulop T Jr, Wagner JR, Khalil A, Weber J, Trottier L, Payette H. Relationship between the response to influenza vaccination and the nutritional status in institutionalized elderly subjects. J Gerontol A Biol Sci Med Sci. 1999;54(2):M59–64.
256. Johnson NPAS, Mueller J. Updating the accounts: global mortality of the 1918–1920 "Spanish" influenza pandemic. Bull Hist Med. 2002;76(1):105–15.
257. Karlsson EA, Beck MA. The burden of obesity on infectious disease. Exp Biol Med (Maywood). 2010;235(12):1412–24.

# Chapter 6
# Nutrition and Protozoan Pathogens of Humans: A Primer

**Mark F. Wiser**

## Abbreviations

AIDS    Acquired immunodeficiency syndrome
Th      T helper

**Key Points**
- Several human diseases are caused by pathogenic protozoa.
- Dietary factors can influence transmission as many protozoal diseases are acquired via ingestion.
- Undernutrition, due to its adverse effect on immunity, generally increases the virulence of protozoal diseases.
- Diarrheal diseases caused by intestinal protozoa lead to malabsorption and contribute to undernutrition.
- Blood-borne protozoa including malaria cause hypoglycemia and acidosis.

## Introduction

Protozoa are ubiquitous eukaryotic microbes that are found in nearly all ecological niches. In the taxonomic sense, protozoa do not represent a monophylogenetic group but are a convenient grouping of a diverse array of unicellular eukaryotic organisms. In fact, organisms that have been historically classified as protozoa are found in all eukaryotic supergroups [1]. This diversity is also accompanied by a wide range of metabolisms including autotrophic, heterotrophic, and mixotrophic. Although most protozoa are free-living, a large number exist in symbiotic or parasitic relationships with other organisms. Of particular relevance to human health, several protozoa are human pathogens and cause important human diseases (Table 6.1).

Among the major pathogenic protozoan of humans, there are two major routes of infection: ingestion of the pathogen and transmission via a blood-feeding arthropod vector. One exception is *Trichomonas*

M. F. Wiser (✉)
Department of Tropical Medicine, Tulane University School of Public Health and Tropical Medicine,
New Orleans, LA, USA
e-mail: wiser@tulane.edu

© Springer Nature Switzerland AG 2021
D. L. Humphries et al. (eds.), *Nutrition and Infectious Diseases*, Nutrition and Health,
https://doi.org/10.1007/978-3-030-56913-6_6

**Table 6.1** Major protozoan pathogens infecting humans

| Protozoan | Disease | Transmission | Importance |
|---|---|---|---|
| *Trichomonas vaginalis* | Inflammation of the urogenital tract | Sexually transmitted | Most common nonviral sexually transmitted infection with >140 million cases per year worldwide |
| *Entamoeba histolytica* | Amebic dysentery | Fecal-oral | An estimated 50 million symptomatic cases with 100,000 deaths per year |
| *Giardia duodenalis* | Diarrhea | Fecal-oral | Common intestinal infection causing 180 million clinical cases per year |
| *Cryptosporidium* species | Acute watery diarrhea | Fecal-oral and water-borne outbreaks | Prevalence ranges from 1% to 10%; life-threatening in AIDS patients |
| *Plasmodium falciparum* | Malaria, acute febrile disease | Mosquito | Approximately 200 million clinical cases with 500,000 deaths per year |
| *Leishmania* species | Cutaneous or visceral disease | Sand fly | 1.5–2 million new cases and 70,000 deaths per year |
| *Trypanosoma cruzi* | Chagas disease | Triatomine bug | Major cause of cardiac disease in South and Central America with at least 6 million infected |
| *Trypanosoma gambiense* | African sleeping sickness | Tse-tse fly | 70–80,000 new cases with 30,000 deaths per year |
| *Toxoplasma gondii* | Neurological and vision defects | Ingestion of undercooked meat | A common infection that can cause birth defects; seroprevalence ranges from 6% to 75% depending on the region |

*vaginalis,* which is sexually transmitted. Numerous protozoa inhabit the gastrointestinal tract of humans, and these are all transmitted via ingestion of the organism. Many intestinal protozoa are considered nonpathogenic commensals or only cause mild disease symptoms. However, *Entamoeba histolytica*, *Giardia duodenalis*, and *Cryptosporidium* are well-documented pathogens that cause diarrhea. *Toxoplasma gondii,* while also being transmitted via ingestion, affects internal organs rather than the gastrointestinal tract. Toxoplasmosis is initiated by the ingestion of undercooked meat containing the parasite or food or water that has been contaminated with feces from an infected cat.

Several major protozoan pathogens of humans are transmitted via arthropod vectors. Most notable is the malaria parasite, transmitted by mosquitoes, that is a very common infection in some tropical regions. Other notable vector-transmitted pathogens include *Leishmania*, *Trypansoma cruzi*, and the African trypanosomes, which are all phylogenetically related and form a group called the kinetoplastids. Vector-transmitted pathogens can gain access to the circulatory system and disseminate throughout the body, affecting various internal organs.

The biology of human protozoan pathogens and the diseases they cause have been described in detail [2]. This chapter covers the salient features of transmission and pathology for the major protozoal pathogens of humans. The major protozoal diseases include trichomoniasis, amebiasis, giardiasis, cryptosporidiosis, malaria, African sleeping sickness, Chagas disease, leishmaniasis, and toxoplasmosis. For each of these diseases, aspects of the pathogen's physiology are discussed in relation to human nutrition and the pathophysiology of the disease.


# Nutrition and Infection

The relationship between nutrition and infection can be viewed as a two-way street. Nutrition can affect pathogens, and at the same time pathogens can impact nutritional status. Currently we have limited knowledge about the mutual influences between pathogenic protozoa and nutrition. Broadly speaking, however, undernutrition can increase the success of a pathogen, while at the same time nutritional deficiencies may be antagonistic to a pathogen and have a protective effect. In particular, undernutrition has a major negative impact on immunity [3] and can exacerbate infections in ways that promote disease progression and slow recovery [4]. Similarly, many pathogens are opportunistic in that severe disease is primarily associated with an immunocompromised state. Thus, there is a synergism between undernutrition and infectious disease since the immunological impairment associated with undernutrition promotes parasite proliferation and increases disease virulence.

Enteric infections, as discussed in detail in Chap. 8 [5], are another example of synergism between undernutrition and infectious disease. The inflammation and diarrhea associated with intestinal infections—especially in the small intestine—result in malabsorption [6]. This malabsorption results in decreased uptake of nutrients and contributes to undernutrition. In the case of systemic infections, the resulting fever and inflammation increase the metabolic rate and lead to an increase in energy expenditure. This diversion of energy and nutrients away from normal processes means less energy is available for growth and normal physiological processes. This decrease in absorption and diversion of energy worsens the nutritional status and in resource-poor settings leads to a vicious cycle between infection and nutrition, especially in children.

On the other hand, as pathogens are highly dependent on the host for nutrients, it is certainly feasible that the nutritional status of the host might negatively impact pathogen proliferation and disease progression. For example, deficiencies in certain nutrients may limit the ability of a pathogen to proliferate [7]. In particular, iron presents a bit of an enigma since it is an important nutrient for immune function and especially innate immunity. However, at the same time, iron is also an essential nutrient for most, if not all, pathogens [8]. Thus, deficiencies in certain minerals and vitamins may be antagonistic to pathogen proliferation and disease progression. Limitations in energy-yielding nutrients probably do not greatly impact pathogen proliferation and disease progression, given that the total biomass of a pathogen will generally be a small percentage of that of the total microbiome. Exceptions would include a localized effect on nutrient availability due to the tropism of a pathogen for a particular organ or tissue.

# Trichomoniasis

*Trichomonas vaginalis* is a common sexually transmitted infection [9]. Despite the name, the parasite readily infects both men and women and is likely the most prevalent nonviral sexually transmitted infection. The parasite is transmitted from person-to-person during sexual intercourse. The life cycle of *Trichomonas* is rather simple, with a single stage called the trophozoite. *Trichomonas* trophozoites are flagellated and mobile, and they replicate by binary fission. The parasite can adhere to epithelial cells of the urogenital tract.

*T. vaginalis* is a relatively non-virulent pathogen, and generally infections are asymptomatic or produce a rather mild disease. Women are more likely to exhibit symptoms than men. The infection in women is primarily associated with the vagina and usually causes a mild inflammation. This vaginitis is often associated with a vaginal discharge that is accompanied by burning and itching. The urethra and prostate are the most common sites of infection in men. More than half of the infections in men are asymptomatic, and symptoms when present are generally mild urethral discharge, painful urination, and itching.

## *Trichomonad Metabolism*

The trophozoites of *T. vaginalis* readily grow in rather simple media and do not have any exceptional metabolic requirements. *T. vaginalis* does secrete a glucosidase that breaks glycogen into simple sugars and thus exploits the glycogen-rich environment of the vaginal mucosa [10]. These simple sugars are also available for other microbes of the vaginal microbiome which are unable to use glycogen as an energy source. Trichomonads exhibit a unique anaerobic metabolic feature involving a specialized organelle called the hydrogenosome [11]. This hydrogenosome is a remnant of the mitochondrion that lacks the enzymes of the tricarboxylic acid cycle and oxidative phosphorylation. Instead, the pyruvate produced during glycolysis is converted to acetate and carbon dioxide, and the electrons released during this reaction are ultimately transferred to hydrogen ions to produce molecular hydrogen ($H_2$) via the action of a hydrogenase within the hydrogensome. Thus, molecular oxygen is not the terminal electron acceptor, as is the case in typical aerobic metabolism.

As is true for most organisms, *Trichomonas* requires an exogenous source of iron for survival and proliferation. In response to the constant flux in vaginal iron concentrations, *Trichomonas* has evolved mechanisms to prevent intracellular depletion or overload of iron. Iron depletion upregulates the expression of genes for the assembly of iron-sulfur proteins but downregulates the expression of genes associated with carbohydrate metabolism in the hydrogenosome [12]. In addition, nitric oxide accumulates in the hydrogenosome and maintains hydrogenosomal functions under iron-poor conditions [13]. The host has also evolved mechanisms to interfere with the bioavailability of iron. For example, lactoferrin binds iron and reduces its availability to microbes at mucosal sites. Accordingly, lactoferrin concentrations are higher in women infected with *T. vaginalis*, and this may affect iron homeostasis for the parasite [14].

## Intestinal Protozoan Infections

Several protozoan species infect the human gastrointestinal tract (Table 6.2). Many of these protozoa do not cause severe disease, and some are no longer commonly found in human stools. Considering both prevalence and clear evidence of human disease, *Entamoeba histolytica*, *Giardia duodenalis*, and *Cryptosporidium* are the most important human pathogens. Diarrhea is a major clinical manifestation for all three of these pathogens and can be quite profuse in the case of giardiasis and cryptosporidiosis. Profuse diarrhea can certainly contribute to protein-energy malnutrition and electrolyte imbalances, as well as deficiencies in vitamins, minerals, and other micronutrients [5]. Intestinal infections can also result in dehydration. This intestinal dysfunction can lead to weight loss and a failure to thrive, especially in malnourished children.

Although the protozoa that infect the human gastrointestinal tract are quite diverse, they all exhibit a similar life cycle and mode of transmission referred to as fecal-oral transmission (Fig. 6.1). The infection is acquired through the ingestion of food or water that has been contaminated with fecal matter. In most cases a specialized stage called the cyst initiates the infection. After ingestion the cyst converts into a trophozoite. The trophozoite is often motile and exhibits an active metabolism. Most importantly, the trophozoite is the replicative form of the parasite and leads to an expansion of the population. Some of the trophozoites convert back into cyst stages which are passed in the feces. The

**Table 6.2** Protozoa infecting the human gastrointestinal tract (major pathogens in bold face)

| Ameba | Flagellates | Apicomplexa | Other |
|---|---|---|---|
| **Entamoeba histolytica** | **Giardia duodenalis** | **Cryptosporidium hominis** | *Blastocystis hominis* (stramenopile) |
| *Entamoeba dispar* | *Dientamoeba fragilis* | **Cryptosporidium parvum** | *Balantidium coli* (ciliate) |
| *Entamoeba coli* | *Chilomastix mesnili* | *Cyclospora cayetanensis* | Microsporidia (now considered to be highly derived fungi) |
| *Entamoeba hartmanni* | *Pentatrichomonas hominis* | *Isospora belli* | |
| *Endolimax nana* | *Enteromonas hominis* | | |
| *Iodamoeba bütschlii* | *Retortamonas intestinalis* | | |

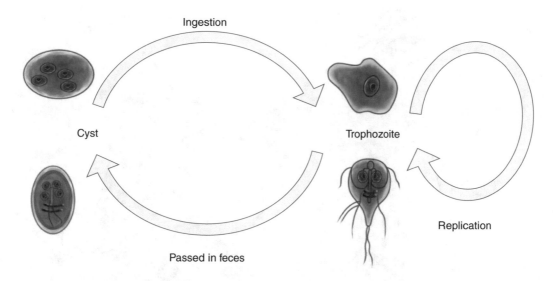

**Fig. 6.1** Typical protozoan fecal-oral life cycle. Cysts are highly infectious forms that convert to trophozoites following the ingestion of contaminated food or water. Trophozoites are feeding stages that replicate within the intestinal tract and are often motile. Some trophozoites convert back into cysts and are passed in the feces. Cysts have a thick wall and can survive outside of the host until ingested by another host

cyst stage is characterized by a cyst wall that makes the parasite more resilient to environmental elements such as desiccation. Many protozoan cysts can survive for months outside of the body if kept moist and cool. Furthermore, the cysts are highly infectious in that ingestion of only a few cysts can initiate an infection.

## Amebiasis

Disease manifestations associated with *E. histolytica* infections can range from asymptomatic in the case of a cyst passer, to death [15]. In regard to pathogenesis, the disease is often characterized as being either noninvasive or invasive. During noninvasive disease, the trophozoites establish a colony of ameba in the colon and exhibit the typical fecal-oral life cycle. The trophozoites ingest bacteria and fecal matter as a food source and replicate by binary fission. Noninvasive disease is often asymptomatic but can be associated with diarrhea and other gastrointestinal symptoms such as cramping or pain. Most infections exhibit no severe clinical manifestations and self-resolve in weeks to months.

However, in some cases the infection does not resolve and progresses into a severe invasive disease (Fig. 6.2). *E. histolytica* trophozoites can kill intestinal epithelial cells in a contact-dependent manner resulting in the formation of colonic ulcers that can progress to colitis and dysentery. The lesions can expand through the submucosa and occasionally through the colon wall leading to a perforation of the colon wall and peritonitis. In addition, the trophozoites in the submucosa can enter the circulatory system and metastasize throughout the body and cause extraintestinal amebiasis. Since the mesentery blood vessels and portal vein system go directly from the intestines to the liver, the liver is the most common site of extra-intestinal amebiasis. From the liver the trophozoites can continue spreading throughout the body and affecting other organs. The pathology associated with amebiasis is due to a contact-dependent killing of host cells by the trophozoites. Severe disease such as fulminant amebic colitis, peritonitis, or extraintestinal amebiasis can be fatal if not treated.

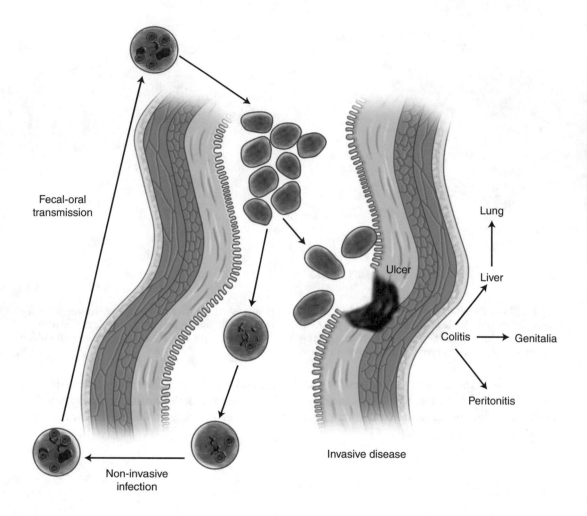

**Fig. 6.2** Noninvasive versus invasive amebiasis. During noninvasive disease, the trophozoites of *Entamoeba histolytica* form a colony on the mucosa of the large intestine and exhibit a typical fecal-oral life cycle. Invasion of the epithelial layer of the colon by trophozoites results in ulcers and colitis. Trophozoites in the submucosa can enter the portal vein system and travel to the liver and other organs, such as the lung. The lesion can also expand and perforate the colon wall leading to peritonitis or spread to the genitalia

The severity of amebiasis is increased under conditions that lower immunity such as in neonates and young children, pregnant and postpartum women, those using corticosteroids, those with malignancies, and malnourished individuals. In particular, protein-energy malnutrition adversely affects immunity and plays a role in susceptibility to amebiasis and the progression to severe disease [16].

## Giardiasis

*Giardia duodenalis*, formerly known as *G. lamblia*, is a common protozoan of the intestinal tract [17]. As implied by the name, the parasites have a strong tropism for the duodenum. The prevalence in low resource countries ranges from 4 to 43% and 1 to 7% in high-resource countries. It exhibits a typical

**Fig. 6.3** Adhesive disk of *Giardia*. A scanning electron micrograph showing the ventral surface of a *Giardia* trophozoite. The suction cup-like structure is the adhesive disk (AD) that attaches to the intestinal epithelium. The circle to the left (arrowhead) is an imprint left in the brush border (microvilli) of the intestinal epithelium following the detachment of the trophozoite. (Courtesy of the Public Health Image Library and attributed to Dr. Stan Erlandsen and the CDC)

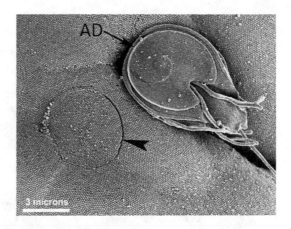

fecal-oral life cycle and is periodically associated with water-borne outbreaks. *Giardia* trophozoites have a unique structure on their ventral surface called the adhesive disk (Fig. 6.3). This disk is composed of cytoskeletal elements and contractile proteins and is involved in the attachment of the trophozoite to the epithelium of the small intestine. The attached trophozoites absorb nutrients from the intestinal milieu via pinocytosis.

Most infections with *Giardia* are either asymptomatic or go undiagnosed. The most common symptom associated with giardiasis is acute diarrhea. Initially the stools are watery and profuse but later may become greasy and foul-smelling. Abdominal cramping, bloating, and flatulence are also common symptoms. The symptoms usually clear spontaneously after 5–7 days. A small number of people develop a chronic infection that can last for several months or even years. Chronic giardiasis is characterized by intermittent diarrheal episodes and progresses to weight loss and a failure to thrive.

No mortality or severe pathology is associated with giardiasis. In some patients villus blunting, crypt cell hyperplasia, and an increased rate of enterocyte apoptosis are observed. The increased crypt cell proliferation leads to a repopulation of the intestinal epithelium by immature enterocytes with reduced absorptive capabilities. This malabsorption, combined with increased secretion of chloride and water, results in an osmotic type of diarrhea. Damage to the brush border and microvillus shortening is also sometimes observed. This is accompanied by a decrease in metabolite transport function and a reduction in enzymes, particularly disaccharidases, on the surface of epithelial cells. In fact, some patients present with lactose intolerance that can persist for months after parasite clearance. This reduced digestion and absorption of metabolites and electrolytes increase the fluid retention in the intestinal lumen and contribute to watery diarrhea.

## Cryptosporidiosis

*Cryptosporidium* is another common intestinal protozoan of humans [17, 18]. Two *Cryptosporidium* species infect humans: *C. hominis* is strictly a human pathogen, and *C. parvum* is a parasite of cattle that infects a wide range of mammals including humans. *Cryptosporidium* is a member of the Apicomplexa and exhibits an apicomplexan life cycle. Although the details of the *Cryptosporidium* life cycle are more complex than other protozoal pathogens of the intestinal tract, it still exhibits a basic fecal-oral life cycle. The infection is initiated upon the ingestion of the oocyst stage. Like the cyst, the oocyst is covered with a thick cyst wall and can survive for extended periods in the environment. The oocysts contain forms known as sporozoites that are released from the oocyst after passing through the stomach.

The sporozoites are motile forms that interact with epithelial cells of the small intestine. As part of this interaction, the sporozoites induce the microvilli of the enterocytes to expand, flatten, and fuse together so

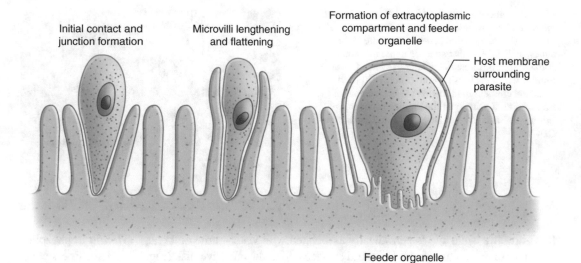

Fig. 6.4 Extracytoplasmic location of *Cryptosporidium*. Upon initial interaction between the sporozoite or merozoite and the intestinal epithelial cell, a junction forms between the parasite and the host cell. The microvilli of the intestinal epithelial cells lengthen, flatten, and fuse to surround the parasite. The junction between the parasite and the epithelial cell develops into the feeder organelle

that the parasite is completely surrounded by a double membrane of host origin (Fig. 6.4). This is referred to as an extracytoplasmic location since the parasite is not intracellular, but yet it is surrounded by membranes of host origin. A junction forms between the parasite and epithelial cell called either the feeder organelle or the adhesive zone. The parasite derives nutrients from the host cell via this junction.

After attachment and formation of the extracytoplasmic space, the parasite undergoes an asexual replication producing four or eight progeny called merozoites. These merozoites are functionally equivalent to the sporozoites and infect intestinal epithelial cells and repeat this replicative process to maintain the infection. Some of the parasites, instead of undergoing replication, differentiate into sexual forms that ultimately produce the oocyst containing the sporozoites. After maturation the oocyst is released from the intestinal epithelial cell and passed with the feces to complete the life cycle.

The most common clinical manifestation of cryptosporidiosis is a mild to profuse watery diarrhea. Generally, the infection is self-resolving and the symptoms persist for a few days. However, recrudescence is common and the infection can persist for weeks to months. The symptoms are generally more severe in immunocompromised persons, and the disease can be life-threatening in AIDS patients [19]. In AIDS patients diarrhea can be voluminous and is often described as being cholera-like. As is common in other intestinal infections, undernutrition intensifies the disease manifestations, and *Cryptosporidium* infection contributes to undernutrition [20]. The pathogenesis associated with cryptosporidiosis is primarily due to superficial damage to the intestinal epithelium and in general is quite similar to that of giardiasis. In immunocompetent persons, the infection is primarily confined to the jejunum and ileum of the small intestine. However, the infection spreads to the duodenum, biliary tract, colon, and stomach in immunocompromised persons.

## Malaria

Among the diseases caused by protozoa, malaria is clearly the most important in terms of human morbidity and mortality. Even though control efforts over the past two decades have been relatively successful at decreasing the incidence of malaria, there are still approximately 200 million cases per

**Table 6.3** Human malarial parasites

| Species | Key features |
|---------|-------------|
| P. falciparum | Found throughout the tropics and subtropics<br>Mortality associated with disease complications due to sequestration of infected erythrocytes in deep tissues |
| P. vivax | Found in most tropical areas and can extend into temperate zones<br>Lower prevalence in Africa due to Duffy-negative phenotype<br>Can cause severe febrile attacks but very low mortality<br>Relapses from liver stage possible |
| P. malariae | Spotty distribution throughout tropics<br>Causes a rather benign disease<br>Can produce sub-patent infection lasting for decades |
| P. ovale | Occurs primarily in tropical west Africa<br>Causes a rather benign disease<br>Relapses from the liver stage possible |
| P. knowlesi | Natural parasite of macaque monkeys<br>A limited number of human infections reported in Malaysia and Southeast Asia<br>Some mortality associated with infection |

year with nearly a half million deaths. The mortality associated with malaria is predominantly due to *Plasmodium falciparum* as the other species of human malaria parasites rarely cause death (Table 6.3). Most of the deaths associated with malaria are among children in sub-Saharan Africa.

## Life Cycle

The malaria parasite has a complex life cycle that includes features found in other apicomplexans [21]. Infection in humans is initiated via the bite of a mosquito (Fig. 6.5). Sporozoite stages in the mosquito saliva are injected as the mosquito takes a blood meal and enter the circulatory system. The sporozoites invade liver cells and undergo an asexual replication that results in the production of thousands of merozoites that are released into the circulation. The merozoites then invade erythrocytes and undergo additional rounds of asexual replication to produce more merozoites. The newly produced merozoites repeat the erythrocyte invasion and replication and thus maintain the infection in the human host. It is this blood stage of the infection that is responsible for the disease pathology.

As an alternative to this asexual replication, some of the merozoites differentiate into sexual forms that are infective to the mosquito. When these forms are taken up by a mosquito during feeding, they undergo a complex differentiation process called sporogony which culminates in the production of sporozoites. The sporozoites migrate to the salivary glands in anticipation of infecting a new host.

## The Food Vacuole and Digestion of Hemoglobin

During the erythrocytic stage, the malaria parasite takes up the host cell cytoplasm and breaks down the hemoglobin to amino acids. The digestion of hemoglobin takes place within a lysosome-like organelle called the food vacuole (Fig. 6.6). Various proteases acting in sequential fashion break down the globin polypeptide chains into peptides and amino acids [22]. During its erythrocytic stage cycle, the parasite digests 60–80% of the host's hemoglobin. The resulting amino acids and peptides are transported to the parasite cytoplasm and utilized by the parasite for the synthesis of parasite proteins and as an energy source.

**Fig. 6.5** The life cycle of malaria parasite. The *Anopheles* mosquito bites a human and injects sporozoites with the saliva. The sporozoites invade liver cells and undergo an asexual replication culminating in the production of merozoites. Merozoites invade erythrocytes and undergo repeated rounds of asexual replication producing more merozoites. It is the blood stage of the infection that is responsible for the disease. Instead of continuing to replicate, some merozoites differentiate into sexual forms that are infective for the mosquito. The parasite undergoes a process called sporogony in the mosquito that results in sporozoites in the salivary glands

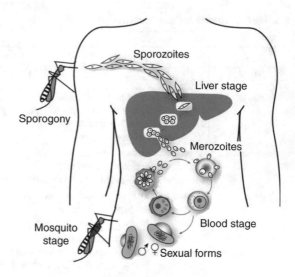

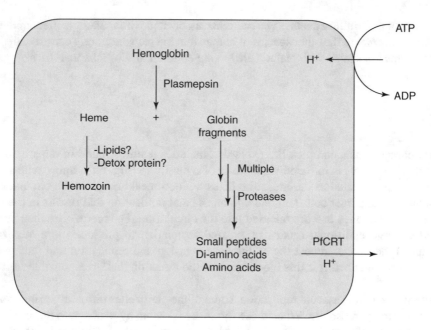

**Fig. 6.6** The food vacuole and digestion of hemoglobin. The *Plasmodium* food vacuole is an acidic lysosome-like organelle specialized in the digestion of hemoglobin. An initial cleavage of hemoglobin by plasmepsin results in an unfolding of the molecule exposing it to other proteases. The resulting amino acids and peptides are transported to the cytoplasm via the chloroquine resistance transporter (PfCRT). The free heme that is released during the degradation of hemoglobin is detoxified via a biocrystallization process that forms hemozoin

One consequence of breaking down hemoglobin is the release of free heme. Free heme is toxic due to its ability to destabilize and lyse membranes. The parasite detoxifies the heme via a biocrystallization process converting the heme into hemozoin [23]. Hemozoin is also known as the malarial pigment. The deposition of this malarial pigment in tissues has long been associated with malaria and was described even before the parasite was identified. In fact, the malarial pigment played a role in the identification of the malaria parasite. The formation of hemozoin is also important in that chloroquine and other anti-malarials block its formation resulting in high levels of free heme and parasite death.

The fact that the biocrystallization of heme is a rather unique process accounts for the high therapeutic index of chloroquine and other related drugs.

This sequestration of the iron into hemozoin means that it is not available for the parasite, and the parasite needs an exogenous source of iron. Paradoxically, iron deficiency appears to protect against severe malaria, while iron supplementation increases the risks of infection and progressing to severe disease [24]. Thus, there is controversy about iron supplementation in malaria-endemic areas as populations with high rates of iron deficiency are often at the highest risks of malaria [25].

## Sequestration and Severe Falciparum Malaria

Approximately 10% of falciparum malaria cases develop into a severe disease with complications and a mortality rate of 10–50%. The increased severity associated with falciparum malaria is due in large part to the higher parasitemia as compared to the other species. In addition, erythrocytes infected with *P. falciparum* cytoadhere to endothelial cells and sequester in the deep tissues [26]. This cytoadherence is mediated by structures induced on the erythrocyte membrane by the parasite called knobs (Fig. 6.7). Several parasite proteins are associated with the knobs, and one of these is a transmembrane protein called PfEMP1 [27]. This protein corresponds to members of the *var* gene family, and there are approximately 60 paralogs (i.e., alleles) of this gene in the parasite's genome. PfEMP1 has a large extracellular domain, and the various PfEMP1 proteins bind to a wide range of receptors found on endothelial cells. Sequential expression of the various *var* genes results in antigenic variation as well as a change in the binding phenotype of the infected erythrocyte.

The sequestration of the infected erythrocytes also has pathological consequences. One obvious consequence is the blockage of capillaries in the tissues, and some of the pathology is ischemic in nature due to the mechanical blockage of the blood vessels. In addition, the parasite exhibits a high level of glycolysis that can cause localized hypoglycemia and lactic acidosis (Box 6.1). Furthermore, there is some inflammation that affects endothelial cell function and leads to vascular leakage and hemorrhaging. One potential complication of falciparum malaria is cerebral malaria which is characterized by impaired consciousness and other neurological manifestations. The ischemia, metabolic effects, vascular leakage, and hemorrhaging in the brain all contribute to the severe disease symptoms associated with cerebral malaria. Respiratory distress is another complication associated with severe

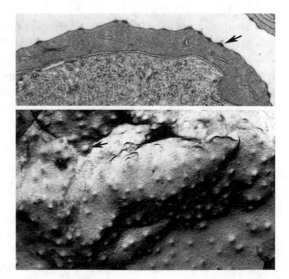

**Fig. 6.7** *Plasmodium falciparum* knobs. Transmission electron micrograph (upper panel) showing electron-dense knobs on the surface of infected erythrocytes (lower panel). A carbon replica scanning electron micrograph (lower panel) showing the distribution of knobs protruding from the surface of the infected erythrocyte. Arrows denote examples of knobs. (Micrographs kindly provided by Dr. H. Norbert Lanners)

**Box 6.1 Glucose Metabolism by Blood Parasites**

Hypoglycemia has long been associated with severe malaria, and some of this hypoglycemia is likely due to glucose consumption by the parasite [28]. The parasite essentially only utilizes anaerobic glycolysis for the conversion of glucose into energy, and this anaerobic metabolism results in excess glucose consumption. In other words, the pyruvate produced as a result of glycolysis is not subjected to aerobic metabolism involving the tricarboxylic acid cycle and oxidative phosphorylation in the generation of ATP. This is rather wasteful in that glycolysis of one molecule of glucose results in the net synthesis of two ATP molecules, whereas the complete aerobic metabolism of a single glucose molecule produces 38 molecules of ATP. The extreme abundance of glucose in the blood and tissues of the host means that the parasite can be rather wasteful in the generation of ATP. Another consequence of glycolysis without the tricarboxylic acid cycle is that pyruvate is converted to lactic acid as a final product of glucose metabolism. This can result in acidosis, another clinical manifestation of malaria. If one also considers the phenomenon of sequestration observed in *P. falciparum*, the hypoglycemia and acidosis can be quite extreme in a localized area in the deep tissues.

This phenomenon of hypoglycemia and acidosis due to anaerobic metabolism is also observed in other vector-transmitted protozoa, such as African trypanosomes. Both the African trypanosomes and malaria parasites have the full complement of genes for the tricarboxylic acid pathway and oxidative phosphorylation. However, these genes are not expressed during the blood stage of the infection. During the vector stage of the infection, though when glucose is much less abundant, these parasites switch to an aerobic metabolism and oxidize glucose completely to carbon dioxide and water. In addition, in the case of the African trypanosomes, proline is the major fuel source during the vector stage [29]. Proline is an abundant amino acid in the tsetse fly and is the main energy source used by the fly for egg production, lactation, and to fuel flight muscles.

malaria and is a good predictor of death. Metabolic acidosis in the lungs due to parasite sequestration and a high rate of glycolysis is the likely cause of the lung injury that can lead to respiratory failure.

# Kinetoplastids

The kinetoplastids are a monophyletic group of flagellated protozoa. The original unifying feature of this group was a Giemsa-staining structure distinct from the nucleus that was named the kinetoplast due to its proximity to the base of the flagellum. Despite its name and location, the kinetoplast is not involved in the movement, although it contains an abundance of mitochondrial DNA. Kinetoplastids parasitize virtually all animal groups—ranging from fish to humans—as well as plants and insects. Three distinct human diseases are caused by kinetoplastids: human African trypanosomiasis, Chagas disease, and leishmaniasis [30]. All three are transmitted by arthropod vectors (Table 6.1).

## *Human African Trypanosomiasis*

Human African trypanosomiasis, also called African sleeping sickness, is a parasitic infection that is almost always fatal if not treated [31]. African trypanosomiasis exhibits a patchy distribution in equatorial Africa that is determined by the distribution of the tse-tse vector. Two species of African trypanosomes infect humans: *Trypanosoma gambiense* and *T. rhodesiense*. *T. gambiense* is the more common cause of human African trypanosomiasis and exhibits an anthroponotic type of transmission, whereas *T. rhodesiense* is a common parasite of animals and exhibits a zoonotic transmission cycle in humans.

The infection is initiated when forms known as metacyclic trypomastigotes are introduced via the bite wound as the tse-tse is taking a blood meal. The trypomastigotes are extracellular parasites that reside in the blood and tissue fluids of the host. A sophisticated antigenic variation involving a surface coat protein allows the parasite to avoid elimination by the host immune system [32]. These bloodstream forms exhibit a high rate of replication with a doubling time as short as 6 h. Associated with this high rate of replication is a high rate of glycolysis (Box 6.1). After bloodstream forms are taken up by the tse-tse, they convert into a stage known as the procyclic trypomastigote. The procyclic forms replicate within the gut of the tse-tse and then later migrate to the salivary glands, where they convert into metacyclic trypomastigotes in preparation for infecting another human or mammalian host.

African trypanosomiasis is often broken down into two stages: early and late. During the early stage, parasites are found in the bloodstream and lymphatics. Clinical manifestations of this stage include intermittent fevers and swollen lymph nodes. The late stage is marked by the invasion of the central nervous system, and clinical manifestations become neurological in nature. Initially the symptoms are subtle behavioral changes that progress to more serious symptoms, eventually leading to convulsions, coma, and death. A notable neurological manifestation is severe sleep disturbances, thus the name African sleeping sickness. Little has been done in humans on the impact of nutrition on African trypanosomiasis. Studies using rodent models have demonstrated that vitamin deficiencies increase parasitemia and infection duration (Box 6.2).

## Chagas Disease

Another trypanosome that infects humans is *Trypanosoma cruzi* [37]. The disease caused by this pathogen is called Chagas disease in reference to Carlos Chagas who first discovered the parasite and vector and described the salient features of the disease. The vectors in this case are blood-feeding insects known as triatomine bugs. *T. cruzi* infects a wide range of vertebrates, and transmission to humans generally involves close proximity of domiciliary or peri-domiciliary triatomine bugs and animal reservoirs. Chagas disease is found in foci throughout South and Central America where sufficient contact between humans and vectors exists.

---

**Box 6.2 Vitamin Deficiencies and Trypanosomiasis**

Lab studies using rodent models related to the African trypanosomes have explored the impact of low dietary vitamins A, $B_{12}$, and E on parasite proliferation. Vitamin A-deficient diets were associated with earlier and prolonged parasitemia in *T. musculi*-infected mice [33]. Similarly, rats deficient in vitamin $B_{12}$ suffered earlier and higher parasitemia followed by persistent infection when infected with *T. lewisi* [34]. This increase in susceptibility to *T. lewisi* was accompanied by a decrease in antibody production. Similarly, reduced macrophage activity was observed in vitamin $B_{12}$-deficient rats infected with *T. lewisi* [35]. In contrast, knockout of the alpha-tocopherol transfer protein gene in mice, which creates a vitamin E deficiency, conferred resistance to *T. congolense* [36]. This is likely due to the free radical scavenger activity of vitamin E and the hypersensitivity of trypanosomes to oxidative stress. In other words, without vitamin E the parasites are not able to completely detoxify reactive oxygen species.

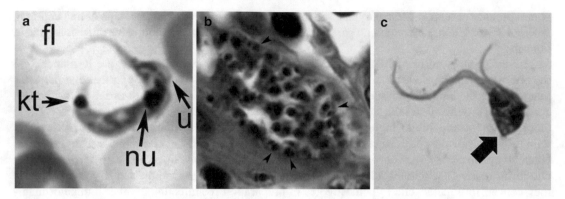

**Fig. 6.8** *Trypanosoma cruzi* life cycle stages. (**a**) A trypomastigote found in blood with kinetoplast (kt), nucleus (nu), flagellum (fl), and undulating membrane (u) denoted with arrows. This is a nonreplicating form capable of infecting various host cells or the triatomine vector. (**b**) A heart muscle cell infected with amastigotes which replicate by binary fission. The arrows denote individual amastigotes in which the nucleus and kinetoplast are both visible. (**c**) A replicating epimastigote form with two nuclei and two kinetoplasts. This stage is found in the midgut of the triatomine vector

Infection is initiated by metacyclic trypomastigotes excreted in the feces of the infected triatomine bug as it takes a blood meal. This happens at night while the person is sleeping. The trypomastigote gains entry via the bite wound or penetrating mucous membranes, especially the conjunctiva of the eyes. After gaining entry into the host, the trypomastigotes invade host cells and convert into amastigotes (Fig. 6.8). The parasite is capable of invading a wide range of host cells. Within the cytoplasm of the host cell, the amastigotes replicate by binary fission. Following replication the amastigotes convert back into trypomastigotes which are released from the infected cell. The trypomastigotes then invade other cells and continue these replicative cycles.

Alternatively, some trypomastigotes enter the blood where they can be ingested when a triatomine bug takes a blood meal. These ingested trypomastigotes convert into epimastigotes in the midgut of the triatomine and replicate. Some of the epimastigotes migrate to the hindgut and convert into metacyclic trypomastigotes to complete the life cycle.

Chagas disease is characterized by three phases: an acute stage, a long latent or indeterminate period, and chronic disease. The acute phase lasts a few weeks to months and is most often asymptomatic. If symptoms are present, they are generally typical of systemic infections such as fever, malaise, and swollen lymph nodes. The acute phase is followed by a decades-long asymptomatic latent period that is characterized by seropositivity, but no detectable parasitemia. During this latent period, the immune system controls the parasitemia, but does not eliminate the parasites. Approximately one-third of those seropositive individuals in the long latent phase will develop symptomatic Chagas disease.

Symptomatic Chagas disease most often manifests as either cardiomyopathy or megaviscera (Table 6.4). Myocardial involvement associated with Chagas disease includes arrhythmias, conduction defects, cardiomegaly, congestive heart failure, and thromboembolic events. All parts of the heart, including the endocardium, myocardium, and pericardium, can be affected. Autonomic ganglia and cardiac nerves are also frequently affected. Dilation of the digestive tract, especially the esophagus and colon, is also sometimes observed in chronic Chagas disease. The dilation of these organs is possibly due to the loss of autonomic ganglia associated with these organs. Pathogenesis is likely due to the persistence of *T. cruzi* at a low parasitemia that results in the foci of cellular damage and inflammation. Over time the accumulation of these small areas of damage may reach a clinically relevant level and produce the symptoms of cardiomyopathy and megaviscera.

In that the pathophysiology of Chagas disease includes a major chronic inflammation component, it is likely that both protein-energy and micronutrient undernutrition affects the infection. A low-

**Table 6.4** Pathophysiology of chronic Chagas disease

| Pathology | Clinical symptoms or possible outcomes |
|---|---|
| Heart | |
| Arrhythmias and conduction defects | Abnormal ECG, palpitations, lightheadedness, fainting |
| Enlargement of the heart | Aneurysm due to thinning heart wall |
| Inflammation and fibrosis | Congestive heart failure and thromboembolic events |
| Gastrointestinal tract | |
| Megaesophagus | Difficult swallowing, regurgitation, heartburn, hiccups, increased salivation, and speech impairments |
| Megacolon | Prolonged constipation |

---

**Box 6.3 Undernutrition and Chagas Disease**

Results from experimental *Trypanosoma cruzi* models generally show that undernutrition is accompanied by a lower immunity and higher parasitemia. In that the acute stage of Chagas disease is often asymptomatic and usually goes undetected, it is difficult to discern if undernutrition has a major impact on parasitemia in humans. Furthermore, the decades-long latent period would likely mask any effect of undernutrition on the development and progression of symptomatic chronic Chagas disease. However, infection with *T. cruzi* may impact nutritional status. De Andrade and Zicker [44] compared anthropometric measurements in Brazilian school children in seropositive individuals and seronegative individuals. Seropositive children had a 2.4-fold higher risk of being stunted and a 2.8-fold higher risk of being underweight suggesting a potential impact of infection on nutrition or metabolism.

---

protein diet results in an earlier appearance of parasitemia and higher parasitemia and mortality in experimental rodent models [38, 39]. Similarly, deficiencies in iron and vitamins A, E, $B_1$, $B_5$, and $B_6$ exacerbate *T. cruzi* infections in experimental models [reviewed in 40]. In addition, rats fed a low-protein diet exhibited a slower recovery of noradrenaline levels in the heart following *T. cruzi* infection, as compared to rats fed a normal diet [41].

However, despite the higher parasitemias and slower recovery, the inflammatory lesions associated with the heart were less extensive in the mice fed on a restricted protein diet [39]. Similarly, Martins et al. [42] observed higher parasitemias associated with a low-protein diet but at the same time, less infiltration of inflammatory cells into the heart. Therefore, despite the higher parasitemia, there was less inflammation and pathogenesis. Similarly, a marked leukopenia was observed in infected vitamin E-deficient rats as compared to infected control rats [43]. However, this leukopenia was accompanied by a monocytosis and increased differentiation into macrophages resulting in enhanced pathology. At this time our knowledge about the relationship between Chagas disease and nutrition is quite limited, and there have been very few studies in humans (Box 6.3).

## *Leishmaniasis*

Several species of *Leishmania* infect humans and cause a wide range of disease manifestations (Table 6.5). Leishmaniasis is found in tropical and subtropical regions throughout the world. The disease is transmitted by two different genera of phlebotomine sandflies: *Phlebotomus* in the eastern hemisphere (i.e., Old World including Africa, Asia, and Europe) or *Lutzomyia* in the western

**Table 6.5** Major *Leishmania* species infecting humans

| Species | Clinical manifestations | Geographical distribution |
|---|---|---|
| *L. mexicana* complex | CL and rare cases of DCL | Central America, northern and central South America; very rare in southern USA |
| *L. braziliensis* complex | CL with some cases developing into MCL | Central and South America |
| *L. major* | CL | Northern and Central Africa, Middle East, Southern Asia |
| *L. tropica* | CL and rare cases of relapses | Middle East and Southern Asia |
| *L. aethiopica* | CL and some cases of DCL | Highlands of Ethiopia and Kenya |
| *L. donovani* | VL with rare cases of posttreatment CL | East Africa, Sub-Saharan Africa, Southern Asia including India and Iran |
| *L. infantum* | VL or CL according to strain | North Africa and Southern Europe |
| *L. (infantum) chagasi* | VL and some CL | Foci in Brazil, Venezuela, and Colombia; isolated cases throughout South America |

*CL* cutaneous leishmaniasis, *MCL* mucocutaneous leishmaniasis, *DCL* diffuse cutaneous leishmaniasis, *VL* visceral leishmaniasis

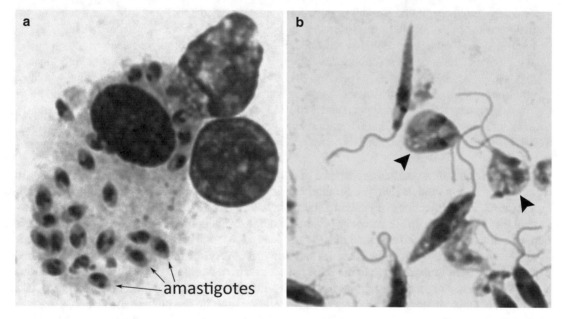

**Fig. 6.9** *Leishmania* life cycle stages. (**a**) An infected macrophage containing numerous amastigotes. Amastigotes are the replicating form in the vertebrate host. (**b**) Promastigote forms are the replicating form found in the sand fly vector. Arrowheads denote parasites actively dividing as indicated by two nuclei and kinetoplasts

hemisphere (i.e., New World including South and Central America). Leishmaniasis is often a zoonotic infection involving either a rodent or dog reservoir. Clinical manifestations associated with leishmaniasis can range from simple benign cutaneous lesions to a fatal systemic disease [45]. The clinical manifestation depends largely on the species causing the infection, as well as the nature of the immune response against the pathogen. Strong T helper type 1 (Th1) responses combined with weak T helper type 2 (Th2) responses are associated with a self-healing cutaneous lesion [46]. A strong Th2 response is generally associated with more severe pathology.

During vector feeding a stage known as the promastigote is introduced into the bite wound (Fig. 6.9). The promastigotes are then phagocytosed by macrophages or other professional phagocytic cells. The parasite cannot actively invade host cells and is dependent on the phagocytic activity of the host cell to gain entry. The promastigote converts into an amastigote and replicates within the macrophage. The *Leishmania* amastigote has several adaptations that allow it to survive in the phagolysosome of the macrophage [46]. Newly formed amastigotes are released via lysis of the host macrophage and re-phagocytosed by other macrophages to continue the replicative cycle. If the infected macrophage is ingested by a sand fly, the amastigotes are released and convert back into promastigotes. The promastigotes replicate in the gut of the fly and develop into the promastigote form that is infective for the mammalian host.

The most common clinical manifestation associated with leishmaniasis is a self-healing skin lesion referred to as simple cutaneous leishmaniasis. The lesions are typically ulcerated with raised borders. Generally, the lesion starts as a papule at the bite site. Replication of the amastigotes destroys the macrophages, and the localized inflammation leads to tissue destruction and ulceration. The lesion expands outward with the repeated cycles of parasite replication at the boundary between the ulcerated tissue and healthy tissue. With the onset of the Th1 response, the macrophages begin to eliminate the parasite, and the lesion stops expanding and retracts until it completely heals. This process generally takes weeks to months. On rare occasions the infected macrophages can metastasize and cause diffuse cutaneous leishmaniasis or mucocutaneous leishmaniasis. These clinical manifestations heal more slowly and are associated with a high level of pathogenesis.

Visceral leishmaniasis is due to infection of macrophages in the reticuloendothelial system including the spleen, liver, bone marrow, and lymph nodes. It is a disseminated disease characterized by a weak Th1 response and a strong Th2 response. This results in a slowly progressing systemic infection that is often fatal if not treated. The three most common species associated with visceral leishmaniasis are *L. donovani*, *L. infantum*, and *L. chagasi*. All three species are closely related, and *L. chagasi* and *L. infantum* are especially closely related. Some data suggest that *L. chagasi* was introduced to the Americas by the early Spanish and Portuguese colonists and thus is sometimes designated at *L. infantum chagasi*. The immune status of the host also influences the development of visceral leishmaniasis in that immune suppression can result in normally cutaneous species or strains causing a visceral disease. Likewise, more severe disease manifestations are associated with undernutrition (Box 6.4).

---

**Box 6.4 Protein Deficiency and Leishmaniasis**

Nutritional status plays a critical role in the clinical manifestations of leishmaniasis [reviewed in 47]. Epidemiological studies have shown that protein-energy malnutrition is a major determinant of both the progression and severity of leishmaniasis and undernutrition increases the case fatality rate. Studies in laboratory models consistently find that mice fed protein-deficient diets develop long-term chronic infections instead of self-resolving infections. The failure to resolve infections is generally associated with impaired innate and adaptive immune responses and especially the Th1 response. One consequence of this immune impairment is an increased likelihood of visceral disease [48]. Specifically, protein deficiency has been shown to impair monocyte and polymorphonuclear leukocyte function [49], to reduce phagocytes in the lymph nodes and lower skin lymph node barrier function [50], to reduce chemotaxis of T cells to the spleen [51], and to dysregulate T cell and cytokine responses against the parasite [52]. Furthermore, an increase in arginase activity in monocytes and macrophages is also associated with protein deficiency, and this likely provides a more permissive environment for parasite replication [53]. In general, these changes in T-cell and phagocyte function would increase parasite dissemination and reduce parasite killing, thereby increasing visceralization and severe disease manifestations.

## Toxoplasmosis

*Toxoplasma gondii* is an apicomplexan parasite that infects a wide range of mammals and birds. Estimates based on seropositivity suggest that up to one-third of the human population may be infected with *Toxoplasma*. However, toxoplasmosis in adults and children beyond the neonatal stage is usually benign and symptomless. Severe disease is generally only observed in immunocompromised persons or associated with congenitally acquired infections.

### *Transmission*

*Toxoplasma* exhibits a complex predator-prey life cycle [54, 55]. Felines, including domestic cats, are the definitive host in which sexual reproduction of the parasite occurs. Cats acquire the infection by eating an infected intermediate host. The parasite infects the intestinal epithelium of the cat and exhibits a coccidian life cycle similar to *Cryptosporidium* resulting in the production of oocysts that are excreted with the feces. Intermediate hosts such as rodents become infected by ingesting the mature oocysts. Within the intermediate host, the parasite disseminates throughout the body and establishes a life-long chronic infection. The immune response restrains the parasite in a latent form called the tissue cyst. These tissue cysts are highly infectious to felines, as well as other intermediate hosts, if ingested.

Humans generally acquire *Toxoplasma* infections by one of three routes: (1) ingestion of oocysts via contaminated food or water, (2) ingestion of undercooked meat containing tissue cysts, or (3) congenitally (Fig. 6.10). Thus, diet increases potential exposure to *Toxoplasma* (Box 6.5). Historically, infections were sometimes acquired via organ transplants. However, screening of organ donors and recipients has essentially eliminated organ transplants as a source of toxoplasmosis. Children of the crawling and dirt eating age may be particularly susceptible to infections via oocysts. Similarly, gardening or ingesting raw vegetables may be a risk factor for acquiring toxoplasmosis. It is generally believed that the ingestion of undercooked meat is the major source of human infections. Presumably, livestock that graze in areas contaminated with cat feces become infected and are carriers of latent toxoplasmosis. In addition, during pregnancy, the acute stage of the parasite can be transmitted from mother to fetus.

### *Pathogenesis*

The progression of toxoplasmosis is the same regardless of whether infections are acquired by ingestion of oocysts or tissue cysts. Immediately following infection there is an acute phase of the infection involving rapid parasite replication and dissemination throughout the body [54, 55]. Most acute infections are asymptomatic, and when symptoms do occur, they are generally described as being mononucleosis-like with fever, headache, muscle ache, fatigue, and swollen lymph nodes. After a few weeks and coinciding with immunity, the parasite converts to the slowly replicating tissue cysts to mark the beginning of a life-long latent chronic phase without symptoms. Immunosuppression such as the development of AIDS can lead to a reactivation of the acute phase of the infection (Fig. 6.11). The most common clinical manifestation associated with this reactivation is toxoplasmic encephalitis [60]. Early symptoms associated with toxoplasmic encephalitis include headache, lethargy, and minor personality changes. As the disease progresses, the neurological symptoms increase in severity leading to disturbances in speech and coordination and ultimately to seizures and convulsions. It has been

**Fig. 6.10** Transmission cycles of *Toxoplasma*. A natural transmission cycle between cats and small animals and birds exists in nature. Humans become infected primarily through three routes: (1) the ingestion of food or water contaminated with oocysts from cat feces, (2) ingestion of tissue cysts in undercooked meat from infected intermediate hosts, or (3) congenital infection from mother to fetus

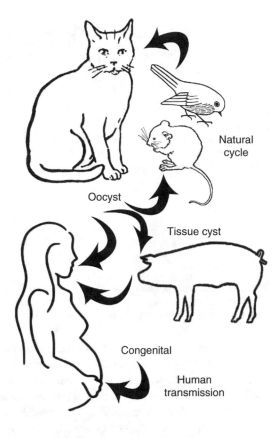

### Box 6.5 Diet and Toxoplasmosis

Animal source foods are an important source of high-quality nutrients. However, production and consumption of animal source foods do entail some potential food safety risks [56]. *Toxoplasma* is well documented in the food supply [57], and consumption of raw or under-cooked meat is a major source of human toxoplasmosis. An estimated 30–60% of newly acquired toxoplasmosis in European pregnant women is due to the consumption of inadequately cooked or cured meat [58]. Cultural differences in the consumption of raw or cured meat obviously impact the risk of acquiring toxoplasmosis. In addition, there may be an increased risk of infection in regions where fuel for cooking is limited. Contact with soil contaminated with cat feces is another risk factor for toxoplasmosis. This includes activities such as gardening and the ingestion of raw unwashed fruit and vegetables [59].

suggested that the neurological manifestations may be due in part to the parasite acquiring folate and/or vitamin $B_{12}$ from the host neural cells to such an extent that it affects cognitive function [61].

Infections acquired congenitally are more likely to be symptomatic than postnatal infections and can be quite severe [62]. Possible outcomes include spontaneous abortion and stillbirth or live birth with neurological or vision problems ranging from moderate to severe. The most common outcome is to be asymptomatic at birth and develop retinochoroiditis or neurological symptoms later in childhood or adolescence. Ocular disease is a common sequela of congenital infection. In addition, ocular toxoplasmosis is sometimes observed in immunocompetent persons. Generally, ocular toxoplasmosis is self-resolving in immunocompetent persons, and vision problems are transient. However, there can be

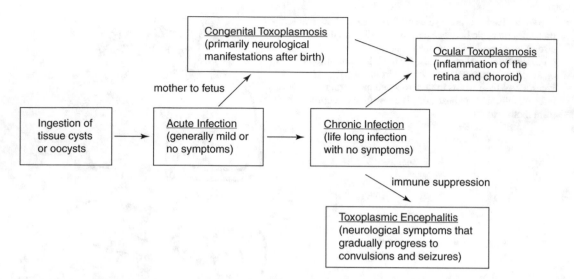

**Fig. 6.11** Disease progression and clinical manifestations associated with toxoplasmosis. Following infection there is a relatively asymptomatic acute phase followed by a life-long asymptomatic chronic phase. Disease manifestations are primarily due to immune suppression, congenital transmission, and ocular disease

scarring of the retina leading to longer-lasting vision problems. In AIDS patients the retinochoroiditis continues to progress and results in severe eye damage.

As symptomatic toxoplasmosis is generally associated with an immunocompromised state, such as AIDS or congenital infection, one might think undernutrition would have a negative impact on disease outcome as it does in most other diseases. However, there are no studies clearly showing a link between nutritional deficiencies and the severity of toxoplasmosis. Nonetheless, *Toxoplasma* may induce immune-metabolic interactions. For example, *Toxoplasma*- infected mice lose 20% of their body mass, including both adipose and muscle tissue [63]. A transient anorexia and an elevation in cachexia inflammatory cytokines accompany this weight loss. In contrast, patients seropositive for *Toxoplasma* infection may have a higher prevalence of nonalcoholic fatty liver disease [64] and may be at higher risk for obesity [65]. At the cellular level, *Toxoplasma* alters lipid metabolism within the host cell [66]. Thus, at this time it is not clear exactly how the chronic toxoplasmosis affects inflammation and metabolism and how these effects impact the nutritional status of the host.

## Conclusion

Protozoa are a diverse group of eukaryotic microbes and include several major human pathogens. Several of these protozoan pathogens cause diarrheal disease which contributes to undernutrition and lowers immunity. Similarly fever and inflammation associated with systemic infections divert energy and negatively impact nutritional status. In general, undernutrition, and especially protein deficiency, lowers immunity and leads to more severe disease. This creates a snowball effect in which undernutrition worsens the outcomes of infections and infections worsen the nutritional status of the individual. This is especially true in resource-poor settings where undernutrition and infectious diseases are both prevalent. In general, we have little specific knowledge about the interactions of protozoan pathogens and nutritional status and how specifically host nutritional status may affect the immune response against protozoan pathogens.

# References

1. Simpson AGB, Roger AJ. The real 'kingdoms' of eukaryotes. Curr Biol. 2004;14(17):R693–6.
2. Wiser MF. Protozoa and human disease. London/New York: Garland Science; 2011.
3. Stephenson CB. Primer on immune response and interface with malnutrition. In: Humphries DL, Scott ME, Vermund SH, editors. Nutrition and infectious diseases – shifting the clinical paradigm. Cham: Springer Nature; 2020.
4. Katona P, Katona-Apte J. The interaction between nutrition and infection. Clin Infect Dis. 2008;46(10):1582–8.
5. Siddiqui F, Belayneh G, Bhutta ZA. Nutrition and diarrheal disease and enteric pathogens. In: Humphries DL, Scott ME, Vermund SH, editors. Nutrition and infectious diseases – shifting the clinical paradigm. Cham: Springer Nature; 2020.
6. Ramakrishna BS, Venkataraman S, Mukhopadhya A. Tropical malabsorption. Postgrad Med J. 2006;82(974):779–87.
7. Ezwena VO. Co-infection and nutrition: integrating ecological and epidemiological perspectives. In: Humphries DL, Scott ME, Vermund SH, editors. Nutrition and infectious diseases – shifting the clinical paradigm. Cham: Springer Nature; 2020.
8. Cassat JE, Skaar EP. Iron in infection and immunity. Cell Host Microbe. 2013;13(5):509–19.
9. Meites E. Trichomoniasis: the "neglected" sexually transmitted disease. Infect Dis Clin N Am. 2013;27(4):755–64.
10. Huffman RD, Nawrocki LD, Wilson WA, Brittingham A. Digestion of glycogen by a glucosidase released by *Trichomonas vaginalis*. Exp Parasitol. 2015;159:151–9.
11. Hrdy I, Tachezy J, Müller M. Metabolism of trichomonad hydrogenosomes. In: Tachezy J, editor. Hydrogenosomes and mitosomes: mitochondria of anaerobic euakryotes. Berlin, Heidelberg: Springer-Verlag; 2008. p. 114–45.
12. Beltrán NC, Horváthová L, Jedelský PL, Sedinová M, Rada P, Marcinčiková M, et al. Iron-induced changes in the proteome of *Trichomonas vaginalis* hydrogenosomes. PLoS ONE. 2013;8:e65148.
13. Cheng WH, Huang KY, Huang PJ, Hsu JH, Fang YK, Chiu CH, et al. Nitric oxide maintains cell survival of *Trichomonas vaginalis* upon iron depletion. Parasit Vectors. 2015;8:393.
14. Roberts SA, Brabin L, Diallo S, Gies S, Nelson A, Stewart C, et al. Mucosal lactoferrin response to genital tract infections is associated with iron and nutritional biomarkers in young Burkinabé women. Eur J Clin Nutr. 2019; https://doi.org/10.1038/s41430-019-0444-7.
15. Haque R, Huston CD, Hughes M, Houpt E, Petri WA. Amebiasis. N Engl J Med. 2003;348(16):1565–73.
16. Verkerke HP, Petri WA, Marie CS. The dynamic interdependence of amebiasis, innate immunity, and undernutrition. Semin Immunopathol. 2012;34(6):771–85.
17. Cama VA, Mathison BA. Infections by intestinal coccidia and *Giardia duodenalis*. Clin Lab Med. 2015;35(2):423–44.
18. Bouzid M, Hunter PR, Chalmers RM, Tyler KM. *Cryptosporidium* pathogenicity and virulence. Clin Microbiol Rev. 2013;26(1):115–34.
19. Hunter PR, Nichols G. Epidemiology and clinical features of *Cryptosporidium* infection in immunocompromised patients. Clin Microbiol Rev. 2002;15(1):145–54.
20. Coutinho BP, Oriá RB, Vieira CM, Sevilleja JE, Warren CA, Maciel JG, et al. *Cryptosporidium* infection causes undernutrition and, conversely, weanling undernutrition intensifies infection. J Parasitol. 2008;94(6):1225–32.
21. Greenwood BM, Fidock DA, Kyle DE, Kappe SHI, Alonso PL, Collins FH, et al. Malaria: progress, perils, and prospects for eradication. J Clin Invest. 2008;118(4):1266–76.
22. Goldberg DE. Hemoglobin degradation. Curr Top Microbiol Immunol. 2005;295:275–91.
23. Egan TJ. Haemozoin formation. Mol Biochem Parasitol. 2008;157(2):127–36.
24. Spottiswoode N, Duffy PE, Drakesmith H. Iron, anemia and hepcidin in malaria. Front Pharmacol. 2014;5:125.
25. Kim HH, Bei AK. Nutritional frameworks in malaria. In: Humphries DL, Scott ME, Vermund SH, editors. Nutrition and infectious diseases – shifting the clinical paradigm. Cham: Springer Nature; 2020.
26. Cunnington AJ, Riley EM, Walther M. Stuck in a rut? Reconsidering the role of parasite sequestration in severe malaria syndromes. Trends Parasitol. 2013;29(12):585–92.
27. Smith JD. The role of PfEMP1 adhesion domain classification in *Plasmodium falciparum* pathogenesis research. Mol Biochem Parasitol. 2014;195(2):82–7.
28. White NJ, Warrell DA, Chanthavanich P, Looareesuwan S, Warrell MJ, Krishna S, et al. Severe hypoglycemia and hyperinsulinemia in falciparum malaria. N Engl J Med. 1983;309(2):61–6.
29. Mantilla BS, Marchese L, Casas-Sánchez A, Dyer NA, Ejeh N, Biran M, et al. Proline metabolism is essential for *Trypanosoma brucei brucei* survival in the tsetse vector. PLoS Pathol. 2017;13(1):e1006158.
30. Filardy AA, Guimarães-Pinto K, Nunes MP, Zukeram K, Fliess L, Pereira L, et al. Human Kinetoplastid protozoan infections: where are we going next? Front Immunol. 2018;9:1493.
31. Büscher P, Cecchi G, Jamonneau V, Priotto G. Human African trypanosomiasis. Lancet. 2017;390(10110):2397–409.
32. Horn D. Antigenic variation in African trypanosomes. Mol Biochem Parasitol. 2014;195(2):123–9.
33. Lee CM, Aboko-Cole F, Fletcher J. Effect of malnutrition on susceptibility of mice to *Trypanosoma musculi*: vitamin A-deficiency. Z Parasitenkd. 1976;49:1–10.

34. Thomaskutty KG, Lee CM. Interaction of nutrition and infection: effect of vitamin $B_{12}$ deficiency on resistance to *Trypanosoma lewisi*. J Natl Med Assoc. 1985;77:289–99.
35. Thomaskutty KG, Lee CM. Interaction of nutrition and infection: macrophage activity in vitamin $B_{12}$-deficient rats infected with *Trypanosoma lewisi*. J Natl Med Assoc. 1987;79:441–6.
36. Herbas MS, Thekisoe OM, Inoue N, Xuan X, Arai H, Suzuki H. The effect of alpha-tocopherol transfer protein gene disruption on *Trypanosoma congolense* infection in mice. Free Radic Biol Med. 2009;47:1408–13.
37. Rassi A. American trypanosomiasis (Chagas disease). Infect Dis Clin N Am. 2012;26(2):275–91.
38. Carlomagno M, Leer G, Esteva M, Hansen D, Segura EL. Role of protein deficiency on the course of *Trypanosoma cruzi* infection and on the degree of protection conferred by a flagellar fraction. J Nutr Immunol. 1996;4(4):37–45.
39. Gomes NG, Pereira FE, Domingues GC, Alves JR. Effects of severe protein restriction in levels of parasitemia and in mortality of mice acutely infected with *Trypanosoma cruzi*. Rev Soc Bras Med Trop. 1994;27:19–24.
40. Malafaia G, Talvani A. Nutritional status driving infection by *Trypanosoma cruzi*: lessons from experimental animals. J Trop Med. 2011;2011:981879.
41. Machado CR, Moraes-Santos T, Machado AB. Cardiac noradrenalin in relation to protein malnutrition in chronic experimental Chagas' disease in the rat. Am J Trop Med Hyg. 1984;33:835–8.
42. Martins RF, Martinelli PM, Guedes PM, da Cruz PB, Dos Santos FM, Silva ME, et al. Protein deficiency alters CX3CL1 and endothelin-1 in experimental *Trypanosoma cruzi*-induced cardiomyopathy. Tropical Med Int Health. 2013;18(4):466–76.
43. Carvalho LS, Camargos ER, Almeida CT, Peluzio Mdo C, Alvarez-Leite JI, Chiari E, et al. Vitamin E deficiency enhances pathology in acute *Trypanosoma cruzi*-infected rats. Trans R Soc Trop Med Hyg. 2006;100(11):1025–31.
44. de Andrade AL, Zicker F. Chronic malnutrition and *Trypanosoma cruzi* infection in children. J Trop Pediatr. 1995;41(2):112–5.
45. McGwire BS, Satoskar AR. Leishmaniasis: clinical syndromes and treatment. Q J Med. 2014;107(1):7–14.
46. Rossi M, Fasel N. How to master the host immune system? Leishmania parasites have the solutions! Int Immunol. 2018;30(3):103–11.
47. Malafaia G. Protein-energy malnutrition as a risk factor for visceral leishmaniasis: a review. Parasite Immunol. 2009;31(10):587–96.
48. Carrillo E, Jimenez MA, Sanchez C, Cunha J, Martins CM, da Paixão SA, et al. Protein malnutrition impairs the immune response and influences the severity of infection in a hamster model of chronic visceral leishmaniasis. PLoS ONE. 2014;9(2):e89412.
49. Kumar V, Bimal S, Singh SK, Chaudhary R, Das S, Lal C, et al. *Leishmania donovani*: dynamics of *L. donovani* evasion of innate immune cell attack due to malnutrition in visceral leishmaniasis. Nutrition. 2014;30:449–58.
50. Ibrahim MK, Barnes JL, Osorio EY, Anstead GM, Jimenez F, Osterholzer JJ, et al. Deficiency of lymph node-resident dendritic cells (DCs) and dysregulation of DC chemoattractants in a malnourished mouse model of *Leishmania donovani* infection. Infect Immun. 2014;82:3098–112.
51. Losada-Barragán M, Umaña-Pérez A, Cuervo-Escobar S, Berbert LR, Porrozzi R, Morgado FN, et al. Protein malnutrition promotes dysregulation of molecules involved in T cell migration in the thymus of mice infected with *Leishmania infantum*. Sci Rep. 2017;7:45991.
52. Cuervo-Escobar S, Losada-Barragán M, Umaña-Pérez A, Porrozzi R, Saboia-Vahia L, Miranda LH, et al. T-cell populations and cytokine expression are impaired in thymus and spleen of protein malnourished BALB/c mice infected with *Leishmania infantum*. PLoS ONE. 2014;9(12):e114584.
53. Corware K, Yardley V, Mack C, Schuster S, Al-Hassi H, Herath S, et al. Protein energy malnutrition increases arginase activity in monocytes and macrophages. Nutr Metab. 2014;11:51.
54. Halonen SK, Weiss LM. Toxoplasmosis. Handb Clin Neurol. 2013;114:125–45.
55. Montoya JG, Liesenfeld O. Toxoplasmosis. Lancet. 2004;363(9425):1965–76.
56. Li M, Havelaar AH, Hoffmann S, Hald T, Kirk MD, Torgerson PR, et al. Global disease burden of pathogens in animal source foods, 2010. PLoS ONE. 2019;14:e0216545.
57. Hussain MA, Stitt V, Szabo EA, Nelan B. *Toxoplasma gondii* in the food supply. Pathogens. 2017;26;6(2):21.
58. Cook AJC, Gilbert RE, Buffolano W, Zufferey J, Petersen E, Jenum PA, et al. Sources of toxoplasma infection in pregnant women: European multicentre case-control study. Br Med J. 2000;321(7254):142–7.
59. Alvarado-Esquivel C, Estrada-Martínez S, Liesenfeld O. *Toxoplasma gondii* infection in workers occupationally exposed to unwashed raw fruits and vegetables: a case control seroprevalence study. Parasit Vectors. 2011;4:235.
60. Nissapatorn V. Toxoplasmosis in HIV/AIDS: a living legacy. SE Asian J Trop Med Public Health. 2009;40(6):1158–78.
61. Berrett AN, Gale SD, Erickson LD, Brown BL, Hedges DW. *Toxoplasma gondii* moderates the association between multiple folate-cycle factors and cognitive function in U.S. adults. Nutrients. 2017;9(6):564.
62. Hampton MM. Congenital toxoplasmosis: a review. Neonatal Netw. 2015;34(5):274–8.
63. Hatter JA, Kouche YM, Melchor SJ, Ng K, Bouley DM, Boothroyd JC, et al. *Toxoplasma gondii* infection triggers chronic cachexia and sustained commensal dysbiosis in mice. PLoS ONE. 2018;13(10):e0204895.

64. Huang J, Zhang H, Liu S, Wang M, Wan B, Velani B, et al. Is *Toxoplasma gondii* infection correlated with nonalcoholic fatty liver disease? – a population-based study. BMC Infect Dis. 2018;18(1):629.
65. Reeves GM, Mazaheri S, Snitker S, Langenberg P, Giegling I, Hartmann AM, et al. A positive association between *T. gondii* seropositivity and obesity. Front Public Health. 2013;1:73.
66. Hu X, Binns D, Reese ML. The coccidian parasites *Toxoplasma* and *Neospora* dysregulate mammalian lipid droplet biogenesis. J Biol Chem. 2017;292(26):11009–20.

# Chapter 7
# Human Helminth Infections: A Primer

**Timothy G. Geary and Manjurul Haque**

## Abbreviations

| | |
|---|---|
| ABZ | Albendazole |
| DEC | Diethylcarbamazine |
| GI | Gastrointestinal tract |
| IVM | Ivermectin |
| L | Larval stage |
| LF | Lymphatic filariasis |
| MBZ | Mebendazole |
| MDA | Mass drug administration |
| MF | Microfilariae |
| NTD | Neglected tropical disease |
| PZQ | Praziquantel |
| STH | Soil-transmitted helminths |

---

**Key Points**
- Helminth infections remain common in resource-limited regions, particularly in tropical areas.
- These parasites contribute to the cycle of poverty that restrains economic development in tropical areas.
- Helminth parasitism limits growth, development, and physical and cognitive abilities, especially in individuals bearing large numbers of these pathogens.
- Although anthelmintic-based control programs have limited the numbers of heavily infected individuals and have decreased the morbidity associated with many parasitic helminths, more than a billion people remain infected.

---

T. G. Geary (✉)
Institute of Parasitology, McGill University, Ste-Anne-de-Bellevue, QC, Canada

School of Biological Sciences, Queen's University – Belfast, Belfast, UK
e-mail: timothy.g.geary@mcgill.ca

M. Haque
Institute of Parasitology, McGill University, Ste-Anne-de-Bellevue, QC, Canada
e-mail: manjurul.haque@mail.mcgill.ca

© Springer Nature Switzerland AG 2021
D. L. Humphries et al. (eds.), *Nutrition and Infectious Diseases*, Nutrition and Health,
https://doi.org/10.1007/978-3-030-56913-6_7

# Introduction

Infectious diseases commonly found in people living in resource-limited areas are often termed "tropical diseases," the most prominent of which, based on mortality, are tuberculosis, HIV/AIDS, and malaria. The pathogens responsible for these diseases wreak enormous tolls in morbidity and mortality in regions of poverty, but also threaten health in wealthier countries, and consequently have attracted significant funding to develop and support research and control programs. In contrast, helminth infections fall into a group of diseases of poverty that are chronic rather than acutely lethal and consequently have attracted much less interest and funding; these are termed "Neglected Tropical Diseases" (NTDs) [1]. Prominent among the NTDs are the human helminthiases that are the subjects of this chapter.

Once essentially ubiquitous in human populations, helminth infections have been largely eliminated as threats to public health in areas that enjoy adequate infrastructure for housing and sanitation or areas where pathogen transmission is limited to at least some degree by climate and the ready availability of safe and effective medicines (anthelmintics). Nonetheless, helminth parasites are thought to infect 1.5–2 billion people, almost all of whom live in regions characterized by limited resources for infrastructure and health care [2–4]. Many of these people are infected with more than one species of parasite ("polyparasitism" or "co-infection") as well as by bacterial and/or viral pathogens. The intersection of limited resources and common infectious diseases contributes to physical and economic underdevelopment, leading to a cycle of poverty that is challenging to break.

Parasitic helminths of humans are primarily classified into three general groups: nematodes (roundworms) in the phylum Nematoda and trematodes (flatworms or flukes) and cestodes (tapeworms) in the phylum Platyhelminthes. These macroscopic pathogens are among the most important factors that sustain the cycle of poverty; helminth infections have been associated with reductions in birthweight, reduced physical and educational development, anemia, and reduced work output [2, 5]. Measurable effects are more common in individuals who harbor larger numbers of adult parasites, but detrimental effects cannot be ruled out in individuals who have lower worm burdens. Helminthiases pose continuing challenges for human health, particularly in tropical areas in which transmission is favored by environmental conditions. However, it must be stressed that parasitic helminths are also enormously detrimental to animal health and plant agriculture on a global scale, seriously limiting the production of livestock, poultry, and crops in the absence of control programs, which are primarily based on chemical treatments. Notwithstanding the important extent to which these parasites limit food security in many regions of the world, the focus of this chapter is on the biology and health impacts of the most common human helminth infections.

Helminth NTDs include infections by nematodes that reside in systemic tissues (filariae), which cause lymphatic filariasis (LF) and onchocerciasis (river blindness) [6], and those that inhabit the gastrointestinal (GI) tract, commonly referred to as soil-transmitted helminths (STHs) [2, 4]. As noted, some 1.5–2 billion people harbor parasitic nematodes (Table 7.1), many being infected with more than one species. The infectious larval stages of filarial parasitic nematodes are transmitted from one infected human to another by the bite of an arthropod vector (in which the parasite undergoes development), while the infectious larval stages of STH species are acquired directly from environments contaminated by fecal material excreted by infected people. Among trematode NTDs, parasites in the genus *Schistosoma* cause urinary or intestinal schistosomiasis in hundreds of millions of people [7], and other species of parasitic trematodes infect tens of millions of humans via food-borne infections [8] (Table 7.1). Several cestode species cause intestinal infections in humans, while larval stages of two species encyst in systemic tissues and can cause serious pathology (Table 7.1). Among the NTDs is the tapeworm *Taenia solium*, a parasite of pigs; following ingestion of eggs, cysts of this parasite often localize in the human brain (neurocysticercosis) and are a common cause of epilepsy in endemic areas [9, 10]. It should be stressed that estimates of the prevalence of these infections are

**Table 7.1** Varying estimates of global prevalence of some human helminth infections

| | Estimated prevalence (2008)[e] | Estimated prevalence (2018)[f] |
|---|---|---|
| *Soil-transmitted nematodes* | | |
| *Ascaris lumbricoides* | 820,000,000 | 450,000,000 |
| Hookworms | | |
| *Necator americanus, Ancylostoma* spp. | 439,000,000 | 230,000,000 |
| *Trichuris trichiura* | 465,000,000 | 300,000,000 |
| *Strongyloides stercoralis*[a] | 30–100,000,000 | |
| *Filarial nematodes* | | |
| *Wuchereria bancrofti* (LF)[b] | 36,000,000 | 65,000,000 |
| *Onchocerca volvulus* | 30,000,000 | 21,000,000 |
| *Trematodes* | | |
| *Schistosoma* spp. | 250,000,000 | 145,000,000 |
| Food-borne trematodes[c] | 16,000,000 | 85,000,000 |
| *Cestodes* | | |
| Adult tapeworms[d] | | |
| Cysticercosis | 1,400,000 | 5,500,000 |
| Echinococcosis | 1,100,000 | 600,000 |

[a]From Ref. [19]
[b]Includes *B. malayi* and *B. timori*
[c]Includes *Clonorchis sinensis, Paragonimus* spp., *Opisthorchis* spp., and *Fasciola hepatica*
[d]Reliable estimates not available
[e]From Ref. [2]
[f]From Ref. [18]

based on incomplete datasets and vary depending on geographical region. However, they serve to illustrate that very large numbers of people are infected, justifying the need for better understanding and control measures.

Human helminthiases are chronic infections, with some species of parasites surviving more than a decade in a human host. In general, immunity against helminths develops slowly and often incompletely [11], and ongoing transmission allows worm numbers to accumulate within an individual over time. Indeed, for some of these pathogens, the immune response directly contributes to the pathology associated with infection (see below). For many of these parasites, highly evolved transmission strategies make re-infection an expected occurrence following chemotherapeutic intervention in the absence of adequate infrastructure and sanitation practices. A common feature of many helminthiases is that the distribution of the number of worms per host is highly skewed, with a few individuals harboring large number of parasites while most of the population is moderately or lightly infected [12]. Importantly, the symptomatic and pathological consequences of helminth infection are highly dependent on the number of parasites present in the host ("worm burden"); health consequences are often not explicitly demonstrable in individuals who harbor few parasites. However, data from the use of anthelmintic chemotherapy in livestock supports the conclusion that even light infections can affect host performance. Routine treatment with anthelmintics consistently leads to measurable productivity benefits (meat, milk, wool), even in animals that bear low worm burdens and show no overt symptoms (subclinical infections) [13–15].

Our ability to precisely define the effects of helminth infections on humans is challenged by diverse factors that are difficult to control. These include a lack of appropriate field-compatible methods to measure long-term changes in health or performance following the removal of parasites by chemotherapy, unlike the case in livestock animals. The situation is further complicated by the fact that our ability to measure adult worm burdens in people is based on indirect measures (egg output in excreta, for example, or the presence of a parasite antigen) and that the rate of re-infection following treatment may be very high, meaning that the duration of parasite-free periods following treatment can be quite short. Finally, we have made insufficient progress in resolving the influence of confounding variables on the health of helminth-infected children or adults living in resource-limited regions, including chronic malnutrition, periodic undernutrition, helminth-induced changes in the microbiome, parasite-induced changes in host immune response, and frequent co-infections with other pathogens (parasites, fungi, bacteria, and viruses).

# Nematode Infections

## *Gastrointestinal Infections*

Although many species of nematodes can infect humans, this discussion focuses on those categorized as NTDs (Table 7.1). The most common human nematode infections are STHs, prominently including *Ascaris lumbricoides*; the hookworms *Ancylostoma duodenale*, *A. ceylanicum*, and *Necator americanus*; and the whipworm *Trichuris trichiura*. These species have been estimated to infect up to 2 billion people combined [2, 4, 16, 17], although lower estimates have also been reported [18]. *Strongyloides stercoralis* is an additional species of interest; while the prevalence of infection is imprecisely known, perhaps 30–100 million humans may be infected, and this is likely an underestimate [19, 20]. Much less is known about the impacts of this parasite on human health and nutrition (except for disseminated infections in immunocompromised individuals) (see Chap. 12) [20, 21], and it will not be a focus of the current discussion.

STHs are globally distributed in areas of poverty, with significant variations in local abundance of particular species. Parasites are directly acquired from environments contaminated with infective eggs or larvae, which are shed in human feces. The infective stages can persist in the environment, sometimes for several years, depending on variables such as temperature and relative humidity. Environmental persistence greatly complicates control measures that rely on sporadic interventions, since re-infection can readily occur in the absence of co-incident improvements in sanitation infrastructure and practices.

*Ascaris lumbricoides* is the most prevalent human STH, with estimates of up to 800,000,000 infections [2, 4]. Eggs shed into the environment in feces develop in a few weeks to the infective stage (embryonated eggs) (Fig. 7.1). After ingestion in contaminated food or water, or transfer from person to person via unclean hands, the eggs hatch in the duodenum. $L_3$-stage larvae penetrate the gut wall and migrate to the liver and reach the lungs in approximately 10 days. During this transition, the larvae molt to the $L_4$ stage before exiting the lung into the trachea, from which they are coughed up and swallowed. Back in the intestine, the worms undergo a final molt to the adult stage and grow to sexual maturity in a few months. Females can be up to 30 cm in length, with males about half as long. Adults are usually found in the jejunum, where they feed on gut contents and are motile to resist peristalsis and the flow of gastrointestinal (GI) contents. Adults can live at least 2 years, and immunity slowly develops; infections are more common in children than in adults. This is a very fertile parasite; a female may produce and excrete as many as 200,000 eggs per day.

A complicating factor is the zoonotic potential of a very closely related species, *Ascaris suum*, which preferentially infects pigs but can also infect people. These species are virtually identical in morphology and life cycle and are so closely related at the genomic level that the possibility that they are the same species has been advanced [22]. However, some differences have been observed, and there appears to be at least a degree of host preference for the two [23]. Nonetheless, to the extent that *A. suum* can infect people, the control of ascariasis in populations that live in proximity to pigs may not be attainable without some veterinary intervention.

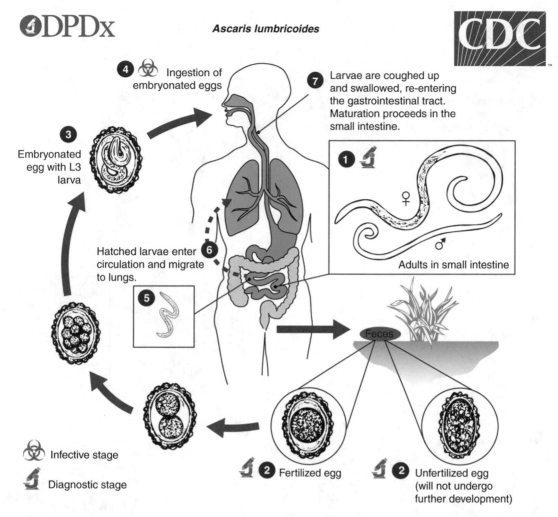

**Fig. 7.1** Life cycle of *Ascaris lumbricoides*. Adult worms (1) live in the lumen of the small intestine. A female may produce approximately 200,000 eggs per day, which are passed with the feces (2). Unfertilized eggs may be ingested but are not infective. Larvae develop to infectivity within fertile eggs after 18 days to several weeks (3), depending on the environmental conditions (optimum: moist, warm, shaded soil). After infective eggs are swallowed (4), the larvae hatch (5), invade the intestinal mucosa, and are carried via the portal, then systemic circulation to the lungs (6). The larvae mature further in the lungs (10 to 14 days), penetrate the alveolar walls, ascend the bronchial tree to the throat, and are swallowed (7). Upon reaching the small intestine, they develop into adult worms. Between 2 and 3 months are required from ingestion of the infective eggs to oviposition by the adult female. Adult worms can live 1 to 2 years. (Source: CDC Parasites Ascariasis: https://www.cdc.gov/parasites/ascariasis/biology.html. Accessed 10 Oct 2019)

Like *A. lumbricoides*, whipworm infections are acquired by oral ingestion of embryonated eggs that develop in an environment contaminated by feces shed from an infected person (Fig. 7.2). Development in the environment from the egg to the infectious embryonated egg ($L_2$ larva) takes 2–4 weeks, depending mostly on temperature. Ingested embryonated eggs hatch in the small intestine and undergo two additional molts to become adults, at which point they have migrated to the cecum and ascending colon and have inserted their anterior end into the gastric mucosa. Adults are about 4 cm in length and resemble a whip (hence the name), with a slender anterior end and a relatively enlarged posterior. Adults may live a year and a female can shed 20,000 eggs per day. Partial immunity is thought to develop, as infections are more common in children than adults. Estimates of the

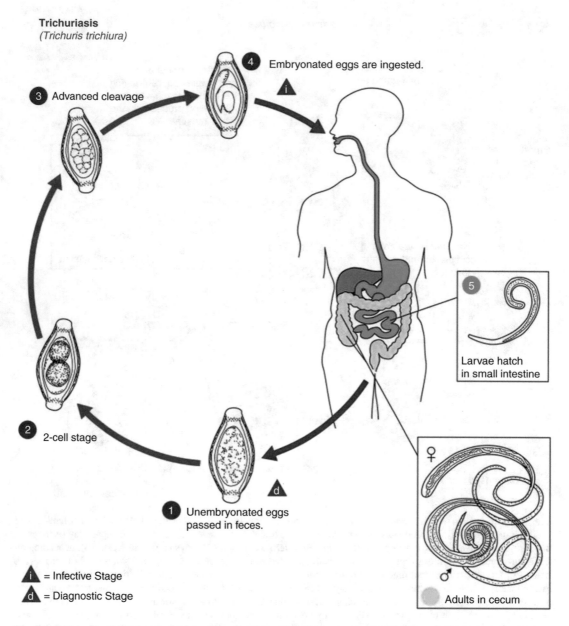

**Trichuriasis**
*(Trichuris trichiura)*

4 Embryonated eggs are ingested.

3 Advanced cleavage

i

5 Larvae hatch
in small intestine

2 2-cell stage

d

1 Unembryonated eggs
passed in feces.

♀
♂
Adults in cecum

i = Infective Stage

d = Diagnostic Stage

**Fig. 7.2** Life cycle of *Trichuris trichiura*. The unembryonated eggs are passed with the stool (1). In the soil, the eggs develop into a two-cell stage (2), an advanced cleavage stage (3), and then they embryonated (4); eggs become infective in 15 to 30 days. After ingestion (soil-contaminated hands or food), the eggs hatch in the small intestine and release larvae (5) that mature and establish themselves as adults in the colon (6). The adult worms (approximately 4 cm in length) live in the cecum and ascending colon. The adult worms are fixed in that location, with the anterior portions threaded into the mucosa. The females begin to oviposit 60 to 70 days after infection. Female worms in the cecum shed between 3000 and 20,000 eggs per day. The life span of the adults is about 1 year. (Source: CDC Parasites: Trichuriasis [Whipworm Infection]: https://www.cdc.gov/parasites/whipworm/biology.html. Accessed 10 Oct 2019)

number of infected humans range from 500 to 1000 million. Pathology, like that from ascariasis, is primarily evident in individuals bearing heavy infections [24].

As for the other STHs, hookworm eggs are shed into the environment in infected feces and develop to the infectious larval stage (L$_3$). Unlike *Ascaris* and *Trichuris*, hookworm infective larvae are free-living (not in the eggshell) and not transmitted orally. Instead, they directly penetrate bare skin. Unprotected by a shell, hookworm infectious larvae may survive only about a month in the environment in favorable conditions of temperature and humidity. Following penetration, the larvae migrate through tissues until reaching the lungs, enter the airspace, and are coughed up and swallowed, a process that takes about 10 days. During this period, a molt to the L$_4$ stage occurs. These larvae begin to ingest blood in the GI tract, undergoing the final molt to the fertile adult stage in about a month (Fig. 7.3). Hookworms are hematophagous and acquire blood meals by cutting small holes in the intestinal epithelium. Adult *N. americanus* can live up to 5 years, whereas *Ancylostoma* spp. typically

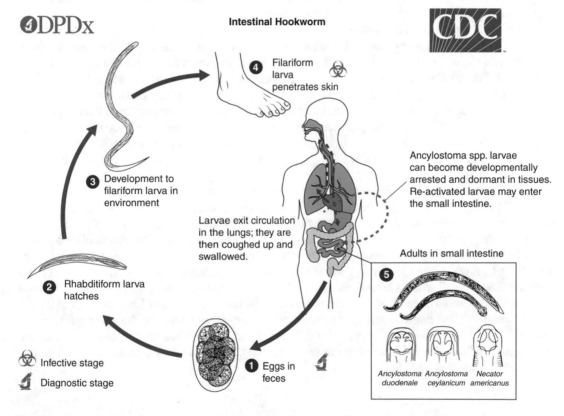

**Fig. 7.3** Life cycle of human hookworms. Eggs are passed in the stool (1), and under favorable conditions (moisture, warmth, shade), larvae hatch in 1 to 2 days. The released larvae grow in the feces and/or the soil (2), and after 5 to 10 days (and two molts), they become infective third-stage larvae (3). These infective larvae can survive 3 to 4 weeks in favorable environmental conditions. On contact with the human host, the larvae penetrate the skin and are carried through the blood vessels to the heart and then to the lungs. They penetrate into the pulmonary alveoli, ascend the bronchial tree to the pharynx, and are swallowed (4). The larvae reach the small intestine, where they reside and mature into adults. Adult worms live in the lumen of the small intestine, where they attach to the intestinal wall with resultant blood loss by the host (5). Most adult worms are eliminated in 1 to 2 years, but the longevity may reach several years. (Source: CDC Parasites: Intestinal Hookworm: https://www.cdc.gov/parasites/hookworm/biology.html. Accessed 10 Oct 2019)

survive less than a year (but dormant parasites in tissue can reactivate to continue the infection). Females can produce as many as 30,000 eggs per day. Immunity to hookworms develops slowly; adults as well as children may harbor significant and clinically relevant worm burdens [25].

## Systemic Infections

Tissue-dwelling filarial nematodes include *Onchocerca volvulus*, the cause of river blindness, with approximately 21 million current infections, and *Wuchereria bancrofti*, *Brugia malayi*, and *B. timori*, the causes of LF, with perhaps 60 million current cases (the considerable majority due to *W. bancrofti*) [6, 18]. These infections are transmitted by arthropod vectors (black flies in the genus *Simulium* for the former and a variety of mosquito species for LF) (Fig. 7.4). Adult *O. volvulus* reside in nodules located around the body, some of which are palpable and which do not cause much overt pathology. Larval stages called microfilariae (mf or $L_1$) are produced by fertilized females and circulate in the skin. Immune responses that eventually develop against the mf lead to their death in dermal (and sometimes optical) tissues; bystander damage associated with immune-mediated killing events causes pathology in the skin and eye, leading to the characteristic symptoms of intense itching, skin pathology, and blindness [26]. The infection is spread when a black fly ingests mf while feeding on an infected person; in the black fly intermediate host, the larvae molt to the infective $L_3$ stage and are then transmitted to a human during a blood meal, where they resume development through the $L_4$ stage to adults over several months. These parasites may live up to 15 years, producing around 1000 mf per day. Adult females, which can exceed 0.5 meters in length, reside in a nodule in which movement is restricted; adult males (much smaller) travel among nodules to inseminate the females. Immunity against the adult stage develops very slowly.

The life cycle of parasites that cause LF resembles that of *O. volvulus*. Adult worms, which live around 5 years, reside in lymph vessels, often in the groin region. Adult females are up to 10 cm in length, and males are no more than half this length. Fertile females produce around 10,000 mf per day. After migrating to the blood stream, mf can be ingested by a suitable mosquito intermediate host during a blood meal. The larvae undergo two molts in the mosquito over about a 2-week period to the infectious $L_3$ stage. Upon transfer to a host during a blood meal, larvae undergo two additional molts over a period of 6–12 months before becoming adults in a "worm nest" in a lymph vessel. Unlike the case for onchocerciasis, the primary cause of pathology is the adult stages of LF parasites, not the mf. Adult worms and the immune response to them cause long-term changes in lymph vessel structure and function, leading to lymphedema downstream of the worm nest, with potentially profound enlargement of the affected limb or tissue (elephantiasis), and secondary infections, which can be severe and incapacitating [27].

## Pathogenesis

Parasitic nematodes cause pathology in several ways. The damage observed in the skin, eyes, and lymphatic tissues due to filariases can be attributed in large part to the host immune response to mf (onchocerciasis) or adults (LF) . These parasites, like other helminths, induce a T-regulatory phenotype that retards inflammatory responses and enables chronic infection [11, 26, 27]. As the infection proceeds, the host response gradually begins to evolve beyond this state, and inflammation-related "bystander" damage to host tissues commences in areas in which the parasites reside. Skin damage, blindness, and the classic lymphedema and associated sequelae of LF ensue.

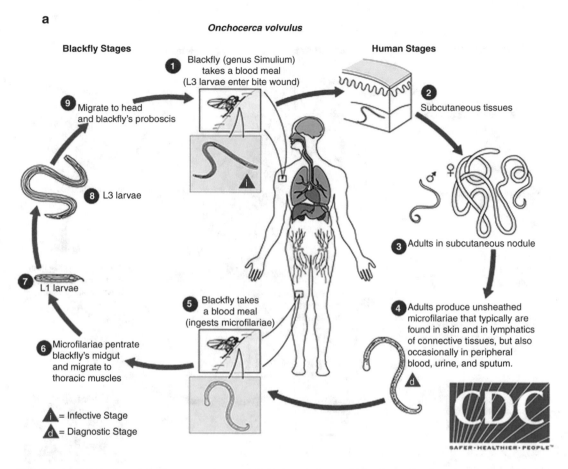

**Fig. 7.4** (**a**) Life cycles of *Onchocerca volvulus* and *Wuchereria bancrofti*. During a blood meal, an infected blackfly (genus *Simulium*) introduces third-stage filarial larvae onto the skin of the human host, where they penetrate into the bite wound (1). In subcutaneous tissues the larvae (2) develop into adult filariae, which commonly reside in nodules in subcutaneous connective tissues (3). Adults can live in the nodules for approximately 15 years. Some nodules may contain numerous male and female worms. Females measure 33 to 50 cm in length and 270 to 400 μm in diameter, while males measure 19 to 42 mm by 130 to 210 μm. In the subcutaneous nodules, the female worms are capable of producing microfilariae for approximately 9 years. The microfilariae, measuring 220 to 360 μm by 5 to 9 μm and unsheathed, have a life span that may reach 2 years. They are occasionally found in peripheral blood, urine, and sputum but are typically found in the skin and in the lymphatics of connective tissues (4). A blackfly ingests the microfilariae during a blood meal (5). After ingestion, the microfilariae migrate from the blackfly's midgut through the hemocoel to the thoracic muscles (6). There the microfilariae develop into first-stage larvae (7) and subsequently into third-stage infective larvae (8). The third-stage infective larvae migrate to the blackfly's proboscis (9) and can infect another human when the fly takes a blood meal (1). (Source: CDC Parasites: Onchocerciasis [River Blindness]: https://www.cdc.gov/parasites/onchocerciasis/biology.html. Accessed 10 Oct 2019). (**b**) Different species of the following genera of mosquitoes are vectors of *W. bancrofti* filariasis depending on geographical distribution. During a blood meal, an infected mosquito introduces third-stage filarial larvae onto the skin of the human host, where they penetrate into the bite wound (1). They develop in adults that commonly reside in the lymphatics (2). The female worms measure 80 to 100 mm in length and 0.24 to 0.30 mm in diameter, while the males measure about 40 mm by 0.1 mm. Adults produce microfilariae measuring 244 to 296 μm by 7.5 to 10 μm, which are sheathed and have nocturnal periodicity, except the South Pacific microfilariae which have the absence of marked periodicity. The microfilariae migrate into lymph and blood channels moving actively through lymph and blood (3). A mosquito ingests the microfilariae during a blood meal (4). After ingestion, the microfilariae lose their sheaths, and some of them work their way through the wall of the proventriculus and cardiac portion of the mosquito's midgut and reach the thoracic muscles (5). There the microfilariae develop into first-stage larvae (6) and subsequently into third-stage infective larvae (7). The third-stage infective larvae migrate through the hemocoel to the mosquito's proboscis (8) and can infect another human when the mosquito takes a blood meal (1). (Source: CDC Parasites: Lymphatic Filariasis https://www.cdc.gov/parasites/lymphaticfilariasis/biology_w_bancrofti.html. Accessed 10 Oct 2019)

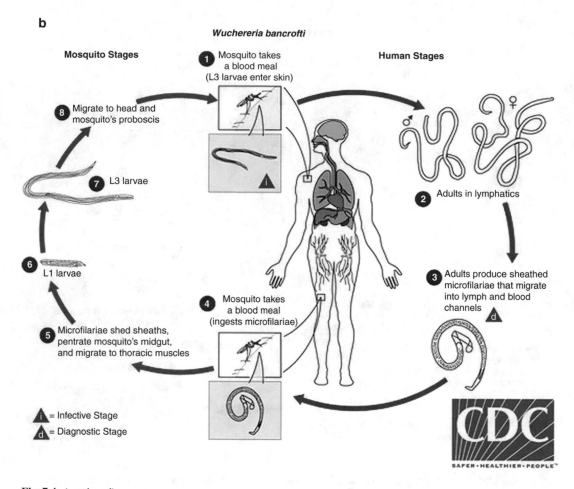

**b**

**Wuchereria bancrofti**

**Mosquito Stages**

**Human Stages**

1 Mosquito takes a blood meal (L3 larvae enter skin)

8 Migrate to head and mosquito's proboscis

7 L3 larvae

2 Adults in lymphatics

6 L1 larvae

3 Adults produce sheathed microfilariae that migrate into lymph and blood channels

4 Mosquito takes a blood meal (ingests microfilariae)

5 Microfilariae shed sheaths, pentrate mosquito's midgut, and migrate to thoracic muscles

i = Infective Stage
d = Diagnostic Stage

**Fig. 7.4** (continued)

Larval stages of *A. lumbricoides* and hookworms cause acute pathology, including fever and cough, as they migrate through host tissues on their way to the gut [2, 4]. The symptoms may be severe if large numbers of larvae are present. Adult STH species cause chronic pathology via several mechanisms. Mechanical damage to the intestinal surface occurs and increases with increasing worm burdens. Higher worm burdens put greater stress on the absorptive surface of the intestinal wall and cause changes in its cellular structure and function. Large numbers of *A. lumbricoides* can physically cause intestinal blockage, and large numbers of *T. trichiura* can lead to rectal prolapse. Adult *Ascaris* can migrate out of the lumen into the bile ducts and elsewhere, causing multiple complications. However, thanks to control campaigns (see below), few people now harbor large worm burdens, and these sequelae are more rarely observed.

The most significant STH pathology is the anemia caused by hookworms, which are hematophagous; these parasites use oral cutting plates or teeth to rip small holes in the intestinal epithelium and consume the blood that emerges [2, 4, 25]. An adult *N. americanus* may consume 30 ul of blood per day, while the larger *Ancylostoma* adults may ingest 10 times that amount. It is therefore not surprising that anemia is a consequence of hookworm infection and that the risk of clinically significant anemia increases as the worm burden and duration of infection increase [21].

As noted, it has long been observed that STH infections are associated with growth and developmental delays and suboptimal productivity in humans [2–5, 28]. The anemia induced by hookworm infections is an obvious cause of these long-term effects, but they also can result from a combination of myriad, difficult-to-unravel factors which are of variable and imprecisely defined importance in each individual. These factors include parasite-dependent reduced nutrient absorption, loss of appetite, diarrhea, recently recognized changes in the host microbiome [29–33], and the effects of parasite-induced altered host immune responses [11, 34]. The additional complicating factors associated with parasitism in resource-limited areas, including chronic malnutrition and concomitant infections, make it challenging to define the precise contribution of STH to the growth, developmental, and behavioral phenotypes too frequently observed in children who live in endemic areas [5, 35].

The proliferation of anthelmintic-based control programs has markedly reduced the number of people who harbor high worm burdens, in whom the consequences of infection are more apparent [36–39]. Double-blind, placebo-controlled long-term studies that monitor growth and performance in children provided with regular (e.g., quarterly) anthelmintic treatments in a cohort of at at-risk individuals are not possible for many reasons, including the unethical denial of treatment to infected individuals. Studies that measure before-and-after indicators in individuals following a single anthelmintic treatment are problematic from a design perspective (since each individual has a different background of ill-defined complicating factors and re-infection occurs rapidly after treatment), and such studies have perhaps unsurprisingly provided conflicting results [35]. Against this background, it is prudent to revisit the commonly accepted concept in veterinary medicine that the presence of even small numbers of gastrointestinal helminths leads to reduced measures of performance. It is unwise to presume that humans are an exception in this regard.

## Effects on Human Nutritional Status

It is essential to distinguish direct from indirect impacts of nematode infections on human nutritional status. For example, the pathological consequences of symptomatic onchocerciasis and LF clearly reduce the ability of the affected individual to contribute to household activities and economic productivity, limiting familial food security and hence detracting from general nutritional status. In this regard, the nutritional consequences of these systemic infections are similar to those due to other physical disabilities or limitations and will not be discussed further.

In contrast, most STH infections do not cause acute, obvious physical limitations in an infected person that could lead to food insecurity. Nonetheless, as noted above, it has generally been accepted that STH are associated with growth impairment, developmental delays, and reduced productivity, especially in heavily infected individuals. Although the pathophysiological causes may be imprecisely defined, STH infections have been associated with nutritional deficiencies in humans [5, 28, 40, 41]. Most prominent is iron deficiency associated especially with hookworm infections (due to blood-feeding), but this condition may also arise during infection with other STH species. Malabsorption and reduced appetite can lead to reduced energy and fat intake, resulting in reduced vitamin A levels; intake of essential micronutrients may also be reduced [21].

As discussed above, simple surveys of the health and nutritional impacts of human STH face challenges in quantification and causality due to the difficulty of controlling the confounding variables. Unfortunately, it is also difficult to extrapolate from studies in helminth-infected laboratory animals to humans. Animal models typically explore impacts of a single infection on nutritional variables of inbred strains of rodents. In contrast, human nutrition in regions of poverty, as noted, is affected by myriad factors that are challenging to replicate in the laboratory environment, not least of which is concurrent infection with other pathogens. A complicating factor that is only recently being addressed is the effect of helminth infections on the composition and metabolic profile of the gut microbiota; the influence of the microbiome on human nutrition has become clear [42], but how helminth infections affect this complex ecosystem remains an urgent subject for research, particularly in chronically infected individuals in whom microbiome alterations may persist after removal of the parasites by chemotherapy (see section, Understanding Microbiome-Helminth Interactions, below).

# Trematode Infections

Schistosomes are the most prevalent parasitic trematodes of humans. Three species, *Schistosoma mansoni*, *S. haematobium*, and *S. japonicum*, account for almost all human infections, with *S. mansoni* being the most prevalent. Estimates of prevalence typically range around 200 million infections [2, 43], with recent estimates somewhat lower [18]. However, prevalence is likely underestimated, as the diagnostic tests are not optimally sensitive [44]. Schistosomes are acquired from water bodies that harbor specific species of snails that serve as intermediate hosts (Fig. 7.5). Infective larvae

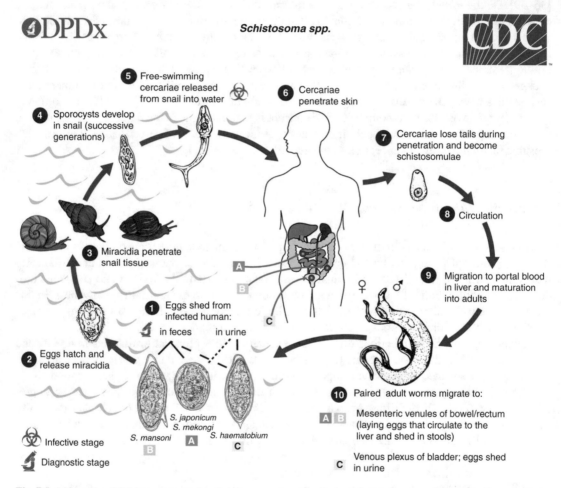

**Fig. 7.5** Life cycle of *Schistosoma* species. *Schistosoma* eggs are eliminated with feces or urine, depending on species (1). Under appropriate conditions the eggs hatch and release miracidia (2), which swim and penetrate specific snail intermediate hosts (3). The stages in the snail include two generations of sporocysts (4) and the production of cercariae (5). Upon release from the snail, the infective cercariae swim, penetrate the skin of the human host (6), and shed their forked tails, becoming schistosomulae (7). The schistosomulae migrate via venous circulation to lungs, then to the heart, and then develop in the liver, exiting the liver via the portal vein system when mature (8,9). Male and female adult worms copulate and reside in the mesenteric venules, the location of which varies by species (with some exceptions) (10). *S. japonicum* is more frequently found in the superior mesenteric veins draining the small intestine (A), and *S. mansoni* occurs more often in the inferior mesenteric veins draining the large intestine (B). However, both species can occupy either location and are capable of moving between sites. *S. haematobium* most often inhabits the vesicular and pelvic venous plexus of the bladder (C), but it can also be found in the rectal venules. The females deposit eggs in the small venules of the portal and perivesical systems. The eggs are moved progressively toward the lumen of the intestine and of the bladder and ureters and are eliminated with feces or urine, respectively (1). (Source: CDC Parasites: Schistosomiasis: https://www.cdc.gov/parasites/schistosomiasis/biology.html. Accessed 10 Oct 2019)

("cercariae") emerge from snails to seek an appropriate host; they enter through the skin and mature into adult male and female parasites which live for many years in veins surrounding the intestine or bladder, depending on the species of parasite. Eggs produced by fertilized females (thousands per day) must travel to the feces or urine in order to reach the external environment and so must pass through tissue barriers to be evacuated. Once shed into the water, the eggs hatch and release larval stages ("miracidia") that infect snails, where they undergo additional rounds of development and replication. The pathology of schistosomiasis is almost entirely due to the host response to eggs trapped in tissues [45]. Acute lethality is rare, but—like nematode infections—these parasites cause chronic symptoms that reduce growth and productivity. Chronic untreated schistosomiasis is associated with mortality due to liver damage, esophageal varices, and bladder cancer, among other pathologies.

In addition to schistosomes, parasitic trematodes that inhabit the lungs or liver are also considered NTDs [1, 2]. These parasites are typically acquired from undercooked or raw freshwater fish, amphibians, or crustaceans and are estimated to infect in aggregate almost 100,000,000 people, with highly regional patterns of distribution of the various species involved. Pathology induced by these foodborne parasites includes chronic cough, lung damage, and liver cancer [8]. Their effects on growth, development, and nutritional status have been little studied and remain unresolved.

## Cestode Infections

All cestodes are parasitic and have life cycles that require infection of more than one host animal (like schistosomes but unlike gastrointestinal nematodes). Tapeworms are hermaphrodites and most contain a long string of connected segments ("proglottids"), each with its own ovary and testes that allow both self-fertilization and cross-fertilization with nearby adults. Humans are important definitive hosts for a few species in the genus *Taenia*, of which the most globally important are *T. solium* (acquired from pigs) and *T. saginata* (acquired from cattle); infectious larval stages in these intermediate hosts (pigs or cattle) are ingested by humans in undercooked meat, leading to the development of adult stages in the intestinal tract that shed infectious eggs into the environment (Fig. 7.6). In addition, humans who ingest the eggs of *T. solium* may develop larval stage infections in tissues (cysticercosis; Fig. 7.6); these infections cause by far the greatest health burden of tapeworm parasites in humans. Because of this, *T. solium* is considered to be an NTD. Of particular concern is encystation of larvae in the brain (neurocysticercosis), a leading cause of epilepsy in people who live in close proximity to pigs in regions with inadequate sanitary infrastructure [46].

A much less common but even more devastating human infection by larval tapeworms is associated with ingestion of eggs shed by *Echinococcus granulosus* or *E. multilocularis*. These tapeworms normally cycle between canids as definitive hosts and a variety of other mammals as intermediate hosts; humans become accidental hosts when they ingest the eggs following close contact with infected dogs. Larval stages of *Echinococcus* spp. cause serious and difficult-to-treat infections in people that have high fatality rates [9].

In addition to infection with adult *T. solium* and *T. saginata*, humans can be infected with adult *Hymenolepis nana* (the dwarf tapeworm) by eating infected insects and *Diphyllobothrium latum* (the fish tapeworm) by eating larval stages in undercooked fish [10]. The most common human infection appears to be *H. nana* because in addition to infection from insects, this infection can also recur in an infected human via autoinfection. In these cases, eggs can be retained in the intestinal tract and develop from larvae to adults in situ. The other human tapeworms may reach lengths of many meters in the GI tract, but adult *H. nana* are much smaller. Remarkably, adult tapeworms cause little overt pathology in humans unless present in large numbers [10]. Occasionally, inappetence, nausea, diarrhea, and/or gastric discomfort may coincide with the presence of adult tapeworms; infections with *D.*

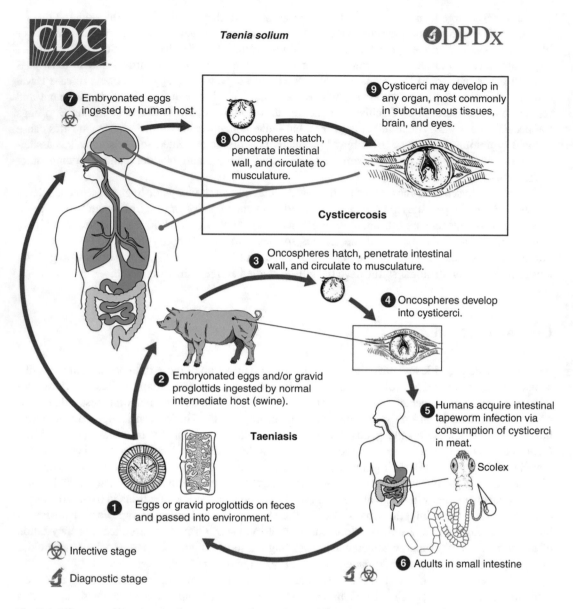

**Fig. 7.6** Life cycle of *Taenia solium. Cysticercosis* is an infection of both humans and pigs with the larval stages of the parasitic cestode, *Taenia solium.* This infection is caused by ingestion of eggs shed in the feces of a human tapeworm carrier (1). These eggs are immediately infectious and do not require a developmental period outside the host. Pigs and humans become infected by ingesting eggs or gravid proglottids (2,7). Humans are usually exposed to eggs by ingestion of food/water contaminated with feces containing these eggs or proglottids or by person-to-person spread. Tapeworm carriers can also infect themselves through fecal-oral transmission (e.g., caused by poor hand hygiene). Once eggs or proglottids are ingested, oncospheres hatch in the intestine (3,8) invade the intestinal wall, enter the bloodstream, and migrate to multiple tissues and organs where they mature into cysticerci over 60–70 days (4,9). Some cysticerci will migrate to the central nervous system, causing neurocysticercosis. This differs from *taeniasis*, which is an intestinal infection with the adult tapeworm. Humans acquire intestinal infections with *T. solium* after eating undercooked pork containing cysticerci (5). Cysts evaginate and attach to the small intestine. Adult tapeworms develop to maturity and may reside in the small intestine for years (6). (Source: CDC Parasites: Cysticercosis https://www.cdc.gov/parasites/cysticercosis/biology.html. Accessed 10 Oct 2019)

*latum* were historically associated with vitamin $B_{12}$ deficiency and consequent anemia in the human host due to scavenging by the parasite [47], but this symptom is now rarely noted. The folkloric concept that the presence of adult tapeworms can lead to weight reduction in people has long been disproven, and there is little evidence of a major impact of intestinal tapeworms on human development or performance.

## Helminth Feeding Strategies

Little recent work has been reported on how parasitic helminths acquire nutrients in the host milieu. Although the host provides the sole source of nutrients for parasitic stages, the mechanisms of acquisition and subsequent metabolism vary, primarily depending on the location.

### *Systemic Nematodes*

Adult filarial parasites primarily absorb small-molecule nutrients from the host by transport across their outer cuticle ("transcuticular uptake"); glucose, nucleotide precursors, and amino acids are absorbed across the cuticle of the worm [48]. Microfilariae lack a gut and therefore obtain all nutrients via transcuticular absorption. This strategy is understandable in light of the fact that these parasites are continuously bathed in a solution rich in nutrients, maintained by the host at constant osmotic pressure. Because glucose is so readily available, filariae are nominally homolactate fermenters and do not need to engage mitochondrial electron transport for energy generation. However, adult filariae are capable of oxidative phosphorylation and can survive in culture, for example, with glutamine as the sole energy source [49]. In the context of the current discussion, it is important to recognize that the biomass of these parasites is usually too small, especially in areas with chemotherapy-based control programs, to deprive a human host of key nutrients by competition. An exception may be vitamin A, which filarial parasites acquire from the host; humans with high burdens of *O. volvulus* may show hypovitaminosis A [50]. However, high parasite loads are also associated with reduced work performance, and it can be challenging to control for inadequate diet in heavily infected individuals who lack the capacity to contribute to the economics of the household or community.

The exception to the transcuticular nutrient absorption paradigm is iron acquisition. Large quantities of iron are needed for the production of larvae, but the only iron available in the host is complexed to proteins that are too large to cross the cuticle. This is proposed to underlie the need for oral ingestion, which can be directly observed in situ, and potentially for the anti-reproductive effects of the anthelmintic ivermectin, which paralyzes the pharynx and could therefore restrict the availability of iron necessary for the formation of mf [51].

### *Soil-Transmitted Helminths*

Few recent studies have been reported on nutrition and intermediary metabolism of adult STH species. Two species residing in the gastrointestinal tract primarily utilize anaerobic pathways for energy generation, a process that has been most intensively explored in *A. suum* [52]. Adults of *Ascaris* spp. ingest luminal contents of the intestinal tract, including digesta and bacteria, but also obtain nutrients by transcuticular absorption [53, 54]. The proportion of nutrients acquired by oral ingestion vs.

transcuticular absorption by *Ascaris* adults in situ is unknown, but—as for adult filariae—iron acquisition is almost certainly by the oral route.

In contrast, adult *Trichuris* spp. have a distinct feeding strategy; the anterior end of these nematodes is encased in a tunnel of intestinal epithelial cells, leading to its characterization as a macroscopic intracellular parasite. The mouth is very small, and the parasite lacks teeth and a muscular pharynx, suggesting that oral ingestion is not an important route for nutrient acquisition. Instead, the parasite is characterized by an unusual bacillary band in the anterior region that contains a large number of pores overlaying cells that are specialized for absorption. It appears that secreted digestive enzymes produce pools of nutrients from host epithelial cells which are then absorbed through the bacillary band [55–57]. This system can absorb proteins as large as 100 kDa, suggesting that iron absorption can also occur through this pathway. The intermediary metabolism of *Trichuris* is primarily anaerobic, consistent with its niche environment [52].

Finally, adult hookworms employ a different strategy. These parasites, as noted above, ingest large quantities of oxygenated blood and have the capacity for aerobic as well as anaerobic metabolism in culture [58], although this has not been confirmed in vivo. The proportion of nutrients absorbed orally vs. across the cuticle by these parasites is unknown. Nonetheless, the blood loss induced by their feeding strategy, including the amounts ingested and lost to the intestinal lumen, constitutes by far the greatest nutritional consequence of helminth parasites on human health.

## Schistosomes

Adult schistosomes ingest blood and thus have access to all the nutrients contained therein; they also are able to transport a variety of nutrients across their outer tegument [48, 52, 59]. Adult females ingest about 10 times more blood than males, reflecting the increased demand for iron for the formation of viable eggs. Nonetheless, both sexes can acquire essential nutrients by absorption across the tegument; the proportion of nutrients acquired by ingestion vs. tegumental absorption in situ has not been defined. Despite living in a highly oxygenated environment, adult schistosomes exhibit a primarily anaerobic type of intermediary metabolism, generating energy primarily through glycolysis and excreting primarily lactose back into the host circulation. However, these parasites are clearly capable of aerobic metabolism, and how these pathways are coordinated and integrated remains the subject of research [60].

## Cestodes

Cestodes lack a mouth and an anatomically distinct digestive system, and acquisition of nutrients occurs by absorption across the tegument [48, 52]. In the course of host-parasite co-evolution, cestodes have adapted to compete with the intestinal epithelium of the host for nutrients. The tegument is characterized by numerous finger-like projections called microtriches, which increase the surface area by ten-fold, providing for efficient nutrient absorption [61]. Microtriches contain transporters for low molecular weight nutrients present in the intestinal lumen. *Hymenolepis diminuta* has six transporters for amino acids, three for purine/pyrimidines, and at least two for nucleosides. Carbohydrates such as glucose, galactose, and glycerol are transported either by carrier molecules or by diffusion. Additionally, distinct transporters exist for short-chain and long-chain fatty acids [62, 63]. Microtriches also express extrinsic digestive enzymes (such as glucose-6-phosphatase) which cleave nutrients for absorption by the worms [52]. The important zoonotic cestode *D. latum* absorbs vitamin $B_{12}$ from the host and can cause megaloblastic anemia [64]. Another zoonotic species, *H. diminuta*, may utilize vitamin $B_6$ from the host [65], although evidence for clinically significant deficiency in humans is not available.

Developing, but probably not mature, proglottids also exhibit endocytosis, which may be necessary for the acquisition of iron to fuel the development of eggs. Adult stages are anaerobic in their intermediary metabolism [52], reflecting the low-oxygen tension in their environment.

## Influence of Human Nutritional Status on Helminth Infections

Human susceptibility to helminth infection, measured as the number of worms present in a person and the pathological consequences of those worms, is controlled by many hard to quantify factors. As discussed above, the effects of chronic malnutrition, microbiome composition, and concomitant infections all influence the outcome of infection, and it is difficult to investigate all these conditions simultaneously in animal models. Evidence from studies in humans supports a conclusion that malnutrition (protein, energy, and micronutrient insufficiency) can be a risk factor for helminth infections, possibly by impairing the immune response to them [21, 66], leading to a negative spiral given the infections also lead to malnutrition.

Like nematode infections, concurrent schistosomiasis and malnutrition are widely prevalent, and animal studies have shown that host nutritional status influences pathogenesis of the infection, likely correlated with altered immune responses [67]. Other studies in animal models have demonstrated that host nutritional status influences multiple aspects of reproduction of *Schistosoma* [68–70], but whether these findings can be extrapolated to parasites in humans is unknown.

As for nematode infections, studies in humans with schistosome infections are difficult to interpret, as the vast majority are cross-sectional surveys that associate anthropometric indices with the presence or absence of schistosomes, with sometimes conflicting results. A recent meta-analysis indicated that micronutrient supplementation reduced the risk of infection with *S. mansoni* and *S. haematobium* [71], and an earlier analysis of the STH and schistosome infections of children in the Philippines found evidence that low energy and nutrient intake was associated with increased risks of infection with schistosomes, hookworms, and whipworms [72]. Whether these risks were associated with altered immune responses was not investigated.

## Impact of Control Programs

The consequences of chronic helminth infections led to the development and implementation of programs designed to limit the prevalence and intensity of these infections, with the primary intention of improving child development and population health. Initial efforts were based on environmental interventions, including the construction of sanitation infrastructure and vector control methods for snails and black flies to address schistosomiasis and onchocerciasis, respectively [73, 74]. The introduction of ivermectin (IVM) for onchocerciasis control revolutionized these efforts, particularly because the drug was donated for this indication (see below). The success of the program led to donations of medicines for other helminth control programs [75, 76]. These interventions have reduced the morbidity of human helminth infections on a global scale and to a remarkable (although incomplete) extent. Success has led to the adoption of ambitious goals to eliminate these parasites as threats to public health in the next decade, although challenges unquestionably remain.

Treatment options for helminthiases can be divided into two principal strategies: mass drug administration (MDA) and diagnosis-driven therapy (sometimes referred to as "test and treat"). MDA) programs directed at filariases, schistosomiasis, and STH are summarized in Table 7.2. These campaigns

**Table 7.2** MDA control programs for human helminthiases

| Indication | Drugs | Donor/number of doses per year |
|---|---|---|
| Onchocerciasis | Ivermectin | Merck & Co./>700,000,000 |
| Lymphatic filariasis | Ivermectin[a] | Merck & Co./>700,000,000 |
| | Diethylcarbamazine | Eisai/2,000,000,000 total by 2020 |
| | Albendazole | GSK/600,000,000 |
| Schistosomiasis | Praziquantel | Merck KGaA/250,000,000 |
| STH | Albendazole | GSK/400,000,000 |
| | Mebendazole | Johnson & Johnson/200,000,000 |

Data from WHO: https://www.who.int/neglected_diseases/Medicine_Donation_June_2016.pdf
[a]Donations for the filarial diseases combined in this total

are triggered by epidemiological surveys of the prevalence and intensity of infection [77]. These surveys typically measure the abundance of larval stages of filarial parasites (mf) in skin snips (onchocerciasis) or blood samples (LF), although antigen detection tests have become more common and new diagnostic assays have been the subject of research [78]. STH and schistosome infections are typically detected by counting parasite eggs in feces (or urine) using microscopy, although antigen detection assays are becoming more common for schistosome infections [43]. Communities that exceed prevalence/intensity thresholds can be targeted for MDA campaigns. These programs rely on donated anthelmintics which are given as a single dose once or twice yearly to as many residents as possible in these communities (often targeting school-age children) without individual diagnosis prior to treatment [77, 79, 80]. The goals of MDA programs are complex and depend on the target parasite, and progress varies; considerable progress has been achieved for many helminth parasites, but challenges remain.

Test and treat regimens are employed following individual diagnosis and, as noted, may be more intensive than the treatment received as part of MDA campaigns. However, this strategy will have to be extended to the field as control programs move closer to elimination or eradication; it will be challenging to sustain MDA programs in areas where incidence has dropped. In these areas, it will be important to identify and treat the remaining infected people to prevent resurgence of the infection as MDA ceases. The unabated presence of competent vectors and inadequate sanitation infrastructure will be of continuing concern.

## Filarial Infections

The first helminth MDA campaign was for onchocerciasis, motivated and sustained by donations of IVM by Merck and Co. IVM was discovered and developed for veterinary use by this company; based on its extraordinary potency and efficacy in preventing infections with the canine heartworm, *Dirofilaria immitis*, which is closely related to *O. volvulus*, trials were initiated in onchocerciasis patients [81]. A single low oral dose of IVM removes all or almost all mf from the skin and sterilizes adult worms for 6–9 months; the removal of mf and prevention of their re-appearance for many months limits the development of dermal and ocular pathology and blocks transmission. This drug does not kill adult *O. volvulus*, necessitating yearly or biannual treatments with IVM for 10–15 years, which can locally eliminate the parasite as transmission ceases and the adults eventually die [80, 82, 83].

MDA programs for onchocerciasis have made notable progress in eliminating these infections; a remarkable success story is the near-eradication of this parasite from sites in Central and South America through intensive rounds of IVM-based MDA [84, 85]. Impressive gains have been made in Africa as well, although the availability of field-friendly macrofilaricides (anthelmintics that kills adult filarial worms) would help achieve elimination goals. Moxidectin, a macrocyclic lactone in the milbemycin class structurally related to IVM, was recently approved by the US Food and Drug Administration for treatment of onchocerciasis. Moxidectin has a much longer half-life than IVM in humans and causes a more prolonged suppression of microfilaridermia than the standard once-yearly dose of IVM [86]. Inclusion of this drug in MDA campaigns could reduce the time required for elimination [87]; whether cumulative doses have macrofilaricidal effects and are safe for use in regions that are co-endemic for the filarial parasite *Loa loa* (see below) remains to be determined.

MDA programs were subsequently introduced for LF, based on annual treatment of people in endemic areas with single doses of diethylcarbamazine (DEC) plus albendazole (ABZ). In areas in which LF is co-endemic with onchocerciasis, DEC is contraindicated, and a yearly dose of IVM + ABZ was used [80, 88]. As for onchocerciasis, this strategy removes mf from the circulation and provides long-term suppression of new mf production, blocking transmission but not pathology. Annual treatments for 5 years have eliminated LF from some areas [80, 88–90], depending on the underlying epidemiology and degree of population coverage.

Recently, high macrofilaricidal efficacy has been reported for a "triple therapy" regimen, simultaneous administration of single doses of DEC + ABZ + IVM [91]. This strategy appears to kill adult LF parasites, and the regimen is now being introduced for this purpose [92]. This strategy should dramatically accelerate the elimination of LF as a threat to public health by killing adult parasites, reducing the duration of treatment required. Extension of triple therapy to onchocerciasis is challenging because of the danger of serious adverse events posed by DEC-induced killing of mf in onchocerciasis patients. Filarial parasites respond differently to anthelmintic drugs, and evidence of efficacy of the combination against adult *O. volvulus* is not available. As mentioned above, a complicating factor is the use of IVM or DEC in regions where recipients may also be infected with *L. loa* [93]. Patients harboring high numbers of *L. loa* mf are at risk of severe adverse CNS events following administration of DEC or IVM, a situation that poses a challenge in the field unless prescreening can guarantee patient safety.

Patients presenting in a clinical setting with a diagnosis of onchocerciasis or LF can be treated with the same regimens used in MDA, though dosing may be more frequent. In the case of onchocerciasis, surgical removal of palpable nodules, in which adult female parasites reside, may be helpful. An additional therapeutic option is treatment with standard antibiotic doses of doxycycline daily for 4–6 weeks, a regimen which slowly kills adult filarial parasites through elimination of the essential *Wolbachia* symbiotic bacteria present in most filarial species that parasitize humans [94]. It is not clear that the duration of daily dosing needed for efficacy is compatible with use in all endemic areas, but finding new anti-*Wolbachia* chemotherapeutics that act more rapidly is a highly promising area of drug discovery [95].

## Soil-Transmitted Helminths

MDA programs for STH primarily rely on single doses of the benzimidazole anthelmintics ABZ or mebendazole (MBZ), given quarterly, semiannually, or yearly [77, 79, 80]. ABZ is donated for this purpose by GlaxoSmithKline, and MBZ is donated by Johnson & Johnson; each company provides hundreds of millions of tablets every year [75, 76] (Table 7.2). The single-dose regimen of either drug provides excellent efficacy against *A. lumbricoides*, less complete but still notable efficacy against hookworms, and suboptimal efficacy against whipworms [96–99]. In diagnosed patients in a clinic, three doses of either drug given once per day provide excellent efficacy against all STH species, but this regimen (although standard for treatment of pets in veterinary clinics) is thought not to be compatible with MDA. The persistence of infective stages of these parasites in the environment means that re-infection following treatment is expected, and benefits are not equivalent for all STH species, notably for hookworms [25], or in areas of high transmission, where successful control is particularly challenging. Nonetheless, MDA reduces adult worm burdens in treated populations, reducing the consequences of parasitism, even if elimination remains a challenge without concomitant improvements in sanitation [98–101]. Several other anthelmintics have been approved for use in human STH infections in at least some countries, most notably the nicotinic cholinergic agonists pyrantel (as the pamoate salt), levamisole, and oxantel; none has particular advantages over ABZ or MBZ in the absence of drug resistance, which, while undoubtedly threatening, has not yet emerged as an impediment to STH control.

## Trematodes

Treatment of schistosome infections relies almost entirely on MDA programs that administer a single dose of praziquantel (PZQ) once or twice a year (sometimes more frequently) to populations in endemic areas [77, 79, 80]. PZQ, hundreds of millions of doses of which are donated annually for MDA programs by Merck KGaA [75, 76], has reasonably high efficacy against adult schistosomes but not against juvenile parasites during their tissue migration, and re-treatment approximately 6 weeks after the first dose may be needed to clear the parasites [102, 103]. Continued contact with contaminated water means that re-infection in highly endemic areas is to be expected. As for STH, MDA programs have reduced adult worm burdens in treated populations, resulting in fewer eggs produced and less pathology [37, 80, 100]. However, PZQ in single dose regimens is typically not 100% efficacious, and its bitter taste and sometimes unpleasant side effects may lead to reduced compliance. As with many MDA programs, challenges remain, particularly in areas of high transmission [104]. In addition, as worm burdens are reduced, the health benefits of continuing to adhere to treatment may become less obvious, and coverage may become more difficult to sustain [105].

Most food-borne trematode infections are susceptible to PZQ. For GI parasites, a single oral dose of 25 mg/kg is used; for liver and lung flukes, the same dose is given three times a day for 2 days. PZQ is not effective for the treatment of fasciolosis; instead one or two doses of 10 mg/kg triclabendazole is used [8]. MDA strategies have not been deployed for control of these infections.

## Cestodes

Infections with adult *T. solium*, *H. nana*, or *D. latum* in the GI tract of humans can be cured with a single 10–25 mg/kg dose of PZQ [102]. Treatment of infected pigs with a single 30 mg/kg dose of oxfendazole eliminates muscle cysts [106], thereby preventing transmission to humans from undercooked pork, and a highly effective recombinant vaccine called TSOL 18 is commercially available that prevents infection in pigs [107]. Insufficient economic gain is realized by pig owners via use of this vaccine to motivate control programs in the field targeted to swine. Nonetheless, a combination strategy of TSOL 18 vaccination and oxfendazole treatment of pigs is a promising strategy to eliminate *T. solium* as a significant cause of human disease if the case for investment of public health resources can be made [107, 108].

Treatment of neurocysticercosis is much more challenging [9, 10, 46]. Cysts typically reside in an inflammatory matrix in the CNS, and killing of the parasites may exacerbate the inflammation, leading to greater pathology. Long courses of either ABZ or PZQ, generally co-administered with a steroid to control inflammation, are the current standard of care; neither option is reliably completely curative.

## Challenges, Gaps, and Unmet Needs

Helminth infections, once ubiquitous in human populations, have been eliminated from many areas of the world. Despite notable success of MDA-driven control programs, helminths remain depressingly common in areas of the world that lack the economic resources to provide adequate sanitation and housing infrastructure. The provision of healthcare resources has reduced the global health burden associated with these parasites, and this may be helping to break the cycle of poverty in at least some regions. In that context, we have identified challenges that limit our ability to remove parasitic helminths as a barrier to healthy human development and performance.

### *Climate Change*

The incidence and prevalence of human helminth infections are strongly influenced by environmental conditions, which are changing as a result of human-induced global warming [109]. Arthropod, molluscan, and aquatic animal species that serve as vectors for these parasites are all dependent upon water bodies, and climate changes that influence rainfall patterns and water body stability will both limit and expand their territories, depending on altered rainfall and temperature patterns (see Chap. 15) [110]. Temperature and humidity influence the longevity of STH egg and larval stages in the environment, and changes in these factors as the world warms will alter the distribution and intensity of these parasites. These changes will be felt locally and will vary from species to species; it is essential that control programs be adaptable to address new realities and that potential expansion of helminth distribution be actively monitored.

### *Impacts of Elimination Programs*

As heavy helminth infections diminish due to overall economic development and the effects of control campaigns, the consequences of these pathogens for human health, development, and productivity will diminish. Because of their environmental persistence, migration of untreated populations, and the ability of some vector species to travel long distances, it is essential that investments in control continue until the risks of resurgence are eliminated. It is possible that some pathogens may be eradicated through MDA campaigns, especially those which lack zoonotic potential (onchocerciasis, *W. bancrofti*, some STH species). Monitoring populations in which these infections have been eliminated as public health threats, but not eradicated, is necessary to prevent re-emergence. Sustainability of progress to date will also depend on availability of low-cost drugs, and both global and local political will. Implementing improved sanitation infrastructure and practices will be an essential part of sustaining and expanding the gains made by ongoing control programs. The investment of resources into this endeavor would be strengthened if better methods to document the beneficial effects of helminth control could be devised.

### *Understanding Microbiome-Helminth Interactions*

STH species and trillions of microbes, including viruses, bacteria, and protozoa/fungi, co-habit the GI tract. As part of this co-existence, microbes and worms constantly interact. GI nematode infections of humans, livestock, and laboratory animals alter/modify the GI microbiome, and these alterations can have positive impacts on the host [111]. For example, nematode infection in mice increased the abundance of *Lactobacillus* [112], a beneficial and health-promoting bacteria. Nematode-mediated microbiome alterations may have ameliorative effects on inflammatory bowel disease [113]. Nonetheless, adverse effects are also possible [114], and the complex interactions among helminths, the microbiome, and the host remain incompletely understood. This is particularly vexing in the context of defining the effects of chronic helminth infections on human nutritional status. This area clearly warrants increased research funding to better understand the therapeutic interventions that may be needed to reverse the effects of chronic helminthiases on human growth and development.

## *The Hygiene Hypothesis*

The hygiene hypothesis proposes that the presence of helminth infections (and infections with other pathogens) reduces the occurrence of chronic inflammatory autoimmune diseases [115]. A multitude of epidemiological and experimental studies involving both human populations and experimental animal models support the hypothesis. For example, exposure to parasitic infection during early childhood reduces the risk of allergic diseases in later life [116]. Given that helminth parasites induce strong Th2 responses similar to those seen in allergic reactions, the idea that exposure to helminths minimizes allergic and autoimmune response may seem counterintuitive. However, besides inducing Th2 responses, helminths also induce regulatory T cells, leading to immune suppression which can reduce the risk of autoimmune and allergic diseases. Intriguingly, the therapeutic potential of GI nematodes and their products for amelioration of autoimmune diseases is a subject of active investigation [117, 118]. A comparison between incidence of autoimmune and allergic cases and prevalence of helminths among developed and developing country clearly showed an inverse relationship, supporting the validity of the hygiene hypothesis. From the co-evolutionary point of view, it is imperative to appreciate the importance of our "old friends" (parasitic nematodes) while formulating control strategies. Thus, given uncertainties about the benefits and potential adverse consequences of eradicating these organisms, questions remain about whether long-term goals should be eradication of infection or control of disease.

## Conclusions

Parasitic helminths have been the almost constant companions of humans (and all other metazoan animals) throughout evolution and have shaped many aspects of physiology, metabolism, and immunology. For the most part, they impose relatively minor burdens on their hosts, unless present in large numbers or in individuals who react badly to them. Capable of creating profound pathology, even death, and of limiting growth, development, and physical and mental performance, these pathogens have attracted investment for control and eradication. Comparatively little has been invested in understanding their precise impacts on human nutritional status and performance. Their elimination from much of the wealthy areas of the globe via vector control and sanitation now restricts their distribution to poorer and more tropical regions. Despite support for MDA-based control campaigns, including the donation of several essential medicines for these operations, these parasites remain prevalent, even if the burden of disease is generally lifting. We do not yet understand enough about their effects on human children, particularly with regard to individual variation and the effects of comorbidity factors, to assume that we can relax control efforts once most people in an area are free from infection. Instead, in the absence of adequate economic development, the environmental conditions that favor their transmission will remain poised to enable a resurgence of disease if we are not vigilant. Breaking the cycle of poverty is a hard task. Removing helminths as contributing factors is an important step toward that goal.

# References

1. World Health Organization Neglected Tropical Diseases. https://www.who.int/neglected_diseases/diseases/en/. Accessed 12 Aug 2019.
2. Hotez PJ, Brindley PJ, Bethony JM, King CH, Pearce EJ, Jacobson J. Helminth infections: the great neglected tropical diseases. J Clin Invest. 2008;118:1311–21.
3. Mitra AK, Mawson AR. Neglected tropical diseases: epidemiology and global burden. Trop Med Infect Dis. 2017;2:36.
4. Jourdan PM, Lamberton PHL, Fenwick A, Addiss SG. Soil-transmitted helminth infections. Lancet. 2018;391:252–65.
5. Hall A, Hewitt G, Tuffrey V, de Silva N. A review and meta-analysis of the impact of intestinal worms on child growth and nutrition. Mat Child Nutr. 2008;4:118–236.
6. Taylor MJ, Hoerauf A, Bockarie M. Lymphatic filariasis and onchocerciasis. Lancet. 2010;376:1175–85.
7. Colley DG, Bustinduy AL, Secor WE, King CH. Human schistosomiasis. Lancet. 2014;383:2253–64.
8. Keiser J, Utzinger J. Food-borne trematodiases. Clin Microbiol Rev. 2009;22:466–83.
9. Brunetti E, White AC Jr. Cestode infections: hydatid disease and cysticercosis. Inf Dis Clinics N Am. 2012;26:421–35.
10. Webb C, Cabada MM. Intestinal cestodes. Curr Opin Infect Dis. 2017;30:504–10.
11. McSorley HJ, Maizels RM. Helminth infections and host immune regulation. Clin Microbiol Rev. 2012;25:585–608.
12. Anderson RM, May RM. Infectious diseases of humans. Dynamics and control. Oxford: Oxford University Press; 1991.
13. Gross SJ, Ryan WG, Ploeger HW. Anthelmintic treatment of dairy cows and its effect on milk production. Vet Rec. 1999;144:581–7.
14. Forbes AB, Huckle CA, Gibb MJ, Rook AJ, Nuthall R. Evaluation of the effects of nematode parasitism on grazing behaviour, herbage intake and growth in young grazing cattle. Vet Parasitol. 2000;90:111–8.
15. Miller CM, Waghorn TS, Leathwick DM, Candy PM, Oliver A-MB, Watson TG. The production costs of anthelmintic resistance in lambs. Vet Parasitol. 2012;186:376–81.
16. World Health Organization. Soil-transmitted helminthiases: eliminating soil-transmitted helminthiases as a public health problem in children: progress report 2001–2010 and strategic plan 2011–2020. Geneva: WHO; 2012.
17. Pullan RL, Smith JL, Jasrasaria R, Brooker SJ. Global numbers of infection and disease burden of soil transmitted helminth infections in 2010. Parasit Vectors. 2014;7:37.
18. Global Burden of Disease 2017 Disease and Injury Incidence and Prevalence Collaborators. Global, regional, and national incidence, prevalence and years lived with disability for 354 diseases and injuries for 195 countries and territories. 1990-2017: a systematic analysis for the global burden of disease study 2017. Lancet. 2018;392:1789–858.
19. Schär F, Trostdorf U, Giardina F, Khieu V, Muth S, Marti H, et al. Strongyloides stercoralis: global distribution and risk factors. PLoS Negl Trop Dis. 2013;7:e2288.
20. Bisoffi Z, Buofrate D, Montresor A, Requena-Méndez A, Muñoz J, Krolewiecki AJ, et al. Strongyloides stercoralis: a plea for action. PLoS Negl Trop Dis. 2013;7:e2214.
21. Scott ME, Koski KG. Soil-transmitted helminths – does nutrition make a difference? In: Humphries DL, Scott ME, Vermund SH, editors. Nutrition and infectious diseases – shifting the clinical paradigm. Switzerland: Springer Nature; 2020.
22. Leles D, Gardner SL, Reinhard K, Iñiguez A, Araujo A. Are *Ascaris lumbricoides* and *Ascaris suum* a single species? Parasit Vectors. 2012;5:42.
23. Anderson TJ. The dangers of using single locus markers in parasite epidemiology: *Ascaris* as a case study. Trends Parasitol. 2001;17:183–8.
24. Izurieta R, Reina-Ortiz M, Ochoa-Capello, T. Trichuris trichiura. In: JB Rose, B Jiménez-Cisneros (eds) Global Water Pathogen Project. http://www.waterpathogens.org (Robertson, L (ed) Part 4 Helminths). Michigan State University, East Lansing, MI, UNESCO 2018. http://www.waterpathogens.org/book/trichuris-trichiura.
25. Bartsch SM, Hotez PJ, Asti L, Zapf KM, Bottazzi ME, Diemert DJ, et al. The global economic and health burden of human hookworm infection. PLoS Negl Trop Dis. 2016;10:e0004922.
26. Ottesen EA. Immune responsiveness and the pathogenesis of human onchocerciasis. J Infect Dis. 1995;171:659–71.
27. Babu S, Nutman TB. Immunopathogenesis of lymphatic filarial disease. Semin Immunopathol. 2012;34:847–61.

28. Stephenson LS, Latham MC, Ottesen EA. Malnutrition and parasitic helminth infections. Parasitology. 2000;121(Suppl):S23–38.

29. Glendinning L, Nausch N, Free A, Taylor DW, Mutapi F. The microbiota and helminths: sharing the same niche in the human host. Parasitology. 2014;141:1255–71.

30. Jenkins TP, Rathnayaka Y, Perera PK, Peachey LE, Nolan MJ, Krause L, et al. Infections by human gastrointestinal helminths are associated with changes in faecal microbiota diversity and composition. PLoS One. 207(12):e0184719.

31. Rosa BA, Supali T, Gankpala L, Djuardi Y, Sartono E, Zhou Y, et al. Differential human gut microbiome assemblages during soil-transmitted helminth infections in Indonesia and Libya. Microbiome. 2018;6:33.

32. Schneeberger PHH, Coulibaly JT, Panic G, Daubenberger C, Gueuning M, Frey JE, et al. Investigations on the interplay between *Schistosoma mansoni*, praziquantel and the gut microbiome. Parasit Vectors. 2018;11:168.

33. Easton AV, Quiñones M, Vukkovic-Cvijin I, Oliveira RG, Kepha S, Odiere MR, et al. The impact of anthelmintic treatment on human gut microbiota based on cross-sectional and pre- and postdeworming comparisons in western Kenya. MBio. 2019;10:e–00519-19.

34. Varyani F, Fleming O, Maizels RM. Helminths in the gastrointestinal tract as modulators of immunity and pathology. Am J Gastrointest Liver Physiol. 2017;312:G537–49.

35. Majid MH, Kang SJ, Hotez PJ. Resolving "worm wars": an extended comparison review of findings from key economics and epidemiological studies. PLoS Negl Trop Dis. 2019;13:e0006940.

36. Webster JP, Molyneux DH, Hotez PJ, Fenwick A. The contribution of mass drug administration to global health: past, present and future. Phil Trans Roy Soc B. 2014;369:20130434.

37. Andrade G, Bertsch DJ, Gazzinelli A, King CH. Decline in infection-related morbidities following drug-mediated reductions in the intensity of *Schistosoma* infection: a systematic review and meta-analysis. PLoS Negl Trop Dis. 2017;11:e0005372.

38. Marocco C, Bangert M, Joseph SA, Fitzpatrick C, Montresor A. 2017. Preventative chemotherapy in one year reduces by over 80% the number of individuals with soil-transmitted helminthiases causing morbidity: results from meta-analysis. Trans Roy Soc Trop Med Hyg. 2017;111:12–7.

39. Lo NC, Addiss DG, Hotez PJ, King CH, Stothard JR, Evans DS, et al. A call to strengthen the global strategy for schistosomiasis and soil-transmitted helminthiasis: the time is now. Lancet Infect Dis. 2017;17:e64–9.

40. Solomons NW. Pathways to the impairment of human nutritional status by gastrointestinal pathogens. Parasitology. 1993;107(Suppl):S19–35.

41. Crompton DWT, Nesheim MC. Nutritional impact of intestinal helminthiasis during the human life cycle. Ann Rev Nutr. 2002;22:35–59.

42. Robertson RC, Manges AR, Finlay BB, Prendergast AJ. The human microbiome and child growth – first 1000 days and beyond. Trends Microbiol. 2018;27:131–47.

43. McManus DP, Dunne DW, Sacko M, Utzinger J, Vennervald BJ, Zhou X-N. Schistosomiasis. Nature Rev Dis Primer. 2018;4:13.

44. Colley DG, Andros TS, Campbell CH Jr. Schistosomiasis is more prevalent than previously thought: what does it mean for public health goals, policies, strategies, guidelines and intervention programs? Infect Dis Poverty. 2017;6:63.

45. Burke ML, Jones MK, Gobert GN, Li YS, Ellis MK, McManus DP. Immunopathogenesis of human schistosomiasis. Parasite Immunol. 2009;31:163–76.

46. Nash TE, Mahanty S, Garcia HH. Neurocysticercosis – more than a neglected disease. PLoS Negl Trop Dis. 2013;7:e1964.

47. Nyberg W, Grasbeck R, Saarni M, von Bonsdorff B. Serum vitamin $B_{12}$ levels and incidence of tapeworm anemia in a population heavily infected with *Diphyllobothrium latum*. Am J Clin Nutr. 1961;9:606–12.

48. Thompson DP, Geary TG. Helminth surfaces: structural, molecular and functional properties. In: Marr JJ, Komuniecki R, editors. Molecular medical parasitology. Oxford: Academic Press; 2003. p. 297–338.

49. MacKenzie NE, VandeWaa EA, Gooley PR, Williams JF, Bennett JL, Bjorge SM, et al. Comparison of glycolysis and glutaminolysis in *Onchocerca volvulus* and *Brugia pahangi* by $^{13}$C NMR spectroscopy. Parasitology. 1989;99:427–35.

50. Storey DM. Filariasis: nutritional interactions in human and animal hosts. Parasitology. 1993;107:S147–58.

51. Geary TG, Moreno Y. Macrocyclic lactone anthelmintics: spectrum of activity and mechanism of action. Curr Pharmaceut Biotechnol. 2012;13:866–72.

52. Saz HJ. Energy metabolism of parasitic helminths. Annu Rev Physiol. 1981;43:323–41.

53. Fleming MW, Fetterer RH. *Ascaris suum*: continuous perfusion of the pseudocoelom and nutrient absorption. Exp Parasitol. 1984;57:142–8.

54. Halton DW. Nutritional adaptations to parasitism. Int J Parasitol. 1997;27:693–704.

55. Tilney LG, Connelly PS, Guild GM, Vranich KA, Artis D. Adaptation of a nematode parasite to living with the mammalian epithelium. J Exp Zool A Comp Exp Biol. 2005;303:927–45.

56. Hansen TVA, Hansen M, Nejsum P, Mejer H, Denwood M, Thamsborg SM. Glucose absorption by the bacillary band of *Trichuris muris*. PLoS Negl Trop Dis. 2016;10:e0004971.

57. Hüttemann M, Schmahl G, Mehlhorn H. Light and electron microscopic studies on two nematodes, *Angiostrongylus cantonensis* and *Trichuris muris*, differing in their mode of nutrition. Parasitol Res. 2007;101:S225–32.

58. Warren LG. Biochemistry of the dog hookworm. III. Oxidative phosphorylation. Exp Parasitol. 1970;27:417–23.

59. Skelly PJ, Da'dara AA, Li X-H, Castro-Borges W, Wilson RA. Schistosome feeding and regurgitation. PLoS Pathog. 2014;10:e1004246.

60. You H, Stephenson RJ, Gobert GN, McManus DP. Revisiting glucose uptake and metabolism in schistosomes: new molecular insights for improved schistosomiasis therapies. Front Genetics. 2014;5:1.

61. Hayunga EG. Morphological adaptations of intestinal helminths. J Parasitol. 1991;77:865–73.

62. Pappas PW, Read CP. Membrane transport in helminth parasites-a review. Exp Parasitol. 1975;33:469–530.

63. Insler GD. Population and developmental changes in thymidine uptake kinetics of *Hymenolepis diminuta* (Cestoda: Cyclophyllidea). Comp Biochem Physiol. 1981;70B:697–702.

64. Nyberg W. *Diphyllobothrium latum* and human nutrition, with particular reference to vitamin $B_{12}$ deficiency. Proc Nutr Soc. 1963;22:8–14.

65. Platzer EG, Roberts LS. Developmental physiology of cestodes. V. Effects of vitamin deficient diets and host coprophagy prevention on development of *Hymenolepis diminuta*. J Parasitol. 1969;55:1143–52.

66. Koski KG, Scott ME. Gastrointestinal nematodes, nutrition and immunity: breaking the negative spiral. Ann Rev Nutr. 2001;21:297–321.

67. Marques DVB, Felizardo AA, Souza RLM, Pereira AAC, Gonçalves RV, Novaes RD. Could diet composition modulate pathological outcomes in schistosomiasis mansoni? A systematic review of in vivo preclinical evidence. Parasitology. 2018;145:1127–36.

68. Neves RH, Machado-Silva JR, Pelajo-Machado M, Oliveira SA, Coutinho EM, Lenzi HL, et al. Morphological aspects of *Schistosoma mansoni* adult worms isolated from nourished and undernourished mice: a comparative analysis by confocal laser scanning microscopy. Memòrias Instituto Oswaldo Cruz. 2001;96:1013–6.

69. Okumura-Noji K, Sasai K, Zhan R, Kawaguchi H, Maruyama H, Tada T, et al. Cholesteryl ester transfer protein deficiency causes slow egg embryonation of *Schistosoma japonicum*. Biochem Biophys Res Comm. 2001;286:305–10.

70. Oliveira SA, Barbosa AA Jr, Gomes DC, Machado-Silva JR, Barros AF, Neves RH, et al. Morphometric study of *Schistosoma mansoni* adult worms recovered from undernourished infected mice. Memòrias Instituto Oswaldo Cruz. 2003;98:623–7.

71. Morales-Suarez-Varela M, Peraita-Costa I, Llopis-Morales A, Llopis-Gonzalez A. Supplementation with micronutrients and schistosomiasis: systematic review and meta-analysis. Pathogens Glob Health. 2019;113:101–8.

72. Papier K, Williams GM, Luceres-Catubig R, Ahmed F, Olveda RM, McManus DP, et al. Childhood malnutrition and parasitic helminth interactions. Clin Infect Dis. 2014;59:234–43.

73. Sokolow SH, Wood CL, Jones IJ, Swartz SJ, Lopez M, Hsieh MH, et al. Global assessment of schistosomiasis control over the past century shows targeting the snail intermediate host works best. PLoS Negl Trop Dis. 2016;10:e0004794.

74. Cupp EW, Sauerbrey M, Richards F. Elimination of human onchocerciasis: history of progress and current feasibility using ivermectin (Mectizan®) monotherapy. Acta Trop. 2011;120(Suppl. 1):S100–8.

75. World Health Organization. NTD donation program. 2016. https://www.who.int/neglected_diseases/Medicine_Donation_June_2016.pdf. Accessed 10 Oct 2019.

76. Cohen JP, Silva L, Cohen A, Awatin J, Sturgeon R. Progress report on neglected tropical disease drug donation programs. Clin Therapeut. 2016;38:1193–204.

77. World Health Organization. Preventive chemotherapy in human helminthiasis: coordinated use of anthelminthic drugs in control interventions: a manual for health professionals and programme managers. Geneva: World Health Organization; 2006.

78. Alhassan A, Li Z, Poole CB, Carlow CKS. Expanding the MDx toolbox for filarial diagnosis and surveillance. Trends Parasitol. 2015;31:391–400.

79. World Health Organization. Accelerating work to overcome the global impact of neglected tropical diseases—a roadmap for implementation. Geneva: World Health Organization; 2012.

80. World Health Organization. Crossing the billion: lymphatic filariasis, onchocerciasis, schistosomiasis, soil-transmitted helminthiases and trachoma: preventative chemotherapy for neglected tropical diseases. Geneva: WHO; 2017.

81. Campbell WC. Ivermectin as an antiparasitic agent for use in humans. Ann Rev Microbiol. 1991;45:445–74.

82. Boatin BA, Richards FO. Control of onchocerciasis. Adv Parasitol. 2006;61:349–94.

83. Lawrence J, Sodahlon YK, Ogoussan KT, Hopkins AD. Growth, challenges and solutions over 25 years of Mectizan and the impact on onchocerciasis control. PLoS Negl Trop Dis. 2015;9:e0003507.

84. Sauerbrey M, Rakers LJ, Richards FO. Progress toward elimination of onchocerciasis in the Americas. Int J Health. 2018;10(suppl 1):i71–8.
85. World Health Organization. Progress report on the elimination of human onchocerciasis, 2017-2018. Weekly Epidemiol Rec. 2018;93:633–48.
86. Opoku NO, Bakajika DK, Kanza EM, Howard H, Mambandu GL, Nyathirombo A, et al. Single dose moxidectin versus ivermectin for *Onchocerca volvulus* infection in Ghana, Liberia, and the Democratic Republic of the Congo: a randomised, controlled, double-blind phase 3 trial. Lancet. 2018;392:1207–16.
87. Boussinesq M, Fobi G, Kuesel AC. Alternative treatment strategies to accelerate the elimination of onchocerciasis. Int Health. 2018;10:i40–8.
88. Gyapong JO, Owusu IO, da Costa Vroom FB, Mensah EO, Gyapong M. Elimination of lymphatic filariasis: current perspectives on mass drug administration. Res Rep Trop Med. 2018;9:25–33.
89. Ramaiah KD, Ottesen EA. Progress and impact of 13 years of the global Programme to eliminate lymphatic Filariasis on reducing the burden of filarial disease. PLoS Negl Trop Dis. 2014;8:e3319.
90. World Health Organization. Global programme to eliminate lymphatic filariasis: progress report, 2017. Weekly Epidemiol Rec. 2018;93:589–604.
91. King CH, Suamani J, Sanuku N, Cheng YC, Satofan S, Mancuso B, et al. A trial of a triple-drug treatment for lymphatic filariasis. N Engl J Med. 2018;379:1801–10.
92. World Health Organization. WHO guideline: alternative mass drug administration regimens to eliminate lymphatic filariasis. Geneva: World Health Organization; 2017.
93. Herrick JA, Legrand F, Gounoue R, Nchinda G, Montavon C, Bopda J, et al. Posttreatment reactions after single-dose diethylcarbamazine or ivermectin in subjects with *Loa loa* infection. Clin Infect Dis. 2017;64:1017–25.
94. Hoerauf A. Filariasis: new drugs and new opportunities for lymphatic filariasis and onchocerciasis. Curr Opin Infect Dis. 2008;21:673–81.
95. Bakowski MA, McNamara CW. Advances in antiwolbachial drug discovery for treatment of parasitic filarial worm infections. Trop Med Infect Dis. 2018;4:E108.
96. Becker SL, Liwanag HJ, Snyder JS, Akogun O, Belizario V Jr, Freeman MC, et al. Toward the 2020 goal of soil-transmitted helminthiasis control and elimination. PLoS Negl Trop Dis. 2018;12:e0006606.
97. Farrell SH, Coffeng LE, Truscott JE, Werkman M, Toor J, de Vlas SJ, et al. Investigating the effectiveness of current and modified World Health Organization guidelines for the control of soil-transmitted helminth infections. Clin Infect Dis. 2018;66(S4):S253–9.
98. Schulz JD, Moser W, Hürlimann E, Keiser J. Preventative chemotherapy in the fight against soil-transmitted helminthiasis: achievements and limitations. Trends Parasitol. 2018;34:590–602.
99. Freeman MC, Akogun O, Belizario Jr. V, Broker SJ, Gyorkos TW, Imtiaz R, et al. Challenges and opportunities for control and elimination of soil-transmitted helminth infection beyond 2020. PLoS Negl Trop Dis 2019;13:e0007201.
100. World Health Organization. Schistosomiasis and soil-transmitted helminthiases: number of people treated in 2016. Weekly Epid Record. 2017;92:749–60.
101. World Health Organization. NTD elimination roadmap. https://www.who.int/neglected_diseases/news/NTD-Roadmap-targets-2021-2030.pdf. Accessed 1 Aug 2019.
102. Chai J-Y. Praziquantel treatment in trematode and cestode infections: an update. Inf Chemotherapy. 2013;45:32–43.
103. LoVerde PT. Schistosomiasis. Adv Exp Biol Med. 2019;1154:45–70.
104. Toor J, Alsallaq R, Truscott J, Turner HC, Werkman M, Gurarie D, et al. Are we on our way to achieving the 2020 goals for schistosomiasis morbidity control using current WHO guidelines? Clin Infect Dis. 2018;66(S4):S245–2.
105. Mutapi F, Maizels R, Fenwick A, Woolhouse M. Human schistosomiasis in the post mass drug administration era. Lancet Infect Dis. 2017;17:e42–8.
106. Sikasunge CS, Johansen MV, Willingham ALIII, Leifsson PS, Phiri IK. *Taenia solium* porcine cysticercosis: viability of cysticerci and persistency of antibodies and cysticercal antigens after treatment with oxfendazole. Vet Parasitol. 2008;158:57–66.
107. Lightowlers MW. Control of *Taenia solium* taeniasis/cysticercosis: past practices and new possibilities. Parasitology. 2013;140:1566–77.
108. Lightowlers MW, Donadeu M. Designing a minimal intervention strategy to control *Taenia solium*. Trends Parasitol. 2017;33:426–34.
109. Blum AJ, Hotez PJ. Global "worming": climate change and its projected its projected general impact on human helminth infections. PLoS Negl Trop Dis. 2018;12:e0006370.
110. Rocklov J, et al. Climate change pathways and potential future risks to nutrition and infection. In: Humphries DL, Scott ME, Vermund SH, editors. Nutrition and infectious diseases: shifting the clinical paradigm. Switzerland: Springer Nature; 2020.

111. Jenkins TP, Rathnayaka Y, Perera PK, Peachey LE, Nolan MJ, Krause L, et al. Infections by human gastrointestinal helminths are associated with changes in faecal microbiota diversity and composition. PLoS One. 2017;12:e0184719.
112. Reynolds LA, Smith KA, Filbey KJ, Harcus Y, Hewitson JP, Redpath SA, et al. Commensal-pathogen interactions in the intestinal tract: lactobacilli promote infection with, and are promoted by, helminth parasites. Gut Microbes. 2014;5:522–32.
113. Zaiss MM, Rapin A, Lebon L, Dubey LK, Mosconi I, Sarter K, et al. The intestinal microbiota contributes to the ability of helminths to modulate allergic inflammation. Immunity. 2015;43:998–1010.
114. Reynolds LA, Redpath SA, Yurist-Doutsch S, Gill N, Brown EM, van der Heijden J, et al. Enteric helminths promote *Salmonella* coinfection by altering the intestinal metabolome. J Infect Dis. 2017;215:1245–54.
115. Greenwood BM. Autoimmune disease and parasitic infections in Nigerians. Lancet. 1968;2(7564):380–2.
116. Cooper PJ. Interactions between helminth parasites and allergy. Curr Opin Allergy Clin Immunol. 2009;9:29–37.
117. Fleming JO, Weinstock JV. Clinical trials of helminth therapy in autoimmune diseases: rationale and findings. Parasite Immunol. 2015;37:277–92.
118. Stiemsma L, Reynolds L, Turvey S, Finlay B. The hygiene hypothesis: current perspectives and future therapies. ImmunoTargets Therapy. 2015;4:143–57.

# Part III
# Nutrition Issues During Major Infections: Case Studies of Nutrition and Infectious Diseases

# Chapter 8
# Nutrition and Diarrheal Disease and Enteric Pathogens

**Fahad Javaid Siddiqui, Grace Belayneh, and Zulfiqar A. Bhutta**

## Abbreviations

| | |
|---|---|
| AhR | Aryl Hydrocarbon Receptor |
| APP | Acute phase protein |
| C | Complement |
| CD2 | Cluster of Differentiation 2 |
| CD69 | Cluster of Differentiation 69 |
| CRP | C-reactive protein |
| DALY | Disability Adjusted Life Year |
| DC | Dendritic cell |
| DNA | Deoxyribonucleic acid |
| EED | Environment Enteric Dysfunction |
| EPEC | Enteropathogenic *Escherichia coli* |
| ETEC | Enterotoxigenic *Escherichia coli* |
| GALT | Gut Associated Lymphoid Tissue |
| IFN-$\gamma$ | Interferon gamma |
| IgA | Immunoglobulin A |
| IL | Interleukin |
| ILC | Innate Lymphoid Cell |
| IMCI | Integrated management of childhood illnesses |
| LPS | Lipopolysaccharide |
| MAM | Moderate acute malnutrition |

F. J. Siddiqui
SickKids Centre for Global Child Health, Toronto, ON, Canada

Duke-NUS Medical School, Singapore, Singapore

G. Belayneh
Duke-NUS Medical School, Singapore, Singapore

Z. A. Bhutta (✉)
Robert Harding Chair in Global Child Health & Policy, SickKids Centre for Global Child Health, The Hospital for Sick Children, Toronto, ON, Canada

Departments of Paediatrics, Nutritional Sciences and Public Health, University of Toronto, Toronto, ON, Canada
e-mail: zulfiqar.bhutta@sickkids.ca

© Springer Nature Switzerland AG 2021
D. L. Humphries et al. (eds.), *Nutrition and Infectious Diseases*, Nutrition and Health,
https://doi.org/10.1007/978-3-030-56913-6_8

MHC     Major histocompatibility complex molecules
NK      Natural Killer cell
NO      Nitric oxide
PEM     Protein-energy malnutrition
PGE2    Prostaglandin E2
RUTF    Ready to use therapeutic food
SAM     Severe acute malnutrition
SDG     Sustainable development goal
SDI     Sociodemographic Index
SIgA    Serum Immunoglobulin A
Th1     Helper T cell (Type 1)
WHO     World Health Organization

**Key Points**
- Malnutrition, as protein calorie and micronutrient deficiency, still remains a formidable challenge for public health experts.
- Malnutrition increases the exposure to diarrhea causing pathogens, adversely affects the components of gut barrier including the gut microbiome and gut mucosa.
- Malnutrition generally reduces the ability of the immune system to mount adequate responses against pathogens although some components of the immune system remain unaffected or are enhanced in response to infection.
- Disease progresses faster, leads to more severe symptoms, takes longer to resolve, and has worse outcomes in malnourished individuals.
- Antibiotics, though lifesaving, have detrimental effects on the gut microbiome, a key defense mechanism against gut pathogens.
- Infection by some pathogens (e.g., *Entamoeba histolytica*) becomes less likely in malnourished individuals.
- More research will help identify newer intervention targets.

# Introduction

## *Definitions*

Diarrhea is defined by the World Health Organization (WHO) as "the passage of three or more loose or liquid stools per day (or more frequent passage than is normal for the individual) [1]. It is one of the most common symptoms of gut infection, frequently caused by bacteria, viruses, and parasites (see Chaps. 4–7) [2–5]. Diarrhea is classified clinically into various types, which are not necessarily mutually exclusive: acute watery diarrhea which lasts several hours or days, and includes cholera; acute bloody diarrhea, also called dysentery; prolonged acute diarrhea which lasts for 7–13 days; and persistent diarrhea which lasts 14 days or longer. Enteric infections refer to a group of disorders that affect gut function but may or may not cause diarrhea [6]. The term "diarrheal diseases" is used for the collection of diseases that frequently result in diarrhea caused by infectious agents [7].

## *Epidemiology*

Diarrhea ranked fifth among the most common causes of death in 2017 globally and is the third leading cause of death and disability in countries with a low social development index (SDI) [8]. Out of 2.3 billion diarrheal episodes estimated for the year 2015 globally, 957 million occurred in children younger than 5 years (yrs) and caused nearly half a million deaths in this age group. Diarrhea also resulted in loss of over 71 million disability adjusted life years (DALYs), 63% of which were among children younger than 5 yrs. [9]. These children are more likely to develop malnutrition [10].

The burden of enteric infections estimated by the Global Burden of Disease project provides the following figures for 2017: globally there were over 6.3 billion diarrheal episodes resulting in 1.7 million deaths; children younger than 5 yrs. experienced 1.1 billion episodes that resulted in 589,000 deaths. Almost all of these deaths occurred in low- and low-middle and middle-SDI countries [11]. While there has been significant reduction in diarrhea mortality and morbidity in the last decade owing to various interventions, such mortality and morbidity are still a major public health problem [9].

## *Etiology*

Thirteen organisms have been identified as causing diarrheal episodes [11]. If all age groups are considered, rotavirus, *Shigella* and *Salmonella* spp. are the top three leading causes of death. However, the etiology of diarrheal disease is slightly different for children younger than 5 yrs., where rotavirus caused 29.3% of deaths, *Cryptosporidium* spp. caused 1.1% and *Shigella* spp. 5.5%. Table 8.1 provides a list of the microbial agents that are the most important contributors to enteric infection-related deaths [9, 11]. Use of advanced diagnostic techniques for identifying causes of diarrhea implicated six pathogens in 75% of the diarrhea burden in seven countries, including *Shigella* spp., rotavirus, adenovirus 40/41, enterotoxigenic *Escherichia coli* (ETEC), *Cryptosporidium* spp., and *Campylobacter* spp. [12].

## Risk Factors and Determinants of Diarrhea

During the first decade of the twenty-first century, large reductions in child mortality have been observed. Yet the burden of child mortality is still high, with diarrhea and pneumonia as the leading causes [13]. Reduction rates are slower than that required to meet the relevant Sustainable Development Goals (SDGs) [14, 15]. Increasing the reduction rates in order to achieve the SDGs requires a better

**Table 8.1** Commonly implicated microbial agents in enteric infections

| Bacteria | Viruses | Protozoan Parasites |
|---|---|---|
| *Campylobacter* spp | Adenoviruses | *Entamoeba histolytica* |
| *Vibrio cholerae* | Rotavirus | *Cryptosporidium* |
| Enterotoxigenic *Escherichia coli* (ETEC) | Norovirus | *Giardia* |
| Enteropathogenic *Escherichia coli* (EPEC) | | |
| *Shigella* spp. | | |
| *Salmonella* spp. | | |
| *Aeromonas* spp. | | |
| *Clostridium difficile* | | |

understanding of the risk factors and determinants of the major killers of children under 5 yrs. The most common, but non-modifiable, factors are age and gender. Over 80% of the mortality associated with diarrhea in children under 5 yrs. occurs in children under 2 yrs. [13]. There is some evidence indicating a higher risk of diarrhea in boys compared to girls of the same age [13]. The pathogens involved in the diarrheal burden also differ with age [13].

Modifiable risk factors for both morbidity and mortality include absence of breastfeeding, being underweight, stunted, or wasted and being vitamin A deficient [13]. Intensity of exposure is also directly associated with outcomes [13]. A systematic review from India identified several other risk factors [16], including low socioeconomic status, low mother's education, unsafe drinking water, and anemia. This combination of factors suggests sociodemographic improvements as an important avenue for further reduction of morbidity and mortality due to diarrheal diseases.

## Ways in Which Malnutrition Contributes to Enteric Infection

The importance of malnutrition as an underlying cause of childhood deaths has been long established [17]. Undernutrition plays a significant role in enteric infections and diarrheal diseases through a variety of pathways, and the relationship is bidirectional. In order to appreciate the phenomenon, we have chosen to begin with malnutrition, then to explore the impact of nutritional status on diarrheal diseases and enteric infections, and finally to circle back to the impact of diarrheal diseases on nutritional status.

While significant steps are being taken to address malnutrition globally, undernutrition still underlies 45% of childhood deaths, and 20 million babies are born underweight each year. Simultaneously, overweight and obesity among children are growing and have reached record high levels among adults [18]. This double burden of malnutrition can coexist in the same country, community, household, and even in the same person—all at the same time [18].

Undernutrition is particularly problematic for low- and middle-income countries where the socioeconomic environment restricts access to resources needed to meet basic nutritional requirements. In this context, malnourished mothers give birth to malnourished children with compromised immunity (see Chap. 3) [19] and diminished developmental potential, outcomes that have lifelong consequences for the child and intergenerational consequences for society.

The impact of socioeconomic context can be clearly seen in the disease burden disparities that exist and persist between countries. While noncommunicable diseases have become the leading cause of early death in the most socioeconomically developed countries, communicable diseases, like diarrheal diseases, remain the biggest problems where development indicators are lowest [20]. Notably, undernutrition is a primary underlying risk factor for deaths caused by communicable diseases and also the most important risk factor for diarrheal disease-related mortality, accounting for nearly 3 in 4 deaths [20, 21]. Hidden hunger, referring to invisible micronutrient deficiencies (see Chap. 2) [22], also plays a role. Children with micronutrient deficiencies have increased rates and severity of diarrheal episodes, and studies investigating the effects of micronutrient supplementation (specifically, iron, zinc, and vitamin A) have consistently demonstrated significant benefits [23–27].

Malnutrition has wide-ranging deleterious impacts on the immune system (see Chap. 3) [19]. The complex mechanisms involved have yet to be fully elucidated although a few explanations have been put forth as no theory completely explains all immune system events observed during malnutrition. Following are the salient features of current explanations. Rytter et al. can be referred for finer details [28].

*Lack of energy and building blocks*: Due to lack of energy and nutrients, immune system-related proteins cannot be produced leading to a subnormal immune response. However, this fails to explain why all parameters of the immune system are not equally affected. Rather, some immune response pathways appear to become more pronounced in malnutrition.

*Mixed hormonal profile*: Changes in hormones that activate or suppress immune system components lead to elevated positive acute phase proteins (APP) among malnourished children, signaling subclinical inflammation resulting in catabolism which exacerbates malnutrition. However, numbers of activated T cells and dendritic cells (DCs) do not correspond to the acute phase reaction, and their numbers remain either unaffected or lower than expected.

*Tolerance*: This mechanism hypothesizes that, to avoid an autoimmune reaction against self-antigens released due to ongoing catabolism, the body downregulates the immune response. A counter argument to this theory is that one would expect to see some breakthrough of autoimmune reactions among malnourished children. However, research to explore this has not yet been conducted.

*Hormonal interplay*: This mechanism suggests that thymus-stimulating hormones such as leptin, prolactin, and growth hormones are deficient with malnutrition, and thymus-suppressing hormones such as adrenaline and cortisol are high in malnourished children. This is consistent with other observed immune system events in malnourished children like elevated APP and depressed negative APP. However, why growth hormone is low when needed by the body needs is unexplained.

In this chapter, we will consider how undernutrition increases the risk of exposure and susceptibility to enteric infections, contributes to suboptimal immune responses, and can lead to more rapid disease progression, increased severity of disease, and slower or delayed responses to treatment, all of which result in the high morbidity and mortality associated with what remains a leading cause of death in children under 5 yrs. Figure 8.1 provides an overview of the complex relationship between malnutrition and diarrhea. The vicious cycle frequently begins with inadequate nutrition, either in utero or after birth, initiating a cascade of events all augmented by a worsening of malnutrition throughout the cycle. At other times, repeated infections push a well-nourished child into this cycle. In the following sections, we will describe mechanisms whereby malnutrition as a trigger.

## *Increased Risk of Exposure*

Malnutrition, once established, increases a child's risk of exposure to enteric pathogens through several potential mechanisms. Malnutrition-related hospitalizations for severe acute malnutrition increase a child's exposure to hospital-acquired enteric infections [29, 30]. Another sequence of events that leads to increased risk of exposure starts with the difficulty of feeding malnourished children, as they are often irritable, anorexic, and intolerant of larger amounts of food. As a result, caregivers make more frequent feeding attempts, increasing the number of opportunities of exposure to pathogens if personal and environmental hygiene is sub-optimal—which is frequently the case. There are also significant challenges associated with food storage, as protecting food from microbes is a formidable task in resource-constrained environments. Access to clean water is yet another challenge that can lead to contamination of many of the foods recommended for malnourished children, whether cattle milk, homemade meals, or ready-to-use therapeutic foods (RUTF) [31]. The WHO identifies all the above as avoidable risks that can prevent microbial contamination of foods, especially during complementary feeding, and thus reduce a major cause of gastrointestinal illnesses in childhood [32].

Cultural beliefs and practices related to malnutrition have been reported to influence risk of exposure as well. These reports are mostly anecdotal. However, one study from Talensi district in the Upper East Region of Ghana documented a traditional treatment of malnourishment using water in which avian feces had been soaked, a practice that can obviously increase risk of exposure to bird pathogens that also infect humans [33]. There are likely to be other common but undocumented beliefs and practices related to malnutrition in different communities which, when practiced, can put malnourished children at higher risk of exposure to enteric pathogens.

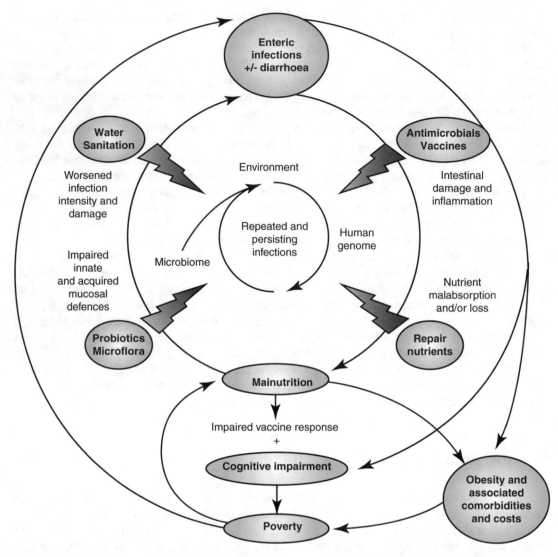

**Fig. 8.1** The complex interconnections among factors that perpetuate the malnutrition-infection cycle. Enteric infections, especially in the first 2–3 years of life, with or without overt diarrhea, can predispose an individual to malnutrition and stunted growth through multiple mechanisms. Stunting by 2 years of age, in turn, is associated with impaired cognitive development that extends into later childhood and even adulthood and adult productivity. In addition, malnourished children experience both greater frequency and duration of diarrheal illnesses, and, documented in animal models, heavier infections. The latter is documented with *Cryptosporidium* and with enteroaggregative *Escherichia coli*. Finally, enteric infections or stunting can predispose to obesity and its comorbidities of diabetes, hypertension, cardiovascular disease, metabolic syndrome, and burgeoning health-care expenditures, contributing to individual and societal poverty in vicious cycles. Reprinted from Guerrant et al. [162] with permission from Springer Nature

On the other hand, there is evidence of an association between decreased risk of certain gut infections and malnutrition. This is particularly observed for rotavirus and *Giardia* [34, 35]. Although the mechanisms have not been fully elucidated, malnourished hosts may not be able to provide the energy and nutrients needed by pathogens (see Chap. 14) [36]. Similarly, iron deficiency affords protection against *Entamoeba histolytica* infection, as both adherence and cytotoxicity of this protozoan pathogen have been found to be lower in children with iron deficiency [37, 38]. No such effect was observed with other mineral deficiencies that were tested [38]. Further research is needed to learn the exact mechanisms.

## Reduced Immune Response Increases Susceptibility to Pathogens

Malnutrition adversely affects immune functioning, preventing the maintenance of core functions critical for survival. Reduced functionality has wide-ranging effects on both innate and adaptive immunity (see Chap. 3) [19]. Effects are particularly pronounced in the first 1000 days of life when development of the immune system is most sensitive to nutritional status [39]. If the immune system has been weakened by malnutrition either in utero or postnatally, susceptibility to infections can be increased through a number of pathways. These include weakening or alteration of the gastrointestinal mucosal barrier, defects in immune function in both the innate and humoral arms, impaired inflammatory response, and changes in the microbiome. All are discussed in detail below. Figure 8.2 shows the interlinks between malnutrition, immune function, and susceptibility to infections [39].

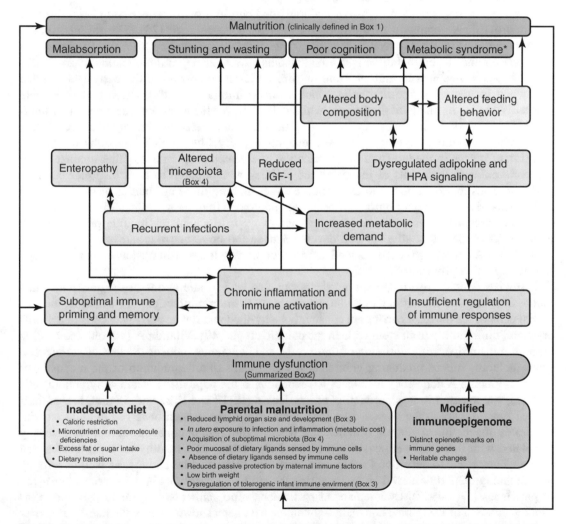

**Fig. 8.2** Conceptual framework for immune dysfunction as a cause and consequence of malnutrition. Immune dysfunction can arise before birth via developmental pathways (purple), compounded by environmental and behavioral factors (yellow), particularly those experienced during early life. Immune dysfunction (blue) can contribute both directly and indirectly to a range of causal pathways (green) that lead to clinical malnutrition (red). HPA, hypothalamus–pituitary–adrenal axis; IGF-1, insulin-like growth factor 1; *, refers to predisposition to metabolic syndrome in adulthood following exposure to undernutrition in infancy. Reprinted from Bourke et al. [39]; Creative Commons CC-BY license

## Alterations of the Gastrointestinal Mucosal Barrier

The gastrointestinal tract houses the largest mucosal surface in the human body. With a single epithelial layer, the intestinal lining protects the interior of the body from the large and diverse population of bacteria that inhabit the gut [40, 41]. The same epithelial layer is also responsible for nutrient absorption and waste secretion, and, as such, a healthy gastrointestinal mucosal barrier is selectively permeable. Permeability is primarily mediated by tight junctions that seal the paracellular spaces and thus maintain the barrier's integrity (see Chap. 6) [4, 40]. The epithelial layer is made up of a variety of cells. Goblet cells produce a mucus layer that covers the surface of the epithelium and functions to protect the epithelium from harmful substances and to bind and flush away pathogenic bacteria. Other epithelial cells secrete salts, hormones, cytokines, proteins, and antibodies to maintain a neutral pH at the epithelium despite acidic surroundings, regulate cell proliferation and differentiation, protect against toxins, bind bacteria, and repair lesions [42].

Structural changes to the mucosa of malnourished children include decreased height of villi and microvilli, lymphocytic infiltration, and increased vascularity [28]. The thinned mucus layer, sometimes referred to as a "tissue paper intestine," increases opportunities for pathogens to adhere and invade epithelial cells. Animal models have shown that the intestinal barrier loses its functional robustness in malnutrition. In vitro research conducted in the early 1990s found that when incubated with *Salmonella typhimurium* epithelial cell destruction and lysis were markedly higher in malnourished mice, while cells from well-nourished mice remained unaffected [43]. Another consequence of a thinned mucosa is decreased production of mucus, likely through interruption of cyclooxygenase 2 enzyme activity [44], which interrupts the barrier function of mucus in the intestine [45]. Detection of elevated titers of antibodies against bacterial endotoxins in the stools of malnourished children as compared to their healthier counterparts indicates that malnourished children are either making more antibodies against bacterial endotoxins or have a greater burden of bacterial endotoxins than their well-nourished peers [46, 47]. More recent studies confirm these findings as well. Mechanisms include protein energy malnutrition (PEM) that alters B-cell development in the bone marrow and increases the frequency of IgA-secreting B cells, as well as IgA secretion by long-lived plasma cells in the small intestinal lamina propria [48].

Likewise, deficiencies in specific nutrients can also lead to alterations of the gastrointestinal mucosal barrier and thus affect a child's susceptibility to enteric infection. For example, the epithelial cells of the mucosal barrier are constantly being shed and replaced by new cells that proliferate and differentiate from stem cells in the colonic crypts [49]. Vitamin A (via retinoic acid) is critical to the proper differentiation of these cells, and deficiency induces the loss of various cell types including mucus-producing goblet cells, which leads to a degradation of the mucus layer [50–52]. Vitamin A deficiency also leads to reductions in the population of innate lymphoid cells (ILC3s), which result in less production of interleukin (IL)17 and IL22 and, in turn, less antimicrobial functionality in the mucus layer [51]. Such impacts have been observed in children with high rates of subclinical vitamin A deficiency, where serum retinol concentrations were inversely correlated with intestinal permeability [53]. Zinc also promotes a healthy mucosal barrier, and its deficiency leads to defective Paneth cells, with less antimicrobial activity, as well as atrophy of villi and lymphoid tissues, thereby impairing the epithelial barrier's ability to prevent invasion of pathogens [51, 54–57]. Deficiencies of particular amino acids also appear to play a role, as supplementation of L-arginine and alanyl-glutamine hass been shown to improve intestinal barrier function in an animal model and in infants [58, 59]. In contrast, iron supplementation is associated with increased permeability of the small intestine and increased susceptibility to diarrheal disease and enteric infection [25].

## Environmental Enteric Dysfunction

Environmental enteric dysfunction (EED) is a subclinical chronic intestinal disorder that, once established, erodes the mucosal barrier function that is important for immunity. It, however, has been demonstrated that dysbiosis of the normal microflora precedes the actual invasion of gut mucosa by microbes, leading to EED, which can in turn lead to subclinical harmful effects even without manifesting as diarrhea [60]. EED was first named as an entity in 2014 by Keusch and colleagues who cited functional deficits as prominent features of the condition [61]. While the definition of EED is still being crafted, the hallmark morphological features (villous flattening, crypt hyperplasia, local and systemic inflammatory biomarkers, lymphocytic infiltration of the lamina propria) all indicate pathophysiological changes and morphological injury to the gut mucosa [62, 63]. Shortening of villi reduces the surface available for nutrient absorption, contributing to malnutrition. This has been supported by indirect evidence, where complementary feeding interventions were less effective in children with EED [47]. Such changes can also lead to malabsorption, further enhancing malnutrition [47]. Observational studies have found associations of stunting with EED, suggesting a potential role for EED in chronic malnutrition [64, 65]. Hypercellularity of the gut mucosa in EED is a sign of chronic inflammation of the intestines, and the chronic inflammation is associated with appetite suppression [66]. The role of appetite suppression leading to reduced food intake may be an important contributor to chronic malnutrition in children [67]. Hormonal disturbances leading to adverse inflammatory events have also been proposed as a mechanism of growth failure in EED, although evidence is limited [68].

As the gut is a potential site of entry for pathogens, it is critical to have a functioning intact barrier. Components of gut barrier functions are impaired in EED. With the thinned mucous layer, capacity for trapping and blocking invasion of harmful microbes is reduced. The presence of an increased number of inflammatory cells suggests the failure of the epithelial barrier to restrict luminal contents from crossing the epithelium and activating an inflammatory response. These effects have been shown to result in linear growth retardation [69]. Finally, sub-optimal response to oral polio and rotavirus vaccines has also been associated with EED [70–73].

## Defects in Immune Function

Malnutrition impacts both innate and adaptive immunity (see Chap. 3) [19]. Innate immunity is comprised of cell and complement complex-mediated immunity that is not specific to the pathogen. Leukocytes, T cells, and cytokines, together with the complement complex, are the main drivers of this arm of the immune system [74]. Adaptive immunity is largely based on T cells, B cells, plasma cells, and antibodies that are produced in response to a particular pathogenic agent and that create immunological memory with the thymus as the central coordinating organ [74]. As highlighted in Fig. 8.3, the responses of the gut epithelium to malnutrition alone and to specific deficiencies when combined with different pathogens can be quite distinctive. Other components play role in protecting the body from infections. Research to date has demonstrated that not all immune functions are adversely affected by malnutrition, although many important functions are [28]. Figure 8.4 summarizes the evidence based on a systematic review of studies on children where the underlying cause of the immune response was not considered. The following details explain how components of immune system are affected by protein calorie or micronutrient deficiencies.

Compounds in saliva and acid production in the stomach are some of the innate mechanisms that protect the body from infection (see Chap. 3) [19]. In malnutrition, primarily due to lack of energy and protein, the quantity and quality of these secretions deteriorate, allowing increased invasion of enteric

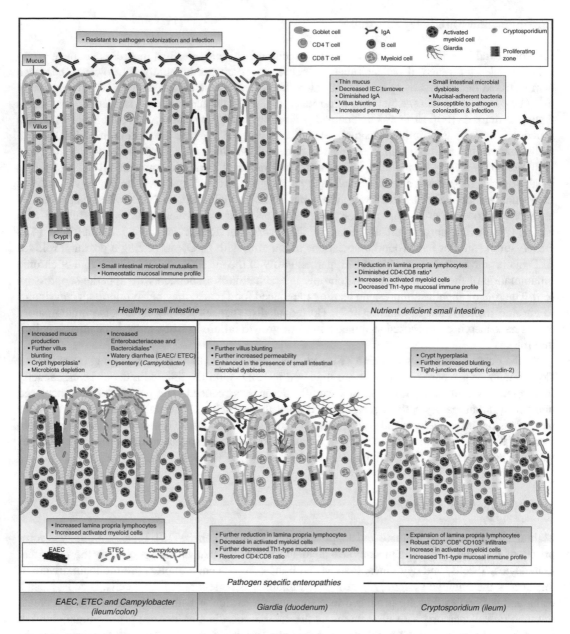

**Fig. 8.3** Schematic diagram contrasting the pathology and immune responses in the intestinal epithelium during a healthy state (green boxes) to that of malnourished individuals (yellow boxes) to the combination of zinc deficiency and bacterial infections (pink boxes) to that of protein deficiency and *Giardia* or *Cryptosporidium* infection. Reprinted from Bartelt et al. [62]; Creative Commons CC-BY License

microbes. Salivary IgA (SIgA) has been found to be reduced in severely malnourished children [75]. Other studies have identified lower gastric secretions in malnourished children with higher (less acidic) pH contributing to reduced protection against infections [76–79].

The total number of immune cells has generally been found to be higher in malnourished children, although some functions were adversely affected, including adherence and ingestion of foreign material [28]. More of the leukocytes show signs of damage to DNA [28]. Levels of APPs such as C-reactive protein (CRP) and haptoglobin were found to be higher in malnourished children with clinical infec-

**Fig. 8.4** Impact of malnutrition in children on components of immune system, without consideration of underlying factors generating an immune response. Reprinted from Rytter et al. [28]; Creative Commons CC-BY License

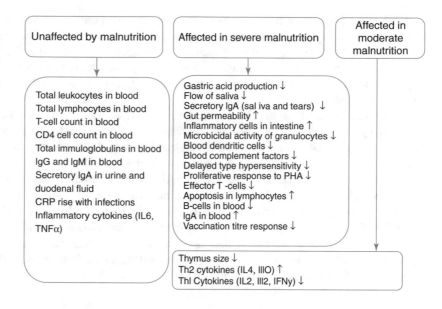

| Unaffected by malnutrition | Affected in severe malnutrition | Affected in moderate malnutrition |

Unaffected by malnutrition:
Total leukocytes in blood
Total lymphocytes in blood
T-cell count in blood
CD4 cell count in blood
Total immuloglobulins in blood
IgG and IgM in blood
Secretory IgA in urine and duodenal fluid
CRP rise with infections
Inflammatory cytokines (IL6, TNFα)

Affected in severe malnutrition:
Gastric acid production ↓
Flow of saliva ↓
Secretory IgA (sal iva and tears) ↓
Gut permeability ↑
Inflammatory cells in intestine ↑
Microbicidal activity of granulocytes ↓
Blood dendritic cells ↓
Blood complement factors ↓
Delayed type hypersensitivity ↓
Proliferative response to PHA ↓
Effector T -cells ↓
Apoptosis in lymphocytes ↑
B-cells in blood ↓
IgA in blood ↑
Vaccination titre response ↓

Thymus size ↓
Th2 cytokines (IL4, IIIO) ↑
Thl Cytokines (IL2, III2, IFNγ) ↓

tions, and results were mixed in children without apparent infections. Proteins of the complement system were largely found to be lower in malnourished children, particularly serum levels of complement (C)3. Insufficiency of C3, the central pillar of this system, significantly reduces microbicidal capacity of leukocytes, especially against gram-negative bacteria, early in the infection [61, 80]. The reduction in complement proteins has mainly been attributed to reduced production although increased utilization due to infections also plays a role [81, 82]. While malnutrition has been found to be associated with reduced production of interferon (IFN)γ, above average IFNγ production has been found to have protective effect against *E. histolytica* [83]. IL10 similarly has a protective effect against *E. histolytica* in mice, but malnourished mice had less IL10 and hence were more susceptible to this infection [84].

Thymus size was found to be reduced in even mild malnutrition and partially reversed after treatment for malnutrition [28]. Extreme malnutrition may cause "nutritional thymectomy" as has been seen upon autopsy of malnourished children [85]. Other defects in adaptive immune function include reduced levels of soluble IgA in saliva and tears, elevated levels of soluble IgA in blood, largely no effect on IgG or IgM antibodies, reduced delayed-type hypersensitivity responses, fewer circulating B cells, a shift from T helper (Th)1-associated to Th2-associated cytokines, and lymphocyte hyporesponsiveness to phytohemagglutinin, with preserved lymphocyte and immunoglobulin levels in peripheral blood [28, 39]. In children with severe malnutrition, seroconversion rates have been found to be either reduced or delayed for typhoid and measles [86–94]. In children that achieved seroconversion following vaccination, titers remained lower than normal among severely malnourished children [28, 86–91, 95–97]. While the evidence strongly suggests sub-optimal development of acquired immunity after vaccination, the results are not consistent as some studies have reported normal antibody titers among severely malnourished children (see Fig. 8.4) [28].

## Impaired Inflammatory Response

The inflammatory response is a reaction of the body that occurs when tissues are injured due to any harmful exposure. The response can lead to a number of signs or symptoms, including pain, localized warmth, redness, swelling, and loss of function-mediated through various cytokines including histamine, bradykinin, and prostaglandins. The cytokines cause blood vessels to leak fluid into the tissues, and when this happens in the gut, it results in diarrhea.

Evidence of impact of malnutrition on inflammatory response is inconsistent both across studies and across the components of cell-mediated immunity. A generalized dampening of the inflammatory response on a low protein diet has been demonstrated in rats [98]. In contrast, in malnourished pigs, local T lymphocyte expansion, enhanced intestinal major histocompatibility class (MHC) I and MHC II gene expression, and elevated tissue concentrations of prostaglandin E2 were observed after rotavirus infection [99, 100].

As above, malnutrition related to specific nutrients can also influence susceptibility to enteric infection by impairment of the inflammatory response. In rats, zinc deficiency led to reduced capacity to quench free oxidative radicals which cause cell injury and also resulted in inadequate handling of nitric oxide which is a diarrhea-triggering messenger [101]. The ileum of such mice demonstrated reduced leukocyte infiltration indicating an impaired inflammatory response [102]. Although the mechanism is not fully understood, intestinal contents of zinc-deficient mice exposed to enteroaggressive *E.coli* also had higher expression of *E. coli* virulence factors than was observed in control mice, indicating that zinc deficiency may increase disease severity [102]. In another animal study, mice deficient in vitamin D developed chronic low-grade intestinal inflammation and had a more severe inflammatory response when challenged with enteric pathogens, despite elevated levels of both pro-inflammatory and anti-inflammatory cytokines [103].

## Changes in the Microbiota

The gastrointestinal tract is home to a large and heterogeneous community of bacteria that protects the gut from colonization by pathogenic bacteria while simultaneously facilitating nutrient and drug metabolism, vitamin production, and development and maintenance of the mucosal barrier [39]. Acquired or adaptive immunity is permissive to nonpathogenic bacteria in the gut, allowing the creation and maintenance of a protective microbiome [74]. We are increasingly realizing that this microbiota is an important mediator of the relationship between nutrition and host.

The microbiota is highly dynamic in composition and sensitive to dietary changes due to its intimate contact with ingested food and environmental contaminants that reach the intestinal lumen. The bacterial composition of a microbiota differs from person to person and even within the same person from day to day [49]. Studies in mice have shown that modifications in dietary protein, fat, polysaccharide, and simple sugars alter the microbiota's composition in a systematic fashion [39]. This sensitivity allows for quick return to normal composition when diets return to normal. However, sustained consumption of a high-fat diet induces proliferation of gram-negative bacteria in the gut [104], and there appears to be a tipping point at which dysbiosis ensues [105]. This is especially problematic in neonatal and pediatric populations, as the microbiota and the immune system are most sensitive to diet during those periods [106]. Dysbiosis at this critical time can have lifelong, if not intergenerational, consequences. Mouse models demonstrate that introduction of the dysbiotic microbiota from malnourished children into the gut of "germ-free" mice produced wide-ranging pathological changes [107]. In contrast, introduction of healthy microbiota helped in recovery from these effects in the mice previously inoculated with dysbiotic microbiota. Such studies demonstrate the critical nature and impact of a healthy microbiome on gut function [108].

Antimicrobial therapy, and even nonantibiotic drugs, can also produce detrimental effects on the microbiome, and yet the WHO recommends antibiotics for children with severe acute malnutrition [109–116]. It is known that antibiotics can disrupt the healthy microbiota while acting on harmful microbes [117]. Silverman and colleagues have reviewed the evidence and conclude that even short courses of antibiotics can disrupt the microbiota [118]. Though most microbial strains recover in a few weeks, depending upon the antibiotic administered, others may take up to 6 months, while still others may not recover at all. Age at the time of disruption also plays an important role, as antibiotic exposure among infants and young children results in a less diverse, less stable microbiome that

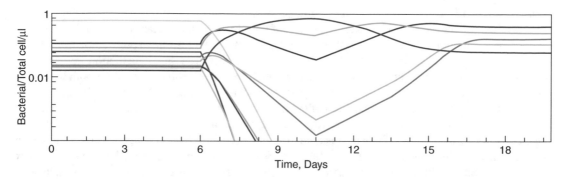

**Fig. 8.5** Impact of a 4-day course of antibiotic (days 6–10) on the relative frequencies of eight of the most abundant bacteria genera (each represented by a different color) in a human gut microbiome. The five that are presumably more sensitive to the antibiotic are eliminated from the gut during antibiotic treatment. The remaining bacteria genera regrow and readapt to the new environment and are able to different but stable microbiota at around day 18. Reprinted from Nogueira et al. [119] with permission from John Wiley and Sons

matures later and shows signs of greater antibiotic resistance [118]. Therefore, disrupting the remaining healthy microbiota of malnourished children can be harmful. Figure 8.5 shows the impact of antibiotics on the microbiota. With the commencement of antibiotics at day 6, the different colonies were either eliminated or adversely affected, and, after antibiotics were stopped, some colonies regrew and readapted to the new environment while others did not [119]. Oral administration of an appropriate mix of bacteria, that have a probiotic effect, can help repair the damage done and recovery from malnourishment [120, 121].

Some pathogens are significantly more prevalent among malnourished children because of the harmful changes in the microbiota due to malnutrition. When malnutrition reduces the number of commensal bacteria, the predominant residents of the gut, it allows for increased growth of pathogenic microbes with increased epithelial adherence and mucosal uptake [122–124]. Compared to their healthy counterparts, malnourished children have microbiomes that are less mature and less diverse [39, 123, 125, 126].

While there are a variety of viruses, bacteria, and parasites associated with diarrheal diseases and enteric infections, globally, greater than 50% of all diarrheal deaths among children under 5 yrs. are attributable to rotavirus, calicivirus, enteropathogenic *Escherichia coli* (EPEC), and ETEC [125, 127, 128]. The Global Enteric Multicenter Study (GEMS), a seven-country case-control study to identify the etiology and population-based burden of pediatric diarrheal disease in sub-Saharan Africa and south Asia, found that rotavirus, *Cryptosporidium*, and ETEC were the most common diarrheal pathogens [129]. Furthermore, a study in Bangladesh found that stool samples from children with malnutrition included ETEC, *Cryptosporidium* sp., and *E. histolytica* more often than those from children without malnutrition [46]. The Malnutrition as an Enteric Disorder (MAL-ED) study, an eight-country birth cohort study investigating risk factors and interactions of enteric infections and malnutrition and the consequences for child health and development, reported that children with high enteropathogen exposure, mainly *E.coli*, and low energy and protein intake, were at higher risk of stunting [130, 131]. Disruption of the microbiota of these malnourished children may explain increased colonization and invasion of pathogenic bacteria, such as *E. coli* and pathogenic protozoan infections.

Deficiencies in specific nutrients can also cause harmful changes to the microbiome. Lv and colleagues [132] found that the gut microbiota differed significantly based on children's vitamin A status. Children with normal vitamin A levels had greater community diversity than their vitamin A-deficient counterparts, and their key phylotypes were *E. coli* and *Clostridium butyricum*, while the microbiome of children with vitamin A deficiency was dominated by *Enterococcus*, a common opportunistic pathogen [132]. Vitamin A also reduces the number of butyrate-producing bacteria, which may be a contributing factor to increased growth of pathogenic strains as butyrate plays a role in suppressing growth of pathogenic strains [132]. Mouse models of protein, zinc, and dietary fiber deficiencies have all been shown to modulate the microbial community, with the latter leading to proliferation of mucus-degrading bacteria [133]. In contrast, both iron deficiency and iron supplementation appear to be associated with detrimental changes in the microbiome. Iron is an essential nutrient for both beneficial commensal bacteria and harmful enteropathogens. As a result, changes in the availability of iron can lead to significant shifts in the composition of the microbiome that can create favorable conditions for pathogenic strains [25]. This may explain why an iron fortification trial in Ghana resulted in increased hospitalizations and another in Pakistan resulted in an increase in diarrheal prevalence [134]. However, while studies in animal and in vitro models support this pathway, iron fortification has not consistently led to increased diarrheal disease or enteric infections across human trials [25, 134]. As such, it is possible that this pathway is only dominant where people live without improved water, sanitation, and hygiene and/or where gut microbiota already include opportunistic pathogens [25].

The microbiome also plays a significant role as an intermediary between host nutritional status and inflammatory response. For example, anaerobic fermentation of dietary fiber by commensal bacteria produces short-chain fatty acids such as butyrate and propionic acid, which, among other immunosuppressive functions, counter inflammation in the gut [133]. Moreover, catabolism of tryptophan, an essential amino acid, by commensal bacteria produces ligands that drive aryl hydrocarbon receptor activation, which also plays a role in protection against intestinal inflammation [135]. Diets deficient in these specific nutrients may result in impairment of the inflammatory response.

## Impact of Malnutrition on Disease Progression, Resolution, and Recovery

We know that enteric infections generally progress in four phases: incubation, prodromal, invasion, and convalescence. Malnourished mice, when exposed to mouse rotavirus, became infected with a lower minimal dose, had a shorter incubation period, reached fecal viral shedding earlier, and experienced more severe disease [136]. Other studies also identified greater penetration of the virus into distant organs of malnourished mice [137]. In humans, no similar studies addressing intestinal infections have been found. However, length of hospital stay, measured as a proxy of disease severity, was longer in European children ages 1 month to 18 yrs. with moderate or severe malnutrition compared with well-nourished children [138]. These malnourished children were also more likely to experience diarrhea and vomiting when compared to their healthy counterparts [138]. Convalescence was also slower, and life-threatening events (LTEs) including deaths, severe pneumonia, severe diarrhea, were more frequent in Kenyan children with severe acute malnutrition (SAM) who were followed for 12 mo for LTEs after being stabilized and discharged from hospitals. Those who did not respond well to the treatment had a higher risk of post-discharge life-threatening events when compared to those who responded well in terms of anthropometric measurements [139]. Figure 8.6 shows the impact of severe acute malnutrition (SAM) following treatment among Kenyan children hospitalized for SAM even after treatment for enteric infections. While the number of children with WHZ < -3 decreases at each time point, children who continue to have low WHZ have significantly shorter survival times without LTEs even 6–12 months after hospital discharge [139]. An in-patient rehabilitation study of Bolivian children with severe malnutrition found that anthropometric indicators recovered in 4–5 weeks, although recovery from immune system damage took 8–9 weeks [140].

Deficiencies of particular nutrients can also contribute to intensified progression of diarrheal disease and delayed resolution and recovery. Studies in animals and humans have demonstrated that vitamin A deficiency is associated with decreased villous surface area and increased intestinal permeability leading to more severe intestinal injury during enteric infections [141]. This may explain why Colombian children with vitamin A deficiencies had an increased risk of diarrhea with vomiting and

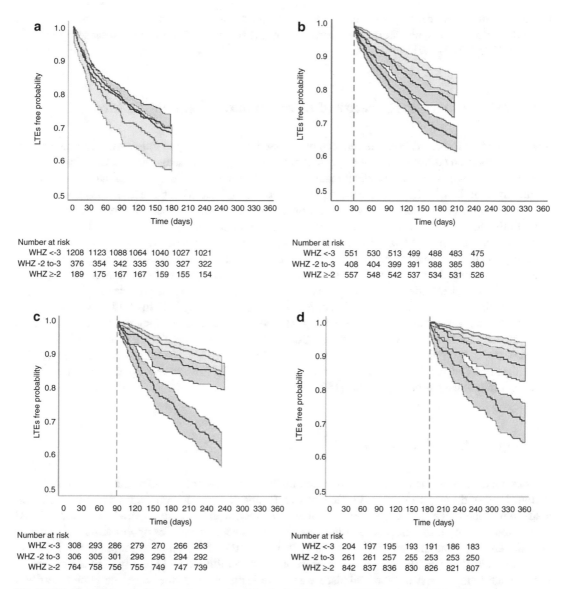

**Fig. 8.6** Kaplan-Meier graphs of the impact of weight-for-height z score (WHZ) on probabilities of remaining free of life-threatening events (LTE) (death, severe pneumonia, and diarrhea) among 1778 HIV-uninfected Kenyan children ages 2–59 mos who were treated for severe acute malnutrition (SAM) at study entry. Figures show the risk of LTEs based on WHZ for 6 months following four different time points: study enrollment (0–180 days) (A), month 1 (30–210 days) (B), month 3 (90–270 days) (C), and month 6 (180–360 days) (D). WHZ with 95%: <−3 (red); −2 to −3 (blue), and ≥ −2 (green). Numbers at risk represent the number of children in the specified WHZ range at each of the indicated time points. Reprinted from Ngari et al. [139]; Creative Commons CC-BY License

why vitamin-A supplemented Ghanaian children had fewer clinic visits and hospital admissions for diarrhea even though the actual rate of diarrheal incidence had not decreased [23, 142, 143]. However, the role of vitamin A in disease progression and resolution appears to be pathogen specific. Long and colleagues found that vitamin A supplemented children had prolonged EPEC infections but faster resolution of infections by ETEC and *G. lamblia*, a difference that is likely mediated by whether the pathogen is cleared via pro- or non-inflammatory immune responses [144]. On the other hand, studies have consistently found that zinc supplementation slows disease progression and improves resolution including reduced incidence, duration (by 12–24 hrs), fluid loss, and recurrence of diarrheal episodes, as well as reduced hospitalization and mortality rates associated with diarrheal disease by an estimated 23% [52, 145–147].

## Malnutrition Increases Severity of Infection and Treatment Failure

Severity of infection or treatment failure can be assessed using a variety of indicators, including severity of symptoms and development of complications. The Integrated Management of Childhood Illness (IMCI) danger signs is one such indicator, and malnourished children exhibit IMCI danger signs more frequently than their healthy counterparts [35]. Penetration of gut microbes across the gut is another indicator, suggesting greater severity of infection or greater risk of treatment failure. Deeper penetration of infectious agents has long been reported in animal models of enteric infections. In the study of malnourished mice infected with murine rotavirus discussed previously, the malnourished mice also had a higher susceptibility to hepatitis caused by the rotavirus, more frequently reaching the liver than in the well-nourished mice [137]. Studies in a humanized pig model show that malnourished pigs with human microbiota experienced a more severe rotavirus infection when compared with the well-nourished pigs [148]. Similarly, detection of *E. coli* in blood is more likely in children with malnutrition, suggesting deeper invasion of gut pathogens [149]. As far as development of complications is concerned, intestinal perforation and enteric septicemia with *Salmonella*, *Shigella*, and *Staphylococcus aureus* are seen more frequently in malnourished children [150, 151]. Kwashiorkor increased the risk of death in hospitalized Botswanan children, another indicator of greater severity of infection although treatment failure cannot be discounted [152].

## Cycling Back to Malnutrition

As mentioned earlier, the relationship between malnutrition and enteric infection is cyclical, where malnutrition and enteric infection create positive feedback loops within themselves. Malnutrition leads to morphological changes in the gastrointestinal tract, with increased permeability and reduced absorption capacity [50]. The resulting increased stool frequency increases opportunities to contaminate the environment and food which, in turn, increases risk of exposure to more enteric infection [153]. Malnutrition can drive increased exposure and susceptibility to and severity of infection, which in turn leads to higher risk of diarrheal disease and enteric infection, further perpetuating malnutrition [10]. Not only do these infections directly affect the integrity and absorptive capacity of the gastrointestinal barrier, but also diarrhea causes nutrients to transit through the gut more rapidly, reducing availability for absorption, thereby contributing to malabsorption [101].

Diarrheal disease pathogens cause malnutrition in different ways. Some, like *Vibrio* spp. or rotavirus, predominantly cause malnutrition through a net loss of nutrients from the body. Others, such as *E. histolytica* and *Giardia*, also deprive the host of nutrients because of intestinal damage that impairs absorption [154–157]. Malnutrition is also a result of the increased nutrient need for immune response and tissue repair that can ultimately lead to a negative nitrogen balance [158].

Infrequent mild to moderate episodes of enteric infection, even in an undernourished child, do not have lasting impacts as long as there is enough time for catchup growth. In contrast, the moderate or severe malnutrition caused by repeated or prolonged episodes of diarrhea that are frequently caused by enteric infections has cumulative effects that are long-lasting even for a well-nourished child [10, 159, 160]. Repeated infections are not an uncommon occurrence in lower resource settings, particularly areas with limited access to safe water, sanitation, and hygiene facilities. Each infectious episode leads to a period of sub-optimal nutrition that can lead to a vicious cycle of malnutrition and infection [71].

The immune system, when triggered by enteric (and other) infections, consumes more energy and causes anorexia in ways that impact both cognition and body composition. Reduced supply and increased demand of energy contribute to inability to mount an adequate immune response against infections thereby perpetuating the cycle of malnutrition (see Fig. 8.3).

## Closing Thoughts

Although we have come a long way in deciphering the interactions between malnutrition and enteric infections, much remains to be learned. Advances in our understanding of the broader malnutrition-infection interaction will undoubtedly shed light on some of what happens in the gut but may be insufficient to fully explain interactions that are driven largely by the gut microbiota, by mucosal barrier function, and by adhesion and invasion of gut pathogens.

Given the complex network of both modifiable and non-modifiable factors that influence gut health, nutritional status, and exposure and response to diarrheal pathogens, it is not surprising that inconsistencies emerge among studies. The challenge is to recognize where specific interventions can reliably be expected to reduce malnutrition and diarrheal disease and to identify the contexts under which their use is recommended. As the malnutrition-diarrhea cycle occurs more frequently in limited resource settings where low-cost interventions are needed, identification of appropriate, and possibly novel, interventions requires a more nuanced understanding of the complex interactions between various gut infections and malnutrition, so that interventions can be tailored to a given environment.

While at the individual level, malnutrition and diarrheal disease cause morbidity, mortality, and reduced productivity, at the large scale, they contribute to poverty and lack of equal access to opportunities resulting in friction between various sections of a society that can lead to political instability. In turn, political instability adversely affects nutrition. Thus malnutrition and diarrheal diseases cycle from the individual level to the local, regional, and national levels and then back to the individuals. Research on this topic is not merely an academic question but carries serious economic, political, and ethical implications [161]. Given the contribution of malnutrition and infection generally, and diarrheal disease more specifically, to the global burden of diseases, both research and interventions should be a global priority and funded commensurately.

## References

1. WHO. Diarrhoeal disease 2017. Available from: https://www.who.int/news-room/fact-sheets/detail/diarrhoeal-disease.
2. Berkley JA. Bacterial infections and nutrition - a primer. In: Humphries DL, Scott ME, Vermund SH, editors. Nutrition and infectious disease: shifting the clinical paradigm: Humana Press; 2020.
3. Green WD, Karlsson EA, Beck MA. Viral infections and nutrition: influenza virus as a case study. In: Humphries DL, Scott ME, Vermund SH, editors. Nutrition and infectious disease: shifting the clinical paradigm: Humana Press; 2020.
4. Wiser MF. Nutrition and protozoan pathogens of humans -- a primer. In: Humphries DL, Scott ME, Vermund SH, editors. Nutrition and infectious diseases: shifting the clinical Paradigm2020.
5. Geary TG, Haque M. Human helminth infections. In: Humphries DL, Scott ME, Vermund SH, editors. Nutrition and infectious disease: shifting the clinical paradigm: Humana Press; 2020.

6. Defeat DD. Diarrhea and enteric illnesses 2017. Available from: https://www.defeatdd.org/article/diarrhea-and-enteric-illnesses.
7. Emory Institute of Drug Development. What is Diarrheal Diseases 2019. Available from: http://www.global-healthprimer.emory.edu/diseases/diarrheal-diseases.html.
8. Institute for Health Metrics and Evaluation. Findings from the Global Burden of Disease Study 2017. Seattle: IHME, 2018.
9. Collaborators GBDDD. Estimates of global, regional, and national morbidity, mortality, and aetiologies of diarrhoeal diseases: a systematic analysis for the global burden of disease study 2015. Lancet Infect Dis. 2017;17(9):909–48.
10. Checkley W, Buckley G, Gilman RH, Assis AM, Guerrant RL, Morris SS, et al. Multi-country analysis of the effects of diarrhoea on childhood stunting. Int J Epidemiol. 2008;37(4):816–30.
11. Global burden of disease collaborative network. Global burden of disease study 2017 (GBD 2017) results. In: Institute for Health Metrics and Evaluation (IHME). Seattle; 2018.
12. Liu J, Platts-Mills JA, Juma J, Kabir F, Nkeze J, Okoi C, et al. Use of quantitative molecular diagnostic methods to identify causes of diarrhoea in children: a reanalysis of the GEMS case-control study. Lancet. 2016;388(10051):1291–301.
13. Walker CLF, Rudan I, Liu L, Nair H, Theodoratou E, Bhutta ZA, et al. Global burden of childhood pneumonia and diarrhoea. Lancet. 2013;381(9875):1405–16.
14. Glass RI, Guttmacher AE, Black RE. Ending preventable child death in a generation. JAMA. 2012;308(2):141–2.
15. Rudan I, El Arifeen S, Black RE, Campbell H. Childhood pneumonia and diarrhoea: setting our priorities right. Lancet Infect Dis. 2007;7(1):56–61.
16. Ganguly E, Sharma PK, Bunker CH. Prevalence and risk factors of diarrhea morbidity among under-five children in India: a systematic review and meta-analysis. Indian J Child Health (Bhopal). 2015;2(4):152–60.
17. Rice AL, Sacco L, Hyder A, Black RE. Malnutrition as an underlying cause of childhood deaths associated with infectious diseases in developing countries. Bull World Health Organ. 2000;78(10):1207–21.
18. Initiatives D. Global nutrition report: shining a light to spur action on nutrition. Bristoal; 2018. p. 2018.
19. Stephensen CB. Primer on immune response and Interface with malnutrition. In: Humphries DL, Scott ME, Vermund SH, editors. Nutrition and infectious disease: shifting the clinical paradigm: Humana Press; 2020.
20. DALYs GBD, Collaborators H. Global, regional, and national disability-adjusted life-years (DALYs) for 359 diseases and injuries and healthy life expectancy (HALE) for 195 countries and territories, 1990–2017: a systematic analysis for the Global Burden of Disease Study 2017. Lancet. 2018;392(10159):1859–922.
21. WHO. Global Health Risks: Mortality and burden of disease attributable to selected major risks. Geneva, Switzerland: WHO, 2009 Contract No.: ISBN 978 92 4 156387 1.
22. Barffour MA, Humphries DL. Core principles: infectious disease risk in relation to macro and micronutrient status. In: Humphries DL, Scott ME, Vermund SH, editors. Nutrition and infectious disease: shifting the clinical paradigm: Humana Press; 2020.
23. Brown KH. Diarrhea and malnutrition. J Nutr. 2003;133(1):328S–32S.
24. Bailey RL, West KP Jr, Black RE. The epidemiology of global micronutrient deficiencies. Ann Nutr Metab. 2015;66(Suppl 2):22–33.
25. Paganini D, Uyoga MA, Zimmermann MB. Iron fortification of foods for infants and children in low-income countries: effects on the gut microbiome, gut inflammation, and diarrhea. Nutrients. 2016;8(8):494.
26. Imdad A, Mayo-Wilson E, Herzer K, Bhutta ZA. Vitamin a supplementation for preventing morbidity and mortality in children from six months to five years of age. Cochrane Database Syst Rev. 2017;3(3):CD008524.
27. Levy A, Fraser D, Rosen SD, Dagan R, Deckelbaum RJ, Coles C, et al. Anemia as a risk factor for infectious diseases in infants and toddlers: results from a prospective study. Eur J Epidemiol. 2005;20(3):277–84.
28. Rytter MJ, Kolte L, Briend A, Friis H, Christensen VB. The immune system in children with malnutrition--a systematic review. PLoS One. 2014;9(8):e105017.
29. Schneider SM, Hebuterne X. Is malnutrition a risk factor for nosocomial infections? Rev Med Interne. 2006;27(7):515–8.
30. Woerther PL, Angebault C, Jacquier H, Hugede HC, Janssens AC, Sayadi S, et al. Massive increase, spread, and exchange of extended spectrum beta-lactamase-encoding genes among intestinal Enterobacteriaceae in hospitalized children with severe acute malnutrition in Niger. Clin Infect Dis. 2011;53(7):677–85.
31. Manary MJ. Local production and provision of ready-to-use therapeutic food for the treatment of severe childhood malnutrition. 2005.
32. World Health O. Complementary feeding: family foods for breastfed children. 2000.
33. Boatbil C, Guure C, Ayoung A. Impact of belief systems on the management of child malnutrition: the case of talensis of northern ghana 2014.
34. Verkerke H, Sobuz S, Ma JZ, Petri SE, Reichman D, Qadri F, et al. Malnutrition is associated with protection from rotavirus diarrhea: evidence from a longitudinal birth cohort study in Bangladesh. J Clin Microbiol. 2016;54(10):2568–74.

35. Tickell KD, Pavlinac PB, John-Stewart GC, Denno DM, Richardson BA, Naulikha JM, et al. Impact of childhood nutritional status on pathogen prevalence and severity of acute diarrhea. Am J Trop Med Hyg. 2017;97(5):1337–44.

36. Ezenwa VO. Co-infection and nutrition: integrating ecological and epidemiological perspectives. In: Humphries DL, Scott ME, Vermund SH, editors. Nutrition and infectious disease: shifting the clinical paradigm: Springer; 2020.

37. Murray MJ, Murray A, Murray CJ. The salutary effect of milk on amoebiasis and its reversal by iron. Br Med J. 1980;280(6228):1351–2.

38. Lee J, Park SJ, Yong TS. Effect of iron on adherence and cytotoxicity of Entamoeba histolytica to CHO cell mono-layers. Korean J Parasitol. 2008;46(1):37–40.

39. Bourke CD, Berkley JA, Prendergast AJ. Immune dysfunction as a cause and consequence of malnutrition. Trends Immunol. 2016;37(6):386–98.

40. Turner JR. Intestinal mucosal barrier function in health and disease. Nat Rev Immunol. 2009;9(11):799–809.

41. Murch S. Gastrointestinal Mucosal Immunology and Mechanisms of Inflammation. In: Wyllie Robert, Jeffery S. Hyams, Kay M, editors. Pediatric gastrointestinal and liver disease. 4th ed: Saint Louis: W.B. Saunders; 2011. p. 50.

42. Genton L, Cani PD, Schrenzel J. Alterations of gut barrier and gut microbiota in food restriction, food deprivation and protein-energy wasting. Clin Nutr. 2015;34(3):341–9.

43. Omoike I, Lindquist B, Abud R, Merrick J, Lebenthal E. The effect of protein-energy malnutrition and refeeding on the adherence of Salmonella typhimurium to small intestinal mucosa and isolated enterocytes in rats. J Nutr. 1990;120(4):404–11.

44. Bansal D, Ave P, Kerneis S, Frileux P, Boche O, Baglin AC, et al. An ex-vivo human intestinal model to study Entamoeba histolytica pathogenesis. PLoS Negl Trop Dis. 2009;3(11):e551.

45. Cornick S, Tawiah A, Chadee K. Roles and regulation of the mucus barrier in the gut. Tissue Barriers. 2015;3(1–2):e982426.

46. Mondal D, Minak J, Alam M, Liu Y, Dai J, Korpe P, et al. Contribution of enteric infection, altered intestinal bar-rier function, and maternal malnutrition to infant malnutrition in Bangladesh. Clin Infect Dis. 2012;54(2):185–92.

47. Campbell DI, Elia M, Lunn PG. Growth faltering in rural Gambian infants is associated with impaired small intes-tinal barrier function, leading to endotoxemia and systemic inflammation. J Nutr. 2003;133(5):1332–8.

48. Rho S, Kim H, Shim SH, Lee SY, Kim MJ, Yang BG, et al. Protein energy malnutrition alters mucosal IgA responses and reduces mucosal vaccine efficacy in mice. Immunol Lett. 2017;190:247–56.

49. Martens EC, Neumann M, Desai MS. Interactions of commensal and pathogenic microorganisms with the intesti-nal mucosal barrier. Nat Rev Microbiol. 2018;16(8):457–70.

50. Rodriguez L, Cervantes E, Ortiz R. Malnutrition and gastrointestinal and respiratory infections in children: a pub-lic health problem. Int J Environ Res Public Health. 2011;8(4):1174–205.

51. Ibrahim MK, Zambruni M, Melby CL, Melby PC. Impact of childhood malnutrition on host defense and infection. Clin Microbiol Rev. 2017;30(4):919–71.

52. Semba RD. The role of vitamin A and related retinoids in immune function. 1998.

53. Maciel AA, Oria RB, Braga-Neto MB, Braga AB, Carvalho EB, Lucena HB, et al. Role of retinol in protecting epithelial cell damage induced by Clostridium difficile toxin a. Toxicon. 2007;50(8):1027–40.

54. Lazzerini M, Wanzira H. Oral zinc for treating diarrhoea in children. Cochrane Database Syst Rev. 2016;(12, 12):CD005436.

55. Tuerk MJ, Fazel N. Zinc deficiency. Curr Opin Gastroenterol. 2009;25(2):136–43.

56. Podany AB, Wright J, Lamendella R, Soybel DI, Kelleher SL. ZnT2-mediated zinc import into Paneth cell gran-ules is necessary for coordinated secretion and Paneth cell function in mice. Cell Mol Gastroenterol Hepatol. 2016;2(3):369–83.

57. Hughes S, Kelly P. Interactions of malnutrition and immune impairment, with specific reference to immunity against parasites. Parasite Immunol. 2006;28(11):577–88.

58. Castro IC, Oliveira BB, Slowikowski JJ, Coutinho BP, Siqueira FJ, Costa LB, et al. Arginine decreases Cryptosporidium parvum infection in undernourished suckling mice involving nitric oxide synthase and arginase. Nutrition. 2012;28(6):678–85.

59. Lima NL, Soares AM, Mota RM, Monteiro HS, Guerrant RL, Lima AA. Wasting and intestinal barrier function in children taking alanyl-glutamine-supplemented enteral formula. J Pediatr Gastroenterol Nutr. 2007;44(3):365–74.

60. Denno DM, Tarr PI, Nataro JP. Environmental enteric dysfunction: a case definition for intervention trials. Am J Trop Med Hyg. 2017;97(6):1643–6.

61. Keusch GT, Denno DM, Black RE, Duggan C, Guerrant RL, Lavery JV, et al. Environmental enteric dysfunction: pathogenesis, diagnosis, and clinical consequences. Clin Infect Dis. 2014;59(Suppl 4):S207–12.

62. Bartelt LA, Bolick DT, Guerrant RL. Disentangling microbial mediators of malnutrition: modeling environmental enteric dysfunction. Cell Mol Gastroenterol Hepatol. 2019;7(3):692–707.

63. Crane RJ, Jones KD, Berkley JA. Environmental enteric dysfunction: an overview. Food Nutr Bull. 2015;36(1 Suppl):S76–87.

64. Goto R, Panter-Brick C, Northrop-Clewes CA, Manahdhar R, Tuladhar NR. Poor intestinal permeability in mildly stunted Nepali children: associations with weaning practices and Giardia lamblia infection. Br J Nutr. 2002;88(2):141–9.
65. Weisz AJ, Manary MJ, Stephenson K, Agapova S, Manary FG, Thakwalakwa C, et al. Abnormal gut integrity is associated with reduced linear growth in rural Malawian children. J Pediatr Gastroenterol Nutr. 2012;55(6):747–50.
66. Ballinger A, El-Haj T, Perrett D, Turvill J, Obeid O, Dryden S, et al. The role of medial hypothalamic serotonin in the suppression of feeding in a rat model of colitis. Gastroenterology. 2000;118(3):544–53.
67. Garcia SE, Kaiser LL, Dewey KG. Self-regulation of food intake among rural Mexican preschool children. Eur J Clin Nutr. 1990;44(5):371–80.
68. Prendergast AJ, Rukobo S, Chasekwa B, Mutasa K, Ntozini R, Mbuya MN, et al. Stunting is characterized by chronic inflammation in Zimbabwean infants. PLoS One. 2014;9(2):e86928.
69. Kosek M, Haque R, Lima A, Babji S, Shrestha S, Qureshi S, et al. Fecal markers of intestinal inflammation and permeability associated with the subsequent acquisition of linear growth deficits in infants. Am J Trop Med Hyg. 2013;88(2):390–6.
70. Korpe PS, Petri WA Jr. Environmental enteropathy: critical implications of a poorly understood condition. Trends Mol Med. 2012;18(6):328–36.
71. Guerrant RL, Oria RB, Moore SR, Oria MO, Lima AA. Malnutrition as an enteric infectious disease with long-term effects on child development. Nutr Rev. 2008;66(9):487–505.
72. Patriarca PA, Wright PF, John TJ. Factors affecting the immunogenicity of oral poliovirus vaccine in developing countries: review. Rev Infect Dis. 1991;13(5):926–39.
73. Soares-Weiser K, Maclehose H, Bergman H, Ben-Aharon I, Nagpal S, Goldberg E, et al. Vaccines for preventing rotavirus diarrhoea: vaccines in use. Cochrane Database Syst Rev. 2012;11:CD008521.
74. Murphy K, Travers P, Walport M, Janeway C. Janeway's immunobiology. New York: Garland Science; 2008.
75. Bhutta ZA, Das JK, Walker N, Rizvi A, Campbell H, Rudan I, et al. Interventions to address deaths from childhood pneumonia and diarrhoea equitably: what works and at what cost? Lancet. 2013;381(9875):1417–29.
76. Gilman RH, Partanen R, Brown KH, Spira WM, Khanam S, Greenberg B, et al. Decreased gastric acid secretion and bacterial colonization of the stomach in severely malnourished Bangladeshi children. Gastroenterology. 1988;94(6):1308–14.
77. Shashidhar S, Shah SB, Acharya PT. Gastric acid, pH and pepsin in healthy and protein calorie malnourished children. Indian J Pediatr. 1976;43(341):145–51.
78. Adesola AO. The influence of severe protein deficiency (kwashiorkor) on gastric acid secretion in Nigerian children. Br J Surg. 1968;55(11):866.
79. Maffei H, Nobrega F. Gastric pH and microflora of normal and diarrhoeic infants. Gut. 1975;16(9):719–26.
80. Peters-Golden M, Canetti C, Mancuso P, Coffey MJ. Leukotrienes: underappreciated mediators of innate immune responses. J Immunol. 2005;174(2):589–94.
81. Jahoor F, Badaloo A, Reid M, Forrester T. Protein metabolism in severe childhood malnutrition. Ann Trop Paediatr. 2008;28(2):87–101.
82. Haller L, Zubler RH, Lambert PH. Plasma levels of complement components and complement haemolytic activity in protein-energy malnutrition. Clin Exp Immunol. 1978;34(2):248–52.
83. Haque R, Mondal D, Shu J, Roy S, Kabir M, Davis AN, et al. Correlation of interferon-gamma production by peripheral blood mononuclear cells with childhood malnutrition and susceptibility to amebiasis. Am J Trop Med Hyg. 2007;76(2):340–4.
84. Hamano S, Asgharpour A, Stroup SE, Wynn TA, Leiter EH, Houpt E. Resistance of C57BL/6 mice to amoebiasis is mediated by nonhemopoietic cells but requires hemopoietic IL-10 production. J Immunol. 2006;177(2):1208–13.
85. Schonland M. Depression of immunity in protein-calorie malnutrition: a post-mortem study. J Trop Pediatr Environ Child Health. 1972;18(3):217–24.
86. Pretorius PJ, De Villiers LS. Antibody response in children with protein malnutrition. Am J Clin Nutr. 1962;10:379–83.
87. Salimonu LS, Johnson AO, Williams AI, Adeleye GI, Osunkoya BO. Lymphocyte subpopulations and antibody levels in immunized malnourished children. Br J Nutr. 1982;48(1):7–14.
88. Awdeh ZL, Kanawati AK, Alami SY. Antibody response in marasmic children during recovery. Acta Paediatr Scand. 1977;66(6):689–92.
89. el-Gamal Y, Aly RH, Hossny E, Afify E, el-Taliawy D. Response of Egyptian infants with protein calorie malnutrition to hepatitis B vaccination. J Trop Pediatr. 1996;42(3):144–5.
90. Hafez M, Aref GH, Mehareb SW, Kassem AS, El-Tahhan H, Rizk Z, et al. Antibody production and complement system in protein energy malnutrition. J Trop Med Hyg. 1977;80(2):36–9.
91. Powell GM. Response to live attenuated measles vaccine in children with severe kwashiorkor. Ann Trop Paediatr. 1982;2(3):143–5.
92. Brown RE, Katz M. Failure of antibody production to yellow fever vaccine in children with kwashiorkor. Trop Geogr Med. 1966;18(2):125–8.

93. Brown RE, Katz M. Antigenic stimulation in undernourished children. East Afr Med J. 1965;42:221–32.
94. Wesley A, Coovadia HM, Watson AR. Immunization against measles in children at risk for severe disease. Trans R Soc Trop Med Hyg. 1979;73(6):710–5.
95. Idris S, El Seed AM. Measles vaccination in severely malnourished Sudanese children. Ann Trop Paediatr. 1983;3(2):63–7.
96. Suskind R, Sirishinha S, Vithayasai V, Edelman R, Damrongsak D, Charupatana C, et al. Immunoglobulins and antibody response in children with protein-calorie malnutrition. Am J Clin Nutr. 1976;29(8):836–41.
97. el-Molla A, el-Ghoroury A, Hussein M, Badr-el-Din MK, Hassen AH, Aref GH, et al. Antibody production in protein calorie malnutrition. J Trop Med Hyg. 1973;76(9):248–50.
98. Taylor PE, Tejada C, Sanchez M. The effect of malnutrition on the inflammatory response as exhibited by the granuloma pouch of the rat. J Exp Med. 1967;126(4):539–56.
99. Zijlstra RT, McCracken BA, Odle J, Donovan SM, Gelberg HB, Petschow BW, et al. Malnutrition modifies pig small intestinal inflammatory responses to rotavirus. J Nutr. 1999;129(4):838–43.
100. Baek O, Fabiansen C, Friis H, Ritz C, Koch J, Willesen JL, et al. Malnutrition predisposes to endotoxin-induced edema and impaired inflammatory response in parenterally fed piglets. JPEN J Parenter Enteral Nutr. 2019;
101. Wapnir RA. Zinc deficiency, malnutrition and the gastrointestinal tract. J Nutr. 2000;130.(5S Suppl:1388S–92S.
102. Bolick DT, Kolling GL, Moore JH 2nd, de Oliveira LA, Tung K, Philipson C, et al. Zinc deficiency alters host response and pathogen virulence in a mouse model of enteroaggregative Escherichia coli-induced diarrhea. Gut Microbes. 2014;5(5):618–27.
103. Ooi JH, Chen J, Cantorna MT. Vitamin D regulation of immune function in the gut: why do T cells have vitamin D receptors? Mol Asp Med. 2012;33(1):77–82.
104. Bibbo S, Ianiro G, Giorgio V, Scaldaferri F, Masucci L, Gasbarrini A, et al. The role of diet on gut microbiota composition. Eur Rev Med Pharmacol Sci. 2016;20(22):4742–9.
105. Reimer RA. Establishing the role of diet in the microbiota-disease axis. Nat Rev Gastroenterol Hepatol. 2019;16(2):86–7.
106. Jain N, Walker WA. Diet and host-microbial crosstalk in postnatal intestinal immune homeostasis. Nat Rev Gastroenterol Hepatol. 2015;12(1):14–25.
107. Blanton LV, Charbonneau MR, Salih T, Barratt MJ, Venkatesh S, Ilkaveya O, et al. Gut bacteria that prevent growth impairments transmitted by microbiota from malnourished children. Science. 2016;351(6275)
108. Raman AS, Gehrig JL, Venkatesh S, Chang HW, Hibberd MC, Subramanian S, et al. A sparse covarying unit that describes healthy and impaired human gut microbiota development. Science. 2019;365(6449)
109. Favier CF, Vaughan EE, De Vos WM, Akkermans AD. Molecular monitoring of succession of bacterial communities in human neonates. Appl Environ Microbiol. 2002;68(1):219–26.
110. Kolida S, Tuohy K, Gibson GR. Prebiotic effects of inulin and oligofructose. Br J Nutr. 2002;87(Suppl 2):S193–7.
111. Hurley BW, Nguyen CC. The spectrum of pseudomembranous enterocolitis and antibiotic-associated diarrhea. Arch Intern Med. 2002;162(19):2177–84.
112. Sullivan A, Edlund C, Nord CE. Effect of antimicrobial agents on the ecological balance of human microflora. Lancet Infect Dis. 2001;1(2):101–14.
113. Lizko NN. Problems of microbial ecology in man space Mission. Acta Astronaut. 1991;23:163–9.
114. Alverdy JC, Laughlin RS, Wu L. Influence of the critically ill state on host-pathogen interactions within the intestine: gut-derived sepsis redefined. Crit Care Med. 2003;31(2):598–607.
115. WHO. Updates on the management of severe acute malnutrition in infants and children. Guideline: Updates on the Management of Severe Acute Malnutrition in Infants and Children. WHO Guidelines Approved by the Guidelines Review Committee. Geneva 2013.
116. Maier L, Pruteanu M, Kuhn M, Zeller G, Telzerow A, Anderson EE, et al. Extensive impact of non-antibiotic drugs on human gut bacteria. Nature. 2018;555(7698):623–8.
117. Gibson MK, Crofts TS, Dantas G. Antibiotics and the developing infant gut microbiota and resistome. Curr Opin Microbiol. 2015;27:51–6.
118. Silverman MA, Konnikova L, Gerber JS. Impact of antibiotics on necrotizing Enterocolitis and antibiotic-associated diarrhea. Gastroenterol Clin N Am. 2017;46(1):61–76.
119. Nogueira T, David PHC, Pothier J. Antibiotics as both friends and foes of the human gut microbiome: the microbial community approach. Drug Dev Res. 2019;80(1):86–97.
120. Guo Q, Goldenberg JZ, Humphrey C, El Dib R, Johnston BC. Probiotics for the prevention of pediatric antibiotic-associated diarrhea. Cochrane Database Syst Rev. 2019;4:CD004827.
121. Gehrig JL, Venkatesh S, Chang HW, Hibberd MC, Kung VL, Cheng J, et al. Effects of microbiota-directed foods in gnotobiotic animals and undernourished children. Science. 2019;365(6449)
122. Lutgendorff F, Akkermans LM, Soderholm JD. The role of microbiota and probiotics in stress-induced gastrointestinal damage. Curr Mol Med. 2008;8(4):282–98.
123. Gupta SS, Mohammed MH, Ghosh TS, Kanungo S, Nair GB, Mande SS. Metagenome of the gut of a malnourished child. Gut Pathog. 2011;3:7.

124. Monira S, Nakamura S, Gotoh K, Izutsu K, Watanabe H, Alam NH, et al. Gut microbiota of healthy and malnourished children in Bangladesh. Front Microbiol. 2011;2:228.
125. Subramanian S, Huq S, Yatsunenko T, Haque R, Mahfuz M, Alam MA, et al. Persistent gut microbiota immaturity in malnourished Bangladeshi children. Nature. 2014;510(7505):417–21.
126. Smith MI, Yatsunenko T, Manary MJ, Trehan I, Mkakosya R, Cheng J, et al. Gut microbiomes of Malawian twin pairs discordant for kwashiorkor. Science. 2013;339(6119):548–54.
127. Lanata CF, Fischer-Walker CL, Olascoaga AC, Torres CX, Aryee MJ, Black RE, et al. Global causes of diarrheal disease mortality in children <5 years of age: a systematic review. PLoS One. 2013;8(9):e72788.
128. Gracey M, Stone DE, Suharjono S. Isolation of Candida species from the gastrointestinal tract in malnourished children. Am J Clin Nutr. 1974;27(4):345–9.
129. Kotloff KL, Nataro JP, Blackwelder WC, Nasrin D, Farag TH, Panchalingam S, et al. Burden and aetiology of diarrhoeal disease in infants and young children in developing countries (the global enteric multicenter study, GEMS): a prospective, case-control study. Lancet. 2013;382(9888):209–22.
130. Rogawski ET, Liu J, Platts-Mills JA, Kabir F, Lertsethtakarn P, Siguas M, et al. Use of quantitative molecular diagnostic methods to investigate the effect of enteropathogen infections on linear growth in children in low-resource settings: longitudinal analysis of results from the MAL-ED cohort study. Lancet Glob Health. 2018;6(12):e1319–e28.
131. M-EN I. Relationship between growth and illness, enteropathogens and dietary intakes in the first 2 years of life: findings from the MAL-ED birth cohort study. BMJ Glob Health. 2017;2(4):e000370.
132. Lv Z, Wang Y, Yang T, Zhan X, Li Z, Hu H, et al. Vitamin a deficiency impacts the structural segregation of gut microbiota in children with persistent diarrhea. J Clin Biochem Nutr. 2016;59(2):113–21.
133. Blander JM, Longman RS, Iliev ID, Sonnenberg GF, Artis D. Regulation of inflammation by microbiota interactions with the host. Nat Immunol. 2017;18(8):851–60.
134. Jaeggi T, Kortman GA, Moretti D, Chassard C, Holding P, Dostal A, et al. Iron fortification adversely affects the gut microbiome, increases pathogen abundance and induces intestinal inflammation in Kenyan infants. Gut. 2015;64(5):731–42.
135. Marinelli L, Martin-Gallausiaux C, Bourhis JM, Beguet-Crespel F, Blottiere HM, Lapaque N. Identification of the novel role of butyrate as AhR ligand in human intestinal epithelial cells. Sci Rep. 2019;9(1):643.
136. Offor E, Riepenhoff-Talty M, Ogra PL. Effect of malnutrition on rotavirus infection in suckling mice: kinetics of early infection. Proc Soc Exp Biol Med. 1985;178(1):85–90.
137. Riepenhoff-Talty M, Uhnoo I, Chegas P, Ogra PL. Effect of nutritional deprivation on mucosal viral infections. Immunol Investig. 1989;18(1–4):127–39.
138. Hecht C, Weber M, Grote V, Daskalou E, Dell'Era L, Flynn D, et al. Disease associated malnutrition correlates with length of hospital stay in children. Clin Nutr. 2015;34(1):53–9.
139. Ngari MM, Mwalekwa L, Timbwa M, Hamid F, Ali R, Iversen PO, et al. Changes in susceptibility to life-threatening infections after treatment for complicated severe malnutrition in Kenya. Am J Clin Nutr. 2018;107(4):626–34.
140. Chevalier P, Sevilla R, Sejas E, Zalles L, Belmonte G, Parent G. Immune recovery of malnourished children takes longer than nutritional recovery: implications for treatment and discharge. J Trop Pediatr. 1998;44(5):304–7.
141. De Santis S, Cavalcanti E, Mastronardi M, Jirillo E, Chieppa M. Nutritional keys for intestinal barrier modulation. Front Immunol. 2015;6:612.
142. Countdown Coverage Writing G, Countdown to Core G, Bryce J, Daelmans B, Dwivedi A, Fauveau V, et al. Countdown to 2015 for maternal, newborn, and child survival: the 2008 report on tracking coverage of interventions. Lancet. 2008;371(9620):1247–58.
143. de Medeiros P, Pinto DV, de Almeida JZ, Rego JMC, Rodrigues FAP, Lima AAM, et al. Modulation of intestinal immune and barrier functions by vitamin a: implications for current understanding of malnutrition and enteric infections in children. Nutrients. 2018;10(9)
144. Long KZ, Santos JI, Rosado JL, Estrada-Garcia T, Haas M, Al Mamun A, et al. Vitamin a supplementation modifies the association between mucosal innate and adaptive immune responses and resolution of enteric pathogen infections. Am J Clin Nutr. 2011;93(3):578–85.
145. Iannotti LL, Trehan I, Clitheroe KL, Manary MJ. Diagnosis and treatment of severely malnourished children with diarrhoea. J Paediatr Child Health. 2015;51(4):387–95.
146. Walker CL, Black RE. Zinc for the treatment of diarrhoea: effect on diarrhoea morbidity, mortality and incidence of future episodes. Int J Epidemiol. 2010.;39 Suppl 1(Supplement 1:i63–9.
147. Hoque KM, Sarker R, Guggino SE, Tse CM. A new insight into pathophysiological mechanisms of zinc in diarrhea. Ann N Y Acad Sci. 2009;1165:279–84.
148. Kumar A, Vlasova AN, Deblais L, Huang HC, Wijeratne A, Kandasamy S, et al. Impact of nutrition and rotavirus infection on the infant gut microbiota in a humanized pig model. BMC Gastroenterol. 2018;18(1):93.
149. Berkley JA, Lowe BS, Mwangi I, Williams T, Bauni E, Mwarumba S, et al. Bacteremia among children admitted to a rural hospital in Kenya. N Engl J Med. 2005;352(1):39–47.

150. Smythe PM. Changes in intestinal bacterial flora and role of infection in kwashiorkor. Lancet. 1958;2(7049):724–7.
151. Mogasale V, Desai SN, Mogasale VV, Park JK, Ochiai RL, Wierzba TF. Case fatality rate and length of hospital stay among patients with typhoid intestinal perforation in developing countries: a systematic literature review. PLoS One. 2014;9(4):e93784.
152. Creek TL, Kim A, Lu L, Bowen A, Masunge J, Arvelo W, et al. Hospitalization and mortality among primarily nonbreastfed children during a large outbreak of diarrhea and malnutrition in Botswana, 2006. J Acquir Immune Defic Syndr. 2010;53(1):14–9.
153. Motarjemi Y, Kaferstein F, Moy G, Quevedo F. Contaminated weaning food: a major risk factor for diarrhoea and associated malnutrition. Bull World Health Organ. 1993;71(1):79–92.
154. Schaible UE, Kaufmann SH. Malnutrition and infection: complex mechanisms and global impacts. PLoS Med. 2007;4(5):e115.
155. Petri WA Jr, Mondal D, Peterson KM, Duggal P, Haque R. Association of malnutrition with amebiasis. Nutr Rev. 2009;67(Suppl 2):S207–15.
156. Coles CL, Levy A, Dagan R, Deckelbaum RJ, Fraser D. Risk factors for the initial symptomatic giardia infection in a cohort of young Arab-Bedouin children. Ann Trop Paediatr. 2009;29(4):291–300.
157. Mondal D, Petri WA, Sack RB, Kirkpatrick BD, Haque R. Entamoeba histolytica-associated diarrheal illness is negatively associated with the growth of preschool children: evidence from a prospective study. T Roy Soc Trop Med H. 2006;100(11):1032–8.
158. Scrimshaw NS. Historical concepts of interactions, synergism and antagonism between nutrition and infection. J Nutr. 2003;133(1):316S–21S.
159. Moore SR, Lima NL, Soares AM, Oria RB, Pinkerton RC, Barrett LJ, et al. Prolonged episodes of acute diarrhea reduce growth and increase risk of persistent diarrhea in children. Gastroenterology. 2010;139(4):1156–64.
160. Richard SA, Black RE, Gilman RH, Guerrant RL, Kang G, Lanata CF, et al. Diarrhea in early childhood: short-term association with weight and long-term association with length. Am J Epidemiol. 2013;178(7):1129–38.
161. World Bank. Repositioning nutrition as central to development: a strategy for large-scale action. Washington, DC; 2006.
162. Guerrant RL, DeBoer MD, Moore SR, Scharf RJ, Lima AA. The impoverished gut--a triple burden of diarrhoea, stunting and chronic disease. Nat Rev Gastroenterol Hepatol. 2013;10(4):220–9.

# Chapter 9
# Nutrition in HIV and Tuberculosis

Marianna K. Baum, Javier A. Tamargo, and Christine Wanke

## Abbreviations

| | |
|---|---|
| ART | Antiretroviral therapy |
| ATT | Antituberculosis treatment |
| BIA | Bioelectrical impedance analysis |
| BMI | Body mass index |
| CDC | Centers for Disease Control and Prevention |
| CT | Computed tomography |
| DXA | Dual-energy X-ray absorptiometry |
| GI | Gastrointestinal |
| HAART | Highly active antiretroviral therapy |
| HCV | Hepatitis C virus |
| HIV | Human immunodeficiency virus |
| IDU | Injection drug use |
| IL | Interleukin |
| INSTIs | Integrase strand transfer inhibitors |
| MSM | Men who have/had sex with men |
| MUAC | Mid-upper arm circumference |
| NHANES | National Health and Nutrition Examination Survey |
| NRTIs | Nucleoside reverse-transcriptase inhibitors |
| PBMCs | Peripheral blood mononuclear cells |
| PIs | Protease inhibitors |
| PLWH | People living with HIV |
| RCT | Randomized controlled trial |
| REE | Resting energy expenditure |
| TB | Tuberculosis |
| TNF | Tumor necrosis factor |
| WHO | World Health Organization |

M. K. Baum (✉) · J. A. Tamargo
Florida International University, Miami, FL, USA
e-mail: baumm@fiu.edu; jtamargo@fiu.edu

C. Wanke
Professor Emeritus Tufts University School of Medicine, Boston, MA, USA
e-mail: christine.wanke@tufts.edu

© Springer Nature Switzerland AG 2021
D. L. Humphries et al. (eds.), *Nutrition and Infectious Diseases*, Nutrition and Health,
https://doi.org/10.1007/978-3-030-56913-6_9

**Key Points**

- HIV and TB infections increase the risk for nutritional compromise, and, in turn, poor nutritional status may increase risk for infection and worsen health outcomes in individuals living with HIV and/or TB.
- People living with HIV and/or TB, particularly in resource-limited settings and those who are untreated, continue to be at increased risk for malnutrition and wasting and, subsequently, increased risk for disease progression and mortality.
- HIV-associated wasting may result from complications of HIV, opportunistic infections, or other comorbidities, particularly in conjunction with poor dietary intake. Similar complications are seen in TB infection.
- The advent of antiretroviral treatments has made HIV infection a manageable chronic condition; hence, the focus has largely shifted to the prevention and management of noncommunicable diseases, many of which are closely related to nutritional status.
- Gastrointestinal conditions are frequent in people living with HIV, the most common being diarrhea, which contribute to nutritional compromise and wasting via poor dietary intake and malabsorption.
- One of the emergent complications in the era of antiretroviral therapy is the "lipodystrophy syndrome," or fat redistribution, which results in the accumulation of visceral fat and/or losses in peripheral subcutaneous fat and is often accompanied by cardiometabolic abnormalities.
- Numerous factors contribute to obesity in people living with HIV, which may be protective in certain subgroups of the population, but is also associated with poor diet quality, micronutrient deficiencies, immunodeficiency, and increased risk for mortality.
- Drug use is disproportionately prevalent among people living with HIV and a leading factor in HIV transmissions, and is an important consideration for nutritional compromise as it may have direct and indirect effects on appetite, food intake, body composition, and nutrient absorption and utilization.
- Micronutrients play key roles in maintaining innate and acquired immunocompetence, and their deficiency is associated with immunodeficiency. While conflicting evidence exists, micronutrient supplementation may be important for those not receiving treatment, as well as an adjuvant treatment to support immunity.
- A comprehensive nutritional assessment consists of anthropometric measurements, biochemical markers, measurement of dietary intake, and a clinical assessment of nutritional needs and factors that may affect intake. A review of protocols for adequate nutritional assessment is included.

# Introduction

Nutritional compromise is one of the most frequent complications in both human immunodeficiency virus (HIV) and tuberculosis (TB) infections. This is especially true in resource-limited settings and particularly among individuals who have advanced, untreated HIV or TB disease. Individuals living with these infections may experience the full spectrum of nutritional complications, which promote comorbidities and increase mortality. The interaction of nutrition with these infections is bidirectional, as individuals who are malnourished have an increased risk of infection and those infected with HIV or TB are likely to develop nutritional abnormalities [1–3]. Early in the HIV epidemic, nutritional abnormalities ranged from micronutrient deficiencies to severe acute wasting, especially among those who developed the acquired immunodeficiency syndrome (AIDS). On the other hand, the advent

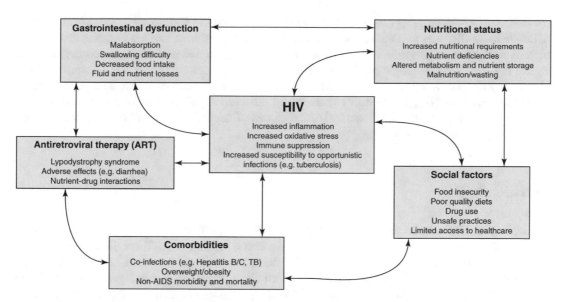

**Fig. 9.1** Relationships between HIV, nutrition, and associated factors. The bidirectional, interconnected relationships between nutritional status, HIV infections, HIV-related complications, and comorbidities

of antiretroviral therapy (ART) has changed HIV from a deadly infection to a chronic, manageable condition. ART is now available worldwide and, following worldwide trends, more and more people living with HIV (PLWH) on ART are now overweight or obese, with metabolic abnormalities or metabolic syndrome. This chapter describes the full spectrum of nutritional compromise in individuals living with HIV, TB, or HIV/TB co-infection and explores the epidemiology, presentation, and etiology of nutritional issues of both infections. The complex relationship between nutritional status and HIV infection, as discussed in this chapter, is visually represented in Fig. 9.1.

In many ways, nutritional compromise is similar in both infections, but there are major differences as well. Many health outcomes, particularly immunity, comorbidities, and response to therapy, are influenced by an individual's nutritional status and vice versa. Weight loss and wasting may be a result of poor dietary intake, malabsorption, or increased metabolic demands, as well as the effects of HIV, TB, and other opportunistic infections. The infections, as well as some of the treatments, may induce gastrointestinal disorders (e.g., nausea, vomiting, and diarrhea), leading to inadequate intake and malabsorption of nutrients. These complications are more pronounced in resource-limited settings, where malnutrition was often endemic prior to the HIV epidemic. Over a quarter of the world's population (≈2 billion people) experienced moderate to severe food insecurity in 2018, with nearly 11% (821.6 million) estimated to be undernourished [4]. Undernutrition itself is a leading cause of immunodeficiency globally [5–7]. Hence, nutritional interventions should be part of all national HIV/AIDS and TB control and treatment programs [8]. In 2018, there were an estimated 37.9 million people in the world living with HIV, two-thirds (67.5%) in sub-Saharan Africa [9], and the World Health Organization (WHO) estimated 1.7 million new HIV infections and 10 million new active TB cases, including ~900,000 who were co-infected with HIV and TB [9]. The co-occurrence of HIV and TB leads to especially severe malnutrition, typically resulting in worse outcomes than would be associated with HIV or TB alone. Malnutrition is associated with increased incidence and severity of HIV-related opportunistic infections, including TB, which in turn can precipitate loss of appetite, weight loss, and wasting [8]. Weight loss and low body weight increase the risk of mortality in individuals with HIV and/or TB, even after initiation of ART or antituberculosis therapy [10–13].

Since the advent of ART in 1996 and its global dissemination from 2004 to the present, PLWH who have access to care have achieved longer life spans, now approaching those of the general population

[14–16]. Along with an aging population of PLWH, there has been a shift in healthcare priorities from AIDS-defining illnesses to noncommunicable diseases and conditions that are associated with HIV, such as cardiometabolic syndrome (e.g., cardiovascular disease and diabetes); respiratory, psychological [17–19], and neurologic conditions [20]; and non-AIDS-defining cancers [21], among others. Moreover, PLWH develop some age-related noncommunicable diseases earlier than the general population [22]. As with HIV, TB mortality rates fell by 42% among HIV-negative people and by 68% among PLWH [23] between 2000 and 2018, and causes of death in this population are increasingly due to non-TB-related causes [24].

## Nutrition in HIV

The history of HIV can be separated into the pre-ART era and the post-ART era that followed the advent and widespread use of highly active ART in 1996. In the pre-ART era, HIV infection progressed to AIDS at a high rate, while post-ART, there has been an expanded landscape of health conditions among PLWH. If HIV is untreated, opportunistic infections and malignancies—similar to the pre-ART era—can manifest, while among PLWH who are virally suppressed, noncommunicable diseases can be accelerated by chronic immune activation. The nutritionally relevant conditions associated with HIV infection have changed with ART use and longer survival of PLWH and now include not only wasting and GI disorders but also lipodystrophy and obesity.

### *HIV-Associated Wasting*

Wasting was among the most common complications of HIV/AIDS in the pre-ART era [25–27] and continues to affect untreated vulnerable populations [28–33]. Precise estimates of the prevalence of wasting in PLWH are lacking due to incongruent definitions in the literature. HIV-associated wasting, or "wasting syndrome," was initially defined by the US Centers for Disease Control and Prevention (CDC) as involuntary weight loss of 10%, accompanied by diarrhea or fever that was not attributable to a condition other than HIV [34]. Using this definition, the CDC estimated that approximately 21% of persons who died with AIDS between 1992 and 1997 had co-occurring wasting [28]. Concerns about the limited scope of the definition led others to propose more comprehensive categorizations. Wanke et al. investigated the prevalence of wasting among PLWH in the Nutrition for Healthy Living cohort ($n = 633$) using the following criteria to define wasting: (1) unintentional loss of >10% body weight since baseline; (2) a body mass index of <20 kg/m$^2$; or (3) unintentional loss of >5% body weight within 6 months that persisted for at least a year [35]. The investigators found that 33.6% of the participants met at least one criterion for wasting. More than 50% of this cohort were receiving ART, and weight loss was seen to occur irrespective of ART, in those treated successfully with ART, in those for whom ART failed, and in those who were ART-naïve [36].

Although weight loss is the simplest clinical marker of wasting, interpretation of unintended weight loss may be confounded by fluid losses from vomiting, diarrhea, rehydration, or metabolic abnormalities such as abnormal fat distribution [37, 38]. As such, others have proposed additional indicators of wasting, such as loss of body cell mass as measured by bioelectrical impedance analysis [39], which is depleted in PLWH disproportionately to weight loss [26, 40]. These confounders and the findings by Wanke et al. suggest that it is likely that HIV-associated wasting in the pre-ART era was underdiagnosed and underestimated [35].

Wasting itself is an AIDS-defining condition [41], and weight loss often precedes other AIDS-defining illnesses [42]. Indeed, weight loss in PLWH predicts clinical progression to AIDS and mortality, both on and off of ART (though AIDS and mortality frequency drop considerably with ART) [11, 42–44]. The etiology of HIV-associated wasting is multifactorial but is likely due to complications of HIV, opportunistic infections, or other comorbidities, particularly in conjunction with poor dietary intake [36, 45, 46]. The strongest predictor of weight loss in HIV-associated wasting is reduced caloric intake [47, 48], which is exacerbated by an 8–12% increase in resting energy expenditure (REE) in PLWH without immunosuppression and 9–34% in PLWH with AIDS as compared to healthy controls [49–52]. These complications are particularly relevant in those with lower CD4+ cell counts reflective of more progressed HIV disease [53, 54]. Furthermore, acute wasting is associated with opportunistic infections, whereas gastrointestinal complications and malabsorption typically result in chronic wasting [55].

While many use the terms interchangeably, a distinction exists between wasting related to dietary insufficiency and "cachexia" which is a systemic syndrome characterized by hypermetabolism, hyper-inflammation, and increased protein catabolism [56, 57]. The pathology of cachexia involves a hyper-active acute-phase response that is mediated by pro-inflammatory cytokines such as tumor necrosis factor (TNF)-α and interleukin (IL)-6, which play pivotal roles in wasting [58]. In one study of PLWH of whom 63% had AIDS and 43% were on highly active antiretroviral therapy (HAART), TNF-α and IL-1β from peripheral blood mononuclear cells (PBMCs) were more significant predictors of increased REE and loss of lean body mass than inadequate dietary intake [59]. Other studies have found that IL-1β, IL-6, and TNF-α levels from PBMCs, but not plasma, were able to differentiate between HIV-infected participants with wasting and those without [60]. In any case, HIV-associated wasting and cachexia result in depletion of lean body mass and fat mass, with the depletion in lean tissue being more pronounced than that of fat mass [61]. Moreover, the depletion of lean body mass is concentrated in the metabolically active cells of muscle and visceral organs [62]. Critical points in depletion of body cell mass (54% of normal) and weight loss (66% of ideal body weight) have been associated with death among individuals with AIDS independently of the underlying cause(s) of wasting [63].

## Gastrointestinal Disorders and HIV Enteropathy

Gastrointestinal (GI) conditions have long been observed in patients with HIV [25, 64, 65] and may affect any part of the GI tract [54]. PLWH may present with one or more GI symptoms such as diarrhea, nausea and vomiting, dysphagia, odynophagia, abdominal pains and discomforts, GI bleeding, jaundice, and hepatomegaly [66–68]. Diarrhea is the most common GI complication in HIV infection [69], which was particularly prevalent among individuals with AIDS in the pre-ART era [70, 71], and contributed to a high burden of diarrheal diseases in resource-limited countries [72]. With the widespread use of ART, the landscape of diarrheal etiology in PLWH has changed from infectious to non-infectious causes [73, 74]. GI-related adverse events, particularly diarrhea, are an important consideration in ART, but a review of clinical trials has shown that GI events were not often attributed to ART [75]. A meta-analysis of 38 HIV clinical trials conducted from 2008 to 2016, covering 21,066 individuals receiving ART, has shown that the incidence of diarrhea (approximately 18%) did not significantly decline during the study period, even among those who were virally suppressed, although it was significantly lower among ART-experienced than ART-naïve individuals (13.7% vs. 19.7%, respectively; $p < 0.001$) [76]. In contrast, others have reported that the probability of adverse events after ART initiation, most commonly GI symptoms, increased over time and was associated with aging, disease progression, female gender, and male-male sex [77]. GI complications also negatively impact quality of life and reduce adherence to ART [78–81].

Malabsorption and diarrhea prior to ART were often related to opportunistic infections of the small intestine [70, 82, 83]. Nonetheless, structural and functional changes in the GI tract were observed even in the absence of opportunistic infections. The morphological changes observed included villus atrophy, crypt hyperplasia, and epithelial hypoproliferation in the small intestine and colon [25, 64, 84, 85], along with depletion of CD4+ lymphocytes within the lamina propria [86, 87]. These GI alterations are more pronounced when an opportunistic infection is involved [88]. The pathology of "HIV enteropathy" involves direct and indirect effects of HIV and includes increased GI inflammation, increased intestinal permeability, diarrhea, and malabsorption [89, 90]. The GI tract is a primary target for HIV infection and a major site of HIV replication, which results in massive depletion of the mucosal immune system [91, 92], where most of the body's T-cells reside [89, 93]. Moreover, studies have shown incomplete reconstitution of mucosal immunity despite viral suppression secondary to ART [94–96].

GI complications contribute to nutritional compromise and wasting in PLWH [55, 97–100] whether they are directly related to HIV or not [54]. Nutritional intake may be affected by oropharyngeal and esophageal disorders, which result in swallowing difficulties [101]. Adding to poor intake, malabsorption of carbohydrates and fats, usually related to diarrhea, is a common complication in PLWH and not always associated with enteric pathogens [84, 97, 99, 102–108]. Fat malabsorption may lead to significant caloric deficits due to the energy density of fats (9 kcal/g) and contribute to nutrient deficiencies due to impaired absorption of fat-soluble vitamins, which further compromise immunity [109] and may persist even among those receiving HAART [110]. Low serum carotene levels, a marker of fat malabsorption, have been reported in 30–70% of PLWH [111]. Malabsorption in PLWH has also been associated with low levels of vitamin $B_{12}$ and zinc [107, 112–114], hypoalbuminemia [115], and anemia from iron, folate, or vitamin $B_{12}$ malabsorption [116]. Interestingly, one study found that malabsorption was associated with weight loss in PLWH, but it was also associated with decreased REE, suggesting a compensatory metabolic response to caloric deficit [117].

## Lipodystrophy Syndrome

With the development and widespread use of HAART, PLWH have experienced improved health outcomes and decreased prevalence of wasting. Yet even with adequate treatment, PLWH may experience metabolic alterations and nutritional abnormalities. ART itself may lead to nutritional complications via metabolic changes, alterations in body composition, and the impact of ART on food intake. One of the emergent complications in the post-ART era is the "lipodystrophy syndrome," or fat redistribution [118]. The syndrome encompasses lipohypertrophy, lipoatrophy, or a combination of the two [119]. Lipohypertrophy is the accumulation of visceral fat in the abdomen, dorsocervical area ("buffalo hump"), or breasts in both men and women. Lipoatrophy is the loss of subcutaneous fat in the peripheral areas, particularly the face and limbs. Lipodystrophy has been associated mainly with therapy using protease inhibitors (PIs) and nucleoside reverse-transcriptase inhibitors (NRTIs) [120, 121]. Lipoatrophy has been particularly related to certain NRTIs and older combinations no longer in use (e.g., indinavir, nelfinavir, and saquinavir/ritonavir) [122–124] that were more commonly associated with mitochondrial toxicity than are more modern drugs (e.g., emtricitabine, lamivudine, tenofovir, and dolutegravir) [125]. Additionally, HIV may play a role in lipodystrophy by promoting localized adipose tissue inflammation and functional dysregulation [126–128]. Indeed, lipodystrophy has also been observed in PLWH naïve to ART, although much less often than in treated individuals [129, 130]. Kotler et al. have proposed that HIV viral load and hypercortisolemia may have a greater impact on body composition than ART itself [131].

Lipodystrophy is often accompanied by metabolic abnormalities such as hyperlipidemia, hypercholesterolemia, hyperinsulinemia, glucose intolerance, and insulin resistance [132–137]. As a result, lipodystrophy contributes to the development of noncommunicable diseases in PLWH, particularly cardiovascular disease and diabetes mellitus, as well as increasing the risk for all-cause mortality [138]. That said, the relationship between lipodystrophy and metabolic comorbidities may be dependent on the particular manifestations of lipodystrophy in an individual. Hadigan et al. found that PLWH with lipodystrophy had a significantly greater 10-year risk for coronary heart disease than HIV-uninfected controls, yet this risk was less pronounced when participants were matched by waist-to-hip ratio [139]. Notably, the study found that the risk for coronary heart disease was greater among PLWH with lipoatrophy than those with lipohypertrophy or with both lipoatrophy and lipohypertrophy.

## HIV, ART, and Obesity

In the post-ART era, overweight and obesity are growing concerns for PLWH, with increasing prevalence even in resource-limited countries [140–149]. Some individuals were overweight or obese before they contracted HIV [141, 149], secondary to the pandemic of global obesity [150]. Interestingly, a higher BMI, reflective of greater fat stores, may be protective for vulnerable groups among PLWH. A higher BMI and fat mass have been associated with slower HIV disease progression in untreated and drug-using PLWH [151–153]. A BMI of 27 kg/m$^2$ or higher was also protective against mortality [152]. Others have found longitudinal improvements in markers of HIV disease progression and immunity with increased BMI [154–157]. That said, BMI likely underestimates obesity in PLWH [158] as it may fail to recognize excess adiposity in those with low muscle mass [159]. Additionally, even among those with normal BMI (18.5–24.9 kg/m$^2$) or higher, lipodystrophy results in PLWH having a greater amount of visceral adiposity in relation to BMI than HIV-uninfected persons [160, 161]. Nonetheless, much of what we know about obesity in the context of HIV is based on the standard criterion for obesity of BMI $\geq$ 30 kg/m$^2$.

The etiology of obesity is complex and multifaceted [162], and PLWH share many behavioral, socioeconomic, and biological risk factors for obesity with the general population. Nutritional factors that are associated with overweight/obesity among PLWH include food insecurity [163, 164] and poor diet quality [165–167]. In PLWH receiving ART, higher rates of overweight and/or obesity were associated with alcohol consumption, non-smoker, or past smoker status, as well as being seronegative for hepatitis C virus (HCV) or cleared HCV status [168]. Women living with HIV are at higher risk for weight gain and obesity than men living with HIV. It is unclear why the risk for obesity in women living with HIV is greater than for women in the general population, while the reverse is true for men [170]. Furthermore, lower CD4+ cell counts and higher HIV viral loads prior to ART have a greater effect on BMI for women than men [169]. Additionally, nutritional status and the state of HIV disease at the time that ART is initiated could play a role in the development of obesity. In a study of Nigerians living with HIV, the development of obesity was associated with a BMI below 20 kg/m$^2$ and a CD4 count below 350 cells/$\mu$L at the time of ART initiation [145]. Similar findings were reported in a study of Brazilians living with HIV, where obesity was more likely to develop in those who, at the time of ART initiation, had lower baseline CD4 cell counts and/or higher baseline HIV viral loads [171]. In contrast to the Nigerian study, the study in Brazil found obesity to be associated with a higher BMI at the time of ART initiation. Nevertheless, it appears that weight gain is accelerated among those with more advanced HIV disease at the time they initiate treatment; this is considered a "return to health" phenomenon like that seen in malnourished patients [172, 173]. Furthermore, specific ART regimens may also contribute to weight gain, predominantly as fat, with the greatest effect seen with integrase strand transfer inhibitors (INSTIs; e.g., raltegravir and dolutegravir) [174]. Although obesity has been shown to affect the pharmacokinetics of some classes of ART drugs, there is no evidence of an effect of obesity on virologic response [175].

Obesity has numerous health implications for PLWH. While obesity is often thought of as a consequence of overnutrition, the poor diet that often accompanies the excess in energy intake also contributes to micronutrient deficiencies among many obese individuals [176–178]. Micronutrient deficiencies and the inflammatory features of obesity can potentiate immunodeficiency in PLWH [179, 180]. Obesity may be a significant cause of immunodeficiency worldwide, contributing to the global burden of infectious diseases and to worse clinical outcomes in infected patients [181–183]. Adipose tissue is also a significant reservoir for latent HIV infection and presents a major barrier for cure efforts [184]. HIV targets CD4+ T-cells and macrophages in the stromal vascular fraction of adipose tissue, making adipose tissue a viral reservoir and a potent source of persistent inflammation in PLWH, irrespective of obesity [126]. Indeed, both HIV infection and obesity result in persistent inflammation; thus, obesity can exacerbate the inflammatory response already present in PLWH. Additionally, obesity contributes to non-AIDS-related mortality among PLWH due to its role in the development of noncommunicable diseases such as cardiovascular disease, diabetes mellitus, non-AIDS cancers, and liver disease [185], now leading causes of death among PLWH who can access ART [186–188].

## Substance Use and Abuse Among PLWH

An additional factor that may lead to nutritional compromise in PLWH is the use and abuse of drugs and alcohol. Drug use, predominantly but not exclusively injection drug use (IDU), contributes to HIV transmission worldwide due to its association with unsafe practices such as sharing needles, bartering sex for drugs, unprotected sex [189–195], and sexualized drug use ("chemsex") [196, 197]. Substance abuse is also a pervasive barrier for care among PLWH, affecting their engagement and retention in care, as well as their adherence and response to ART [198]. Additionally, Baum et al. have reported significant effects of alcohol and cocaine abuse on HIV disease progression, suggesting direct effects on immune function in addition to their contribution to poor adherence to ART [199, 200]. Of particular concern are those who inject drugs, who are up to 22 times more likely to become infected with HIV than the general population [9] and are at increased risk of TB infection, irrespective of their HIV status [201]. In 2018, IDU accounted for an estimated 12% of new HIV infections globally, including 41% in Eastern Europe and Central Asia, 37% in the Middle East and North Africa, and 13% in Asia and the Pacific [202]. In the United States, IDU contributed to 17% of male and 21% of female HIV infections between 2012 and 2016 [203]. Additionally, people who inject drugs have the highest risk for HCV infection, with a 67% global prevalence [204]. As of 2016, there were an estimated 10.6 million injection drug users worldwide [205]. Of these, 11.8% are living with HIV and 5.5 million with HCV, and 1 million are co-infected with HIV and HCV [205]. Other studies have reported higher estimates of 15.6 million injection drug users worldwide, 17.8% of these living with HIV and 52.3% exposed to HCV [206]. Most notably, the incidence rate of HIV among injection drug users is on the rise. Furthermore, TB is a leading cause of mortality among PLWH who inject drugs, and people who use non-injection drugs have also been found to have increased rates of TB [207].

### Nutritional Status and Substance Use

The impact of drug use on nutritional status is complex and reflects lifestyle, behavioral and socioeconomic factors, as well as the impact of drugs on the brain and body. The nutritional concerns of substance abuse include those caused by the effects of drugs on appetite and food-related behaviors–usually leading to poor food intake–and by physiological alterations on digestion, absorption, metabolism, and nutrient utilization. Additionally, eating disorders such as anorexia nervosa and bulimia nervosa are known to co-exist with substance abuse disorders [208, 209]. Not surprisingly, poor eating habits [210–213], nutrient deficiencies [214–217], and wasting [31, 218, 219, 220] have been reported in drug users. Excessive alcohol consumption, for example, can lead to nutritional deficiencies and malnutrition, as the poor diet that often accompanies alcohol addiction results in a displacement of essential nutrients from the diet [221]. Indeed, alcohol abuse is one of the major causes of nutritional deficiencies and malnutrition in high-resource countries [222]; it accounts for 95% of thiamin deficiencies in developed countries [223], and deficiencies in vitamin $B_6$, folic acid, and vitamin C are also common [224, 225]. These deficiencies may also be difficult to correct given metabolic perturbations and alcoholism recidivism rates in the population suffering micronutrient deficiencies. In detoxification unit patients, 73% of whom suffered from alcohol dependence, 50% of patients had an iron or vitamin deficiency, despite multivitamin and thiamin supplementation on admission [226]. Data are lacking with respect to many drugs of abuse [227], but lower serum concentrations of vitamins A, $B_{12}$, C, and E and minerals zinc and selenium have been found in drug users compared to non-user controls [214, 228].

In addition to direct effects on appetite and food intake, drug use is also associated with socioeconomic factors including food insecurity, poverty, and lack of access to treatment [213, 229, 230, 234, 235] particularly prevalent among persons who inject drugs [231]. Food insecurity is associated with poor nutritional status even after accounting for the effect of poverty [232]. The heightened risk for food insecurity among drug users may be due in part to competing priorities of acquiring drugs to feed a drug addiction versus acquiring food for sustenance [233].

Although for many the picture of the emaciated drug user persists, the association between substance use and BMI is complicated, and studies have shown inconsistent results [236, 237]. This is partly due to the mechanism of action of the different substances of abuse, their effects on food-related behaviors [238], and metabolic changes that disrupt energy balance [239]. Drug users tend to have lower body weights than their non-drug-using counterparts [240], and a lower BMI is typically found among injection drug users [241] and/or cigarette smokers [242]. Cocaine use has been associated with lower body weight and body fat than among non-users [243, 244]. IDU in particular is associated with lower body fat percentage compared to non-users, after adjusting for BMI and waist circumference [245]. Heavy drinkers, on the other hand, tend to have a higher BMI due to the energy content of alcohol [246], although a low BMI may be found among the heaviest drinkers [221]. As seen with food insecurity in Western countries, a high BMI in drug users may also be a result of poor diet quality.

Additionally, a growing body of evidence suggests that substance abuse may predispose individuals for weight gain after cessation of use [236]. Weight gain typically occurs during drug recovery programs, increasing the risk for chronic comorbidities [247]. While weight gain might be desirable among malnourished drug users, unhealthy weight gain has also been reported [212, 248, 249]. The reason for this weight gain is multifactorial. Malnutrition and weight loss during substance abuse can make an individual susceptible to weight gain, but also eating may become an alternative addictive behavior [250, 251].

Irrespective of weight, substance use may lead to metabolic perturbations and micronutrient deficiencies that may further impair nutrient absorption and utilization [252]. In addition to poor dietary intake, alcohol use may lead to malnutrition through the damage it causes to digestion, absorption, metabolism, and nutrient utilization [253]. Alcohol and barbiturates deplete vitamin A levels by enhancing the activity of liver enzymes responsible for alcohol breakdown [254]. Alcohol also alters nutrient metabolism by decreasing the secretion of pancreatic enzymes and inhibits nutrient absorption by damaging the lining of digestive organs, impairing nutrient transport into blood [252]. Thiamin deficiency, a hallmark of alcoholism, impairs metabolism of carbohydrates [223]. Folate deficiency, also a consequence of excessive alcohol, alters the cell lining of the small intestine, impairing absorption of water, glucose, sodium, and folate itself, among others [252]. Chronic heavy drinking leads to alcoholic liver disease, which can result in impaired synthesis of vital proteins such as albumin and clotting factors that are produced in the liver [253, 254]. Substance abuse can also contribute to the development or worsening of cardiometabolic diseases [255–259].

## Nutritional Status and Substance Use Among PLWH

Both nutritional disorders and more advanced HIV disease [31, 199, 200, 220] have been reported in drug users. Lower serum concentrations of several vitamins and minerals that are associated with HIV disease progression and mortality [228] have been found in drug users compared to non-user controls [214]. To more fully understand the impact of nutritional deficiencies and drug abuse on HIV disease progression and comorbidities, more research among drug and alcohol users is needed that overcomes barriers inherent in this hard-to-reach population. Active drug users often fail to adhere to nutritional and pharmaceutical interventions. Polysubstance use is common and adds difficulty when attempting to assess the effects of specific drugs.

The risk for food insecurity of PLWH who also use drugs may depend on the drug(s) of choice. Among PLWH, the use of opioids was associated with a greater risk for food insecurity compared to those who used marijuana or cocaine alone, and polysubstance use more than tripled the risk for food insecurity compared to non-use of illicit drugs [234]. Importantly, food insecurity may be particularly detrimental to drug users living with HIV, as it may lead to poorer adherence to treatment than seen with either drug use or food insecurity alone [235]. In PLWH, drug injection may further exacerbate malabsorption and increase resting energy expenditure [255]. Among PLWH, the use of cocaine/crack was associated with a lower BMI, while those who used marijuana tended to have central obesity [244]. Indeed, a high prevalence of wasting among PLWH (17.6%) was associated with heavy alcohol consumption and use of cocaine/crack, despite most of them taking ART [31]. Among drug users living with HIV, users of cocaine/crack were less likely to be on ART, and high viral loads were associated with the metabolic syndrome [244]. Nutritional deficiencies related to drug use may contribute to immunodeficiency, disease progression [228], and the development of comorbidities that could further compromise nutritional status.

## *HIV and Micronutrients*

As of 2018, of all people living with HIV worldwide, 67% were accessing treatment and 58% were virally suppressed [202]. These statistics represent impressive strides in the fight against new HIV infections worldwide; however, those who do not have access or are not engaged in treatment despite having access to ART continue to have HIV viral load, experience HIV disease progression, and may continue to transmit HIV. Micronutrient deficiencies were identified in PLWH early in the epidemic and were shown to be associated with higher risk of progression of HIV disease and increased mortality [217, 260–263]. Infections, no matter how mild, depressed nutritional status, and, in turn, nutritional deficiencies impair resistance to infection [264]. This synergy between nutritional and immune deficits is evident in all stages, during latency, the progression of HIV disease, and in advanced disease [217, 228, 260–271]. The evidence shows that nutritional therapy is important for PLWH who are not on ART, as well as an adjunct therapy to ART in order to support both the acquired and the innate host defenses [264].

As reviewed above, weight loss and wasting, also common in untreated HIV disease, increase the risk of HIV disease progression and independently predict HIV-related morbidity and mortality [42, 63, 272, 273]. The pathogenesis of wasting in PLWH is related to a combination of weight loss and deficiencies of several micronutrients due to reduced food intake, nutrient malabsorption, and increased rate of metabolism in untreated individuals [46, 274]. Micronutrient deficiencies were described in untreated HIV, including low plasma levels of vitamin $B_{12}$, selenium, zinc, vitamin $B_6$, other B vitamins, and fat-soluble vitamins A and D [228, 275, 276]. Studies in Africa noted frequent vitamin A deficiency associated with increased mortality and higher risk of mother-to-child HIV transmission [277] and more rapid HIV progression in adults [278]. Deficiency of selenium occurred in adults and children with HIV infection and was significantly associated with an increased relative risk of HIV-related mortality in cohorts of men who have/had sex with men, substance users, and children [263, 279]. Elevated oxidative stress levels were found by several studies and were related to T-cell exhaustion and impairment of immune response in controlling viral replication [280]. Antioxidant deficiency augments oxidative stress and can contribute to HIV disease progression due to the role of inflammatory mechanisms in HIV replication [281]. Thus, further research on reducing chronic oxidative stress is needed since suppressing such stress may restore antioxidant levels and reestablish the Th1/Th2 balance [282]. Overly low serum concentrations of these micronutrients were associated with low CD4+ cell counts, faster HIV disease progression, and higher HIV-related mortality [263, 267, 276, 279, 283–289].

The introduction of HAART in 1996 suppressed HIV viral load and improved immunological function; however, many patients continued to lose weight and some even continued to suffer from wasting [11, 35, 290]. Nonetheless, the great majority of the patients in the combination ART era have experienced reduced morbidity and, in high-income countries, have life spans that are close to that of the general population [14–16]. However, considering the crucial role that micronutrients play in maintaining functional immunity, research regarding their role and the effects of supplementation on HIV disease progression became a priority, particularly in Africa [291]. Micronutrient deficiencies have persisted even after the initiation of ART and HIV viral load suppression, although some observational studies showed improvement in the plasma levels of some micronutrients [292].

Early in the HIV epidemic, Baum et al. evaluated the relationship between plasma levels of micronutrients and CD4+ cell counts, alone and in combination with a marker of inflammation, beta 2-microglobulin, in 108 men who had sex with men (MSM) and were living with HIV over an 18-month period [286]. Multiple micronutrient deficiencies were detected, specifically in zinc, selenium, and vitamins A, E, $B_2$, $B_6$, and $B_{12}$ in relatively asymptomatic PLWH with adequate diets. Development of deficiency of vitamins A and $B_{12}$ was associated with a significant decline in CD4 cell count, while normalization of vitamin A, vitamin $B_{12}$, and zinc was associated with significantly higher CD4 cell counts. Low vitamin $B_{12}$ status at baseline significantly predicted accelerated HIV disease progression as determined by CD4 cell count, suggesting that micronutrient normalization may increase symptom-free survival. Moreover, selenium deficiency in this cohort was associated with a survival time of 31.4 months, compared with 57.4 months for those who were not selenium deficient [228].

Baum reports on longitudinal studies in two other cohorts of people living with HIV, illicit drug users and children, in addition to the MSM mentioned previously, and observed similar micronutrient deficiencies in all three cohorts [228]. Multiple micronutrient deficiencies were noted in 41% of the drug users, including vitamins A, C, and E and zinc as the most predominant deficiencies due to poor dietary intake and potential drug-nutrient interactions. In this cohort, deficiencies of vitamins A and $B_{12}$, zinc, and selenium were significantly associated with increased mortality. An almost threefold increase in relative risk of mortality was demonstrated with low plasma zinc levels. Low plasma levels of vitamin A were also associated with a threefold increase in relative risk of mortality consistent with reports by Semba et al. [293]. Low plasma vitamin $B_{12}$ levels were also associated with accelerated HIV disease progression and an increased risk of mortality [228], findings also reported earlier by Tang et al. [267]. The micronutrient deficiency associated with the highest risk for mortality, however, was selenium. While only 7% of the cohort of drug users demonstrated overly low levels of plasma selenium, selenium deficiency was associated with almost a 20-fold increase in relative risk of mortality [263]. When all of the micronutrient deficiencies in this cohort were considered, only selenium was an independent predictor of survival [228]. This finding was confirmed by other investigators following other cohorts of PLWH [269, 279].

Campa et al. followed a small cohort of 24 perinatally HIV-infected children for 5 years prior to the era of ART provision; over the course of the study, 12 of the children died of HIV-related causes [279]. Assessment of micronutrient status identified selenium deficiency as an independent cause of faster HIV disease progression and mortality. Thus, multiple micronutrient deficiencies were noted in observational studies with several cohorts of PLWH and were associated with HIV disease progression and mortality. These compelling studies were followed by multiple micronutrient intervention trials, mostly conducted prior to widespread ART, though some trials included PLWH on effective ART regimens.

## Micronutrient Intervention Trials Among PLWH

Micronutrient supplementation studies using randomized controlled trials (RCTs) in PLWH have shown mixed results. Some of the RCTs that enrolled populations with low prevalence of micronutrient deficiencies had insufficient periods of supplementation to demonstrate effects, did not assess baseline micronutrient status, and/or did not adjust for markers of inflammation. Moreover, widely variable doses of micronutrients were supplemented in different RCTs. Several RCTs supplemented various combinations of micronutrients including vitamins A, D, E, C, $B_1$, $B_2$, niacin, $B_6$, $B_{12}$, K, folate, and β-carotene and trace elements including zinc, selenium, magnesium, iron, iodine, copper, manganese, chromium, cobalt, and molybdenum.

In contrast, some RCTs supplemented only one or two micronutrients. Moreover, the clinical trials have been conducted in a variety of different settings and continents, with variable nutritional status among the study participants at the beginning of the trial. The primary outcomes of all the clinical trials were HIV disease progression, morbidity, and/or mortality.

### Trials Comparing a Single Micronutrient Versus Placebo

*Vitamin A* Several studies investigated the effect of vitamin A supplementation among ART-naïve PLWH. Humphrey et al. supplemented 40 women living with HIV with a single oral dose of 9900 μmol (300,000 IU) vitamin A, and follow-up was conducted for 8 weeks [294]. The participants in the trial did not have vitamin A deficiency, and the supplemented dose did not produce signs of toxicity. There were no effects on any lymphocyte subset or activation markers, nor on HIV viral load at any time during follow-up. Similar results were obtained by Semba et al. supplementing 60 mg of retinol (equivalent to 200,000 IU of vitamin A) in a randomized, double-blinded, placebo-controlled clinical trial with ART-naïve injection drug users living with HIV who were followed for 2 and 4 weeks after treatment ($n = 120$, 60 per arm) [295]. None of the participants had vitamin A deficiency, and no significant effects of the high dose of vitamin A were noted on CD4+ cell count or on HIV viral load. A study in Kenya by Baeten et al. assessed the effect of daily oral supplementation with 10,000 IU vitamin A in the form of retinyl palmitate for 6 weeks on vaginal HIV shedding of women living with HIV. The majority of the participants were vitamin A deficient [296]. No effect of the vitamin A supplementation was found on the prevalence of HIV-1 DNA vaginal shedding or the quantity of HIV-1 RNA in vaginal secretions or on HIV viral load and CD4/CD8 cell counts compared to placebo. Whether this is due to a lack of efficacy or due to the short duration of the supplementation is not known.

*Vitamin D* To test a hypothesis that optimal vitamin D status may be associated with more effective immune responses [297], Mehta et al. determined vitamin D levels in a cohort of 677 patients with TB, 51% of whom were co-infected with HIV [298]. All patients were starting anti-TB treatment and were enrolled into a multivitamin supplementation trial without vitamin D. Vitamin D insufficiency was associated with 66% higher risk of TB relapse, but no association with HIV disease progression was noted. An RCT trial was conducted with 52 PLWH aged 8–26 years who had low serum levels of vitamin D [299]. Participants were supplemented with 100,000 IU active vitamin D compared to placebo every 3 months for 12 months. Vitamin D supplementation had no effect on CD4+ cell count, but was associated with an altered CD4+ T-cell phenotype (decreased Th17:Treg ratio) at 3 months. Another RCT of vitamin D and calcium supplementation was conducted for 48 weeks by Overton et al. during the initiation of ART in PLWH [300]. While vitamin D plus calcium supplementation mitigated the loss of bone mineral density and increased markers of bone turnover, there were no differences in inflammatory or immune biomarkers between the supplementation and the placebo groups. Similar findings were noted by Bang et al. in their RCT [301, 302].

***Zinc Deficiency*** Zinc deficiency is highly prevalent in PLWH, particularly among illicit substance users, and is an independent predictor of a threefold increase in HIV-related mortality [216]. Baum et al. conducted an RCT of zinc supplementation at nutritional levels (12 mg of elemental zinc/day for women and 15 mg of elemental zinc/day for men) for 18 months with 231 PLWH who used illicit drugs and had low plasma zinc levels (<0.75 mg/L) [303]. The primary endpoint was immunological failure defined as CD4+ cell count <200 cells/µL monitored every 6 months. Zinc supplementation reduced the likelihood of immunological failure by a factor of four compared to placebo, without affecting HIV viral load control, and reduced the rate of diarrhea by more than half, but no significant differences in mortality between the two groups were noted. The results of this trial support the use of zinc supplementation as an adjunct therapy with ART in PLWH who are zinc deficient. In a small study of 31 PLWH in Bangkok, Thailand, Asdamongkol et al. randomized zinc supplementation (15 mg chelated Zn/day) to 5 of 12 participants with low plasma zinc levels (<75 µg/dL) and 8 of 19 who had adequate levels of plasma zinc [304]. In the group with low plasma zinc levels, median zinc levels rose 29 µg/dL in the supplemented persons compared to 4.5 µg/dL in the placebo recipients. CD4+ cells rose significantly with zinc supplementation in patients with low plasma zinc levels and did not change in supplemented patients with adequate plasma zinc at baseline. In a similar Peruvian study by Cárcamo et al., however, higher doses of zinc (50–100 mg) for 14 days were not effective in reducing the prevalence of diarrhea when given to ART-naïve study participants with persistent diarrhea [305], possibly due to the short duration of the supplementation. In addition, high doses of zinc for 4 weeks did not improve immune response to TB in PLWH who were on ART and were not zinc deficient in Singapore [306].

***Selenium*** Three randomized clinical trials were conducted with selenium supplementation of 200 µg oral dose per day with a duration of 9–24 months, to both ART-naïve and ART-experienced participants [307]. Baum et al. used a factorial RCT design for 24 months among 878 ART-naïve participants in Botswana with CD4 counts >350 cells/µL to assess daily (1) multivitamins (thiamin, riboflavin, niacin, folic acid, vitamins $B_6$, $B_{12}$, C, and E), (2) selenium, (3) multivitamins with selenium, or (4) placebo [307]. The combined supplement of multivitamins plus selenium had a significantly lower risk vs. placebo of reaching a CD4 count of ≤250 cells/µL (adjusted hazard ratio = 0.46; 95% CI, 0.25–0.85), with the multivitamins without selenium and the selenium-alone groups having less impressive results. The four study groups did not differ in viral loads or their incidence of HIV-related and health-related events. Burbano et al. reported the impact of selenium (200 µg/day) supplementation on hospitalizations in 186 PLWH, some of whom were ART-naïve while others were receiving ART in Miami, Florida [308]. A significantly lower risk of CD4 cell decline and a lower rate of hospitalizations were noted in the selenium supplemented group compared to the placebo group, although the participants on ART had a lower rate of hospitalizations. Hurwitz et al. supplemented with 200 µg/day high selenium yeast in an RCT of 450 PLWH for 9 months in Miami, FL [309]. Increased plasma selenium levels predicted decreased HIV viral load, which predicted increased CD4+ cell count. Nonresponding selenium-treated subjects who had less serum selenium change displayed poor selenium treatment adherence and had elevated HIV viral load and lower CD4+ cell count. In contrast, selenium-treated subjects whose serum selenium increased had excellent selenium treatment adherence, no change in HIV viral load, and an increased CD4 count. However, if selenium adherence was associated with ART adherence, conclusions about selenium benefits may be confounded.

***Vitamin E*** In a small RCT of 29 PLWH with a CD4 count <500 cells/µL, vitamin E or placebo was given for 6 months while initiating ART. Vitamin E supplementation did not affect the indices of HIV infection, though increased lymphocyte viability was reported with vitamin E supplementation [310]. Another study by Allard et al. in Canada assessed the effect of daily antioxidant vitamin supplementation with 800 IU DL-alpha-tocopherol acetate (synthetic vitamin E) and 1000 mg vitamin C, or matched placebo for 3 months on HIV viral load and lipid peroxidation, a measure of oxidative stress, in 49 PLWH [311]. The supplementation with the antioxidant vitamins reduced oxidative stress and produced a nonsignificant trend toward a reduced HIV viral load. These small studies were underpowered and do not provide definitive conclusions in the nutrition and HIV/TB field.

## Supplementation with Multiple Micronutrients

RCTs have compared a daily multiple micronutrient supplementation to placebo for widely divergent periods ranging from 2 weeks to 2 years. Most participants in these trials were ART-naïve PLWH, and in three of the trials, all participants were on treatment for active pulmonary TB. The Botswana Baum et al. RCT was discussed earlier with the selenium review with 878 PLWH [307]. The combined supplement of multivitamins plus selenium (200 µg/day) proved to be a promising intervention in these ART-naïve participants with higher CD4 counts.

In Zambia, Kelly et al. compared oral vitamins A and E, selenium, and zinc vs. albendazole plus placebo in 106 PLWH for 2 weeks [312]. The RCT was based on epidemiological evidence that micronutrient deficiencies were predictive of early death in ART-naïve PLWH and that albendazole reduced diarrhea in PLWH [313]. The 2-week supplementation of micronutrients showed no effect on diarrheal duration or mortality. Short-term oral supplementation was not effective in reducing morbidity or mortality. Kelly et al. then conducted an RCT with 500 PLWH in Zambia who were selected in a cluster-randomized (by household) manner [314]. The participants were supplemented with a daily tablet containing 15 micronutrients (at levels just above the recommended nutrient intakes in the United Kingdom) or placebo, and the study followed participants for up to 3.3 years. While the supplementation did not affect the incidence of diarrhea, severe episodes of diarrhea and mortality were significantly reduced with the supplementation.

McClelland et al. supplemented with multivitamins and selenium compared to placebo in 400 women living with HIV for 6 weeks in a clinical trial in Kenya to reduce cervical and vaginal HIV shedding from infected cells [315]. Unexpectedly, the odds of detecting HIV RNA in vaginal secretions actually increased among women who received micronutrients, particularly those women who had normal baseline selenium levels. There was also a significant increase in CD4 and CD8 counts, while the HIV viral load was unchanged. The authors concluded that while there was some personal benefit to PLWH from a relatively short period of 6-week micronutrient supplementation, PLWH might have potentially greater infectivity. Jiamton et al. supplemented 481 PLWH who were ART-naïve with multiple micronutrients for 48 weeks in Thailand [316]. The supplement contained vitamins A, $D_3$, E, K, C, $B_1$, $B_2$, $B_6$, and $B_{12}$, β-carotene, folic acid, pantothenic acid, iron, magnesium, manganese, zinc, iodine, copper, selenium, chromium, and cysteine above the recommended daily allowances (RDA). Unlike most other trials, supplementation significantly increased survival with no change in CD4 count or HIV viral load. In a trial from China, the immune status of 102 PLWH was improved with multiple micronutrient supplementation close to the daily recommended intake (DRI) for 6 months [317].

Daily supplementation of vitamins A, C, and E to 30 PLWH compared to placebo for 6 months increased plasma levels of the supplemented vitamins, prevented oxidative modification of DNA in the lymphocytes, and increased CD4 counts, although the increase in CD4 counts was not significant [318]. Kaiser et al. conducted an RCT of comprehensive vitamin, mineral (in amounts above the RDA), and antioxidant (N-acetylcysteine, acetyl-L-carnitine, lipoic acid) supplementation to 40 PLWH on stable ART for 12 weeks; the supplementation significantly increased CD4 count without affecting fasting levels of glucose, insulin levels, lipids, venous lactate, serum creatinine, alanine aminotransferase, total bilirubin, or alkaline phosphatase [319]. In contrast, an RCT by Isanaka et al. was conducted among 3418 PLWH in Tanzania receiving high-dose compared to standard-dose multivitamin supplementation for 24 months beginning at the time of ART initiation and did not affect HIV disease progression or mortality. However, the high-dose multivitamins reduced the risk of neuropathy, potentially due to the high levels of vitamin E [320]. All RCT participants in Isanaka et al. received micronutrient supplementation, in contrast to other studies where the demonstrated benefits of micronutrient supplementation were evident compared to a placebo. It is possible that the Isanaka et al. study suggests a potential dosing threshold (i.e., a standard dose) with long-term use (24 months in this study) beyond which there is no further benefit. One summary hypothesis is that PLWH who are not on ART may require micronutrient intakes that are above the RDA to slow progression of HIV disease whereas micronutrient supplementation in PLWH on ART should not be supplemented with micronutrients above the RDA. Long-term micronutrient supplementation to PLWH on effective ART in the levels of one RDA thus appears to be beneficial.

## Nutrition in Tuberculosis

### *Epidemiology of Tuberculosis*

*Mycobacterium tuberculosis* is the leading cause of death from an infectious disease worldwide, and the tenth leading cause of death, overall; the largest burden is in Africa and Asia with 83% of all cases [23]. Tuberculosis is transmitted when an infected person spreads the bacteria by coughing, sneezing, or talking, and the bacterium is inhaled by another individual. Cellular immune response is mounted within 2–6 weeks by CD4+ T-lymphocytes; however, in 70–90% of the cases, the individuals fight off the *M. tuberculosis* bacteria and do not become infected [321]. In approximately 30% of the cases, the *M. tuberculosis* infection is contained, but the immune response is not able to "sterilize" the bacteria. This person becomes "latently" infected, and in this state the infection is asymptomatic and non-transmissible [322].

Approximately 80% of all HIV/TB co-infections have occurred in Africa, which has been experiencing the worst TB epidemic since the introduction of antibiotics. This crisis has been driven by the high prevalence of HIV and compounded by malnutrition, weak healthcare systems, drug-resistant strains of *M. tuberculosis*, and occupational, housing, and medical care facility conditions that facilitate transmission [323]. TB is the most common infectious comorbidity in PLWH, and 30–40% of PLWH die from tuberculosis [324]. HIV co-infection with TB greatly increases morbidity and mortality mainly because TB is often undiagnosed and consequently untreated or treated too late. A 2019 WHO report estimates that 10.0 million people were infected with TB in 2018 globally, along with 1.2 million TB deaths among HIV-negative people and 251,000 among PLWH [23]. Most of these individuals died due to lack of diagnosis of either HIV or TB, or delay in providing treatment. Moreover, immunodeficiency caused by HIV increases the risk for reactivation of latent TB infection, as well as facilitating acquisition of new TB infection [325]. Treatment of HIV/TB co-infection is complicated by drug toxicities and drug-drug interactions between ART and antituberculosis therapy. ART is associated with significantly reduced rates of TB [326], confirmed by RCTs [327, 328]. Thus, early diagnosis and treatment are essential for co-infected persons, and prevention of TB is a vital priority for HIV mono-infected persons [329, 330]. Unfortunately, sensitive diagnostic tests like Xpert MTB/RIF and Xpert MTB/RIF Ultra (Cepheid, Sunnyvale, CA, USA), loop-mediated isothermal amplification, and lateral flow lipoarabinomannan are not available in many African or Asian settings such that undiagnosed persons infected with TB remain infectious to others [331]. After TB diagnosis, only 70% of African patients are successfully treated, giving rise to relapse and emergence of drug resistance [323].

## Tuberculosis and Malnutrition

The relationship between TB and malnutrition is complex, with TB causing malnutrition and malnutrition contributing to the development of TB. While most of the individuals who are positive for TB have latent infections, progression to active TB can occur if the immune response weakens, and malnutrition is an important contributor to a weakened immune response.

### Malnutrition as a Consequence of Tuberculosis

Infection with *M. tuberculosis* can lead to wasting. In patients with active TB, REE increases while energy intake declines as a result of anorexia, eventually leading to wasting [332] and premature mortality [12]. A body composition study using dual-energy X-ray absorptiometry (DXA) in wasted patients with TB revealed depletion of both lean and fat tissues in equal proportions. However, lean tissue was more depleted in the limbs, while fat tissue depletion was greater in the trunk, and HIV co-infection did not alter the effects of TB on body composition [333]. In an Indonesian study, 66% of patients with TB were underweight with body mass index (BMI) <18.5 kg/m$^2$ [334]. Similar results were reported from a study in rural Malawi with 57% of 1,161 newly diagnosed TB patients being underweight and accompanied by a twofold increased risk of premature death [12]. A study from the United Kingdom also reported significantly lower BMI, muscle mass, and subcutaneous fat stores among patients who had active TB compared to those who were not infected [335]. A clinical trial providing nutritional supplementation for 6 weeks to wasted patients with newly diagnosed TB showed improved lean body mass and better physical function compared to patients in the control group who received standard nutritional counseling. During subsequent follow-up, patients who were supplemented maintained higher body weight, but the weight increase was due to greater gains in fat mass than lean body mass [336]. Nutritional supplementation may also shorten the convalescent period and improve the survival of patients infected with TB [337]. When active TB is treated with medications, nutritional status improves, most likely due to better appetite and reduced energy and nutrient requirements [338].

### Active Tuberculosis as a Consequence of Malnutrition

Epidemiological studies point to malnutrition as one of the chief factors contributing to an increased risk of primary and latent infection progressing to active TB disease [339] and to nutrient and energy deficiency exacerbating the pathogenesis of TB [340]. Yet there is surprisingly little rigorously controlled evidence, especially in humans, for these conclusions.

Most of the epidemiological evidence comes from observational studies in regions ravaged by war, famine, or natural disasters [341]. A study of TB among British and Russian prisoners of war (POW) during the Second World War showed that 1.2% of the British POW suffered from TB compared to 15–19% of the Russian POW. Both groups of the POW shared the same overcrowding and working conditions, except the British POW uniquely received 30 gm protein within a 1000 kcal/day in Red Cross food supplements [342]. Another example came from the First World War, when Denmark, while remaining neutral, exported the majority of its meat, fish, poultry, and dairy products to the warring countries. The exports created severe shortages of food in Denmark and simultaneously the rates of TB sharply increased. Once Germany blockaded Denmark and did not allow the exports, the rates of malnutrition and TB sharply decreased while the incidence of TB in the warring countries continued to climb [343]. A study conducted in a naval training school in Norway noted a high prevalence of TB among recruits in the early twentieth century. The recruits lived in crowded, inadequate housing with poor hygiene. However, when the training school improved the hygiene and the housing, the rates of TB did not change. Once the diet was fortified with margarine, cod liver oil, whole wheat bread, fresh fruits and vegetables, and milk, the rates of TB fell sharply [344]. Thus, these natural history and quasi-experimental observations support the theory that malnutrition is associated with increased incidence and severity of TB [345].

The first National Health and Nutrition Examination Survey (NHANES 1 of the US Centers for Disease Control and Prevention) Epidemiological Follow-up Study showed a six- to tenfold increase in relative risk for TB among the lowest decile of the representative sample of the US population, who suffered from undernutrition [346]. This finding was consistent with results from an earlier cohort study of 1100 men, TB-free at baseline, which examined the relationship between micronutrient deficiency and the incidence of TB. Despite similar risk of exposure to TB, the 16 men who developed active TB during follow-up had significantly lower plasma levels of vitamins A and C than those who remained free of TB [347]. Lower risk of TB was also found among 26,975 healthy smokers followed for a mean of 6.7 years in Finland, who consumed vitamin C-rich foods and vegetables [348]. Similar findings were shown in a study conducted in New York City in 1941 when 194 families with similar income, housing, crowding, and food habits were randomized into a vitamin/mineral supplement group and a control group and followed for 5 years. Intent-to-treat analyses showed that the participants in the supplementation group had 2.8 times lower risk of TB than the control group [349]. Greatly increased risk for TB was seen for men whose weight was <85% of ideal weight compared to those who had normal weight [350], and in a clinical setting, intestinal or gastric bypass surgery for morbid obesity resulted in rapid postoperative weight loss which may have contributed to several patients contracting TB [351].

It is likely that the increased risk of TB in malnourished individuals comes from the impact of nutrient deficiency on cell-mediated immunity, the principal host defense against TB [345]. Protein-energy malnutrition in particular decreases cell-mediated immunity while increasing susceptibility to infections [352–355]. Experimental studies with animals have shown that protein undernutrition impairs host defense against *M. tuberculosis* and that the risk can be rapidly reversed with nutritional supplementation [356]. Protein-deficient animals have, for example, defects in T-cell trafficking and diminished production of protective cytokines even when infection dose and route are altered [357–359]. In humans, severe protein-energy malnutrition results in atrophy of the thymus and peripheral lymphoid organs, thereby reducing T-cell number and CD4/CD8 ratio and increasing the number of immature T-cells in the peripheral blood [360], as well as the level of circulating pro-inflammatory cytokines [361], all of which increase the possibility that TB will progress.

As summarized by Cegielski and McMurray in 2004 [345], distinguishing whether malnutrition is a cause or consequence of TB is very challenging. Most of the evidence linking nutritional deficiencies with TB is in the area of latent infection progressing to active TB disease, since it is difficult to determine whether malnutrition precedes TB infection or whether TB leads to malnutrition. Hence, it is not clear whether there is a direct relationship between undernutrition and the risk of initial TB infection. Also, it is unclear whether and how much the risk of TB increases with specific types of malnutrition. It is difficult to extrapolate results from experimental models of TB, due to differences in the nature of disease induced and the immune responses among species and due to route and dose of administration in animals compared with humans.

The majority of epidemiological studies investigating the impacts of nutritional status on TB are observational and cross-sectional, with numerous methodological weaknesses that preclude confirming causality, especially as they do not take into consideration potential confounding factors such as overcrowding, psychological stress, collapse of health programs, and trauma [362–364]. Nevertheless, the findings to date suggest that, with TB, multiple simultaneous nutritional deficiencies are encountered more frequently than specific nutritional deficits [362–364].

## Micronutrients and Tuberculosis

Micronutrient deficiency is one of the most frequent causes of immunodeficiency. Vitamins A, C, E, and $B_6$, folic acid, zinc, copper, selenium, and iron have been found to be significantly lower in patients with active TB [337]. These micronutrients play key roles in maintaining innate and acquired immunocompetence, and their deficiency is associated with immunodeficiency [337]. Karyadi et al. showed that the concentrations of plasma levels of retinol and zinc as well as hemoglobin were lower in patients with active pulmonary TB compared with healthy controls [365]. This observational study was followed up with an RCT supplementing zinc and vitamin A for TB patients who were receiving anti tuberculosis medication, compared to a combination of the medication and a placebo, by the same investigators. They noted an improved effect of tuberculosis medication with micronutrient supplementation after 2 months of treatment and earlier sputum conversion compared with the groups that received medication with a placebo [334]. However, a confirmatory clinical trial supplementing vitamin A and zinc to malnourished TB patients 8 years later in a larger study did not show benefit of either single nutrient or combined supplementation of zinc and vitamin A with medications. The disparity in the results may have been due to the patients in the second clinical trial being more severely malnourished than those in the previous supplementation study [366]. Larger studies that supplement protein, other macronutrients, and micronutrients to severely malnourished TB patients are needed to address this question definitively.

While TB is known to contribute to nutritional deficiencies, which in turn may depress immune function and delay recovery, several Cochrane systematic reviews have concluded that currently there is insufficient evidence to show the benefit of any nutritional supplements for people being treated for active TB [367–369]. However, a number of subsequent studies have shown the efficacy of supplementation with micronutrients including vitamin D and combinations of vitamins and minerals in reducing TB-related mortality and decreased incidence of new TB infections [297, 298, 370].

*Vitamin D* Vitamin D deficiency may increase susceptibility and severity of TB since vitamin D is necessary for macrophage activation, which is essential for maintaining TB infection in latency [371, 372]. Observational studies noted a high prevalence of vitamin D deficiency in patients with active TB due to low dietary intake and lack of exposure to sunshine in the winter months [373]. An in vitro study indicated that addition of 1,25-dihydroxyvitamin $D_3$ inhibited multiplication of virulent tubercle bacilli in cultured human macrophages [374, 375]. Indeed, Martineau et al. showed that a single dose of vitamin D enhanced immunity to *M. tuberculosis* in patients with active TB [370], and Mehta et al. demonstrated that adequate vitamin D status was associated with a lower risk of relapse and with improved BMI in patients infected with TB whether they were co-infected with HIV or not [298]. Moreover, in a prospective cohort of 6751 HIV-negative household contacts of TB patients in Peru, Aibana et al. showed that vitamin D status is predictive of TB disease risk in a dose-dependent manner [376]. The population with the highest risk of TB was PLWH with severe vitamin D deficiency, suggesting a potential role for vitamin D supplementation.

***Multiple Micronutrients*** Other micronutrients were found to be lower in patients with pulmonary tuberculosis, including the antioxidant vitamins C, E, and $B_6$ and minerals zinc, copper, and selenium, and were previously reviewed [337]. These micronutrients play key roles in immunocompetence; Kawai et al. showed that micronutrient supplementation in TB patients during the initiation of TB treatment resulted in higher proliferative responses to concanavalin A compared to the placebo group in Tanzania [377]. An RCT of micronutrient supplementation with zinc and multivitamins (vitamins A, C, E, and B complex) in Tanzania did not have an effect on culture conversion, which is the surrogate marker of the efficacy of anti-TB therapy. However, multivitamin supplementation increased weight gain in the patients with TB independently of culture conversion and significantly decreased mortality in HIV-/TB-co-infected patients [378, 379]. The same investigators conducted a double-blind placebo-controlled clinical trial supplementing the same combination of multivitamins, and instead of zinc, they provided selenium in Tanzania among 471 HIV-infected and 416 HIV-uninfected adults with pulmonary TB during initiation of therapy. The supplementation decreased the risk of TB recurrence by 45% in all patients and by 63% in those co-infected with HIV/TB. There was no effect on mortality in the overall sample; however, the HIV-negative patients had a 64% reduction in deaths, although this effect was not statistically significant with the number of deaths in the subcohort. The supplementation increased CD3+ and CD4+ cell counts and decreased the incidence of extrapulmonary and genital ulcers in the HIV-uninfected group. In addition, supplementation with the micronutrients reduced the incidence of peripheral neuropathy by 57% in both HIV-infected and HIV-uninfected patients [380]. Baum et al. conducted a placebo-controlled randomized clinical trial supplementing multivitamins and selenium to 878 HIV-infected adults in Botswana with CD4 cell count >350 cells/µL and BMI >18.5 who did not receive ART [307]. Supplementation with selenium, alone and with multivitamins, significantly decreased the incidence of TB infections in the participants who were ART-naïve. The investigators recommended providing this supplementation to patients who are infected with HIV prior to antiretroviral treatment, particularly in areas where TB and malnutrition are endemic [381].

The improvement of TB infection, however, depends primarily on anti-TB therapy to correct the inflammatory process before any effect of micronutrient supplementation can be noted [382]. Micronutrient supplementation reduces rates of TB recurrence by improving the immune response when added as adjuvant multidrug therapy [334] and appears to improve the efficacy of anti-TB medications [380]. Protein, energy, and micronutrient supplementation increases body weight, total lean body mass, physical function, and clinical improvement and shortens the convalescent period to allow earlier return to productive work [383]. More research is needed to determine the optimal doses of micronutrients provided in conjunction with multidrug therapy and their effectiveness.

## Nutrition Assessment in HIV and TB

In order to characterize nutritional status in the context of PLWH and/or TB infection and to identify nutritional issues of importance that require targeted intervention, a careful and comprehensive nutritional assessment should be performed as detailed below. No one single measure can fully describe the nutritional status of an individual. If a complete assessment is not performed, significant errors in classification may result, which could lead to the development of inappropriate or flawed interventions that could waste or misdirect resources.

A comprehensive nutritional assessment consists of anthropometric measurements, biochemical markers (i.e., plasma or serum levels of protein, micronutrients, and metabolic parameters), measurement of dietary intake, and a clinical assessment of nutritional needs and factors that may affect intake [384, 385, 386]. A number of HIV-specific screening tools have been developed and evaluated for use by healthcare providers [387]. That said, medical nutrition therapy for HIV requires specialized knowledge, and, whenever possible, nutritional assessments should be performed by a registered dietitian with experience on HIV nutrition [387–389]. The following sections provide a brief overview of nutritional assessments as they pertain to HIV, most of which are equally relevant to TB.

## Anthropometric Measurements

Standardized anthropometric measures are inexpensive, noninvasive methods used to monitor nutritional status, including characterizing body fat deposition and screening for nutritional risks. Techniques and protocols for anthropometric measurements can be obtained from the CDC [390]. These measurements are mainly height, weight, body circumferences (waist, hip, and limbs), and skinfold thickness [391]. Weight history, percentage of usual weight, and weight change over time are important when assessing nutritional status [384]. The most common measure used to characterize nutrition status is the calculation of body mass index (BMI) from an individual's height and weight, expressed as $kg/m^2$. Calculation of BMI is preferable to a simple measure of weight as it adjusts for height. BMI is a useful assessment tool that can provide valuable data in individuals from both the resource-sufficient and the resource-limited settings, allowing for comparison with population standards by classifying underweight ($<18.5$ $kg/m^2$), normal weight ($18.5–24.9$ $kg/m^2$), overweight ($25–29.9$ $kg/m^2$), and obesity ($\geq 30$ $kg/m^2$). However, it should be noted that it is possible for people with a "normal" or high BMI to have nutrient deficiencies, which contribute to poor health outcomes.

In situations where determination of BMI is not feasible, measuring mid-upper arm circumference (MUAC) can be substituted to estimate body composition. MUAC is also useful in young children who cannot stand for height measurements with a stadiometer and in pregnant women for whom weight measures may not accurately reflect nutritional status. However, MUAC must be performed in a consistent, standardized fashion so that the results can be interpreted. Measures of waist and hip circumferences, waist-to-hip ratio, and MUAC might also be obtained to permit documentation of longitudinal changes and to determine body fat accumulation and lipodystrophy. A simple waist circumference (WC) measurement is an excellent companion to BMI, as waist circumference over 40 inches (102 cm) in men or 35 inches (88 cm) in women is indicative of abdominal obesity and can be predictive of cardiometabolic comorbidities [393].

Skinfold measures can be used to estimate percent body fat and compare to standardized values. Despite being relatively simple, skinfold measures require well-trained personnel to be performed reliably and are dependent on interpretative equations.

If available, a bioelectrical impedance analysis (BIA) machine can estimate total body water, from which body cell mass, fat-free mass, and fat mass can be calculated. The BIA is safe, noninvasive, easy, and quick to use. However, it does not measure body tissues directly; estimates are based on assumed relationships between the intracellular and extracellular water compartments [394]. It can, therefore, be affected by dehydration, and it cannot identify the regional distribution of lean and fat tissues.

### Anthropometric Measurements in PLWH/TB

Weight history is particularly important in PLWH as weight loss is a key diagnostic criterion of HIV-associated wasting, which in turn is an AIDS-defining illness [392]. BMI might be unreliable in PLWH with lipodystrophies since it may obscure low muscle mass and underestimate visceral adiposity [159]. Early in the HIV epidemic, Kotler et al. showed that measuring body weight alone in PLWH does not detect losses in body cell mass (a marker of lean body mass) that progress to more severe disease and death [63].

Waist circumference cutoffs have not yet been validated in PLWH [121]. A study by Dimala et al. showed significant direct correlations between WC and BMI as continuous variables, but there was no agreement between the standard waist circumference cutoffs and a BMI $\geq 30$ kg/m$^2$ on identifying cardiometabolic risk in PLWH [395]. These findings illustrate the importance of using more than one assessment tool.

Sex-specific models using anthropometric measurements have been suggested for the prediction of lipodystrophy in PLWH [396]. The accuracy of BIA estimates of body cell mass, fat-free mass, and fat mass is dependent on selection of adequate predictive equations, such as those suggested by Kotler et al. for use in PLWH [397]. Other methods for assessing body composition among PLWH/TB such as dual-energy X-ray absorptiometry (DXA), computed tomography (CT), or magnetic resonance elastography (MRE) are more precise but might be better suited to research settings since they are cost- and resource-intensive.

## Biochemical Assessments

Laboratory measurements can be useful in assessing general nutritional status and specific nutrient deficiencies and identifying or monitoring metabolic comorbidities. Serum albumin and prealbumin (transthyretin) are widely used to assess nutritional status in the clinical setting; with a half-life of approximately 20 days, low albumin values can be the result of protein-energy malnutrition, while the 2- to 3-day half-life of prealbumin is reflective of acute changes in nutritional status. However, both albumin and prealbumin are negative acute-phase reactants; thus, they may reflect an inflammatory response rather than nutritional compromise specifically [389, 398, 399]. In a systematic review and meta-analysis of 63 studies, serum albumin and prealbumin failed to identify protein-energy malnutrition in otherwise healthy individuals with acute or chronic starvation, except at the most extremes of cases [400]. Nonetheless, since there is no laboratory test that is sensitive and specific to protein-energy malnutrition, albumin and transthyretin may help identify individuals at severe risk of malnutrition [401].

Plasma levels of micronutrients should be assessed as they may be correctable with treatment. Deficiencies in vitamins A, E, and D, as well as iron, zinc, and selenium, are priorities for testing, and additional micronutrients should be tested as indicated by medical symptoms, such as vitamin B$_{12}$ in peripheral neuropathy. In patients with fat malabsorption, an evaluation of fat-soluble vitamin deficiencies should include prothrombin time (a marker of vitamin K status) and serum concentrations of 25-hydroxyvitamin D, alpha-tocopherol (vitamin E), and β-carotene (vitamin A) [393].

### Biochemical Assessment in PLWH/TB

A biochemical assessment of nutritional status in PLWH should include a complete blood count with differential, fasting lipid profile, fasting blood glucose, liver and renal panels, and serum testosterone [394]. Albumin has been shown to be a good predictor of HIV disease progression [406, 407] and non-AIDS-related events [408]. Given the metabolic abnormalities that may result from HIV infection and/or ART [118, 134], both fasting lipid profile and fasting glucose should be monitored in all PLWH.

Measurement of micronutrient status is an important element of nutritional assessment in PLWH/TB. Particular micronutrients to prioritize include vitamins A and B$_{12}$, selenium, and zinc, as deficiencies of these have been associated with HIV disease progression [216, 217, 263, 267]. Deficiencies in vitamins A, E, and D, as well as iron, zinc, and selenium, are also common among individuals infected with TB [366, 402–405], and measurement of these micronutrients should be prioritized among TB patients.

## Clinical Assessment

Clinical assessment of nutritional status includes a medical history and physical examination for signs and symptoms of nutritional deficiency. The medical history identifies opportunistic infections and comorbid conditions such as diarrhea, malabsorption, coronary heart disease, diabetes mellitus, and renal and liver diseases. In addition, assessment of social status, including financial resources and access to medical care, and psychological status is important in evaluating nutritional risk [384]. A thorough physical examination, in addition to anthropometric measurements, can provide valuable information about an individual's nutritional risks that might be missed with dietary or laboratory methods and that may reveal signs of other diseases [388, 411]. Most notably, anthropometric measurements in combination with a physical examination can be used to evaluate past nutritional history without relying on self-report [412]. Protein-energy malnutrition, a sign of wasting, might be identified with loss of subcutaneous fat and temporal wasting, loss of buccal fat pads, and prominence of ribs, iliac crests, and other bones [393]. Other signs of protein deficiency include ascites, edema, hair loss, and desquamative skin rash. A joint statement by the Academy of Nutrition and Dietetics and the American Society for Parenteral and Enteral Nutrition provides detailed recommendations for standardized assessment of adult [413] and pediatric [414] malnutrition. Gerrior et al. also reviewed the signature physical signs and symptoms of micronutrient deficiencies [393].

### Clinical Assessment with PLWH/TB

Evaluating usual dietary intake and ART or anti-TB treatment regimens is essential in preventing adverse events from drug-drug and food-drug interactions, which may lead to undesirable side effects that affect tolerability and adherence to treatment and can influence drug concentrations in blood [387, 409]. Several gastrointestinal symptoms and disorders may be present as a result of HIV enteropathy, opportunistic infections, comorbidities, or side effects from ART. These complications increase the risk for malnutrition by their impact on dietary intake, malabsorption, and nutrient utilization. A host of factors may affect dietary intake in PLWH, including gastrointestinal symptoms (e.g., anorexia, nausea, vomiting, diarrhea), oral or dental diseases, and psychosocial (e.g., depression, substance abuse) and socioeconomic factors (e.g., food insecurity, poverty). Food safety practices are particularly relevant in immunocompromised groups and should be evaluated, as food- and water-borne illnesses can result in gastrointestinal disorders and chronic diseases, increasing the risk for malnutrition and death [410].

## Food-/Nutrition-Related History

Assessment of typical dietary intake is used to evaluate the adequacy of energy, macronutrient, and micronutrient intake. These tools are mainly 24-hour food recalls, food frequency questionnaires (FFQs), and dietary records. One of the most popular tools is the 24-hour food recall, where a trained interviewer asks the patient/participant to recount all food and beverage consumed in the prior 24 hours, thereby obtaining qualitative and quantitative data on foods and nutrients [412]. The use of visual aids is recommended to improve the accuracy of portion sizes. The advantages of the 24-hour food recall include the following: it is a low burden to respondents, it can be used in individuals with poor literacy, it can be performed either in-person or over the telephone, and since the patients/participants report what they are actually eating, it is possible to obtain preparation methods, ingredients, brand names of products, and culturally relevant nuances [416–418]. On the other hand, the 24-hour food recall is susceptible to intra- and inter-individual variability [418], requires well-trained interviewers and nutritional analysis software, is time- and resource-intensive [415], and is greatly affected if the past 24 hours do not reflect usual dietary patterns. In order to improve the accuracy of the 24-hour food recalls, standardized, multiple-pass methods such as the one developed by the US Department of Agriculture (USDA) [419] can aid in the recall of foods consumed and additional details [420]. The accuracy of this tool for estimating usual dietary intake can also be improved with multiple nonconsecutive 24-hour food recalls, including a weekend day, which can then be averaged.

FFQs can be used to obtain qualitative and semiquantitative information about typical food consumption patterns by assessing the consumption of food groups over a certain timeframe [412]. These tend to be well-suited for large epidemiological studies because they are simple, inexpensive, and less time-intensive than other tools and can be tailored for specific research questions and populations [417, 421]. Drawbacks include the lack of quantitative data regarding specific foods and beverages, the need for comprehensive food lists that are suited to the population (e.g., cultural foods and dishes) and research objectives, and the possibility that particular nutritive ingredients or condiments may be missed [415, 416].

Weighed food records are the most precise method to assess dietary intake; all foods and beverages consumed over a certain time period are weighed and listed in detail, in a similar fashion to 24-hour food recalls [412]. This method has a high respondent burden and requires that they are highly motivated and literate. A similar but less burdensome tool is the dietary record, or food diary (usually a 3-day record with one weekend day), which consists of detailed record-keeping of foods and beverages consumed, where portion sizes are estimated rather than weighed [412, 421]. These, too, have a high burden to respondents and are subject to incorrect portion sizes and incorrect conversions between volumes and weights and greatly depend on the commitment and literacy of respondents [412, 415]. On the other hand, they may be more precise than dietary recalls as they are not reliant on long-term memory.

### Dietary Assessment Among PLWH/TB

Fielden et al. reviewed a range of tools that can be utilized to assess dietary sufficiency and diversity in PLWH, at both the individual and household levels, each with their unique advantages and disadvantages [415]. Generally speaking, the energy and protein requirements for PLWH are as follows: 30–35 kcal/kg and 1.1–1.5 g/kg for asymptomatic PLWH, 35–40 kcal/kg and 1.5–2.0 g/kg for symptomatic PLWH, and 40–50 kcal/kg and 2.0–2.5 g/kg for PLWH who have AIDS (CD4+ cell count <200/μL), respectively [386]. The WHO recommends similar requirements for people living with TB [3].

## Conclusions

The epidemics of HIV and TB pose complex nutritional issues. Effective medical treatment is available for HIV to make it a long-term manageable condition, and TB is curable. Hence, nutritional issues related to HIV have broadened to include obesity, cardiovascular disease, and diabetes mellitus in persons with chronic HIV who are living longer with ART. While treatment of HIV and TB requires drug therapy, there is ample evidence to suggest that nutrition therapy may be of benefit in improving outcomes for both diseases. There are difficulties in some resource-limited settings in providing adequate nutrition, and challenges for the healthcare provider who wants to deliver nutrition as a part of evidence-based comprehensive care for their HIV- or TB-infected patients. In addition to medical treatment, nutrition remains a critical factor in the progression of HIV and TB and in the optimization of care.

The lack of good and useful data that can be used to develop appropriate interventions in HIV and/or TB stems in large part from the lack of awareness from medical providers and policymakers of the importance of nutrition in the optimization of care for these patients. There are too few studies with appropriate study design, rigorously defined endpoints, sample sizes, and study durations to draw definitive conclusions. Endpoints and interventions vary widely and may not be defined in the same way in different studies. A greater awareness of the importance of nutritional assessment and the need to develop targeted interventions would be of benefit for vulnerable populations throughout the world. We posit that attention to nutritional status could permit incremental improvement in overall health of PLWH and/or TB, particularly in resource-limited settings.

# References

1. Schwenk A, Macallan DC. Tuberculosis, malnutrition and wasting. Curr Opin Clin Nutr Metab Care. 2000;3(4):285–91.
2. Case A, Deaton A. Health and wealth among the poor: India and South Africa compared. Am Econ Rev. 2005;95(2):229–33.
3. World Health Organization. Guideline: nutritional care and support for patients with tuberculosis. Geneva: World Health Organization; 2013.
4. FAO, IFAD, UNICEF, WFP, WHO. The state of food security and nutrition in the world 2019. In: Safeguarding against economic slowdowns and downturns. Rome: FAO; 2019.
5. Katona P, Katona-Apte J. The interaction between nutrition and infection. Clin Infect Dis. 2008;46(10):1582–8.
6. Bourke CD, Berkley JA, Prendergast AJ. Immune dysfunction as a cause and consequence of malnutrition. Trends Immunol. 2016;37(6):386–98.
7. Hughes S, Kelly P. Interactions of malnutrition and immune impairment, with specific reference to immunity against parasites. Parasite Immunol. 2006;28(11):577–88.
8. World Health Organization. Nutrient requirements for people living with HIV/AIDS: report of a technical consultation. Geneva: World Health Organization; 2003.
9. UNAIDS. Global HIV and AIDS Statistics: 2019 Fact sheet. https://www.unaids.org/en/resources/fact-sheet. Accessed 29 Apr 2020.
10. Yuh B, Tate J, Butt AA, Crothers K, Freiberg M, Leaf D, et al. Weight change after antiretroviral therapy and mortality. Clin Infect Dis. 2015;60(12):1852–9.
11. Tang AM, Forrester J, Spiegelman D, Knox TA, Tchetgen E, Gorbach SL. Weight loss and survival in HIV-positive patients in the era of highly active antiretroviral therapy. J Acquir Immune Defic Syndr. 2002;31(2):230–6.
12. Zachariah R, Spielmann MP, Harries AD, Salaniponi FM. Moderate to severe malnutrition in patients with tuberculosis is a risk factor associated with early death. Trans R Soc Trop Med Hyg. 2002;96(3):291–4.
13. Yen YF, Chuang P, Yen M, Lin S, Chuang P, Yuan M, et al. Association of body mass index with tuberculosis mortality: a population-based follow-up study. Medicine (Baltimore). 2016;95(1):e2300.
14. Antiretroviral Therapy Cohort Collaboration. Life expectancy of individuals on combination antiretroviral therapy in high-income countries: a collaborative analysis of 14 cohort studies. Lancet. 2008;372(9635):293–9.
15. Marcus JL, Chao CR, Leyden WA, Xu L, Quesenberry CP Jr, Klein DB, et al. Narrowing the gap in life expectancy between HIV-infected and HIV-uninfected individuals with access to care. J Acquir Immune Defic Syndr. 2016;73(1):39–46.
16. Samji H, Cescon A, Hogg RS, Modur SP, Althoff KN, Buchacz K, et al. Closing the gap: increases in life expectancy among treated HIV-positive individuals in the United States and Canada. PLoS One. 2013;8(12):e81355.
17. Serrão R, Piñero C, Velez J, Coutinho D, Maltez F, Lino S, et al. Non-AIDS-related comorbidities in people living with HIV-1 aged 50 years and older: the AGING POSITIVE study. Int J Infect Dis. 2019;79:94–100.
18. Allavena C, Hanf M, Rey D, Duvivier C, BaniSadr F, Poizot-Martin I, et al. Antiretroviral exposure and comorbidities in an aging HIV-infected population: the challenge of geriatric patients. PLoS One. 2018;13(9):e0203895.

19. Fontela C, Castilla J, Juanbeltz R, Martínez-Baz I, Rivero M, O'Leary A, et al. Comorbidities and cardiovascular risk factors in an aged cohort of HIV-infected patients on antiretroviral treatment in a Spanish hospital in 2016. Postgrad Med. 2018;130(3):317–24.
20. Mateen FJ, Shinohara RT, Carone M, Miller EN, McArthur JC, Jacobson LP, et al. Neurologic disorders incidence in HIV+ vs HIV- men: multicenter AIDS Cohort Study, 1996–2011. Neurology. 2012;79(18):1873–80.
21. Casper C, Crane H, Menon M, Money D. HIV/AIDS Comorbidities: impact on cancer, noncommunicable diseases, and reproductive health. In: Holmes KK, Bertozzi S, Bloom B, Jha P, editors. Disease control priorites: major infectious diseases. 3rd ed. Washington, DC: World Bank Group; 2017.
22. Guaraldi G, Orlando G, Zona S, Menozzi M, Carli F, Garlassi E, Berti A, et al. Premature age-related comorbidities among HIV-infected persons compared with the general population. Clin Infect Dis. 2011;53(11):1120–6.
23. World Health Organization. Global tuberculosis report 2019. Geneva: World Health Organization; 2019.
24. Lin CH, et al. Tuberculosis mortality: patient characteristics and causes. BMC Infect Dis. 2014;14:5.
25. Kotler DP, Gaetz HP, Lange M, Klein EB, Holt PR. Enteropathy associated with the acquired immunodeficiency syndrome. Ann Intern Med. 1984;101(4):421–8.
26. Kotler DP, Wang J, Pierson RN. Body composition studies in patients with the acquired immunodeficiency syndrome. Am J Clin Nutr. 1985;42(6):1255–65.
27. Nahlen BL, Chu SY, Nwanyanwu OC, Berkelman RL, Martinez SA, Rullan JV. HIV wasting syndrome in the United States. AIDS. 1993;7(2):183–8.
28. Jones JL, Hanson DL, Dworkin MS, Alderton DL, Fleming PL, Kaplan JE, et al. Surveillance for AIDS-defining opportunistic illnesses, 1992–1997. MMWR CDC Surveill Summ. 1999;48(2):1–22.
29. Lee CY, Tseng YT, Lin WR, Chen YH, Tsai JJ, Wang WH, et al. AIDS-related opportunistic illnesses and early initiation of HIV care remain critical in the contemporary HAART era: a retrospective cohort study in Taiwan. BMC Infect Dis. 2018;18(1):352.
30. Siddiqui J, Phillips AL, Freedland ES, Sklar AR, Darkow T, Harley CR. Prevalence and cost of HIV-associated weight loss in a managed care population. Curr Med Res Opin. 2009;25(5):1307–17.
31. Campa A, Yang Z, Lai S, Xue L, Phillips JC, Sales S, et al. HIV-related wasting in HIV-infected drug users in the era of highly active antiretroviral therapy. Clin Infect Dis. 2005;41(8):1179–85.
32. Keithley JK, Swanson B. HIV-associated wasting. J Assoc Nurses AIDS Care. 2013;24(1 Suppl):S103–11.
33. Koethe JR, Heimburger DC. Nutritional aspects of HIV-associated wasting in sub-Saharan Africa. Am J Clin Nutr. 2010;91(4):1138S–42S.
34. Centers for Disease Control (CDC). Revision of the CDC surveillance case definition for acquired immunodeficiency syndrome. Council of State and Territorial Epidemiologists; AIDS Program, Center for Infectious Diseases. MMWR Suppl. 1987;36(1):1S–15S.
35. Wanke CA, Silva M, Knox TA, Forrester J, Speigelman D, Gorbach SL. Weight loss and wasting remain common complications in individuals infected with human immunodeficiency virus in the era of highly active antiretroviral therapy. Clin Infect Dis. 2000;31(3):803–5.
36. Mangili A, Murman DH, Zampini AM, Wanke CA. Nutrition and HIV infection: review of weight loss and wasting in the era of highly active antiretroviral therapy from the nutrition for healthy living cohort. Clin Infect Dis. 2006;42(6):836–42.
37. Grunfeld C, Kotler DP. Wasting in the acquired immunodeficiency syndrome. Semin Liver Dis. 1992;12(2):175–87.
38. Kotler D. Challenges to diagnosis of HIV-associated wasting. J Acquir Immune Defic Syndr. 2004;37(Suppl 5):S280–3.
39. Polsky B, Kotler D, Steinhart C. HIV-associated wasting in the HAART era: guidelines for assessment, diagnosis, and treatment. AIDS Patient Care STDs. 2001;15(8):411–23.
40. Kotler DP, Thea DM, Heo M, Allison DB, Engelson ES, Wang J, et al. Relative influences of sex, race, environment, and HIV infection on body composition in adults. Am J Clin Nutr. 1999;69(3):432–9.
41. Centers for Disease Control and Prevention (CDC). Revised surveillance case definition for HIV infection--United States, 2014. MMWR Recomm Rep. 2014;63(RR-03):1–10.
42. Palenicek JP, Graham NM, He YD, Hoover DA, Oishi JS, Kingsley L, et al. Weight loss prior to clinical AIDS as a predictor of survival. Multicenter AIDS Cohort Study Investigators. J Acquir Immune Defic Syndr Hum Retrovirol. 1995;10(3):366–73.
43. Malvy E, Thiébaut R, Marimoutou C, Dabis F, Groupe d'Epidemiologie Clinique du Sida en Aquitaine. Weight loss and body mass index as predictors of HIV disease progression to AIDS in adults. Aquitaine cohort, France, 1985–1997. J Am Coll Nutr. 2001;20(6):609–15.
44. Wheeler DA, Gibert CL, Launer CA, Muurahainen N, Elion RA, Abrams DI, et al. Weight loss as a predictor of survival and disease progression in HIV infection. Terry Beirn Community Programs for Clinical Research on AIDS. J Acquir Immune Defic Syndr Hum Retrovirol. 1998;18(1):80–5.
45. Macallan DC. Wasting in HIV infection and AIDS. J Nutr. 1999;129(1S Suppl):238S–42S.
46. Greene JB. Clinical approach to weight loss in the patient with HIV infection. Gastroenterol Clin N Am. 1988;17(3):573–86.

47. Macallan DC, Noble C, Baldwin C, Jebb SA, Prentice AM, Coward WA, et al. Energy expenditure and wasting in human immunodeficiency virus infection. N Engl J Med. 1995;333(2):83–8.

48. Grunfeld C, Pang M, Shimizu L, Shigenaga JK, Jensen P, Feingold KR. Resting energy expenditure, caloric intake, and short-term weight change in human immunodeficiency virus infection and the acquired immunodeficiency syndrome. Am J Clin Nutr. 1992;55(2):455–60.

49. Melchior JC, Salmon D, Rigaud D, Leport C, Bouvet E, Detruchis P, et al. Resting energy expenditure is increased in stable, malnourished HIV-infected patients. Am J Clin Nutr. 1991;53(2):437–41.

50. Melchior JC, Raguin G, Boulier A, Bouvet E, Rigaud D, Matheron S, et al. Resting energy expenditure in human immunodeficiency virus-infected patients: comparison between patients with and without secondary infections. Am J Clin Nutr. 1993;57(5):614–9.

51. Hommes MJ, Romijn JA, Endert E, Sauerwein HP. Resting energy expenditure and substrate oxidation in human immunodeficiency virus (HIV)-infected asymptomatic men: HIV affects host metabolism in the early asymptomatic stage. Am J Clin Nutr. 1991;54(2):311–5.

52. Hommes MJ, Romijn JA, Godfried MH, Schattenkerk JK, Buurman WA, Endert E, et al. Increased resting energy expenditure in human immunodeficiency virus-infected men. Metabolism. 1990;39(11):1186–90.

53. Woods MN, Spiegelman D, Knox TA, Forrester JE, Connors JL, Skinner SC, et al. Nutrient intake and body weight in a large HIV cohort that includes women and minorities. J Am Diet Assoc. 2002;102(2):203–11.

54. Williams B, Waters D, Parker K. Evaluation and treatment of weight loss in adults with HIV disease. Am Fam Physician. 1999;60(3):843–54, 857–60.

55. Macallan DC, Noble C, Baldwin C, Foskett M, McManus T, Griffin GE. Prospective analysis of patterns of weight change in stage IV human immunodeficiency virus infection. Am J Clin Nutr. 1993;58(3):417–24.

56. Koethe JR, Heimburger DC, PrayGod G, Filteau S. From wasting to obesity: the contribution of nutritional status to immune activation in HIV infection. J Infect Dis. 2016;214(Suppl 2):S75–82.

57. Evans WJ, Morley JE, Argilés J, Bales C, Baracos V, Guttridge D, et al. Cachexia: a new definition. Clin Nutr. 2008;27(6):793–9.

58. Kotler DP. Cachexia. Ann Intern Med. 2000;133(8):622–34.

59. Roubenoff R, Grinspoon S, Skolnik PR, Tchetgen E, Abad L, Spiegelman D, et al. Role of cytokines and testosterone in regulating lean body mass and resting energy expenditure in HIV-infected men. Am J Physiol Endocrinol Metab. 2002;283(1):E138–45.

60. Abad LW, Schmitz HR, Parker R, Roubenoff R. Cytokine responses differ by compartment and wasting status in patients with HIV infection and healthy controls. Cytokine. 2002;18(5):286–93.

61. Salomon J, de Truchis P, Melchior JC. Body composition and nutritional parameters in HIV and AIDS patients. Clin Chem Lab Med. 2002;40(12):1329–33.

62. Ott M, Lembcke B, Fischer H, Jäger R, Polat H, Geier H, et al. Early changes of body composition in human immunodeficiency virus-infected patients: tetrapolar body impedance analysis indicates significant malnutrition. Am J Clin Nutr. 1993;57(1):15–9.

63. Kotler DP, Tierney AR, Wang J, Pierson RN Jr. Magnitude of body-cell-mass depletion and the timing of death from wasting in AIDS. Am J Clin Nutr. 1989;50(3):444–7.

64. Batman PA, Miller AR, Forster SM, Harris JR, Pinching AJ, Griffin GE. Jejunal enteropathy associated with human immunodeficiency virus infection: quantitative histology. J Clin Pathol. 1989;42(3):275–81.

65. Gazzard BG. HIV disease and the gastroenterologist. Gut. 1988;29(11):1497–505.

66. Lim SG, Lipman MC, Squire S, Pillay D, Gillespie S, Sankey EA, et al. Audit of endoscopic surveillance biopsy specimens in HIV positive patients with gastrointestinal symptoms. Gut. 1993;34(10):1429–32.

67. Thompson T, Lee MG, Clarke T, Mills M, Wharfe G, Walters C. Prevalence of gastrointestinal symptoms among ambulatory HIV patients and a control population. Ann Gastroenterol. 2012;25(3):243–8.

68. May GR, Gill MJ, Church DL, Sutherland LR. Gastrointestinal symptoms in ambulatory HIV-infected patients. Dig Dis Sci. 1993;38(8):1388–94.

69. Norval DA. Symptoms and sites of pain experienced by AIDS patients. S Afr Med J. 2004;94(6):450–4.

70. Antony MA, Brandt LJ, Klein RS, Bernstein LH. Infectious diarrhea in patients with AIDS. Dig Dis Sci. 1988;33(9):1141–6.

71. Katabira ET. Epidemiology and management of diarrheal disease in HIV-infected patients. Int J Infect Dis. 1999;3(3):164–7.

72. Kelly P, Baboo KS, Wolff M, Ngwenya B, Luo N, Farthing MJ. The prevalence and aetiology of persistent diarrhoea in adults in urban Zambia. Acta Trop. 1996;61(3):183–90.

73. Call SA, Heudebert G, Saag M, Wilcox CM. The changing etiology of chronic diarrhea in HIV-infected patients with CD4 cell counts less than 200 cells/mm3. Am J Gastroenterol. 2000;95(11):3142–6.

74. Mönkemüller KE, Call SA, Lazenby AJ, Wilcox CM. Declining prevalence of opportunistic gastrointestinal disease in the era of combination antiretroviral therapy. Am J Gastroenterol. 2000;95(2):457–62.

75. Hill A, Balkin A. Risk factors for gastrointestinal adverse events in HIV treated and untreated patients. AIDS Rev. 2009;11(1):30–8.

76. Asmuth DM, Clay P, Blick G, Chaturvedi P, MacFarlane K. Incidence and prevalence of diarrhea in HIV clinical trials in the recent post-cART era: analysis of data from 38 clinical trials from 2008–2017 in over 21,000 patients. In: 22nd International AIDS Conference. Amsterdam: National AIDS Treatment Advocacy Project; 2018.

77. Prosperi MCF, Fabbiani M, Fanti I, Zaccarelli M, Colafigli M, Mondi A, et al. Predictors of first-line antiretroviral therapy discontinuation due to drug-related adverse events in HIV-infected patients: a retrospective cohort study. BMC Infect Dis. 2012;12:296.

78. Chubineh S, McGowan J. Nausea and vomiting in HIV: a symptom review. Int J STD AIDS. 2008;19(11):723–8.

79. MacArthur RD, DuPont HL. Etiology and pharmacologic management of noninfectious diarrhea in HIV-infected individuals in the highly active antiretroviral therapy era. Clin Infect Dis. 2012;55(6):860–7.

80. Siddiqui U, Bini EJ, Chandarana K, Leong J, Ramsetty S, Schiliro D, et al. Prevalence and impact of diarrhea on health-related quality of life in HIV-infected patients in the era of highly active antiretroviral therapy. J Clin Gastroenterol. 2007;41(5):484–90.

81. Tramarin A, Parise N, Campostrini S, Yin DD, Postma MJ, Lyu R, et al. Association between diarrhea and quality of life in HIV-infected patients receiving highly active antiretroviral therapy. Qual Life Res. 2004;13(1):243–50.

82. Connolly GM, Shanson D, Hawkins DA, Webster JN, Gazzard BG. Non-cryptosporidial diarrhoea in human immunodeficiency virus (HIV) infected patients. Gut. 1989;30(2):195–200.

83. Colebunders R, Lusakumuni K, Nelson AM, Gigase P, Lebughe I, van Marck E, et al. Persistent diarrhoea in Zairian AIDS patients: an endoscopic and histological study. Gut. 1988;29(12):1687–91.

84. Ullrich R, Zeitz M, Heise W, L'age M, Hoffken G, Riecken EO. Small intestinal structure and function in patients infected with human immunodeficiency virus (HIV): evidence for HIV-induced enteropathy. Ann Intern Med. 1989;111(1):15–21.

85. Cummins AG, LaBrooy JT, Stanley DP, Rowland R, Shearman DJ. Quantitative histological study of enteropathy associated with HIV infection. Gut. 1990;31(3):317–21.

86. Clayton F, Snow G, Reka S, Kotler DP. Selective depletion of rectal lamina propria rather than lymphoid aggregate CD4 lymphocytes in HIV infection. Clin Exp Immunol. 1997;107(2):288–92.

87. Zeitz M, Ullrich R, Schneider T, Kewenig S, Hohloch K, Riecken EO. HIV/SIV enteropathy. Ann N Y Acad Sci. 1998;859:139–48.

88. Francis N. Light and electron microscopic appearances of pathological changes in HIV gut infection. Baillieres Clin Gastroenterol. 1990;4(2):495–527.

89. Brenchley JM, Douek DC. HIV infection and the gastrointestinal immune system. Mucosal Immunol. 2008;1(1):23–30.

90. Crum-Cianflone NF. HIV and the gastrointestinal tract. Infect Dis Clin Pract (Baltim Md). 2010;18(5):283–5.

91. Clayton F, Reka S, Cronin WJ, Torlakovic E, Sigal SH, Kotler DP. Rectal mucosal pathology varies with human immunodeficiency virus antigen content and disease stage. Gastroenterology. 1992;103(3):919–33.

92. Rodgers VD, Fassett R, Kagnoff MF. Abnormalities in intestinal mucosal-T cells in homosexual populations including those with the lymphadenopathy syndrome and acquired-immunodeficiency-syndrome. Gastroenterology. 1986;90(3):552–8.

93. Brenchley JM, Schacker TW, Ruff LE, Price DA, Taylor JH, Beilman GJ, et al. CD4(+) T cell depletion during all stages of HIV disease occurs predominantly in the gastrointestinal tract. J Exp Med. 2004;200(6):749–59.

94. Mehandru S, Poles MA, Tenner-Racz K, Jean-Pierre P, Manuelli V, Lopez P, et al. Lack of mucosal immune reconstitution during prolonged treatment of acute and early HIV-1 infection. PLoS Med. 2006;3(12):e484.

95. Guadalupe M, Sankaran S, George MD, Reay E, Verhoeven D, Shacklett BL, et al. Viral suppression and immune restoration in the gastrointestinal mucosa of human immunodeficiency virus type 1-infected patients initiating therapy during primary or chronic infection. J Virol. 2006;80(16):8236–47.

96. Asmuth DM, Ma ZM, Mann S, Knight TH, Yotter T, Albanese A, et al. Gastrointestinal-associated lymphoid tissue immune reconstitution in a randomized clinical trial of raltegravir versus non-nucleoside reverse transcriptase inhibitor-based regimens. AIDS. 2012;26(13):1625–34.

97. Ehrenpreis ED, Ganger DR, Kochvar GT, Patterson BK, Craig RM. D-xylose malabsorption: characteristic finding in patients with the AIDS wasting syndrome and chronic diarrhea. J Acquir Immune Defic Syndr (1988). 1992;5(10):1047–50.

98. Carbonnel F, Beaugerie L, Rached A, D'Almagne H, Rozenbaum W, Le Quintrec Y, et al. Macronutrient intake and malabsorption in HIV infection: a comparison with other malabsorptive states. Gut. 1997;41(6):805–10.

99. Gillin JS, Shike M, Alcock N, Urmacher C, Krown S, Kurtz RC, et al. Malabsorption and mucosal abnormalities of the small-intestine in the acquired immunodeficiency syndrome. Ann Intern Med. 1985;102(5):619–22.

100. Keating J, Bjarnason I, Somasundaram S, Macpherson A, Francis N, Price AB, et al. Intestinal absorptive-capacity, intestinal permeability and jejunal histology in HIV and their relation to diarrhea. Gut. 1995;37(5):623–9.

101. Rabeneck L, Popovic M, Gartner S, McLean DM, McLeod WA, Read E, et al. Acute HIV infection presenting with painful swallowing and esophageal ulcers. JAMA. 1990;263(17):2318–22.

102. Miller AR, Griffin GE, Batman P, Farquar C, Forster SM, Pinching AJ, et al. Jejunal mucosal architecture and fat absorption in male homosexuals infected with human immunodeficiency virus. Q J Med. 1988;69(260):1009–19.

103. Kapembwa MS, Bridges C, Joseph AE, Fleming SC, Batman P, Griffin GE. Ileal and jejunal absorptive function in patients with AIDS and enterococcidial infection. J Infect. 1990;21(1):43–53.

104. Kotler DP, Reka S, Chow K, Orenstein JM. Effects of enteric parasitoses and HIV infection upon small intestinal structure and function in patients with AIDS. J Clin Gastroenterol. 1993;16(1):10–5.

105. Lim SG, Menzies IS, Lee CA, Johnson MA, Pounder RE. Intestinal permeability and function in patients infected with human immunodeficiency virus. A comparison with coeliac disease. Scand J Gastroenterol. 1993;28(7):573–80.

106. Church DL, Sutherland LR, Gill MJ, Visser ND, Kelly JK. Absence of an association between enteric parasites in the manifestations and pathogenesis of HIV enteropathy in gay men. The GI/HIV Study Group. Scand J Infect Dis. 1992;24(5):567–75.

107. Knox TA, Spiegelman D, Skinner SC, Gorbach S. Diarrhea and abnormalities of gastrointestinal function in a cohort of men and women with HIV infection. Am J Gastroenterol. 2000;95(12):3482–9.

108. Dworkin B, Wormser GP, Rosenthal WS, Heier SK, Braunstein M, Weiss L. Gastrointestinal manifestations of the acquired immunodeficiency syndrome: a review of 22 cases. Am J Gastroenterol. 1985;80(10):774–8.

109. Duggal S, Chugh TD, Duggal AK. HIV and malnutrition: effects on immune system. Clin Dev Immunol. 2012;2012:784740.

110. Poles MA, Fuerst M, McGowan I, Elliott J, Rezaei A, Mark D, et al. HIV-related diarrhea is multifactorial and fat malabsorption is commonly present, independent of HAART. Am J Gastroenterol. 2001;96(6):1831–7.

111. Singhal N, Austin J. A clinical review of micronutrients in HIV infection. J Int Assoc Physicians AIDS Care (Chic). 2002;1(2):63–75.

112. Lambl BB, Federman M, Pleskow D, Wanke CA. Malabsorption and wasting in AIDS patients with microsporidia and pathogen-negative diarrhea. AIDS. 1996;10(7):739–44.

113. Paltiel O, Falutz J, Veilleux M, Rosenblatt DS, Gordon K. Clinical correlates of subnormal vitamin B12 levels in patients infected with the human immunodeficiency virus. Am J Hematol. 1995;49(4):318–22.

114. Ehrenpreis ED, Carlson SJ, Boorstein HL, Craig RM. Malabsorption and deficiency of vitamin B12 in HIV-infected patients with chronic diarrhea. Dig Dis Sci. 1994;39(10):2159–62.

115. Laine L, Garcia F, McGilligan K, Malinko A, Sinatra FR, Thomas DW. Protein-losing enteropathy and hypoalbuminemia in AIDS. AIDS. 1993;7(6):837–40.

116. Kotler DP. Human immunodeficiency virus-related wasting: malabsorption syndromes. Semin Oncol. 1998;25(2 Suppl 6):70–5.

117. Jiménez-Expósito MJ, García-Lorda P, Alonso-Villaverde C, de Vírgala CM, Solà R, Masana L, et al. Effect of malabsorption on nutritional status and resting energy expenditure in HIV-infected patients. AIDS. 1998;12(15):1965–72.

118. Wohl DA, McComsey G, Tebas P, Brown TT, Glesby MJ, Reeds D, et al. Current concepts in the diagnosis and management of metabolic complications of HIV infection and its therapy. Clin Infect Dis. 2006;43(5):645–53.

119. Baril JG, Junod P, Leblanc R, Dion H, Therrien R, Laplante F, et al. HIV-associated lipodystrophy syndrome: a review of clinical aspects. Can J Infect Dis Med Microbiol. 2005;16(4):233–43.

120. Introcaso CE, Hines JM, Kovarik CL. Cutaneous toxicities of antiretroviral therapy for HIV: part I. Lipodystrophy syndrome, nucleoside reverse transcriptase inhibitors, and protease inhibitors. J Am Acad Dermatol. 2010;63(4):549–61; quiz 561–2.

121. Lake JE, Stanley TL, Apovian CM, Bhasin S, Brown TT, Capeau J, et al. Practical review of recognition and management of obesity and lipohypertrophy in human immunodeficiency virus infection. Clin Infect Dis. 2017;64(10):1422–9.

122. Mallal SA, John M, Moore CB, James IR, McKinnon EJ. Contribution of nucleoside analogue reverse transcriptase inhibitors to subcutaneous fat wasting in patients with HIV infection. AIDS. 2000;14(10):1309–16.

123. Carr A, Miller J, Law M, Cooper DA. A syndrome of lipoatrophy, lactic acidaemia and liver dysfunction associated with HIV nucleoside analogue therapy: contribution to protease inhibitor-related lipodystrophy syndrome. AIDS. 2000;14(3):F25–32.

124. Saint-Marc T, Partisani M, Poizot-Martin I, Bruno F, Rouviere O, Lang JM, Gastaut JA, et al. A syndrome of peripheral fat wasting (lipodystrophy) in patients receiving long-term nucleoside analogue therapy. AIDS. 1999;13(13):1659–67.

125. Brinkman K, Smeitink JA, Romijn JA, Reiss P. Mitochondrial toxicity induced by nucleoside-analogue reverse-transcriptase inhibitors is a key factor in the pathogenesis of antiretroviral-therapy-related lipodystrophy. Lancet. 1999;354(9184):1112–5.

126. Damouche A, Lazure T, Avettand-Fènoël V, Huot N, Dejucq-Rainsford N, Satie AP, et al. Adipose tissue is a neglected viral reservoir and an inflammatory site during chronic HIV and SIV infection. PLoS Pathog. 2015;11(9):e1005153.

127. Vidal F, Domingo P, Villarroya F, Giralt M, López-Dupla M, Gutiérrez M, et al. Adipogenic/lipid, inflammatory, and mitochondrial parameters in subcutaneous adipose tissue of untreated HIV-1-infected long-term nonprogressors: significant alterations despite low viral burden. J Acquir Immune Defic Syndr. 2012;61(2):131–7.

128. Agarwal N, Balasubramanyam A. Viral mechanisms of adipose dysfunction: lessons from HIV-1 Vpr. Adipocytes. 2015;4(1):55–9.

129. Miller J, Carr A, Emery S, Law M, Mallal S, Baker D, et al. HIV lipodystrophy: prevalence, severity and correlates of risk in Australia. HIV Med. 2003;4(3):293–301.

130. Palella FJ Jr, Cole SR, Chmiel JS, Riddler SA, Visscher B, Dobs A, et al. Anthropometrics and examiner-reported body habitus abnormalities in the multicenter AIDS cohort study. Clin Infect Dis. 2004;38(6):903–7.

131. Kotler DP, Rosenbaum K, Wang J, Pierson RN. Studies of body composition and fat distribution in HIV-infected and control subjects. J Acquir Immune Defic Syndr Hum Retrovirol. 1999;20(3):228–37.

132. Hadigan C, Meigs JB, Corcoran C, Rietschel P, Piecuch S, Basgoz N, et al. Metabolic abnormalities and cardiovascular disease risk factors in adults with human immunodeficiency virus infection and lipodystrophy. Clin Infect Dis. 2001;32(1):130–9.

133. Mallon PW, Miller J, Cooper DA, Carr A. Prospective evaluation of the effects of antiretroviral therapy on body composition in HIV-1-infected men starting therapy. AIDS. 2003;17(7):971–9.

134. Galescu O, Bhangoo A, Ten S. Insulin resistance, lipodystrophy and cardiometabolic syndrome in HIV/AIDS. Rev Endocr Metab Disord. 2013;14(2):133–40.

135. Grinspoon S. Insulin resistance in the HIV-lipodystrophy syndrome. Trends Endocrinol Metab. 2001;12(9):413–9.

136. Gelpi M, Afzal S, Lundgren J, Ronit A, Roen A, Mocroft A, et al. Higher risk of abdominal obesity, elevated low-density lipoprotein cholesterol, and hypertriglyceridemia, but not of hypertension, in people living with human immunodeficiency virus (HIV): results from the Copenhagen comorbidity in HIV infection study. Clin Infect Dis. 2018;67(4):579–86.

137. Beraldo RA, Santos APD, Guimarães MP, Vassimon HS, Paula FJA, Machado DRL, et al. Body fat redistribution and changes in lipid and glucose metabolism in people living with HIV/AIDS. Rev Bras Epidemiol. 2017;20(3):526–36.

138. Scherzer R, Heymsfield SB, Lee D, Powderly WG, Tien PC, Bacchetti P, et al. Decreased limb muscle and increased central adiposity are associated with 5-year all-cause mortality in HIV infection. AIDS. 2011;25(11):1405–14.

139. Hadigan C, Meigs JB, Wilson PW, D'Agostino RB, Davis B, Basgoz N, et al. Prediction of coronary heart disease risk in HIV-infected patients with fat redistribution. Clin Infect Dis. 2003;36(7):909–16.

140. Hasse B, Iff M, Ledergerber B, Calmy A, Schmid P, Hauser C, et al. Obesity trends and body mass index changes after starting antiretroviral treatment: the Swiss HIV Cohort Study. Open Forum Infect Dis. 2014;1(2):ofu040.

141. Crum-Cianflone N, Roediger MP, Eberly L, Headd M, Marconi V, Ganesan A, et al. Increasing rates of obesity among HIV-infected persons during the HIV epidemic. PLoS One. 2010;5(4):e10106.

142. Pourcher G, Costagliola D, Martinez V. Obesity in HIV-infected patients in France: prevalence and surgical treatment options. J Visc Surg. 2015;152(1):33–7.

143. Jaff NG, Norris SA, Snyman T, Toman M, Crowther NJ. Body composition in the Study of Women Entering and in Endocrine Transition (SWEET): a perspective of African women who have a high prevalence of obesity and HIV infection. Metabolism. 2015;64(9):1031–41.

144. Bärnighausen T, Welz T, Hosegood V, Bätzing-Feigenbaum J, Tanser F, Herbst K, et al. Hiding in the shadows of the HIV epidemic: obesity and hypertension in a rural population with very high HIV prevalence in South Africa. J Hum Hypertens. 2008;22(3):236–9.

145. Ezechi LO, Musa ZA, Otobo VO, Idigbe IE, Ezechi OC. Trends and risk factors for obesity among HIV positive Nigerians on antiretroviral therapy. Ceylon Med J. 2016;61(2):56–62.

146. Nguyen KA, Peer N, de Villiers A, Mukasa B, Matsha TE, Mills EJ, et al. The distribution of obesity phenotypes in HIV-infected African population. Nutrients. 2016;8(6):299.

147. Koethe JR, Jenkins CA, Lau B, Shepherd BE, Justice AC, Tate JP, et al. Rising obesity prevalence and weight gain among adults starting antiretroviral therapy in the United States and Canada. AIDS Res Hum Retrovir. 2016;32(1):50–8.

148. Biggs C, Spooner E. Obesity and HIV: a compounding problem. South Afr J Clin Nutr. 2018;31(4):78–83.

149. Guehi C, Badjé A, Gabillard D, Ouattara E, Koulé SO, Moh R, et al. High prevalence of being overweight and obese HIV-infected persons, before and after 24 months on early ART in the ANRS 12136 Temprano Trial. AIDS Res Ther. 2016;13:12.

150. Swinburn BA, Sacks G, Hall KD, McPherson K, Finegood DT, Moodie ML, et al. The global obesity pandemic: shaped by global drivers and local environments. Lancet. 2011;378(9793):804–14.

151. Martinez SS, Campa A, Bussmann H, Moyo S, Makhema J, Huffman FG, et al. Effect of BMI and fat mass on HIV disease progression in HIV-infected, antiretroviral treatment-naive adults in Botswana. Br J Nutr. 2016;115(12):2114–21.

152. Shor-Posner G, Campa A, Zhang G, Persaud N, Miguez-Burbano MJ, Quesada J, et al. When obesity is desirable: a longitudinal study of the Miami HIV-1-infected drug abusers (MIDAS) cohort. J Acquir Immune Defic Syndr. 2000;23(1):81–8.

153. Jones CY, Hogan JW, Snyder B, Klein RS, Rompalo A, Schuman P, et al. Overweight and human immunodeficiency virus (HIV) progression in women: associations HIV disease progression and changes in body mass index in women in the HIV Epidemiology Research Study cohort. Clin Infect Dis. 2003;37:S69–80.

154. Crum-Cianflone NF, Roediger M, Eberly LE, Ganesan A, Weintrob A, Johnson E, et al. Impact of weight on immune cell counts among HIV-infected persons. Clin Vaccine Immunol. 2011;18(6):940–6.

155. Blashill AJ, Mayer KH, Crane HM, Grasso C, Safren SA. Body mass index, immune status, and virological control in HIV-infected men who have sex with men. J Int Assoc Provid AIDS Care. 2013;12(5):319–24.

156. Tedaldi EM, Brooks JT, Weidle PJ, Richardson JT, Baker RK, Buchacz K, et al. Increased body mass index does not alter response to initial highly active antiretroviral therapy in HIV-1-infected patients. J Acquir Immune Defic Syndr. 2006;43(1):35–41.

157. Koethe JR, Jenkins CA, Shepherd BE, Stinnette SE, Sterling TR. An optimal body mass index range associated with improved immune reconstitution among HIV-infected adults initiating antiretroviral therapy. Clin Infect Dis. 2011;53(9):952–60.

158. Lake JE. The fat of the matter: obesity and visceral adiposity in treated HIV infection. Curr HIV/AIDS Rep. 2017;14(6):211–9.

159. Prado C, Gonzalez MC, Heymsfield SB. Body composition phenotypes and obesity paradox. Curr Opin Clin Nutr Metab Care. 2015;18(6):535–51.

160. Brown TT, Xu X, John M, Singh J, Kingsley LA, Palella FJ, et al. Fat distribution and longitudinal anthropometric changes in HIV-infected men with and without clinical evidence of lipodystrophy and HIV-uninfected controls: a substudy of the Multicenter AIDS Cohort Study. AIDS Res Ther. 2009;6:8–8.

161. Joy T, Keogh HM, Hadigan C, Dolan SE, Fitch K, Liebau J, et al. Relation of body composition to body mass index in HIV-infected patients with metabolic abnormalities. J Acquir Immune Defic Syndr. 2008;47(2):174–84.

162. Sheu NW, Lin YC, Chen CJ. Mechanisms, pathophysiology, and management of obesity. N Engl J Med. 2017;376(15):1490.

163. Sirotin N, Hoover DR, Shi Q, Anastos K, Weiser SD. Food insecurity with hunger is associated with obesity among HIV-infected and at risk women in Bronx, NY. PLoS One. 2014;9(8):e105957.

164. Derose KP, Ríos-Castillo I, Fulcar MA, Payán DD, Palar K, Escala L, et al. Severe food insecurity is associated with overweight and increased body fat among people living with HIV in the Dominican Republic. AIDS Care. 2018;30(2):182–90.

165. Kruzich LA, Marquis GS, Wilson CM, Stephensen CB. HIV-infected US youth are at high risk of obesity and poor diet quality: a challenge for improving short- and long-term health outcomes. J Am Diet Assoc. 2004;104(10):1554–60.

166. Duran AC, Almeida LB, Segurado AA, Jaime PC. Diet quality of persons living with HIV/AIDS on highly active antiretroviral therapy. J Hum Nutr Diet. 2008;21(4):346–50.

167. Hendricks KM, Willis K, Houser R, Jones CY. Obesity in HIV-infection: dietary correlates. J Am Coll Nutr. 2006;25(4):321–31.

168. Obry-Roguet V, Brégigeon S, Cano CE, Lions C, Zaegel-Faucher O, Laroche H, et al. Risk factors associated with overweight and obesity in HIV-infected people: aging, behavioral factors but not cART in a cross-sectional study. Medicine (Baltimore). 2018;97(23):e10956.

169. Bares SH, Smeaton LM, Xu A, Godfrey C, McComsey GA. HIV-infected women gain more weight than HIV-infected men following the initiation of antiretroviral therapy. J Womens Health (Larchmt). 2018;27(9):1162–9.

170. Thompson-Paul AM, Wei SC, Mattson CL, Robertson M, Hernandez-Romieu AC, Bell TK, et al. Obesity among HIV-infected adults receiving medical care in the United States: data from the cross-sectional medical monitoring project and national health and nutrition examination survey. Medicine (Baltimore). 2015;94(27):e1081.

171. Bakal DR, Coelho LE, Luz PM, Clark JL, De Boni RB, Cardoso SW, et al. Obesity following ART initiation is common and influenced by both traditional and HIV-/ART-specific risk factors. J Antimicrob Chemother. 2018;73(8):2177–85.

172. Tate T, Willig AL, Willig JH, Raper JL, Moneyham L, Kempf MC, et al. HIV infection and obesity: where did all the wasting go? Antivir Ther. 2012;17(7):1281–9.

173. Nduka CU, Uthman OA, Kimani PK, Stranges S. Body fat changes in people living with HIV on antiretroviral therapy. AIDS Rev. 2016;18(4):198–211.

174. Sax PE, Erlandson KM, Lake JE, Mccomsey GA, Orkin C, Esser S, et al. Weight gain following initiation of antiretroviral therapy: risk factors in randomized comparative clinical trials. Clin Infect Dis:ciz999. https://doi.org/10.1093/cid/ciz999.

175. Madelain V, Le MP, Champenois K, Charpentier C, Landman R, Joly V, et al. Impact of obesity on antiretroviral pharmacokinetics and immuno-virological response in HIV-infected patients: a case-control study. J Antimicrob Chemother. 2017;72(4):1137–46.
176. Via M. The malnutrition of obesity: micronutrient deficiencies that promote diabetes. ISRN Endocrinol. 2012;2012:103472.
177. Kaidar-Person O, Person B, Szomstein S, Rosenthal RJ. Nutritional deficiencies in morbidly obese patients: a new form of malnutrition? Part A: vitamins. Obes Surg. 2008;18(7):870–6.
178. Kaidar-Person O, Person B, Szomstein S, Rosenthal RJ. Nutritional deficiencies in morbidly obese patients: a new form of malnutrition? Part B: minerals. Obes Surg. 2008;18(8):1028–34.
179. Gregor MF, Hotamisligil GS. Inflammatory mechanisms in obesity. Annu Rev Immunol. 2011;29:415–45.
180. Andersen CJ, Murphy KE, Fernandez ML. Impact of obesity and metabolic syndrome on immunity. Adv Nutr. 2016;7(1):66–75.
181. Huttunen R, Syrjanen J. Obesity and the risk and outcome of infection. Int J Obes. 2013;37(3):333–40.
182. Huttunen R, Syrjanen J. Obesity and the outcome of infection. Lancet Infect Dis. 2010;10(7):442–3.
183. Falagas ME, Athanasoulia AP, Peppas G, Karageorgopoulos DE. Effect of body mass index on the outcome of infections: a systematic review. Obes Rev. 2009;10(3):280–9.
184. Couturier J, Lewis DE. HIV persistence in adipose tissue reservoirs. Curr HIV/AIDS Rep. 2018;15(1):60–71.
185. Lemoine M, Lacombe K, Bastard JP, Sébire M, Fonquernie L, Valin N, et al. Metabolic syndrome and obesity are the cornerstones of liver fibrosis in HIV-monoinfected patients. AIDS. 2017;31(14):1955–64.
186. Croxford S, Kitching A, Desai S, Kall M, Edelstein M, Skingsley A, et al. Mortality and causes of death in people diagnosed with HIV in the era of highly active antiretroviral therapy compared with the general population: an analysis of a national observational cohort. Lancet Public Health. 2017;2(1):e35–46.
187. Masiá M, Padilla S, Álvarez D, López JC, Santos I, Soriano V, et al. Risk, predictors, and mortality associated with non-AIDS events in newly diagnosed HIV-infected patients: role of antiretroviral therapy. AIDS. 2013;27(2):181–9.
188. Pettit AC, Giganti MJ, Ingle SM, May MT, Shepherd BE, Gill MJ, et al. Increased non-AIDS mortality among persons with AIDS-defining events after antiretroviral therapy initiation. J Int AIDS Soc. 2018;21
189. Keen L 2nd, Khan M, Clifford L, Harrell PT, Latimer WW. Injection and non-injection drug use and infectious disease in Baltimore City: differences by race. Addict Behav. 2014;39(9):1325–8.
190. Peng EY, Yeh CY, Cheng SH, Morisky DE, Lan YC, Chen YM, et al. A case-control study of HIV infection among incarcerated female drug users: impact of sharing needles and having drug-using sexual partners. J Formos Med Assoc. 2011;110(7):446–53.
191. Kral AH, Bluthenthal RN, Lorvick J, Gee L, Bacchetti P, Edlin BR. Sexual transmission of HIV-1 among injection drug users in San Francisco, USA: risk-factor analysis. Lancet. 2001;357(9266):1397–401.
192. Strathdee SA, Galai N, Safaiean M, Celentano DD, Vlahov D, Johnson L, et al. Sex differences in risk factors for HIV seroconversion among injection drug users: a 10-year perspective. Arch Intern Med. 2001;161(10):1281–8.
193. Windle M. The trading of sex for money or drugs, sexually transmitted diseases (STDs), and HIV-related risk behaviors among multisubstance using alcoholic inpatients. Drug Alcohol Depend. 1997;49(1):33–8.
194. Persaud N, Klaskala W, Baum M, Duncan R. Sexually transmitted infections, drug use, and risky sex among female sex workers in Guyana. Sex Transm Infect. 2000;76(4):318.
195. Miguez MJ, Page B, Baum MK. Illegal drug use and HIV-1 infection in Columbia. Lancet. 1997;350(9091):1635.
196. Pufall EL, Kall M, Shahmanesh M, Nardone A, Gilson R, Delpech V, et al. Sexualized drug use ('chemsex') and high-risk sexual behaviours in HIV-positive men who have sex with men. HIV Med. 2018;19(4):261–70.
197. Bourne A, Reid D, Hickson F, Torres-Rueda S, Weatherburn P, et al. Illicit drug use in sexual settings ('chemsex') and HIV/STI transmission risk behaviour among gay men in South London: findings from a qualitative study. Sex Transm Infect. 2015;91(8):564–8.
198. Lucas GM. Substance abuse, adherence with antiretroviral therapy, and clinical outcomes among HIV-infected individuals. Life Sci. 2011;88(21–22):948–52.
199. Baum MK, Rafie C, Lai S, Sales S, Page JB, Campa A. Alcohol use accelerates HIV disease progression. AIDS Res Hum Retrovir. 2010;26(5):511–8.
200. Baum MK, Rafie C, Lai S, Sales S, Page B, Campa A. Crack-cocaine use accelerates HIV disease progression in a cohort of HIV-positive drug users. J Acquir Immune Defic Syndr. 2009;50(1):93–9.
201. United Nations Office on Drugs and Crime. HIV Prevention, treatment, care and support for people who use stimulant drugs. Technical guide. Vienna: UNODC; 2019: Vienna. https://www.unodc.org/documents/hiv-aids/publications/People_who_use_drugs/19-04568_HIV_Prevention_Guide_ebook.pdf. Accessed 4 May 2020.
202. UNAIDS. UNAIDS data 2019: reference report. 2019.
203. Centers for Disease Control and Prevention, HIV Surveillance Report, 2017. 2018.
204. Nelson PK, Mathers BM, Cowie B, Hagan H, Des Jarlais D, Horyniak D, et al. Global epidemiology of hepatitis B and hepatitis C in people who inject drugs: results of systematic reviews. Lancet. 2011;378(9791):571–83.

205. United Nations, World Drug Report 2018, in Sales No. E.18.XI.9. 2018.
206. Degenhardt L, Peacock A, Colledge S, Leung J, Grebely J, Vickerman P, et al. Global prevalence of injecting drug use and sociodemographic characteristics and prevalence of HIV, HBV, and HCV in people who inject drugs: a multistage systematic review. Lancet Glob Health. 2017;5(12):e1192–207.
207. World Health Organization. Integrating collaborative TB and HIV services within a comprehensive package of care for people who inject drugs: consolidated guidelines. Geneva: WHO; 2016.
208. Gadalla T, Piran N. Eating disorders and substance abuse in Canadian men and women: a national study. Eat Disord. 2007;15(3):189–203.
209. Cohen LR, Greenfield SF, Gordon S, Killeen T, Jiang H, Zhang Y, et al. Survey of eating disorder symptoms among women in treatment for substance abuse. Am J Addict. 2010;19(3):245–51.
210. Saeland M, Haugen M, Eriksen FL, Wandel M, Smehaugen A, Böhmer T, et al. High sugar consumption and poor nutrient intake among drug addicts in Oslo, Norway. Br J Nutr. 2011;105(4):618–24.
211. Neale J, Nettleton S, Pickering L, Fischer J. Eating patterns among heroin users: a qualitative study with implications for nutritional interventions. Addiction. 2012;107(3):635–41.
212. Cowan J, Devine C. Food, eating, and weight concerns of men in recovery from substance addiction. Appetite. 2008;50(1):33–42.
213. Himmelgreen DA, Pérez-Escamilla R, Segura-Millán S, Romero-Daza N, Tanasescu M, Singer M. A comparison of the nutritional status and food security of drug-using and non-drug-using Hispanic women in Hartford, Connecticut. Am J Phys Anthropol. 1998;107(3):351–61.
214. Nazrul Islam SK, Jahangir Hossain K, Ahsan M. Serum vitamin E, C and A status of the drug addicts undergoing detoxification: influence of drug habit, sexual practice and lifestyle factors. Eur J Clin Nutr. 2001;55(11):1022–7.
215. el-Nakah A, Frank O, Louria DB, Quinones MA, Baker H. A vitamin profile of heroin addiction. Am J Public Health. 1979;69(10):1058–60.
216. Baum MK, Campa A, Lai S, Lai H, Page JB. Zinc status in human immunodeficiency virus type 1 infection and illicit drug use. Clin Infect Dis. 2003;37(Suppl 2):S117–23.
217. Semba RD, Caiaffa WT, Graham NM, Cohn S, Vlahov D. Vitamin A deficiency and wasting as predictors of mortality in human immunodeficiency virus-infected injection drug users. J Infect Dis. 1995;171(5):1196–202.
218. Santolaria-Fernández FJ, Gómez-Sirvent JL, González-Reimers CE, Batista-López JN, Jorge-Hernández JA, Rodríguez-Moreno F, et al. Nutritional assessment of drug addicts. Drug Alcohol Depend. 1995;38(1):11–8.
219. Karajibani M, Montazerifar F, Shakiba M. Evaluation of nutritional status in drug users referred to the center of drug dependency treatment in Zahedan. Int J High Risk Behav Addict. 2012;1(1):18–21.
220. Baum MK, Campa A, Page JB, Lai S, Tsalaile L, Martinez SS, et al. Recruitment, follow-up and characteristics of HIV infected adults who use illicit drugs in Southern Africa. J Drug Abuse. 2015;1(1):7.
221. Foster RK, Marriott HE. Alcohol consumption in the new millennium – weighing up the risks and benefits for our health. Nutr Bull. 2006;31(4):286–331.
222. Bunout D. Nutritional and metabolic effects of alcoholism: their relationship with alcoholic liver disease. Nutrition. 1999;15(7–8):583–9.
223. Thomson AD. Mechanisms of vitamin deficiency in chronic alcohol misusers and the development of the Wernicke-Korsakoff syndrome. Alcohol Alcohol Suppl. 2000;35(1):2–7.
224. Morgan MY, Levine JA. Alcohol and nutrition. Proc Nutr Soc. 1988;47(2):85–98.
225. Glória L, Cravo M, Camilo ME, Resende M, Cardoso JN, Oliveira AG, et al. Nutritional deficiencies in chronic alcoholics: relation to dietary intake and alcohol consumption. Am J Gastroenterol. 1997;92(3):485–9.
226. Ross LJ, Wilson M, Banks M, Rezannah F, Daglish M. Prevalence of malnutrition and nutritional risk factors in patients undergoing alcohol and drug treatment. Nutrition. 2012;28(7–8, 738):–743.
227. Virmani A, Binienda Z, Ali S, Gaetani F. Links between nutrition, drug abuse, and the metabolic syndrome. Ann N Y Acad Sci. 2006;1074:303–14.
228. Baum MK. Role of micronutrients in HIV-infected intravenous drug users. J Acquir Immune Defic Syndr. 2000;25(Suppl 1):S49–52.
229. Whittle HJ, Sheira LA, Frongillo EA, Palar K, Cohen J, Merenstein D, et al. Longitudinal associations between food insecurity and substance use in a cohort of women with or at risk for HIV in the United States. Addiction. 2019;114(1):127–36.
230. Davey-Rothwell MA, Flamm LJ, Kassa HT, Latkin CA. Food insecurity and depressive symptoms: comparison of drug using and nondrug-using women at risk for HIV. J Community Psychol. 2014;42(4):469–78.
231. Strike C, Rudzinski K, Patterson J, Millson M. Frequent food insecurity among injection drug users: correlates and concerns. BMC Public Health. 2012;12:1058.
232. Bhattacharya J, Currie J, Haider S. Poverty, food insecurity, and nutritional outcomes in children and adults. J Health Econ. 2004;23(4):839–62.
233. Romero-Daza N, Himmelgreen DA, Perez-Escamilla R, Segura-Millan S, Singer M. Food habits of drug-using Puerto Rican women in inner-city Hartford. Med Anthropol. 1999;18(3):281–98.

234. Sabrina M, Adriana C, Gustavo Z, Qingyun L, Leslie S, Juphshy J, et al. Food insecurity and substance use in hiv-infected adults in the miami adult studies on hiv (mash) cohort (p04-066-19). Current Developments in Nutrition. 2019;3(1):nzz051. P04–066–19. https://doi.org/10.1093/cdn/nzz051.P04-066-19.

235. Chen Y, Kalichman SC. Synergistic effects of food insecurity and drug use on medication adherence among people living with HIV infection. J Behav Med. 2015;38(3):397–406.

236. Nolan LJ. Shared urges? The links between drugs of abuse, eating, and body weight. Curr Obes Rep. 2013;2(2):150–6.

237. Sansone RA, Sansone LA. Obesity and substance misuse: is there a relationship? Innov Clin Neurosci. 2013;10(9–10):30–5.

238. Meule A. The relation between body mass index and substance use: a true can of worms. Innov Clin Neurosci. 2014;11(3–4):11–2.

239. Crossin R, Lawrence AJ, Andrews ZB, Duncan JR. Altered body weight associated with substance abuse: a look beyond food intake. Addict Res Theory. 2019;27(2):76–84.

240. Forrester JE. Nutritional alterations in drug abusers with and without HIV. Am J Infect Dis. 2006;2(3):173–9.

241. Noble C, McCombie L. Nutritional considerations in intravenous drug misusers: a review of the literature and current issues for dietitians. J Hum Nutr Diet. 1997;10(3):181–91.

242. Chiolero A, Faeh D, Paccaud F, Cornuz J. Consequences of smoking for body weight, body fat distribution, and insulin resistance. Am J Clin Nutr. 2008;87(4):801–9.

243. Ersche KD, Stochl J, Woodward JM, Fletcher PC. The skinny on cocaine: insights into eating behavior and body weight in cocaine-dependent men. Appetite. 2013;71:75–80.

244. Baum MK, Rafie C, Lai S, Xue L, Sales S, Page JB, et al. Coronary heart disease (CHD) risk factors and metabolic syndrome in HIV-positive drug users in Miami. Am J Infect Dis. 2006;2(3):173–9.

245. Tang AM, Forrester JE, Spiegelman D, Flanigan T, Dobs A, Skinner S, et al. Heavy injection drug use is associated with lower percent body fat in a multi-ethnic cohort of HIV-positive and HIV-negative drug users from three U.S. cities. Am J Drug Alcohol Abuse. 2010;36(1):78–86.

246. Suter PM. Is alcohol consumption a risk factor for weight gain and obesity? Crit Rev Clin Lab Sci. 2005;42(3):197–227.

247. Salz A. Substance abuse and nutrition. Today's Dietitian. 2014;16(12):44.

248. Hodgkins C, Frost-Pineda K, Gold MS. Weight gain during substance abuse treatment: the dual problem of addiction and overeating in an adolescent population. J Addict Dis. 2007;26(Suppl 1):41–50.

249. Jackson TD, Grilo CM. Weight and eating concerns in outpatient men and women being treated for substance abuse. Eat Weight Disord. 2002;7(4):276–83.

250. Volkow ND, Wise RA. How can drug addiction help us understand obesity? Nat Neurosci. 2005;8(5):555–60.

251. Krahn D, Grossman J, Henk H, Mussey M, Crosby R, Gosnell B. Sweet intake, sweet-liking, urges to eat, and weight change: relationship to alcohol dependence and abstinence. Addict Behav. 2006;31(4):622–31.

252. National Institute on Alcohol Abuse and Alcoholism. Alcohol alert: alcohol and nutrition. No. 22 PH 346 October 1993. https://pubs.niaaa.nih.gov/publications/aa22.htm. Accessed 4 May 2020.

253. Lieber CS. Relationships between nutrition, alcohol use, and liver disease. Alcohol Res Health. 2003;27(3):220–31.

254. Leo MA, Lowe N, Lieber CS. Potentiation of ethanol-induced hepatic vitamin A depletion by phenobarbital and butylated hydroxytoluene. J Nutr. 1987;117(1):70–6.

255. Hendricks K, Gorbach S. Nutrition issues in chronic drug users living with HIV infection. Addict Sci Clin Pract. 2009;5(1):16–23.

256. Frishman WH, Del Vecchio A, Sanal S, Ismail A. Cardiovascular manifestations of substance abuse part 1: cocaine. Heart Dis. 2003;5(3):187–201.

257. Frishman WH, Del Vecchio A, Sanal S, Ismail A. Cardiovascular manifestations of substance abuse: part 2: alcohol, amphetamines, heroin, cannabis, and caffeine. Heart Dis. 2003;5(4):253–71.

258. Virmani A, Binienda ZK, Ali SF, Gaetani F. Metabolic syndrome in drug abuse. Ann N Y Acad Sci. 2007;1122:50–68.

259. Mohs ME, Watson RR, Leonard-Green T. Nutritional effects of marijuana, heroin, cocaine, and nicotine. J Am Diet Assoc. 1990;90(9):1261–7.

260. Beach RS, Mantero-Atienza E, Shor-Posner G, Javier JJ, Szapocznik J, Morgan R, et al. Specific nutrient abnormalities in asymptomatic HIV-1 infection. AIDS. 1992;6(7):701–8.

261. Baum MK. Nutritional alterations in high-risk groups in relationship to HIV-1 disease progression. Nutrition. 1996;12(2):124–5.

262. Baum MK, Shor-Posner G. Micronutrient status in relationship to mortality in HIV-1 disease. Nutr Rev. 1998;56(1 Pt 2):S135–9.

263. Baum MK, Shor-Posner G, Lai S, Zhang G, Lai H, Fletcher MA, et al. High risk of HIV-related mortality is associated with selenium deficiency. J Acquir Immune Defic Syndr Hum Retrovirol. 1997;15(5):370–4.

264. Beisel WR. AIDS. In: Gershwin ME, German JB, Keen CL, editors. Nutrition and immunology: principles and practices. Totowa: Humana Press; 2000. p. 389–403.

265. Baum MK, Mantero-Atienza E, Shor-Posner G, Fletcher MA, Morgan R, Eisdorfer C, Sauberlich HE, et al. Association of vitamin B6 status with parameters of immune function in early HIV-1 infection. J Acquir Immune Defic Syndr. 1991;4(11):1122–32.

266. Baum MK, Shor-Posner G, Zhang G, Lai H, Quesada JA, Campa A, et al. HIV-1 infection in women is associated with severe nutritional deficiencies. J Acquir Immune Defic Syndr Hum Retrovirol. 1997;16(4):272–8.

267. Tang AM, Graham NM, Chandra RK, Saah AJ. Low serum vitamin B-12 concentrations are associated with faster human immunodeficiency virus type 1 (HIV-1) disease progression. J Nutr. 1997;127(2):345–51.

268. Tang AM, Graham NM, Saah AJ. Effects of micronutrient intake on survival in human immunodeficiency virus type 1 infection. Am J Epidemiol. 1996;143(12):1244–56.

269. Constans J, Pellegrin JL, Sergeant C, Simonoff M, Pellegrin I, Fleury H, et al. Serum selenium predicts outcome in HIV infection. J Acquir Immune Defic Syndr Hum Retrovirol. 1995;10(3):392.

270. Fawzi WW, Hunter DJ. Vitamins in HIV disease progression and vertical transmission. Epidemiology. 1998;9(4):457–66.

271. Fawzi WW, Msamanga GI, Spiegelman D, Urassa EJ, McGrath N, Mwakagile D, et al. Randomised trial of effects of vitamin supplements on pregnancy outcomes and T cell counts in HIV-1-infected women in Tanzania. Lancet. 1998;351(9114):1477–82.

272. Melchior JC, Niyongabo T, Henzel D, Durack-Bown I, Henri SC, Boulier A. Malnutrition and wasting, immuno-depression, and chronic inflammation as independent predictors of survival in HIV-infected patients. Nutrition. 1999;15(11–12):865–9.

273. Maas JJ, Dukers N, Krol A, van Ameijden EJ, van Leeuwen R, Roos MT, et al. Body mass index course in asymptomatic HIV-infected homosexual men and the predictive value of a decrease of body mass index for progression to AIDS. J Acquir Immune Defic Syndr Hum Retrovirol. 1998;19(3):254–9.

274. Mankal PK, Kotler DP. From wasting to obesity, changes in nutritional concerns in HIV/AIDS. Endocrinol Metab Clin N Am. 2014;43(3):647–63.

275. Karter DL, Karter AJ, Yarrish R, Patterson C, Kass PH, Nord J, et al. Vitamin A deficiency in non-vitamin-supplemented patients with AIDS: a cross-sectional study. J Acquir Immune Defic Syndr Hum Retrovirol. 1995;8(2):199–203.

276. Haug CJ, Aukrust P, Haug E, Mørkrid L, Müller F, Frøland SS. Severe deficiency of 1,25-dihydroxyvitamin D3 in human immunodeficiency virus infection: association with immunological hyperactivity and only minor changes in calcium homeostasis. J Clin Endocrinol Metab. 1998;83(11):3832–8.

277. Dreyfuss ML, Fawzi WW. Micronutrients and vertical transmission of HIV-1. Am J Clin Nutr. 2002;75(6):959–70.

278. Camp WL, Allen S, Alvarez JO, Jolly PE, Weiss HL, Phillips JF, et al. Serum retinol and HIV-1 RNA viral load in rapid and slow progressors. J Acquir Immune Defic Syndr Hum Retrovirol. 1998;18(4):401–6.

279. Campa A, Shor-Posner G, Indacochea F, Zhang G, Lai H, Asthana D, et al. Mortality risk in selenium-deficient HIV-positive children. J Acquir Immune Defic Syndr Hum Retrovirol. 1999;20(5):508–13.

280. Allard JP, Aghdassi E, Chau J, Salit I, Walmsley S. Oxidative stress and plasma antioxidant micronutrients in humans with HIV infection. Am J Clin Nutr. 1998;67(1):143–7.

281. Folks TM, Justement J, Kinter A, Dinarello CA, Fauci AS. Cytokine-induced expression of HIV-1 in a chronically infected promonocyte cell line. Science. 1987;238(4828):800–2.

282. Ivanov AV, Valuev-Elliston VT, Ivanova ON, Kochetkov SN, Starodubova ES, Bartosch B, et al. Oxidative stress during HIV infection: mechanisms and consequences. Oxidative Med Cell Longev. 2016;2016:8910396.

283. Abrams B, Duncan D, Hertz-Picciotto I. A prospective study of dietary intake and acquired immune deficiency syndrome in HIV-seropositive homosexual men. J Acquir Immune Defic Syndr. 1993;6(8):949–58.

284. Tang AM, Graham NM, Kirby AJ, McCall LD, Willett WC, Saah AJ. Dietary micronutrient intake and risk of progression to acquired immunodeficiency syndrome (AIDS) in human immunodeficiency virus type 1 (HIV-1)-infected homosexual men. Am J Epidemiol. 1993;138(11):937–51.

285. Allavena C, Dousset B, May T, Dubois F, Canton P, Belleville F. Relationship of trace element, immunological markers, and HIV1 infection progression. Biol Trace Elem Res. 1995;47(1–3, 133):–8.

286. Baum MK, Shor-Posner G, Lu Y, Rosner B, Sauberlich HE, Fletcher MA, et al. Micronutrients and HIV-1 disease progression. AIDS. 1995;9(9):1051–6.

287. Tang AM, Graham NM, Semba RD, Saah AJ. Association between serum vitamin A and E levels and HIV-1 disease progression. AIDS. 1997;11(5):613–20.

288. Baum MK, Shor-Posner G. Nutritional status and survival in HIV-1 disease. AIDS. 1997;11(5):689–90.

289. Visser ME, Maartens G, Kossew G, Hussey GD. Plasma vitamin A and zinc levels in HIV-infected adults in Cape Town, South Africa. Br J Nutr. 2003;89(4):475–82.

290. Tang AM, Jacobson DL, Spiegelman D, Knox TA, Wanke C. Increasing risk of 5% or greater unintentional weight loss in a cohort of HIV-infected patients, 1995 to 2003. J Acquir Immune Defic Syndr. 2005;40(1):70–6.

291. Marston B, De Cock KM. Multivitamins, nutrition, and antiretroviral therapy for HIV disease in Africa. N Engl J Med. 2004;351(1):78–80.

292. Drain PK, Kupka R, Mugusi F, Fawzi WW. Micronutrients in HIV-positive persons receiving highly active antiretroviral therapy. Am J Clin Nutr. 2007;85(2):333–45.
293. Semba RD, Graham NM, Caiaffa WT, Margolick JB, Clement L, Vlahov D. Increased mortality associated with vitamin A deficiency during human immunodeficiency virus type 1 infection. Arch Intern Med. 1993;153(18):2149–54.
294. Humphrey JH, Quinn T, Fine D, Lederman H, Yamini-Roodsari S, Wu LS, et al. Short-term effects of large-dose vitamin A supplementation on viral load and immune response in HIV-infected women. J Acquir Immune Defic Syndr Hum Retrovirol. 1999;20(1):44–51.
295. Semba RD, Lyles CM, Margolick JB, Caiaffa WT, Farzadegan H, Cohn S, et al. Vitamin A supplementation and human immunodeficiency virus load in injection drug users. J Infect Dis. 1998;177(3):611–6.
296. Baeten JM, McClelland RS, Overbaugh J, Richardson BA, Emery S, Lavreys L, et al. Vitamin A supplementation and human immunodeficiency virus type 1 shedding in women: results of a randomized clinical trial. J Infect Dis. 2002;185(8):1187–91.
297. Martineau AR, Timms PM, Bothamley GH, Hanifa Y, Islam K, Claxton AP, et al. High-dose vitamin D(3) during intensive-phase antimicrobial treatment of pulmonary tuberculosis: a double-blind randomised controlled trial. Lancet. 2011;377(9761):242–50.
298. Mehta S, Mugusi FM, Bosch RJ, Aboud S, Urassa W, Villamor E, et al. Vitamin D status and TB treatment outcomes in adult patients in Tanzania: a cohort study. BMJ Open. 2013;3(11):e003703.
299. Giacomet V, Vigano A, Manfredini V, Cerini C, Bedogni G, Mora S, et al. Cholecalciferol supplementation in HIV-infected youth with vitamin D insufficiency: effects on vitamin D status and T-cell phenotype: a randomized controlled trial. HIV Clin Trials. 2013;14(2):51–60.
300. Overton ET, Chan ES, Brown TT, Tebas P, McComsey GA, Melbourne KM, et al. Vitamin D and calcium attenuate bone loss with antiretroviral therapy initiation: a randomized trial. Ann Intern Med. 2015;162(12):815–24.
301. Bang U, Kolte L, Hitz M, Dam Nielsen S, Schierbeck LL, Andersen O, et al. Correlation of increases in 1,25-dihydroxyvitamin D during vitamin D therapy with activation of CD4+ T lymphocytes in HIV-1-infected males. HIV Clin Trials. 2012;13(3):162–70.
302. Bang UC, Kolte L, Hitz M, Schierbeck LL, Nielsen SD, Benfield T, et al. The effect of cholecalciferol and calcitriol on biochemical bone markers in HIV type 1-infected males: results of a clinical trial. AIDS Res Hum Retrovir. 2013;29(4):658–64.
303. Baum MK, Lai S, Sales S, Page JB, Campa A. Randomized, controlled clinical trial of zinc supplementation to prevent immunological failure in HIV-infected adults. Clin Infect Dis. 2010;50(12):1653–60.
304. Asdamongkol N, Phanachet P, Sungkanuparph S. Low plasma zinc levels and immunological responses to zinc supplementation in HIV-infected patients with immunological discordance after antiretroviral therapy. Jpn J Infect Dis. 2013;66(6):469–74.
305. Cárcamo C, Hooton T, Weiss NS, Gilman R, Wener MH, Chavez V, et al. Randomized controlled trial of zinc supplementation for persistent diarrhea in adults with HIV-1 infection. J Acquir Immune Defic Syndr. 2006;43(2):197–201.
306. Green JA, et al. A randomised controlled trial of oral zinc on the immune response to tuberculosis in HIV-infected patients. Int J Tuberc Lung Dis. 2005;9(12):1378–84.
307. Green JA, Lewin SR, Wightman F, Lee M, Ravindran TS, Paton NI. Effect of micronutrient supplementation on disease progression in asymptomatic, antiretroviral-naive, HIV-infected adults in Botswana: a randomized clinical trial. JAMA. 2013;310(20):2154–63.
308. Burbano X, Miguez-Burbano MJ, McCollister K, Zhang G, Rodriguez A, Ruiz P, et al. Impact of a selenium chemoprevention clinical trial on hospital admissions of HIV-infected participants. HIV Clin Trials. 2002;3(6):483–91.
309. Hurwitz BE, Klaus JR, Llabre MM, Gonzalez A, Lawrence PJ, Maher KJ, et al. Suppression of human immunodeficiency virus type 1 viral load with selenium supplementation: a randomized controlled trial. Arch Intern Med. 2007;167(2):148–54.
310. de Souza JO, Treitinger A, Baggio GL, Michelon C, Verdi JC, Cunha J, et al. Alpha-Tocopherol as an antiretroviral therapy supplement for HIV-1-infected patients for increased lymphocyte viability. Clin Chem Lab Med. 2005;43(4):376–82.
311. Allard JP, Aghdassi E, Chau J, Tam C, Kovacs CM, Salit IE, et al. Effects of vitamin E and C supplementation on oxidative stress and viral load in HIV-infected subjects. AIDS. 1998;12(13):1653–9.
312. Kelly P, Musonda R, Kafwembe E, Kaetano L, Keane E, Farthing M. Micronutrient supplementation in the AIDS diarrhoea-wasting syndrome in Zambia: a randomized controlled trial. AIDS. 1999;13(4):495–500.
313. Semba RD. Vitamin A and human immunodeficiency virus infection. Proc Nutr Soc. 1997;56(1b):459–69.
314. Kelly P, Katubulushi M, Todd J, Banda R, Yambayamba V, Fwoloshi M, et al. Micronutrient supplementation has limited effects on intestinal infectious disease and mortality in a Zambian population of mixed HIV status: a cluster randomized trial. Am J Clin Nutr. 2008;88(4):1010–7.

315. McClelland RS, Baeten JM, Overbaugh J, Richardson BA, Mandaliya K, Emery S, et al. Micronutrient supplementation increases genital tract shedding of HIV-1 in women: results of a randomized trial. J Acquir Immune Defic Syndr. 2004;37(5):1657–63.

316. Jiamton S, Pepin J, Suttent R, Filteau S, Mahakkanukrauh B, Hanshaoworakul W, et al. A randomized trial of the impact of multiple micronutrient supplementation on mortality among HIV-infected individuals living in Bangkok. AIDS. 2003;17(17):2461–9.

317. Zhao F, Feng XL, Xu W, Ma YM, Wang Z, Li WJ. Effect of micronutrients on the immune status of human immunodeficiency virus-positive individuals. Zhongguo Yi Xue Ke Xue Yuan Xue Bao. 2010;32(3):340–2.

318. Jaruga P, Jaruga B, Gackowski D, Olczak A, Halota W, Pawlowska M, et al. Supplementation with antioxidant vitamins prevents oxidative modification of DNA in lymphocytes of HIV-infected patients. Free Radic Biol Med. 2002;32(5):414–20.

319. Kaiser JD, Campa AM, Ondercin JP, Leoung GS, Pless RF, Baum MK. Micronutrient supplementation increases CD4 count in HIV-infected individuals on highly active antiretroviral therapy: a prospective, double-blinded, placebo-controlled trial. J Acquir Immune Defic Syndr. 2006;42(5):523–8.

320. Isanaka S, Mugusi F, Hawkins C, Spiegelman D, Okuma J, Aboud S, et al. Effect of high-dose vs standard-dose multivitamin supplementation at the initiation of HAART on HIV disease progression and mortality in Tanzania: a randomized controlled trial. JAMA. 2012;308(15):1535–44.

321. Houben RM, Dodd PJ. The global burden of latent tuberculosis infection: a re-estimation using mathematical modelling. PLoS Med. 2016;13(10):e1002152.

322. Getahun H, Matteelli A, Chaisson RE, Raviglione M. Latent Mycobacterium tuberculosis infection. N Engl J Med. 2015;372(22):2127–35.

323. Chaisson RE, Martinson NA. Tuberculosis in Africa – combating an HIV-driven crisis. N Engl J Med. 2008;358(11):1089–92.

324. Ansari NA, Kombe AH, Kenyon TA, Hone NM, Tappero JW, Nyirenda ST, et al. Pathology and causes of death in a group of 128 predominantly HIV-positive patients in Botswana, 1997–1998. Int J Tuberc Lung Dis. 2002;6(1):55–63.

325. Selwyn PA, Hartel D, Lewis VA, Schoenbaum EE, Vermund SH, Klein RS, et al. A prospective study of the risk of tuberculosis among intravenous drug users with human immunodeficiency virus infection. N Engl J Med. 1989;320(9):545–50.

326. Suthar AB, Lawn SD, del Amo J, Getahun H, Dye C, Sculier D, et al. Antiretroviral therapy for prevention of tuberculosis in adults with HIV: a systematic review and meta-analysis. PLoS Med. 2012;9(7):e1001270.

327. Severe P, Juste MA, Ambroise A, Eliacin L, Marchand C, Apollon S, et al. Early versus standard antiretroviral therapy for HIV-infected adults in Haiti. N Engl J Med. 2010;363(3):257–65.

328. Cohen MS, Chen YQ, McCauley M, Gamble T, Hosseinipour MC, Kumarasamy N, et al. Prevention of HIV-1 infection with early antiretroviral therapy. N Engl J Med. 2011;365(6):493–505.

329. Dierberg KL, Chaisson RE. Human immunodeficiency virus-associated tuberculosis: update on prevention and treatment. Clin Chest Med. 2013;34(2):217–28.

330. Harries AD, Lawn SD, Getahun H, Zachariah R, Havlir DV. HIV and tuberculosis--science and implementation to turn the tide and reduce deaths. J Int AIDS Soc. 2012;15(2):17396.

331. García-Basteiro AL, DiNardo A, Saavedra B, Silva DR, Palmero D, Gegia M, et al. Point of care diagnostics for tuberculosis. Pulmonology. 2018;24(2):73–85.

332. Macallan DC, McNurlan MA, Kurpad AV, de Souza G, Shetty PS, Calder AG, et al. Whole body protein metabolism in human pulmonary tuberculosis and undernutrition: evidence for anabolic block in tuberculosis. Clin Sci (Lond). 1998;94(3):321–31.

333. Paton NI, Ng YM. Body composition studies in patients with wasting associated with tuberculosis. Nutrition. 2006;22(3):245–51.

334. Karyadi E, West CE, Schultink W, Nelwan RH, Gross R, Amin Z, et al. A double-blind, placebo-controlled study of vitamin A and zinc supplementation in persons with tuberculosis in Indonesia: effects on clinical response and nutritional status. Am J Clin Nutr. 2002;75(4):720–7.

335. Onwubalili JK. Malnutrition among tuberculosis patients in Harrow, England. Eur J Clin Nutr. 1988;42(4):363–6.

336. Paton NI, Chua YK, Earnest A, Chee CB. Randomized controlled trial of nutritional supplementation in patients with newly diagnosed tuberculosis and wasting. Am J Clin Nutr. 2004;80(2):460–5.

337. Kant S, Gupta H, Ahluwalia S. Significance of nutrition in pulmonary tuberculosis. Crit Rev Food Sci Nutr. 2015;55(7):955–63.

338. Macallan DC. Malnutrition in tuberculosis. Diagn Microbiol Infect Dis. 1999;34(2):153–7.

339. Chandra RK. Nutrition and immunity: lessons from the past and new insights into the future. Am J Clin Nutr. 1991;53(5):1087–101.

340. Scrimshaw NS, Taylor CE, Gordon JE. Effect of malnutrition on resistance to infection. In: Scrimshaw NS, Taylor CE, Gordon JE, editors. Interactions of nutrition and infection. Geneva: World Health Organization; 1968. p. 60–142.

341. Chandra R, Newberne P. Nutrition, immunity, and infection: mechanisms of interactions. New York: Plenum Press; 1977. p. xiv, 246.
342. Leyton GB. Effects of slow starvation. Lancet. 1946;2(6412):73–9.
343. Faber K. Tuberculosis and nutrition. Acta Tuberc Scand. 1938;12:287ff.
344. Munro WT, Leitch I. Diet and tuberculosis. Proc Nutr Soc. 1945;3:155–64.
345. Cegielski JP, McMurray DN. The relationship between malnutrition and tuberculosis: evidence from studies in humans and experimental animals. Int J Tuberc Lung Dis. 2004;8(3):286–98.
346. Cegielski P, Kohlmeier L, Cornoni-Huntley J. Malnutrition and tuberculosis in a nationally representative cohort of adults in the United States, 1971–1987. In: Proceedings of the 44th Annual Meeting, American Society of Tropical Medicine and Hygiene, vol. 152. San Antonio: American Society of Tropical Medicine and Hygiene; 1995.
347. Getz HR, Long ER, Henderson HJ. A study of the relation of nutrition to the development of tuberculosis; influence of ascorbic acid and vitamin A. Am Rev Tuberc. 1951;64(4):381–93.
348. Hemilä H, Kaprio J, Pietinen P, Albanes D, Heinonen OP. Vitamin C and other compounds in vitamin C rich food in relation to risk of tuberculosis in male smokers. Am J Epidemiol. 1999;150(6):632–41.
349. Downes J. An experiment in the control of tuberculosis among Negroes. Milbank Mem Fund Q. 1950;28(2):127–59.
350. Werbin N. Tuberculosis after jejuno-ileal bypass for morbid obesity. Postgrad Med J. 1981;57(666):252–3.
351. Pickleman JR, Evans LS, Kane JM, Freeark RJ. Tuberculosis after jejunoileal bypass for obesity. JAMA. 1975;234(7):744.
352. Chandra R. Interference of malnutrition with specific immune response. In: Isliker H, Schürch B, editors. The impact of malnutrition on immune defense in parasitic infestation. Bern: Hans Huber; 1981. p. 104–14.
353. Chandra R. Nutritional regulation of immune function at the extremes of life: in infants and the elderly. In: White P, editor. Malnutrition: determinants and consequences. New York: Alan R. Liss; 1984. p. 245–51.
354. Chandra RK. Nutrition, immunity, and infection: present knowledge and future directions. Lancet. 1983;1(8326 Pt 1):688–91.
355. Barffour MA, Humphries DL. Core principles: infectious disease risk in relation to macro and micronutrient status. In: Humphries DL, Scott ME, Vermund SH, editors. Nutrition and infectious disease: shifting the clinical paradigm. Humana Press; 2020. https://www.springer.com/gp/book/9783030569129.
356. Mcmurray DN, Bartow RA. Immunosuppression and alteration of resistance to pulmonary tuberculosis in Guinea-Pigs by protein undernutrition. J Nutr. 1992;122(3):738–43.
357. McMurray DN. Impact of nutritional deficiencies on resistance to experimental pulmonary tuberculosis. Nutr Rev. 1998;56(1):S147–52.
358. McMurray DN, Bartow RA, Mintzer CL. Protein-malnutrition alters the distribution of Fc-Gamma-R+ (T-Gamma) and Fc-Mu-R+ (T-Mu) Lymphocyte-S-T in experimental pulmonary tuberculosis. Infect Immun. 1990;58(2):563–5.
359. Lin YG, et al. Production of monocyte chemoattractant protein 1 in tuberculosis patients. Infect Immun. 1998;66(5):2319–22.
360. Savino W. The thymus gland is a target in malnutrition. Eur J Clin Nutr. 2002;56:S46–9.
361. Dülger H, Arik M, Sekeroğlu MR, Tarakçioğlu M, Noyan T, Cesur Y, et al. Pro-inflammatory cytokines in Turkish children with protein-energy malnutrition. Mediators Inflamm. 2002;11(6):363–5.
362. Roland CG. Courage under siege: starvation, disease, and death in the Warsaw ghetto. Studies in Jewish history. New York: Oxford University Press; 1992.
363. Winick M. Hunger disease: studies by the Jewish physicians in the Warsaw Ghetto. New York: Wiley; 1979.
364. Schechter M. Health and sickness in times of starvation. Harofe Haivri Heb Med J. 1953;2:191–3.
365. Karyadi E, Schultink W, Nelwan RH, Gross R, Amin Z, Dolmans WM, et al. Poor micronutrient status of active pulmonary tuberculosis patients in Indonesia. J Nutr. 2000;130(12):2953–8.
366. Pakasi TA, Karyadi E, Suratih NM, Salean M, Darmawidjaja N, Bor H, et al. Zinc and vitamin A supplementation fails to reduce sputum conversion time in severely malnourished pulmonary tuberculosis patients in Indonesia. Nutr J. 2010;9:41.
367. Abba K, Sudarsanam TD, Grobler L, Volmink J. Nutritional supplements for people being treated for active tuberculosis. Cochrane Database Syst Rev. 2008;4:CD006086.
368. Grobler L, Durao S, Van der Merwe SM, Wessels J, Naude CE. Nutritional supplements for people being treated for active tuberculosis: a technical summary. S Afr Med J. 2018;108(1):16–8.
369. Sinclair D, Abba K, Grobler L, Sudarsanam TD. Nutritional supplements for people being treated for active tuberculosis. Cochrane Database Syst Rev. 2011;11:CD006086.
370. Martineau AR, Wilkinson RJ, Wilkinson KA, Newton SM, Kampmann B, Hall BM, et al. A single dose of vitamin D enhances immunity to mycobacteria. Am J Respir Crit Care Med. 2007;176(2):208–13.
371. Zittermann A. Vitamin D in preventive medicine: are we ignoring the evidence? Br J Nutr. 2003;89(5):552–72.
372. Ustianowski A, Shaffer R, Collin S, Wilkinson RJ, Davidson RN. Prevalence and associations of vitamin D deficiency in foreign-born persons with tuberculosis in London. J Infect. 2005;50(5):432–7.

373. Grange JM, Davies PD, Brown RC, Woodhead JS, Kardjito T. A study of vitamin D levels in Indonesian patients with untreated pulmonary tuberculosis. Tubercle. 1985;66(3):187–91.
374. Crowle AJ, Ross EJ, May MH. Inhibition by 1,25(OH)2-vitamin D3 of the multiplication of virulent tubercle bacilli in cultured human macrophages. Infect Immun. 1987;55(12):2945–50.
375. Rook GA, Steele J, Fraher L, Barker S, Karmali R, O'Riordan J, et al. Vitamin D3, gamma interferon, and control of proliferation of Mycobacterium tuberculosis by human monocytes. Immunology. 1986;57(1):159–63.
376. Aibana O, Huang CC, Aboud S, Arnedo-Pena A, Becerra MC, Bellido-Blasco JB, et al. Vitamin D status and risk of incident tuberculosis disease: a nested case-control study, systematic review, and individual-participant data meta-analysis. PLoS Med. 2019;16(9):e1002907.
377. Kawai K, Meydani SN, Urassa W, Wu D, Mugusi FM, Saathoff E, et al. Micronutrient supplementation and T cell-mediated immune responses in patients with tuberculosis in Tanzania. Epidemiol Infect. 2014;142(7):1505–9.
378. Range N, Andersen AB, Magnussen P, Mugomela A, Friis H. The effect of micronutrient supplementation on treatment outcome in patients with pulmonary tuberculosis: a randomized controlled trial in Mwanza, Tanzania. Tropical Med Int Health. 2005;10(9):826–32.
379. Range N, Changalucha J, Krarup H, Magnussen P, Andersen AB, Friis H. The effect of multi-vitamin/mineral supplementation on mortality during treatment of pulmonary tuberculosis: a randomised two-by-two factorial trial in Mwanza, Tanzania. Br J Nutr. 2006;95(4):762–70.
380. Villamor E, Mugusi F, Urassa W, Bosch RJ, Saathoff E, Matsumoto K, et al. A trial of the effect of micronutrient supplementation on treatment outcome, T cell counts, morbidity, and mortality in adults with pulmonary tuberculosis. J Infect Dis. 2008;197(11):1499–505.
381. Campa A, Baum MK, Bussmann H, Martinez SS, Farahani M, van Widenfelt E, et al. The effect of micronutrient supplementation on active TB incidence early in HIV infection in Botswana. Nutr Diet Suppl. 2017;2017(9):37–45.
382. Shor-Posner G, Miguez MJ, Pineda LM, Rodriguez A, Ruiz P, Castillo G, et al. Impact of selenium status on the pathogenesis of mycobacterial disease in HIV-1-infected drug users during the era of highly active antiretroviral therapy. J Acquir Immune Defic Syndr. 2002;29(2):169–73.
383. Safarian MD, Karagezian KG, Karapetian ET, Avanesian NA. The efficacy of antioxidant therapy in patients with tuberculosis of the lungs and the correction of lipid peroxidation processes. Probl Tuberk. 1990;(5):40–4.
384. Knox TA, Zafonte-Sanders M, Fields-Gardner C, Moen K, Johansen D, Paton N. Assessment of nutritional status, body composition, and human immunodeficiency virus-associated morphologic changes. Clin Infect Dis. 2003;36(Suppl 2):S63–8.
385. Shevitz AH, Knox TA. Nutrition in the era of highly active antiretroviral therapy. Clin Infect Dis. 2001;32(12):1769–75.
386. Coyne-Meyers K, Trombley LE. A review of nutrition in human immunodeficiency virus infection in the era of highly active antiretroviral therapy. Nutr Clin Pract. 2004;19(4):340–55.
387. Nerad J, Romeyn M, Silverman E, Allen-Reid J, Dieterich D, Merchant J, et al. General nutrition management in patients infected with human immunodeficiency virus. Clin Infect Dis. 2003;36(Suppl 2):S52–62.
388. U.S. Department of Health and Human Services, H.R.a.S.A. Guide for HIV/AIDS clinical care – 2014 edition. In: U.S.D.o.H.a.H. Services, editor. Rockville, MD; 2014.
389. Fields-Gardner C, Campa A, American Dietetics Association. Position of the American Dietetic Association: nutrition intervention and human immunodeficiency virus infection. J Am Diet Assoc. 2010;110(7):1105–19.
390. Centers for Disease Control. National Health and Nutrition Examination Survey (NHANES): anthropometry procedures manual. 2017. https://wwwn.cdc.gov/nchs/data/nhanes/2017-2018/manuals/2017_Anthropometry_Procedures_Manual.pdf. Accessed 5 May 2020.
391. Madden AM, Smith S. Body composition and morphological assessment of nutritional status in adults: a review of anthropometric variables. J Hum Nutr Diet. 2016;29(1):7–25.
392. Centers for Disease Control. Revised classification system for HIV infection and expanded surveillance case definition for AIDS among adolescents and adults. Morb Mortal Wkly Rep. 1993;1992:41.
393. Gerrior JL, Neff LM. Nutrition assessment in HIV infection. Nutr Clin Care. 2005;8(1):6–15.
394. Earthman CP. Evaluation of nutrition assessment parameters in the presence of human immunodeficiency virus infection. Nutr Clin Pract. 2004;19(4):330–9.
395. Dimala CA, Ngu RC, Kadia BM, Tianyi F-L, Choukem SP. Markers of adiposity in HIV/AIDS patients: agreement between waist circumference, waist-to-hip ratio, waist-to-height ratio and body mass index. PLoS One. 2018;13(3):e0194653.
396. Dos Santos AP, Navarro AM, Schwingel A, Alves TC, Abdalla PP, Venturini ACR, et al. Lipodystrophy diagnosis in people living with HIV/AIDS: prediction and validation of sex-specific anthropometric models. BMC Public Health. 2018;18(1):806.
397. Kotler DP, Burastero S, Wang J, Pierson RN Jr. Prediction of body cell mass, fat-free mass, and total body water with bioelectrical impedance analysis: effects of race, sex, and disease. Am J Clin Nutr. 1996;64(3 Suppl):489S–97S.

398. Bharadwaj S, Ginoya S, Tandon P, Gohel TD, Guirguis J, Vallabh H, et al. Malnutrition: laboratory markers vs nutritional assessment. Gastroenterol Rep (Oxf). 2016;4(4):272–80.
399. Don BR, Kaysen G. Serum albumin: relationship to inflammation and nutrition. Semin Dial. 2004;17(6):432–7.
400. Lee JL, Oh ES, Lee RW, Finucane TE. Serum albumin and prealbumin in calorically restricted, nondiseased individuals: a systematic review. Am J Med. 2015;128(9):1023.e1–22.
401. Fuhrman MP, Charney P, Mueller CM. Hepatic proteins and nutrition assessment. J Am Diet Assoc. 2004;104(8):1258–64.
402. Ramakrishnan K, Shenbagarathai R, Kavitha K, Uma A, Balasubramaniam R, Thirumalaikolundusubramanian P. Serum zinc and albumin levels in pulmonary tuberculosis patients with and without HIV. Jpn J Infect Dis. 2008;61(3):202–4.
403. Seyedrezazadeh E, Ostadrahimi A, Mahboob S, Assadi Y, Ghaemmagami J, Pourmogaddam M. Effect of vitamin E and selenium supplementation on oxidative stress status in pulmonary tuberculosis patients. Respirology. 2008;13(2):294–8.
404. Kassu A, Yabutani T, Mahmud ZH, Mohammad A, Nguyen N, Huong BT, et al. Alterations in serum levels of trace elements in tuberculosis and HIV infections. Eur J Clin Nutr. 2006;60(5):580–6.
405. Pakasi TA, Karyadi E, Wibowo Y, Simanjuntak Y, Suratih NM, Salean M, et al. Vitamin A deficiency and other factors associated with severe tuberculosis in Timor and Rote Islands, East Nusa Tenggara Province, Indonesia. Eur J Clin Nutr. 2009;63(9):1130–5.
406. Olawumi HO, Olatunji PO. The value of serum albumin in pretreatment assessment and monitoring of therapy in HIV/AIDS patients. HIV Med. 2006;7(6):351–5.
407. Mehta SH, Astemborski J, Sterling TR, Thomas DL, Vlahov D. Serum albumin as a prognostic indicator for HIV disease progression. AIDS Res Hum Retrovir. 2006;22(1):14–21.
408. Ronit A, Sharma S, Baker JV, Mngqibisa R, Delory T, Caldeira L, et al. Serum albumin as a prognostic marker for serious non-AIDS endpoints in the strategic timing of antiretroviral treatment (START) study. J Infect Dis. 2018;217(3):405–12.
409. Gupta KB, Gupta R, Atreja A, Verma M, Vishvkarma S. Tuberculosis and nutrition. Lung India. 2009;26(1):9–16.
410. Hayes C, Elliot E, Krales E, Downer G. Food and water safety for persons infected with human immunodeficiency virus. Clin Infect Dis. 2003;36(Suppl 2):S106–9.
411. Clinical assessment of nutritional status. Am J Public Health. 1973;63(11 Suppl):18–27.
412. Gibson RS. Principles of nutritional assessment. 2nd ed. New York: Oxford University Press; 2005. p. xx, 908.
413. White JV, Guenter P, Jensen G, Malone A, Schofield M, Academy of Nutrition and Dietetics Malnutrition Work Group, et al. Consensus statement of the Academy of Nutrition and Dietetics/American Society for Parenteral and Enteral Nutrition: characteristics recommended for the identification and documentation of adult malnutrition (undernutrition). J Acad Nutr Diet. 2012;112(5):730–8.
414. Becker PJ, Nieman Carney L, Corkins MR, Monczka J, Smith E, Smith SE, et al. Consensus statement of the Academy of Nutrition and Dietetics/American Society for Parenteral and Enteral Nutrition: indicators recommended for the identification and documentation of pediatric malnutrition (undernutrition). J Acad Nutr Diet. 2014;114(12):1988–2000.
415. Fielden SJ, Anema A, Fergusson P, Muldoon K, Grede N, de Pee S. Measuring food and nutrition security: tools and considerations for use among people living with HIV. AIDS Behav. 2014;18(Suppl 5):S490–504.
416. Fowles ER, Sterling BS, Walker LO. Measuring dietary intake in nursing research. Can J Nurs Res. 2007;39(2):146–65.
417. Shim JS, Oh K, Kim HC. Dietary assessment methods in epidemiologic studies. Epidemiol Health. 2014;36:e2014009.
418. Tucker KL. Assessment of usual dietary intake in population studies of gene-diet interaction. Nutr Metab Cardiovasc Dis. 2007;17(2):74–81.
419. Raper N, Perloff B, Ingwersen L, Steinfeldt L, Anana J. An overview of USDA's dietary intake data system. J Food Compost Anal. 2004;17(3):545–55.
420. Moshfegh AJ, Rhodes DG, Baer DJ, Murayi T, Clemens JC, Rumpler WV, et al. The US Department of Agriculture Automated Multiple-Pass Method reduces bias in the collection of energy intakes. Am J Clin Nutr. 2008;88(2):324–32.
421. Ralph JL, Von Ah D, Scheett AJ, Hoverson BS, Anderson CM. Diet assessment methods: a guide for oncology nurses. Clin J Oncol Nurs. 2011;15(6):E114–21.

# Chapter 10
# Nutrition and Arboviral Infections

**Eduardo Villamor and Luis A. Villar**

## Abbreviations

| | |
|---|---|
| 25(OH)D | 25-Hydroxy vitamin D |
| AA | Arachidonic acid |
| BMI | Body mass index |
| CHIKV | Chikungunya virus |
| DBP | Vitamin D binding protein |
| DENV | Dengue virus |
| DF | Dengue fever |
| DGLA | Dihomo-$\gamma$-linolenic acid |
| DHA | Docosahexaenoic acid |
| DHF | Dengue hemorrhagic fever |
| DSS | Dengue shock syndrome |
| EPA | Eicosapentaenoic acid |
| FA | Fatty acids |
| PUFA | Polyunsaturated fatty acids |
| Th | T helper |
| VDR | Vitamin D receptor |
| YFV | Yellow fever virus |
| ZIKV | Zika virus |

E. Villamor (✉)
Department of Epidemiology, University of Michigan School of Public Health, Ann Arbor, MI, USA
e-mail: villamor@umich.edu

L. A. Villar
Departamento de Ciencias Basicas, Universidad Industrial de Santander, Facultad de Medicina, Centro de Investigaciones Epidemiológicas, Bucaramanga, Colombia

© Springer Nature Switzerland AG 2021
D. L. Humphries et al. (eds.), *Nutrition and Infectious Diseases*, Nutrition and Health,
https://doi.org/10.1007/978-3-030-56913-6_10

**Key Points**

- Available evidence on the relations between nutritional factors and arboviral infections focuses on the role of the host's nutritional status on the risk of progression to severe forms of dengue disease, the most common mosquito-borne viral infection worldwide.
- Observational studies suggest that pediatric obesity may be related to adverse dengue disease outcomes.
- Investigators have reported inverse relations between severity of dengue disease and nutrient status biomarkers, including fatty acids, amino acids, vitamin D, and some minerals, but it is unclear whether these relations represent an effect of the nutritional status on the outcome of infection or an effect of the infection on the biomarkers.
- Small randomized trials of vitamin E and zinc supplements to patients with dengue fever have shown protective effects against intermediate outcomes leading to severe disease.
- Dengue and chikungunya infections appear to alter nutrient metabolism acutely. This may be a consequence of the inflammatory response to infection or increased nutrient requirements.
- Obesity during pregnancy has been related to increased seropositivity to chikungunya, but the role of nutrition on clinical outcomes is unknown.
- Studying the interactions between nutrition and arboviral infections is an open area with promising public health and clinical applications.

## Introduction

Arboviruses are infections caused by viruses that are transmitted by arthropods such as mosquitoes and ticks [1]. Of the >500 known arboviruses, only a few from 4 main families (*Flaviviridae*, *Togaviridae*, *Bunyaviridae*, and *Reoviridae*) cause disease in humans. They include dengue virus (DENV), yellow fever virus (YFV), Zika virus (ZIKV), West Nile virus, Japanese encephalitis virus, St. Louis encephalitis virus, and Powassan virus from the *Flaviviridae* family; chikungunya virus (CHIKV), Mayaro virus, Sindbis virus, and Venezuelan, Eastern, and Western equine encephalitis viruses from the *Togaviridae* family; Rift Valley fever virus, Crimean-Congo hemorrhagic fever virus, California encephalitis virus, Jamestown Canyon virus, and La Crosse virus from the *Bunyaviridae* family; and Colorado tick fever virus from the *Reoviridae* family. Most arboviruses are zoonotic pathogens with a nonhuman vertebrate as the primary host that may eventually cross into humans and cause disease. DENV infection, the most common arbovirus worldwide, is an important exception in that humans are the primary host. The arboviral transmission cycle generally consists of the vector's ingestion of blood from an infected host, viral replication within the arthropod's tissue – typically in the salivary glands – during a stage known as the extrinsic incubation period, and viral transmission to a new host when insects take a blood meal. Infected hosts may develop an acute clinical illness with a range of symptoms including febrile syndrome, hemorrhagic fever, encephalitis, and polyarthralgia. Some of the viruses may also cause long-term disease and disability.

## A Framework for the Study of Nutrition and Arboviral Infections

The study of the interactions between factors related to the nutritional status of humans and arboviral infections can be framed in different stages relative to vector, virus, and host characteristics. Some of these stages, which are not mutually exclusive, involve:

1. Effects of food production, transportation, commercialization, and storage systems on:
   • The vector's breeding environment, reproductive success, infectiousness, and geographic distribution.
   • The host's exposure to infected vectors.

It is plausible that habitat changes related to cultivation create new vector breeding grounds, promote vector reproduction [2], and increase vector-host contacts.

2. Effects of arboviral infections on the nutritional and metabolic status of the host. Infections may alter host nutritional status either acutely or chronically through inflammation-related changes in feeding behavior (e.g., anorexia) and metabolic rate, increased energy and essential nutrients requirements, increased oxidative stress, and dehydration.
3. Effects of the host's nutritional status on:
   • Exposure to bites. Mosquitoes rely on olfaction to locate feeding sources, and host factors affecting the secretion of skin compounds related to odor, such as $CO_2$, have been linked to the likelihood of being bitten. The host's body size and alcohol intake are dietary factors that have been associated with the attractiveness of hosts to mosquito bites [3–5].
   • Infectiousness of a bite. Immunological and mechanical factors could in theory limit or amplify infectiousness at the site of a bite. For example, it is conceivable that adipokines produced in subcutaneous fat might modulate a local reaction to the vector's saliva or that subcutaneous fat tissue could affect the distribution of blood capillaries in the dermis from which a mosquito would feed. These possibilities are largely theoretical at present.
   • Immune and inflammatory responses and viral replication after an infective bite. Not all mosquito bites result in detectable infection. Malnutrition could modulate immune and inflammatory responses and thus alter the course of a viral infection from agent replication to the severity and outcome of the clinical presentation.
   • Development of clinical symptoms of infection. In the case of dengue, only a fraction of infections becomes symptomatic. It is plausible that the host's nutritional status influences whether or not an infection will produce symptoms.
   • Risk of progression to severe forms of disease. Most research to date has focused on this area, and the evidence is reviewed in this chapter.
   • Virulence and transmissibility of the virus. The nutritional environment of the host might induce genotypic changes in the virus that change its virulence and potentially its transmissibility. For example, selenium and possibly vitamin E deficiencies in a host increase the virulence of coxsackievirus [6] and may induce more severe clinical forms of the disease caused by infection.
   • Vector reproductive fitness and competence, or ability to become infected and transmit the virus. The nutritional substrate of female mosquitoes relies heavily on blood meals from a host, through which they acquire sugar for glycogen synthesis and fat which is essential for egg development. One might posit that the nutritional quality of the host's blood might affect the vector's fitness with respect to adaptive traits that are strongly driven by nutrient intake, such as reproduction and host-seeking behavior.

Response to vaccines. Host nutritional status may interact with the response to vaccination. For example, vitamin A supplementation enhances some of the immunogenic responses to the yellow fever vaccine [7]. As new anti-DENV vaccines are developed, the potential of host nutritional status to modulate vaccine response deserves the attention of researchers. Not all aspects within this framework have been thoroughly studied in the context of arboviral infections, as most research has focused on the effects of the nutritional status on clinical presentation and the acute effects of infection on the host's metabolism and nutrient status. This evidence is reviewed here for dengue, the most public health-relevant arboviral infection, focusing on the epidemiologic and clinical approaches. We also briefly reference the limited evidence available on other arboviruses.

# Nutrition and Dengue

## *Epidemiology, Pathophysiology, and Clinical Aspects*

Dengue is the most widely distributed mosquito-borne viral infection, producing an estimated 400 million infections in over 100 countries annually (Fig. 10.1) [1]. Approximately a quarter of these infections are symptomatic; half a million result in cases of severe disease, and as many as 20,000 are fatal. The dengue virus is a *Flavivirus* in the *Flaviviridae* family and consists of a single strand of enveloped RNA. There are four antigenically different DENV serotypes that cause disease (DENV1, DENV2, DENV3, and DENV4), and all are transmitted from human to human by species of *Aedes* mosquitoes. *Aedes aegypti* is the most efficient vector; the female mosquito bites an infected host during the day and may infect another person immediately or after an incubation period of 8–10 days. After inoculation, the virus reaches lymph nodes and disseminates to the reticuloendothelial system from which it enters the blood, replicating primarily in mononuclear cells.

The first time a person is infected by any of the four DENV serotypes (primary infection), there is a humoral (antibody) response to that serotype that results in long-lasting immunity to the homologous serotype causing the infection and also generates short-term (2–12 months) cross-reactive heterotypic immunity to all serotypes. A cellular immune response involving activation of T cells with high cytotoxic potential ensues and is fundamental in controlling the infection. When there is a subsequent infection ("secondary") with a dengue serotype different from the first, pre-existing antibodies with cross-reactivity from the primary infection may be insufficient to neutralize replication of the secondary viral infection, resulting in increased cellular uptake through "antibody-dependent enhancement" [8]. The cellular immune response is skewed toward the previous serotype infection rather than

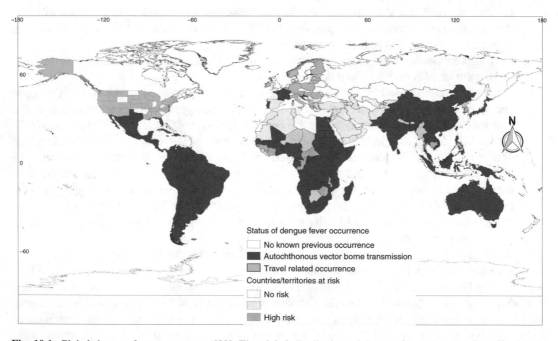

**Fig. 10.1** Global dengue fever occurrence [89]. The global distribution of dengue fever corresponds well with the global dengue risk. The distribution of dengue fever extends to the temperate part of the world, with some European countries reporting its occurrence. It is emphasized that displaying occurrences at the country level overstates the distribution of the virus, especially in China, Argentina, and Chile. (Reprinted from Leta et al. [89], with permission from Elsevier)

the current one and may lead to severe forms of the disease with plasma leakage and tissue damage through unrestrained inflammation.

From a clinical standpoint, dengue can manifest with a wide range of signs and symptoms, from a self-limited febrile illness through a potentially fatal syndrome of hemorrhaging and shock. The clinical evolution is usually divided into three phases: febrile, critical, and recovery. The febrile phase starts after an incubation period of 5–8 days from an infective bite and is characterized by sudden onset of high fever with severe headache and general malaise symptoms. Several other symptoms may occur, including exanthem, anorexia, and mild hemorrhagic signs. The critical phase begins at defervescence, around day 5. While most patients proceed to recovery, in as many as 5% of cases the disease may progress to a severe form characterized by increased vascular permeability and plasma leakage into the extravascular space. Signs and symptoms involve a low (narrow) pulse pressure, thrombocytopenia, hemoconcentration, and shock if plasma volume falls below a critical level. After 24–48 hours, patients enter the recovery phase during which extravascular fluid begins to be resorbed. A few factors, other than secondary infection, are known to increase the risk of severe dengue, although nutritional characteristics may play a role. Identifying these factors is especially important because there is no known prophylaxis to effectively prevent disease progression.

## Relations Between Nutritional Status and the Outcome of Dengue Infection

**Energy Balance** The balance between energy intake and expenditure governs body size and composition, which can be assessed through anthropometry (height, weight, arm circumference, and skinfold thickness) and quantification of the relative sizes of metabolic tissue compartments, such as fat and lean body mass. Most studies on the role of energy balance on risk and outcomes of dengue infection have compared anthropometric indicators between patients admitted to hospital with severe dengue and uninfected persons, and a majority have been conducted among children. Based on observations in dengue endemic regions, experts once thought that protein-energy undernutrition might protect against severe disease through dampening immune and inflammatory responses [9]. Evidence from some pediatric cross-sectional and case-control studies supported this view. For example, underweight (low weight-for-age) and stunted (low height-for-age) children from Vietnam [10] and Thailand [11] were less likely to have severe disease than their better-nourished counterparts, and anthropometric indices of overweight and obesity were positively related to disease severity in children from Thailand [9, 12] and Indonesia [13]. However, findings from other studies contradict the hypothesis, as underweight was positively associated with severe disease in a large case-control investigation of Thai children [14] and unrelated in other studies from India [15], El Salvador [16], Indonesia [17], Thailand [18], Cuba [19], or Sri Lanka [20]. In addition, while overweight was unrelated to disease severity in various settings [14, 16, 18], a meta-analysis of 15 pediatric studies suggested that obesity was associated with a 38% increased risk of severe dengue [21].

Studies in adults are limited by the fact that the seroprevalence of infection in this age group that approaches 100% in endemic regions. Among Indian pregnant women with a history of dengue, those with overweight had a higher risk of preterm delivery than participants without overweight [22]. In Malaysian patients >12 years of age who were hospitalized for dengue, obesity was associated with a more severe clinical course and longer hospital stay [23].

**Macronutrients** The role of energy intake from protein, carbohydrates, fat, or alcohol on dengue-related outcomes has not been well investigated. Most studies have focused on the relations between macronutrient biomarkers and severity of dengue infection using metabolomic techniques. Available evidence prior to 2018 has been previously reviewed [24].

*Fatty Acids (FA)* FA, the basic constituents of dietary fat, are essential to many pathophysiological pathways leading to severe forms of DENV infection. FA influence the organization of cell membranes and the composition of lipid rafts through their incorporation as phospholipids and sphingolipids [25]. Lipid raft microdomains play an essential role in DENV protein synthesis and replication [26]. In addition, some n-3 polyunsaturated fatty acids (PUFA), including eicosapentaenoic acid (EPA, 20:5n-3) and docosahexaenoic acid (DHA, 22:6n-3), could reduce expression of pro-inflammatory cytokines through different mechanisms including downregulated gene expression in mononuclear cells, decreased synthesis of pro-inflammatory eicosanoids derived from n-6 PUFA, reduced chemotaxis and lymphocyte proliferation, enhanced apoptosis of Th-1 cells, and decreased endothelial activation and dysfunction [27]. Some n-6 PUFA, including arachidonic acid (AA, 20:4n-6), are considered pro-inflammatory, while others such as dihomo-γ-linolenic acid (DGLA, 20:3n-6) exhibit anti-inflammatory properties [28]. Some cross-sectional investigations indicate that FA concentrations differ during the acute stages of dengue infection [29, 30], but it is not possible to conclude from them whether FA status prior to the infection had an effect on the outcome since the acute inflammatory process accompanying dengue infection could affect nutrient biomarkers. In two prospective studies of patients diagnosed with dengue fever (DF), higher serum DHA at around the onset of fever predicted an increased risk of progression to severe dengue [31, 32]. This finding was unexpected because DHA contributes to the resolution of inflammation through different pathways [27] and effective resolution of inflammation should be related to less risk of disease progression. The association may not have a causal interpretation if a strong inflammatory response at the time of infection, which independently predicts increased risk of progression, elicits an increase in serum DHA. In one of these studies [31], DGLA and pentadecanoic acid, a saturated FA that reflects dairy intake, were related to a decreased risk of progression to severe dengue among Colombian children and adults. DGLA is a long-chain n-6 PUFA synthesized endogenously from linoleic acid through desaturation and elongation. Even though DGLA can be desaturated into arachidonic acid, a pro-inflammatory FA, it is generally considered anti-inflammatory because it can be converted to prostaglandin $E_1$, a suppressor of chronic inflammation [28]. An increase in DGLA relative to AA could acutely attenuate the synthesis of pro-inflammatory eicosanoids derived from AA, including 4-series leukotrienes, 2-series prostaglandins, and platelet-activating factor, which may be involved in the pathophysiology of severe dengue [32]. In addition, DGLA may exhibit virucidal activity against encapsulated viruses [33, 34]. A potential effect of pentadecanoic acid might be related to its role in regulating gut microbiota signaling through intestinal bacterial synthesis of propionic acid.

**Amino Acids** Serotonin, a product of tryptophan metabolism, was lower in patients with DF compared with uninfected controls and even lower in patients with dengue hemorrhagic fever (DHF), a severe form of the disease, in a metabolomics study of Singaporean adults [35]. These results are valuable as they may highlight the effects of infection on amino acid metabolism; however, they are unlikely to reflect the role of protein on the response against dengue. Low serum proline at the onset of fever predicted a lower risk of progression to severe dengue in Nicaraguan children [32]. Similarly, glutamine concentrations were inversely related to dengue severity in Brazilian patients [36], suggesting that it may be an essential amino acid for viral replication. Finally, serum phenylalanine concentrations were higher in DHF patients compared with those of DF participants in the Singapore study [37], which could be due to decreased conversion into tyrosine due to oxidative stress induced by the infection.

**Micronutrients** Vitamins and minerals play key roles in regulatory and signaling aspects of immunity (see Chap. 3) [38], and their effects on risk and clinical outcome of several non-arboviral infections have been documented in randomized trials [39–43], as described in other chapters of this volume (see Chaps. 8, 9, 10, 11, and 12) [44–46]. In the case of dengue, studies conducted to date have been primarily observational; the evidence published up to 2016 has been reviewed elsewhere [47, 48].

**Vitamin D**  Vitamin D has the potential to modulate immunological events that are involved in the pathophysiology of severe dengue [49], including the downregulation of pro-inflammatory Th1 activity [50]. Vitamin D supplementation has been beneficial in the treatment of infections by hepatitis C virus, an RNA virus that shares some characteristics with dengue virus (DENV) [51]. Epidemiological evidence on the role of vitamin D on progression to severe dengue is scant. In a small cross-sectional study among Indian patients with secondary infections, circulating total 25-hydroxy vitamin D [25(OH)D] was higher in 38 patients with DHF than in 45 controls with DF only [52]; nevertheless, the difference was not statistically significant. It is not possible to discern from cross-sectional studies whether the nutrient influences disease severity or vice versa. In a prospective study of Colombians diagnosed with DF and followed during the acute episode, serum total 25(OH)D and vitamin D binding protein (DBP) concentrations at the onset of fever were compared between 110 cases who progressed to DHF/dengue shock syndrome (DSS) and 235 DF controls who did not progress. There was a strong positive, dose-dependent relation between vitamin D and the risk of progression; vitamin D-deficient patients were 87% less likely to progress to severe dengue compared with those who had adequate 25(OH)D concentrations at baseline [53]. DBP was nonsignificantly lower in cases compared with controls. These findings were contrary to the notion that vitamin D deficiency could worsen dengue-related outcomes, and potential explanatory mechanisms remain speculative. Vitamin D has been related to a decreased anti-inflammatory IL-10 response to viral toll-like receptor-3 stimulation [54]. In addition, some [55] – albeit not all [56] – studies of intracellular infections have suggested that vitamin D may increase dendritic cell expression of CD209, a dengue virus receptor. This could, in theory, enhance cellular susceptibility to infection, viral replication, and inflammation. A different mechanistic path could involve the expression of the vitamin D receptor (VDR) in immune cells. Some studies have found associations between VDR genetic polymorphisms and risk of progression to severe dengue [52, 57, 58], but whether VDR expression differs between progressors and non-progressors has not been investigated. Of note, serum vitamin D concentrations tend to be lower in patients with dengue than in uninfected persons [52, 53] which raises the possibility that the infection elicits an acute increase in circulating vitamin D as part of the body's defense response. In a study of Nicaraguans with DHF/DSS, concentrations of 1,25(OH)D, the active form of the vitamin, were lower compared with those of persons with DF only [32]. An anecdotal report of five cases with DF suggested that the administration of vitamin D and calcium during the acute episode shortened the duration of disease [59]; thus, the potential therapeutic value of enhancing vitamin D bioavailability during acute dengue infection requires careful consideration in future investigations.

**Vitamin A**  Vitamin A may enhance or dampen antibody production against selected antigens and may influence T-cell lymphopoiesis and lymphocyte differentiation [40]. Vitamin A modulates the balance between T helper (Th)1 and Th2 responses and plays a key role in mucosal immunity. Periodic vitamin A supplementation to preschool children [40] decreases morbidity from measles, severe diarrhea, human immune deficiency virus, and possibly malaria and helminthiases [60]. Data on the vitamin's potential effect in the context of arboviral infections are scant. In an observational study of Guatemalan adults, 9 DF patients had significantly lower serum retinol concentrations during the acute phase of the disease than did 12 healthy controls [61]. Retinol levels approached those of controls a week after discharge. These results suggest that clinical dengue infection alters circulating vitamin A levels; notwithstanding, the possible effect of vitamin A on dengue-related outcomes has not been studied.

**Vitamin E**  Vitamin E is a powerful antioxidant with significant effects on different aspects of immunity [62]. In a randomized controlled trial in India, daily administration of 400 mg vitamin E to 33 patients with DF resulted in higher platelet counts during the febrile and critical phases compared to standard treatment without vitamin E among other 33 DF patients [63]. The effect might be attributed to the antioxidant properties of vitamin E.

*Zinc*  Zinc modulates the activity of many immune cells [64], and zinc supplementation to children has positive effects on selected infection outcomes [65]. In a cross-sectional study of 60 Indonesian children <14 years of age, serum zinc concentration was inversely related to the severity of dengue disease; it was substantially lower in children with DSS than in those with DHF or DF [66]. However, in another study of 45 children from Indonesia, serum zinc was not associated with the severity of DHF [67]. In a small cross-sectional study of Thai children, zinc deficiency according to serum concentrations was not significantly related to the duration of hospital stay or duration of fever [68]; nevertheless, in a randomized trial of 50 Thai children admitted to hospital with DF, DHF, or DSS, oral administration of 45 mg elemental zinc for 5 days or until defervescence shortened hospital stay compared to placebo [69]; there was also a nonstatistically significant effect on shorter fever duration. No other outcomes were reported.

*Other Minerals*  In a study of 96 children and adults from India, serum copper concentrations were inversely related to dengue severity at the time of hospital admission but did not differ significantly from those of patients with other febrile illnesses [70]. By the time of defervescence, copper concentrations were significantly higher in dengue patients compared with those with other febrile illnesses. The copper increase paralleled a rise in ceruloplasmin, the copper transport protein [71]. In the same study, serum ferritin concentrations, an iron status indicator, were higher in the most severe dengue group compared with other dengue patients, they increased between hospital admission and defervescence, and they were predictive of severity [71]. Among 177 Thai children, serum ferritin was also positively related to dengue severity [72]. It is not possible to interpret that ferritin contributed to disease severity as it is an acute-phase reactant that increases during acute inflammation, regardless of iron status. Results from animal studies have suggested a potential role for chromium on progression to severe dengue [73, 74], but no data in humans are available.

# Nutrition and Other Arboviral Infections

## Chikungunya

Chikungunya (CHIKV) is an alphavirus in the *Togaviridae* family [1]. From its identification in East Africa in the 1950s, it has spread worldwide and has caused significant outbreaks in Asia and the Americas. CHIKV is transmitted by the same *Aedes* vectors as DENV; thus, both infections overlap geographically. Although CHIKV infections may be asymptomatic, the virus may cause an acute febrile illness after an incubation period of 3–12 days, typically accompanied by incapacitating polyarthralgia in peripheral small joints which can persist for months or years. Arthralgias are likely immune-mediated, caused by increased production of pro-inflammatory cytokines. Rarely, CHIKV disease may progress into a hemorrhagic syndrome, especially in children, or to encephalitis. In utero mother-to-child transmission has been reported, and it may be a cause of neonatal death [75].

Evidence of interactions between nutritional factors and CHIKV infection is limited. In cross-sectional analyses of a CHIKV outbreak among pregnant women in Madagascar [76], body weight >70 kg was associated with a >9 higher odds of seropositivity. Similarly, among pregnant women from Reunion Island, overweight (BMI ≥ 25 kg/m$^2$) was related to a 76% higher odds of seropositivity, compared with BMI <25 kg/m$^2$. In a population representative survey of Reunion Island, obesity (BMI ≥30 kg/m$^2$) was associated with a 29% higher adjusted prevalence of seropositivity to CHIKV compared with BMI <25 kg/m$^2$ [77]. However, BMI was not related to lingering chikungunya rheumatism [78]. CHIKV infection may also alter host metabolism. A metabolomics investigation suggested that CHIKV infection may alter amino acid and carbohydrate metabolism, as well as the tricarboxylic acid cycle [79] that aerobic organisms use to release stored energy through oxidation of acetyl-CoA derived from macronutrients. No study to date has addressed the potential role of micronutrients on CHIKV-related outcomes.

## *Zika*

Zika virus (ZIKV) is a flavivirus from the *Flaviviridae* family that was first discovered in the early 1950s. ZIKV remained contained in Southeast Asia until an epidemic broke out in Micronesia in 2007; it then expanded rapidly through the Americas. The virus is transmitted primarily by *Aedes* vectors, but sexual and mother-to-child transmission can also occur [80–82]. ZIKV infection is typically asymptomatic or involves a mild febrile illness with rash. However, in some rare instances, it can result in Guillain-Barré syndrome or cause severe malformations, particularly microcephalia, when the infection occurs during pregnancy.

No studies relating nutritional factors with ZIKV infection-related outcomes in humans have been published to date. In vitro studies suggest that compounds found in foods might interact with this and other arboviruses. For example, polyphenols like epigallocatechin gallate (abundantly found in tea) and delphinidin (present in grapes and some berries) inhibit ZIKV entry into host cells in vitro (Fig. 10.2) [83–86].

Also, curcumin, a compound found in turmeric, has the potential to inhibit cellular infection by ZIKV [87]. The effect of other nutritional factors on risk and outcome of ZIKV infection remains to be elucidated. Of special interest is whether nutrients involved in one-carbon metabolism (e.g., folic acid, vitamin $B_{12}$) could modulate the risk of neural tube defects associated with intrauterine ZIKV infection.

## Conclusions

Most available evidence on the interactions between nutritional factors and risk and outcome of arboviral infections has focused on dengue, the most significant human mosquito-borne viral infection worldwide. Evidence from anthropometric studies of a potential protective effect of protein-energy malnutrition against severe dengue in children is inconsistent. Pediatric obesity might be related to increased risk of adverse dengue-related outcomes, but most available evidence is from cross-sectional studies without proper adjustment for confounding, and the biological plausibility of a potential effect is unclear. Data on the role of micronutrients also consists predominantly of cross-sectional studies comparing biomarker concentrations between groups of people with dengue infection of varying clinical severity. Because both exposure (e.g., nutrient biomarkers) and outcome (severity of dengue disease) are assessed at the same time, it is impossible to disentangle the temporal sequence of events leading to one another. Rather than representing an effect of nutrient status or stores on the risk of severe dengue, these studies most likely reflect the effect of an acute infection on nutrient biomarkers. This is confirmed in a few studies that assessed the change in biomarker concentrations throughout the acute episode and post-convalescence. Investigations using measures of nutritional status that are stable over the long-term and which are unlikely to be affected by the infection are urgently needed to identify nutrients that might be tested as potential therapeutic targets to prevent progression or treat severe disease. Results from two small randomized trials involving nutrients as therapeutic agents during the acute dengue episode [63, 69] offer hope of the potential of nutraceutical interventions in the context of arboviral infections.

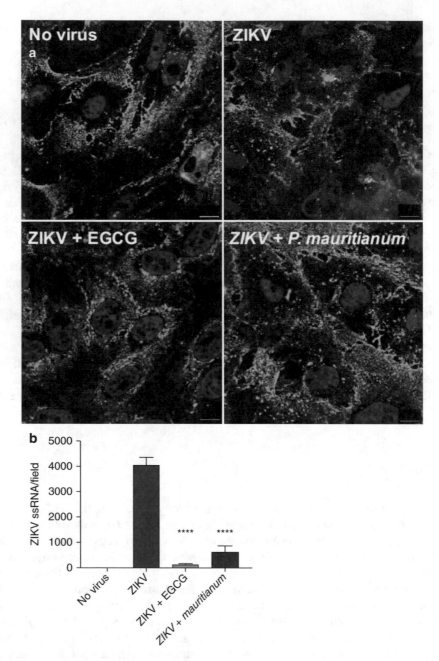

**Fig. 10.2** *P. mauritianum* extract inhibits the production of ZIKV ssRNA. ZIKV-MR766 particles were incubated with the *P. mauritianum* extract for 1 hour at 37 °C [86]. The EGCG treatment (100 μM) was used as a positive control. Vero cells were left uninfected or were infected at an MOI of 1 for 24 hours. (**a**) Cells were processed for FISH using a probe specific for viral RNA (red) and then stained with NucBlue to visualize the nuclei (blue). Cell membranes were stained with AF488-conjugated wheat germ agglutinin. Images are representative of three independent experiments. Scale bars are 20 μm. (**b**) Quantification of ZIKV ssRNA spots counted per field (fields contained on average 300 cells) from the experiments represented in the images. Data are means ± SD of three independent experiments. Statistical analyses were performed using a one-way ANOVA and Dunnett's test for multiple comparisons (**** $p < 0.0001$). (Reprinted from: Clain et al. [86] (Open Access))

Estimating the effect of nutritional factors on the risk of infection, symptomatic or asymptomatic, would require establishing long-term population-based cohorts of uninfected persons with repeated assessments of both the nutritional status and the incidence of new infections. Alternatively, incorporating nutrition measures in ongoing studies of infection dynamics or vaccine efficacy could facilitate the study of nutrition and arboviral infection in a cost-effective manner. Some nutrients could be analyzed in secondary studies of biomarkers in stored biological specimens. Vaccine efficacy trials would offer a unique opportunity to identify vaccine-nutrient interactions, since nutrients could potentiate or interfere with the effect of vaccines [88]. These studies may not be feasible among adults from endemic areas, because most would have a history of infection at the time of recruitment into a cohort.

Metabolomic studies of the effect of acute infections on macro- and micronutrient metabolism may offer valuable information on pathways or nutrients whose demands are increased by the infection, and which may constitute therapeutic targets.

# References

1. Farrar J, Hotez PJ, Junghanss T, Kang G, Lalloo D, White NJ. Manson's tropical diseases. 23rd ed. Philadelphia: Elsevier, 2013.
2. Sarfraz MS, Tripathi NK, Tipdecho T, Thongbu T, Kerdthong P, Souris M. Analyzing the spatio-temporal relationship between dengue vector larval density and land-use using factor analysis and spatial ring mapping. BMC Public Health. 2012;12:853.
3. Port G, Boreham P, Bryan J. The relationship of host size to feeding by mosquitoes of the Anopheles gambiae Giles complex (Diptera: Culicidae). Bull Entomol Res. 1980;70(1):133–44.
4. Shirai O, Tsuda T, Kitagawa S, Naitoh K, Seki T, Kamimura K, et al. Alcohol ingestion stimulates mosquito attraction. J Am Mosq Control Assoc. 2002;18(2):91–6.
5. Lefevre T, Gouagna LC, Dabire KR, Elguero E, Fontenille D, Renaud F, et al. Beer consumption increases human attractiveness to malaria mosquitoes. PLoS One. 2010;5(3):e9546.
6. Beck MA, Shi Q, Morris VC, Levander OA. Rapid genomic evolution of a non-virulent coxsackievirus B3 in selenium-deficient mice results in selection of identical virulent isolates. Nat Med. 1995;1(5):433–6.
7. Ahmad SM, Haskell MJ, Raqib R, Stephensen CB. Men with low vitamin A stores respond adequately to primary yellow fever and secondary tetanus toxoid vaccination. J Nutr. 2008;138(11):2276–83.
8. Halstead SB, O'Rourke EJ. Antibody-enhanced dengue virus infection in primate leukocytes. Nature. 1977;265(5596):739–41.
9. Pichainarong N, Mongkalangoon N, Kalayanarooj S, Chaveepojnkamjorn W. Relationship between body size and severity of dengue hemorrhagic fever among children aged 0–14 years. Southeast Asian J Trop Med Public Health. 2006;37(2):283–8.
10. Nguyen TH, Nguyen TL, Lei HY, Lin YS, Le BL, Huang KJ, et al. Association between sex, nutritional status, severity of dengue hemorrhagic fever, and immune status in infants with dengue hemorrhagic fever. Am J Trop Med Hyg. 2005;72(4):370–4.
11. Thisyakorn U, Nimmannitya S. Nutritional status of children with dengue hemorrhagic fever. Clin Infect Dis. 1993;16(2):295–7.
12. Chuansumrit A, Phimolthares V, Tardtong P, Tapaneya-Olarn C, Tapaneya-Olarn W, Kowsathit P, et al. Transfusion requirements in patients with dengue hemorrhagic fever. Southeast Asian J Trop Med Public Health. 2000;31(1):10–4.
13. Junia J, Garna H, Setiabudi D. Clinical risk factors for dengue shock syndrome in children. Paediatr Indones. 2007;47:7–11.
14. Kalayanarooj S, Nimmannitya S. Is dengue severity related to nutritional status? Southeast Asian J Trop Med Public Health. 2005;36(2):378–84.
15. Kabra SK, Jain Y, Pandey RM, Madhulika ST, Tripathi P, et al. Dengue haemorrhagic fever in children in the 1996 Delhi epidemic. Trans R Soc Trop Med Hyg. 1999;93(3):294–8.
16. Maron GM, Clara AW, Diddle JW, Pleites EB, Miller L, Macdonald G, et al. Association between nutritional status and severity of dengue infection in children in El Salvador. Am J Trop Med Hyg. 2010;82(2):324–9.
17. Anto S, Sebodo T, Sutaryo, Suminta, Ismangoen. Nutritional status of Dengue haemorrhagic fever in children. Paediatr Indones. 1983;23(1–2):15–24.
18. Tantracheewathorn T, Tantracheewathorn S. Risk factors of dengue shock syndrome in children. J Med Assoc Thail. 2007;90(2):272–7.

19. Arguelles JM, Hernandez M, Mazart I. Nutritional evaluation of children and adolescents with a diagnosis of dengue. Bol Oficina Sanit Panam. 1987;103(3):245–51.
20. Malavige GN, Ranatunga PK, Velathanthiri VG, Fernando S, Karunatilaka DH, Aaskov J, et al. Patterns of disease in Sri Lankan dengue patients. Arch Dis Child. 2006;91(5):396–400.
21. Zulkipli MS, Dahlui M, Jamil N, Peramalah D, Wai HVC, Bulgiba A, et al. The association between obesity and dengue severity among pediatric patients: a systematic review and meta-analysis. PLoS Negl Trop Dis. 2018;12(2):e0006263.
22. Nujum ZT, Nirmala C, Vijayakumar K, Saboora Beegum M, Jyothi R. Incidence and outcomes of dengue in a cohort of pregnant women from an endemic region of India: obesity could be a potential risk for adverse outcomes. Trans R Soc Trop Med Hyg. 2019;113(5):242–51.
23. Tan VPK, Ngim CF, Lee EZ, Ramadas A, Pong LY, Ng JI, et al. The association between obesity and dengue virus (DENV) infection in hospitalised patients. PLoS One. 2018;13(7):e0200698.
24. Byers NM, Fleshman AC, Perera R, Molins CR. Metabolomic insights into human arboviral infections: dengue, Chikungunya, and Zika viruses. Viruses. 2019;11(3):225.
25. Turk HF, Chapkin RS. Membrane lipid raft organization is uniquely modified by n-3 polyunsaturated fatty acids. Prostaglandins Leukot Essent Fatty Acids. 2013;88(1):43–7.
26. Garcia Cordero J, Leon Juarez M, Gonzalez YMJA, Cedillo Barron L, Gutierrez CB. Caveolin-1 in lipid rafts interacts with dengue virus NS3 during polyprotein processing and replication in HMEC-1 cells. PLoS One. 2014;9(3):e90704.
27. Calder PC. Omega-3 polyunsaturated fatty acids and inflammatory processes: nutrition or pharmacology? Br J Clin Pharmacol. 2013;75(3):645–62.
28. Wang X, Lin H, Gu Y. Multiple roles of dihomo-gamma-linolenic acid against proliferation diseases. Lipids Health Dis. 2012;11:25.
29. Cui L, Lee YH, Kumar Y, Xu F, Lu K, Ooi EE, et al. Serum metabolome and lipidome changes in adult patients with primary dengue infection. PLoS Negl Trop Dis. 2013;7(8):e2373.
30. Khedr A, Hegazy M, Kamal A, Shehata MA. Profiling of esterified fatty acids as biomarkers in the blood of dengue fever patients using a microliter-scale extraction followed by gas chromatography and mass spectrometry. J Sep Sci. 2015;38(2):316–24.
31. Villamor E, Villar LA, Lozano-Parra A, Herrera VM, Herran OF. Serum fatty acids and progression from dengue fever to dengue haemorrhagic fever/dengue shock syndrome. Br J Nutr. 2018;120(7):787–96.
32. Voge NV, Perera R, Mahapatra S, Gresh L, Balmaseda A, Lorono-Pino MA, et al. Metabolomics-based discovery of small molecule biomarkers in serum associated with dengue virus infections and disease outcomes. PLoS Negl Trop Dis. 2016;10(2):e0004449.
33. Thormar H, Isaacs CE, Kim KS, Brown HR. Inactivation of visna virus and other enveloped viruses by free fatty acids and monoglycerides. Ann N Y Acad Sci. 1994;724:465–71.
34. Villamor E, Koulinska IN, Furtado J, Baylin A, Aboud S, Manji K, et al. Long-chain n-6 polyunsaturated fatty acids in breast milk decrease the risk of HIV transmission through breastfeeding. Am J Clin Nutr. 2007;86(3):682–9.
35. Cui L, Lee YH, Thein TL, Fang J, Pang J, Ooi EE, et al. Serum metabolomics reveals serotonin as a predictor of severe dengue in the early phase of dengue fever. PLoS Negl Trop Dis. 2016;10(4):e0004607.
36. El-Bacha T, Struchiner CJ, Cordeiro MT, Almeida FCL, Marques ET Jr, Da Poian AT. 1H Nuclear magnetic resonance metabolomics of plasma unveils liver dysfunction in dengue patients. J Virol. 2016;90(16):7429–43.
37. Cui L, Pang J, Lee YH, Ooi EE, Ong CN, Leo YS, et al. Serum metabolome changes in adult patients with severe dengue in the critical and recovery phases of dengue infection. PLoS Negl Trop Dis. 2018;12(1):e0006217.
38. Stephensen CB. Primer on immune response and interface with malnutrition. In: Humphries DL, Scott ME, Vermund SH, editors. Nutrition and infectious disease: shifting the clinical paradigm. Switzerland: Springer Nature; 2020.
39. Meydani SN, Leka LS, Fine BC, Dallal GE, Keusch GT, Singh MF, et al. Vitamin E and respiratory tract infections in elderly nursing home residents: a randomized controlled trial. JAMA. 2004;292(7):828–36.
40. Villamor E, Fawzi WW. Effects of vitamin a supplementation on immune responses and correlation with clinical outcomes. Clin Microbiol Rev. 2005;18(3):446–64.
41. Sazawal S, Black RE, Ramsan M, Chwaya HM, Stoltzfus RJ, Dutta A, et al. Effects of routine prophylactic supplementation with iron and folic acid on admission to hospital and mortality in preschool children in a high malaria transmission setting: community-based, randomised, placebo-controlled trial. Lancet. 2006;367(9505):133–43.
42. Lukacik M, Thomas RL, Aranda JV. A meta-analysis of the effects of oral zinc in the treatment of acute and persistent diarrhea. Pediatrics. 2008;121(2):326–36.
43. Martineau AR, Jolliffe DA, Greenberg L, Aloia JF, Bergman P, Dubnov-Raz G, et al. Vitamin D supplementation to prevent acute respiratory infections: individual participant data meta-analysis. Health Technol Assess. 2019;23(2):1–44.

44. Kim HH, Bei AK. Nutritional frameworks in malaria. In: Humphries DL, Scott ME, Vermund SH, editors. Nutrition and infectious disease: shifting the clinical paradigm. Switzerland: Springer Nature; 2020.

45. Scott ME, Koski K. Soil-transmitted helminths – does nutrition make a difference? In: Humphries DL, Scott ME, Vermund SH, editors. Nutrition and infectious disease: shifting the clinical paradigm. Switzerland: Springer Nature; 2020.

46. Siddiqui F, Belayneh G, Bhutta ZA. Nutrition and diarrheal disease and enteric pathogens. In: Humphries DL, Scott ME, Vermund SH, editors. Nutrition and infectious disease: shifting the clinical paradigm. Switzerland: Springer Nature; 2020.

47. Ahmed S, Finkelstein JL, Stewart AM, Kenneth J, Polhemus ME, Endy TP, et al. Micronutrients and dengue. Am J Trop Med Hyg. 2014;91(5):1049–56.

48. Weger-Lucarelli J, Auerswald H, Vignuzzi M, Dussart P, Karlsson EA. Taking a bite out of nutrition and arbovirus infection. PLoS Negl Trop Dis. 2018;12(3):e0006247.

49. Arboleda JF, Urcuqui-Inchima S. Vitamin D-regulated MicroRNAs: are they protective factors against dengue virus infection? Adv Virol. 2016;2016:1016840.

50. Aranow C. Vitamin D and the immune system. J Investig Med. 2011;59(6):881–6.

51. Eltayeb AA, Abdou MA, Abdel-aal AM, Othman MH. Vitamin D status and viral response to therapy in hepatitis C infected children. World J Gastroenterol. 2015;21(4):1284–91.

52. Alagarasu K, Bachal RV, Bhagat AB, Shah PS, Dayaraj C. Elevated levels of vitamin D and deficiency of mannose binding lectin in dengue hemorrhagic fever. Virol J. 2012;9:86.

53. Villamor E, Villar LA, Lozano A, Herrera VM, Herran OF. Vitamin D serostatus and dengue fever progression to dengue hemorrhagic fever/dengue shock syndrome. Epidemiol Infect. 2017;145(14):2961–70.

54. Liao SL, Lai SH, Tsai MH, Hua MC, Yeh KW, Su KW, et al. Maternal vitamin D level is associated with viral toll-like receptor triggered IL-10 response but not the risk of infectious diseases in infancy. Mediat Inflamm. 2016;2016:8175898.

55. Torres C, Sanchez de la Torre M, Garcia-Moruja C, Carrero AJ, Trujillo Mdel M, Fibla J, et al. Immunophenotype of vitamin D receptor polymorphism associated to risk of HIV-1 infection and rate of disease progression. Curr HIV Res. 2010;8(6):487–92.

56. Afsal K, Selvaraj P. Effect of 1,25-dihydroxyvitamin D3 on the expression of mannose receptor, DC-SIGN and autophagy genes in pulmonary tuberculosis. Tuberculosis. 2016;99:1–10.

57. Dettogni RS, Tristao-Sa R, Dos Santos M, da Silva FF, Louro ID. Single nucleotide polymorphisms in immune system genes and their association with clinical symptoms persistence in dengue-infected persons. Hum Immunol. 2015;76(10):717–23.

58. Loke H, Bethell D, Phuong CX, Day N, White N, Farrar J, et al. Susceptibility to dengue hemorrhagic fever in Vietnam: evidence of an association with variation in the vitamin d receptor and Fc gamma receptor IIa genes. Am J Trop Med Hyg. 2002;67(1):102–6.

59. Sanchez-Valdez E, Delgado-Aradillas M, Torres-Martinez JA, Torres-Benitez JM. Clinical response in patients with dengue fever to oral calcium plus vitamin D administration: study of 5 cases. Proc West Pharmacol Soc. 2009;52:14–7.

60. Payne LG, Koski KG, Ortega-Barria E, Scott ME. Benefit of vitamin A supplementation on ascaris reinfection is less evident in stunted children. J Nutr. 2007;137(6):1455–9.

61. Klassen P, Biesalski HK, Mazariegos M, Solomons NW, Furst P. Classic dengue fever affects levels of circulating antioxidants. Nutrition. 2004;20(6):542–7.

62. Meydani SN, Han SN, Wu D. Vitamin E and immune response in the aged: molecular mechanisms and clinical implications. Immunol Rev. 2005;205:269–84.

63. Vaish A, Verma S, Agarwal A, Gupta L, Gutch M. Effect of vitamin E on thrombocytopenia in dengue fever. Ann Trop Med Public Health. 2012;5(4):282–5.

64. Haase H, Rink L. Functional significance of zinc-related signaling pathways in immune cells. Annu Rev Nutr. 2009;29:133–52.

65. Lassi ZS, Moin A, Bhutta ZA. Zinc supplementation for the prevention of pneumonia in children aged 2 months to 59 months. Cochrane Database Syst Rev. 2016;12:CD005978.

66. Yuliana N, Fadil RMR, Chairulfatah A. Serum zinc levels and clinical severity of dengue infection in children. Paediatr Indones. 2009;49(6):309–14.

67. Widagdo. Blood zinc levels and clinical severity of dengue hemorrhagic fever in children. Southeast Asian J Trop Med Public Health. 2008;39(4):610–6.

68. Rerksuppaphol L, Rerksuppaphol S. Zinc deficiency in children with Dengue viral infection. Pediatr Rep. 2019;11(1):7386.

69. Rerksuppaphol S, Rerksuppaphol L. A randomized controlled trial of zinc supplementation as adjuvant therapy for Dengue viral infection in Thai children. Int J Prev Med. 2018;9:88.

70. Soundravally R, Sherin J, Agieshkumar BP, Daisy MS, Cleetus C, Narayanan P, et al. Serum levels of copper and iron in dengue fever. Rev Inst Med Trop Sao Paulo. 2015;57(4):315–20.
71. Soundravally R, Agieshkumar B, Daisy M, Sherin J, Cleetus CC. Ferritin levels predict severe dengue. Infection. 2015;43(1):13–9.
72. Chaiyaratana W, Chuansumrit A, Atamasirikul K, Tangnararatchakit K. Serum ferritin levels in children with dengue infection. Southeast Asian J Trop Med Public Health. 2008;39(5):832–6.
73. Shrivastava R, Srivastava S, Upreti RK, Chaturvedi UC. Effects of dengue virus infection on peripheral blood cells of mice exposed to hexavalent chromium with drinking water. Indian J Med Res. 2005;122(2):111–9.
74. Shrivastava R, Nagar R, Ravishankar GA, Upreti RK, Chaturvedi UC. Effect of pretreatment with chromium picolinate on haematological parameters during dengue virus infection in mice. Indian J Med Res. 2007;126(5):440–6.
75. Contopoulos-Ioannidis D, Newman-Lindsay S, Chow C, LaBeaud AD. Mother-to-child transmission of Chikungunya virus: a systematic review and meta-analysis. PLoS Negl Trop Dis. 2018;12(6):e0006510.
76. Schwarz NG, Girmann M, Randriamampionona N, Bialonski A, Maus D, Krefis AC, et al. Seroprevalence of antibodies against Chikungunya, Dengue, and Rift Valley fever viruses after febrile illness outbreak, Madagascar. Emerg Infect Dis. 2012;18(11):1780–6.
77. Fred A, Fianu A, Beral M, Guernier V, Sissoko D, Mechain M, et al. Individual and contextual risk factors for chikungunya virus infection: the SEROCHIK cross-sectional population-based study. Epidemiol Infect. 2018;146(8):1056–64.
78. Gerardin P, Fianu A, Michault A, Mussard C, Boussaid K, Rollot O, et al. Predictors of Chikungunya rheumatism: a prognostic survey ancillary to the TELECHIK cohort study. Arthritis Res Ther. 2013;15(1):R9.
79. Shrinet J, Shastri JS, Gaind R, Bhavesh NS, Sunil S. Serum metabolomics analysis of patients with chikungunya and dengue mono/co-infections reveals distinct metabolite signatures in the three disease conditions. Sci Rep. 2016;6:36833.
80. Grischott F, Puhan M, Hatz C, Schlagenhauf P. Non-vector-borne transmission of Zika virus: a systematic review. Travel Med Infect Dis. 2016;14(4):313–30.
81. Blohm GM, Lednicky JA, Marquez M, White SK, Loeb JC, Pacheco CA, et al. Evidence for mother-to-child transmission of Zika virus through breast milk. Clin Infect Dis. 2018;66(7):1120–1.
82. Counotte MJ, Kim CR, Wang J, Bernstein K, Deal CD, Broutet NJN, et al. Sexual transmission of Zika virus and other flaviviruses: a living systematic review. PLoS Med. 2018;15(7):e1002611.
83. Carneiro BM, Batista MN, Braga ACS, Nogueira ML, Rahal P. The green tea molecule EGCG inhibits Zika virus entry. Virology. 2016;496:215–8.
84. Sharma N, Murali A, Singh SK, Giri R. Epigallocatechin gallate, an active green tea compound inhibits the Zika virus entry into host cells via binding the envelope protein. Int J Biol Macromol. 2017;104(Pt A):1046–54.
85. Vazquez-Calvo A, Jimenez de Oya N, Martin-Acebes MA, Garcia-Moruno E, Saiz JC. Antiviral properties of the natural polyphenols delphinidin and epigallocatechin gallate against the flaviviruses West Nile virus, Zika virus, and dengue virus. Front Microbiol. 2017;8:1314.
86. Clain E, Haddad JG, Koishi AC, Sinigaglia L, Rachidi W, Despres P, et al. The polyphenol-rich extract from Psiloxylon mauritianum, an endemic medicinal plant from Reunion Island, inhibits the early stages of Dengue and Zika virus infection. Int J Mol Sci. 2019;20(8):1860. https://doi.org/10.3390/ijms20081860.
87. Mounce BC, Cesaro T, Carrau L, Vallet T, Vignuzzi M. Curcumin inhibits Zika and chikungunya virus infection by inhibiting cell binding. Antivir Res. 2017;142:148–57.
88. Benn CS, Aaby P, Nielsen J, Binka FN, Ross DA. Does vitamin A supplementation interact with routine vaccinations? An analysis of the Ghana Vitamin A Supplementation Trial. Am J Clin Nutr. 2009;90(3):629–39.
89. Leta S, Beyene TJ, De Clercq EM, Amenu K, Kraemer MUG, Revie CW. Global risk mapping for major diseases transmitted by Aedes aegypti and Aedes albopictus. Int J Infect Dis. 2018;67:25–35.

# Chapter 11
# Nutritional Frameworks in Malaria

Harry Hyunteh Kim, Morgan M. Goheen, and Amy Kristine Bei

## Abbreviations

| | |
|---|---|
| ACT | Artemisinin-based combination therapy |
| CD | Cluster of differentiation molecule |
| DARC | Duffy antigen/chemokine receptor |
| DDT | Dichloro-diphenyl-trichloroethane |
| DHFR | Dihydrofolate reductase |
| DHPS | Dihydropteroate synthase |
| IDA | Iron deficiency anemia |
| IPTp | Intermittent preventative treatment for malaria in pregnancy |
| LBW | Low birth weight |
| PEM | Protein-energy malnutrition |
| PfHRP2 | *Plasmodium falciparum* histidine-rich protein 2 |
| PS | Phosphatidylserine |
| $R_0$ | Basic reproduction number |
| RBC | Red blood cells |
| SMC | Seasonal malaria chemoprevention |
| SP | Sulfadoxine-pyrimethamine |
| Th | T helper |
| THF | Tetrahydrofolate |
| WHO | World Health Organization |

H. H. Kim (✉) · A. K. Bei
Department of Epidemiology of Microbial Diseases, Yale School of Public Health, New Haven, CT, USA
e-mail: harry.kim@mail.mcgill.ca; amy.bei@yale.edu

M. M. Goheen
Department of Internal Medicine, Yale School of Medicine, New Haven, CT, USA
e-mail: morgan.goheen@yale.edu

© Springer Nature Switzerland AG 2021
D. L. Humphries et al. (eds.), *Nutrition and Infectious Diseases*, Nutrition and Health,
https://doi.org/10.1007/978-3-030-56913-6_11

**Key Points**
- Malaria and malnutrition both display clinically nonspecific symptoms, which make diagnosis and surveillance efforts difficult, especially in low-resource settings.
- The interactions between malaria and malnutrition are complex, and the clinical manifestation may differ based on the species of *Plasmodium*, the type of host malnutrition (micronutrient deficiency, protein-energy malnutrition, iron deficiency), as well as geo-social factors.
- The critical factors to consider when delineating potential pathways between nutritional status and for malaria include definitions of nutritional status, whether hosts are deficient in macro- and/or micronutrients, variability in study designs, and implications of covariates.
- Poor host nutritional status may increase susceptibility to malaria infection, although the implications on severity of pathogenesis and pathology remain unclear when each individual type of nutritional status is considered.
- Public health interventions to combat malnutrition in areas endemic to malaria should consider the possible positive and negative impacts on vulnerable populations from potential malaria infections.
- Standardized metrics and biomarkers common for both malaria and malnutrition are required for effective surveillance of malaria and malnutrition.
- There are many opportunities for public health interventions when approaching these topics holistically, and thus, it is important to consider the possible interactions between the two conditions.

# An Introduction to Malaria and Nutrition

Malaria, a febrile illness caused by species of the *Plasmodium* protozoan parasite, is one of the most important human infectious diseases in history, with a global distribution in 87 countries and 219 million cases and 435,000 deaths in 2017 (see Chap. 6) [1, 2]. Sub-Saharan Africa has the heaviest disease burden, with over 90% of malarial cases and deaths concentrated in that region. *P. falciparum*, the species that generally causes the most severe symptoms, is concentrated in sub-Saharan Africa and Oceania, and *P. vivax* is mostly found in the Americas, and India, with a minor distribution in Africa [3]. Other *Plasmodium* species include *P. ovale*, *P. malariae*, and *P. knowlesi*; these are less common than *P. vivax* and *P. falciparum*, and infection with these species manifests with less severe symptoms. While *P. falciparum* and *P. vivax* represent the majority of the global malaria burden, for the purposes of this chapter, we will focus largely on *P. falciparum*. The burden of malaria is difficult to accurately quantify due to a multitude of factors: endemic areas are also co-endemic with other pathogens that cause nonspecific febrile illnesses, symptoms vary from mild fever to fatal cerebral illness and death, and asymptomatic cases may go undetected as sensitive and specific point-of-care diagnostic tests are often not readily available in low-resource settings. Nevertheless, the field of malaria research has moved away from clinical symptom-based diagnosis and microscopy to more specific detection methods, such as rapid molecular diagnostic tests. Identifying asymptomatic carriers remains a challenge, as they are less likely to present themselves for diagnosis or treatment.

The disease burden of malaria in endemic regions is determined by a mix of extrinsic and intrinsic factors associated with humans, mosquitoes, and the parasite. Of the intrinsic factors, human health and nutritional status, mosquito species, and mosquito behavior (preference for human feeding) are important factors. Of the extrinsic factors, climate and ecology, availability of health resources, prevention and control methods, and political readiness to tackle the disease are the most important [4].

Humans become infected when infected female *Anopheles* mosquitoes transmit sporozoites through their salivary glands when they bite. The parasite's life cycle, described in Chap. 6, is complex and varies slightly by *Plasmodium* species [2]. All species undergo an exoerythrocytic liver stage in the human host, in which asexual replication takes place for 1–2 weeks, resulting in the production of merozoites. For *P. vivax* and *P. ovale*, a subset of sporozoites go through a hypnozoite stage in the liver, remaining dormant for weeks to years after the initial infection. This "latent" stage is associated with the long dormancy and relapse seen in people infected with *P. vivax* or *P. ovale*.

Merozoites are released from liver cells into the bloodstream, where they invade erythrocytes, undergo another round of asexual replication, and form intracellular schizonts. During this blood stage, infected erythrocytes burst, allowing neighboring uninfected erythrocytes to be infected by the newly released merozoites. This is the point where clinical symptoms manifest. The exception is *P. knowlesi*, which can cause high parasitemia and severe symptoms in some cases [5, 6].

*Plasmodium* spp. also display distinct preferences for erythrocytes of different ages [7]. As the erythrocyte ages, it loses surface area and volume, the cluster of differentiation molecule CD71 (cluster of differentiation 71, transferrin receptor) and sialic acid levels decrease, and there is an increase of phosphatidylserine (PS) on the cell surface and an emergence of senescent cell antigen, derived from the oxidation of Band3 [8–10]. These mechanisms make older cells more susceptible to splenic clearance, leading to lower parasitemia. In addition to structural changes, differences in expression levels of certain blood groups have also been described in younger compared to older erythrocytes. Complement receptor (CR)1 [11, 12], decay-accelerating factor (DAF) [13], and the Duffy antigen/chemokine receptor (DARC) [14] have been shown to be expressed more highly on the immature erythrocytes (reticulocytes) than on normocytes. It is thought that such differences in receptor levels might influence the erythrocyte age preference demonstrated by *Plasmodium* species. Of the primate malarias, *Plasmodium knowlesi* (also recognized as the fifth human malaria species) can invade normocytes [15] as can *P. cynomolgi*; however, like *P. falciparum*, *P. cynomolgi* preferentially infects reticulocytes. Of the human malarias, while *P. vivax* [16] and *P. ovale* are restricted to reticulocytes, *P. falciparum* invades erythrocytes of all ages while exhibiting a preference for reticulocytes [17]. *P. malariae* exhibits a preference for aged erythrocytes [18]. This species-specific preference for particular stages of the erythrocyte is a mechanism that can regulate the parasite growth and population levels within the host, and can contribute to their relative pathogenicity. Whether deficiencies of nutrients that interfere with erythropoiesis, such as iron, folate, and vitamin $B_{12}$ [19], alter susceptibility to specific species of *Plasmodium* is not known, but it has been reported that iron supplementation can increase reticulocyte numbers [20] (potentially promoting infection and *Plasmodium* replication).

Among the physiological changes induced by blood stage infection, the production of new erythrocytes in the bone marrow (erythropoiesis) is rendered ineffective. The reduced levels of circulating RBCs, which contribute to the pathology of malarial anemia, are secondary to the parasite's manipulation of host physiology. The observed the suppression of erythropoiesis is thought to be from an imbalance of cytokines secondary to the immune response, rather than from the suppression of the erythropoietic hormone erythropoietin [21, 22]. It may also result from the iron deficiency caused by malaria. Studies have been inconclusive in determining the protective or detrimental roles of pro-inflammatory T helper (Th)1 or Th2 cytokines [23, 24]. Generally, Th1 (type 1) cytokines are important in controlling early-stage infections to reduce parasitemia, while Th2 (type 2) cytokines aid in the production of antibodies for long-term protection (see Chap. 3). The role of pro-inflammatory cytokines in cases of severe disease, such as in cerebral malaria and severe malarial anemia, are less well understood.

Within the erythrocyte, a subset of asexual merozoites will develop into the sexual stages of the parasite—the male and female gametocytes. *P. falciparum* gametocytes have been shown to sequester and accumulate at the extravascular space of the bone marrow and in erythroid precursor cells [25]. Here parasites can avoid phagocytosis from circulating immune cells and utilize alternative adhesion mechanisms to remain in this niche, effectively halting the hematopoiesis process. While immature gametocytes sequester in the bone marrow, mature stage V gametocytes circulate in the peripheral blood waiting to be taken up when a female *Anopheles* mosquito takes a blood meal. This is the only stage of the life cycle that is infectious to the mosquito and thus can transmit infection from an infected human host.

All *Plasmodium* species are transmitted by the mosquitoes of the *Anopheles* genus, which has a worldwide distribution. Over 700 species in the genus have been identified, among which around 70 are potential vectors of the *Plasmodium* species that can be transmitted to humans [26]. *Anopheles* mosquitoes display species-specific habits and habitats, which can affect the time of day when they bite and their host feeding preferences. Breeding sites can include freshwater and saltwater marshes, rice fields, the outskirts of ponds and drainage pits, and urban sites. Further, some species are anthropophilic, preferentially feeding on humans, while others preferentially bite other mammal or non-mammal hosts, with humans being coincidental targets. Among the mosquitoes that readily transmit parasites to humans, *A. gambiense* and *A. funestus* in Africa [27], *A. stephensi* in Asia [28], and *A. darlingi*, and *A. albitarsis* in the Americas [29] are among the most important vectors. Malarial transmission occurs seasonally, with concentrated transmission during rainy seasons in tropical regions. Transmission rates depend on the frequency of interactions between the mosquito and the susceptible human host; these depend on the life expectancy of the mosquito, the number of mosquitoes, the number of times a mosquito bites per day, and the frequency with which a bite results in an infection (Macdonald-Ross Malaria Model) [30, 31].

Once the *Plasmodium* sexual stage gametocyte is ingested by the mosquito vector, its sexual reproduction cycle commences, with haploid gametocytes maturing inside the gut of the mosquito and generating a diploid zygote, the ookinete [32]. If the parasite can overcome the mosquito's immune system and host defense mechanisms, including physical chitin barriers, antimicrobial peptides, and digestive enzymes, the ookinete can develop and rupture to release sporozoites, which migrate to the mosquito salivary glands, ready to be released upon biting a potential host.

In order for *Plasmodium* to survive and be transmitted to another host, it has to overcome the unique defenses of both the mosquito vector and the human host. Interestingly, the nutritional status of not only the host, but the mosquito vector, can have an effect on mosquito physiology and parasite infection, affecting transmission dynamics. When considering the nutritional fitness of the mosquito, body size and macronutrient content, including proteins, lipids, and glycogen levels, are measured. Studies have shown that mosquito nutritional status can modulate both mosquito survival and *Plasmodium* infection rate: nutritionally compromised female *A. gambiae* mosquitoes die earlier and sustain lower levels of *Plasmodium* parasites compared to well-fed females [33], which would reduce risk of a second blood meal transmitting the infection to another human host. Nutritional states can further modulate mosquito avoidance behaviors to insecticides such as dichloro-diphenyl-trichloroethane (DDT), deltamethrin, and lambdacyhalothrin [34], indicating the potential impact of mosquito fitness on the effectiveness of chemical-based insect vector control.

## Critical Factors to Consider in Outlining Pathways Between Nutritional Status and Malaria

The interactions between the *Plasmodium* parasite and the human host or mosquito vector are complex, and the influence of nutritional status is not always a clear unidirectional association (Fig. 11.1). This chapter will seek to define, describe, and illustrate the nutritional frameworks that influence malaria disease. There are some key factors to consider when evaluating the literature and delineating these frameworks, as defined in Box 11.1.

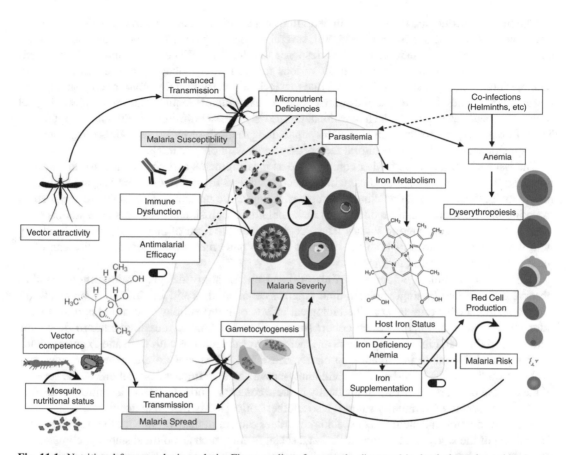

**Fig. 11.1** Nutritional frameworks in malaria. Figure outlines frameworks discussed in depth throughout this chapter involving the impact of nutrition on the interactions between *Plasmodium* parasite-human host-*Anopheles* vector. Solid arrows indicate positive relationships, dotted lines indicate relationships that are less clear or for which more data is needed, and inhibitory or negative relationships are indicated with a barred line. Cyclic arrows indicate feedback loops. Relationships boxed in yellow boxes represent the three major chapter subheadings: Malaria Susceptibility, Malaria Severity, and Malaria Spread

---

**Box 11.1 Considerations in Outlining Pathways by Which Nutritional Status Affects Malaria**

1. Definitions of nutritional status—malnutrition versus protein-energy malnutrition (PEM) versus micronutrient deficiency
2. Measurements—subjective clinical measurements, anthropometric indicators, and reference standards, biologic measurements, and kinetics (single or multiple time points for sampling)
3. Study design—cross-sectional, longitudinal, hospital-based, community-based, randomized control, in vivo versus in vitro, and others
4. Covariates—for example, nutritional status as a marker of socioeconomic status

The first to consider are the nuances in definitions in nutritional status and their relation to malaria infection. As Chaps. 2 and 3 outline [35, 36], several overlapping macro- and micronutrient profiles can affect the immune system and the host response to infections. When discussing nutritional deficiencies, malnutrition can be expressed in various forms, namely, obesity from excessive dietary intake, protein-energy malnutrition (PEM) due to a lack of dietary protein and/or energy, and micronutrient deficiencies due to a lack of essential vitamins and minerals required for proper physiological functioning and development. Each nutritional profile may interact differently with malaria infection. The different malnutrition profiles also affect population groups differently, depending on age, genetic predispositions, and other sociocultural factors associated with dietary intake.

The issue of definitions is further compounded as measurements and benchmarks for these nutritional profiles differ between studies, with subjective clinical measurements and varying anthropometric indicators used to define clinical outcomes. As there are no universal or standardized metrics to define malnutrition, it can be difficult to make definite conclusions based on single studies or to directly compare results among studies. Thus, depending on the rigor of methodology and the clarity with which the definitions of both the variables and the outcomes are described, studies can often yield confusing or contradictory results.

Differences in clinical outcomes can also depend on the study design. Cross-sectional studies observe populations at a single point in time, whereas cohort studies and longitudinal approaches follow populations over time to examine biological effects of interventions or conditions prior to and after the exposure of interest. Such cohort studies allow for kinetic measurements, to determine whether variables and influencing factors are increasing or decreasing with time and exposure. Such studies provide valuable information to clarify cause and effect and dose/response relationships. Whether studies are hospital-based or community-based can also impact associations as the severity of the disease of interest can vary dramatically in these contexts. The selection of a control population in a hospital versus a community study is also another critical study design element.

The identification and inclusion of specific covariates can dramatically influence the study's results. The setting of the study and the geopolitical and social factors, such as political stability, climate, and sociodemographic status, can influence study outcomes. Nutritional status can often be a proxy for higher socioeconomic status, and if these relationships are not identified and controlled for, studies might be capturing the impact of a correlated variable on the outcomes of interest [37–39]. Furthermore, as described below in section "Adding Hookworm to the Mix", the consideration of other infections that co-occur with malaria and that cause (or respond to) anemia is critically important in interpreting epidemiological results.

Currently, while many biomarkers and indicators are used to assess the burden of malaria in a region, there is ongoing debate as to what is the best indicator or measurement of malaria to assess the impact of large-scale interventions on malaria incidence and prevalence. As transmission intensity declines, traditional parasitological measurements of malaria burden may be increasingly difficult to quantify [40]. Recently groups have applied spatiotemporal modeling with increasing resolution of point estimates to measure malaria burden [41–43], using geo-referenced data on the clinical incidence, antimalarial drug treatment coverage, case fatality rate, and population distribution by age to model not only disease burden estimates but also the uncertainty in these estimates [41, 44]. Such analyses have contributed to improvements in surveillance methods in certain countries of the world [45]. A quantitative review of malaria reduction trials in sub-Saharan Africa has shown that in areas of medium-to-high malaria transmission, insecticide-treated bed nets and chemical prophylaxis have been effective in reducing anemia [46]. As the wide implementation of malaria-targeted interventions may reduce the burden of anemia in the same region, modeling the prevalence of both diseases in dually endemic regions may be an effective method to capture the burden of disease in areas of the world where robust surveillance methods are lacking, and to provide valuable knowledge on the interacting effects of malaria on anemia (and vice versa).

## Susceptibility: Ways in Which Diet and Nutrition Influence Infection

In the human host, it is difficult to tease apart the impact of nutrition on malaria infection (susceptibility) independently from the impact of nutrition on pathogenesis (severity), as the clinical symptoms of malaria occur after the parasite leaves the liver and enters the blood stage of the infection. Studies with rodent malaria species in mice or rats have been able to specifically identify factors that influence the process of becoming infected, and longitudinal studies in humans have also elucidated these interactions. This section will focus on the impact of nutritional status on the first stage of malaria susceptibility, the attractivity of uninfected individuals to infected female *Anopheles* mosquitoes.

Mosquito biting rate is a significant factor in vectorial capacity—a measurement of vector transmission efficiency. The mathematical models by Ross and Macdonald were landmark discoveries in the history of malaria mathematical modeling [30, 31] and provided a quantitative framework to evaluate transmission as well as derive strategies and quantitatively evaluate success of vector control measures. The Ross-Macdonald theory of vector control is influenced by the concepts of the basic reproduction ratio ($R_0$) and vectorial capacity, both of which vary spatially and temporally and are influenced by adult mosquito abundance, longevity, biting rates, human blood-feeding behavior, and the parasite's extrinsic incubation period in the mosquito, that is, the time it takes for the parasite to become infectious [47].

Increased host-seeking behavior of *Plasmodium*-infected mosquitoes at the transmissible stage of infection (sporozoites compared to oocysts) has been observed [48]. Conversely, uninfected mosquitoes show increased attraction to the infected human hosts in both controlled laboratory settings [49, 50] and in the field [51–54]. The increased attraction of infected mosquitoes to the human hosts and of uninfected mosquitoes to the infected hosts is likely evolutionary mechanisms exploited by the *Plasmodium* parasite to promote its survival and transmission to both the human host and the mosquito vector. If infection status alone can alter attraction behavior of mosquitoes through volatile substances emitted by the human host, can nutritional status also influence attractivity (see Chap. 1) [55]?

Mosquitoes require and use olfaction to find sources of food. Compounds secreted by humans such as lactic acid and $CO_2$ are released in the skin, sweat, and breath and all serve as mosquito attractants [56]. Nutritional states and dietary components may act to either increase mosquito attractivity or deter biting. Pregnant women have been found to be more attractive to mosquitoes [57] as have individuals performing high-intensity exercise and obese or overweight individuals, possibly due to increased $CO_2$ production and emission [56]. It has been proposed that potassium-rich and salty foods that increase lactic acid production could also increase attractiveness. While many hypotheses have been proposed, clear scientific evidence is lacking that directly links human diet with altered susceptibility to malaria through differences in attraction or repulsion of mosquitoes.

## Severity: The Role of Nutritional Status in Pathogenesis of Malaria Disease

Malaria pathogenesis is determined by a complex set of factors including the parasite, host, geographic, and social factors. Some of the parasite factors include antimalarial drug resistance, merozoite invasion efficiency, multiplication potential, cytoadherence, rosetting, antigenic polymorphism, and antigenic variation. Host factors influencing pathogenesis include immunity, genetic susceptibility, presence of other infections, age, and pregnancy status. Additionally, there are geographic and social factors that influence malaria outcomes such as access to health care, climate (which influences transmission potential and intensity), political stability, and other cultural and economic factors. In this section, we explore how the nutritional status of the host may influence pathogenesis by impacting the parasite, host, and vector determinants of disease severity.

## Malaria Metabolism

When discussing topics in malaria, scientists often study the host and the parasite's biological factors that can contribute to the risk of infection. Meanwhile, the parasite inherently relies on host factors for its growth and survival. Examining the metabolites produced throughout the life cycle of the parasite and the effect on the host's own metabolism can provide insight on downstream effects of infection.

In order to survive in the erythrocytic stage, the parasite requires nutrients from the human host, which it achieves through protease-mediated digestion of the hemoglobin within the erythrocyte. This metabolism provides critical amino acids for protein synthesis by the parasite. Over the course of the 48-hour erythrocytic life cycle, up to 70% of host hemoglobin in infected erythrocytes is digested by the parasite, reducing host capacity for oxygen transportation in the blood [58]. The parasite also relies on the host for nucleotides (purines) for DNA replication, as genomic studies have revealed that protozoan parasites like *Plasmodium* do not have any genes coding for de novo synthesis of purine nucleotides [59]. It is unable to synthesize purine rings de novo and relies on purine salvage pathways for survival. On the other hand, it cannot incorporate exogenous pyrimidines into nucleic acids and relies entirely on de novo synthesis [60].

Throughout the asexual life cycle of the parasite within the host, infected erythrocytes are lost to hemolysis during the blood stage, and neighboring uninfected cells can lose function due to damage and deformation. Erythrocyte clearance when malaria parasites are present is linked to many other parasite-induced physiological changes, such as oxidative damage, reduction in erythropoiesis, and bone marrow function. The loss in number and function of erythrocytes can lead to anemia, a common feature of infection. The severity and specific manifestations of anemia may differ depending on the species of *Plasmodium*.

A recent study used metabolomics and proteomics methodology to determine metabolic networks and examine systems-level changes in metabolic flux when human RBCs were infected with different strains of *P. falciparum* [61]. Describing the metabolic activity of both the host and parasite at a systems-level can reveal important information on host-parasite interaction, as it can show both the overall change in metabolic profile upon infection and changes in individual metabolites. The authors determined that in the presence of infected RBCs, uninfected RBCs' hemoglobin displayed a reduced potential to release oxygen and a decrease in the rate of glycolysis upon parasite-induced oxidative stress. Further, they recognized quantitative differences in flux of metabolic products depending on the *Plasmodium* strain. In future studies, it would be interesting to see differences in host-parasite interaction and respective metabolism depending on the nutritional profile of the host.

## Complex Relationships Between Nutrition and Malaria Morbidity and Mortality

Early literature prior to 1950 indicated that malnutrition resulted in greater susceptibility to malaria [62, 63]. While anecdotal evidence existed to the contrary, the methodology employed was less than quantitative and made drawing scientific conclusions challenging. In the early 1950s, improvements in quantitative epidemiological studies supported the alternative hypothesis that malnutrition was protective for malaria [64–69]. However, the relationship between malaria and nutritional status is now understood to be much more complex. When careful attention is given to definitions of malnutrition as well as clinical diagnosis and study design, the scales have shifted again to malnutrition being a risk factor for increased malaria morbidity and mortality.

# Relationship Between Malaria and Anemia

The discussion that follows will try to put into context these recent findings with special attention to defining the precise contribution of anemia and iron deficiency to malaria infection, pathology, and clinical outcome. We will discuss both the effects of malaria on anemia and vice versa, as each condition can synergize with the other to exacerbate symptoms.

## *General Anemia*

Anemia is defined as hemoglobin below the age, ethnicity, and sex-specific reference values and often occurs when the number of erythrocytes is insufficient or when their function is compromised. Anemia is associated with increased morbidity and mortality in itself, as well as an interaction with other diseases. For many years, the criteria for clinical diagnosis of anemia were based on a WHO report published in 1968 [70], <11 g/dL for children aged 6 months to 6 years, <12 g/dL for children 6–14 years old, <13 g/dL for adult males, <12 g/dL for nonpregnant females, and <11 g/dL for pregnant females. Additionally, the severity of anemia is characterized by the relative level of hemoglobin within these age groups. For example, the most commonly used definitions are as follows: mild anemia ≤11 g/dL, moderate anemia 7–10 g/dL, and severe anemia ≤7 g/dL [71]. However; in studies of malaria and anemia, the ranges are slightly different [72]. Meanwhile, newer studies are challenging the cut-offs for clinical anemia, stating that these values differ widely based on various host factors including host genetics, ethnicity, and nutritional profile, among others [73]. This may be a contributing factor that explains why different research groups employ different cut-off values for clinical anemia in large-scale field studies, thus making it difficult to make direct comparisons in anemia outcomes between study sites. It has been argued that large-scale epidemiological studies are necessary to more accurately capture the burden on health and refine the clinical definition of anemia [74].

Causes of anemia are multifactorial, with the combinatory effects of host genes, micronutrient deficiencies, reproductive history for women, and other infections that cause blood loss or destruction of erythrocytes, such as hookworms (see below section "Adding Hookworm to the Mix") [75]. Most cases of anemia worldwide are understood to be categorized into iron deficiency anemia (IDA) and anemia of chronic disease (or chronic inflammation) [76]. An overview of risk factors for anemia is outlined in Chap. 2 [35]. While some types of anemia are congenital and not preventable, some types can arise with deficiencies in various cofactors and micronutrients due to inadequate nutritional status, such as iron, vitamin $B_{12}$ or folate [77], or from specific physiological states like pregnancy, as iron absorption decreases slightly during the first trimester and increases during the second and third trimesters [78]. Furthermore, because *Plasmodium* ruptures erythrocytes, it is also a major cause of anemia.

In the context of malaria, the precise role of iron has been debated, as varying levels of iron may protect or exacerbate infection, complicating malaria prevention and intervention methods aiming to supply iron supplementation. These topics will be covered later in sections "Contribution of Anemia to Malaria Severity"; "The Iron-Infection Axis, Hepcidin, and Iron Deficiency Anemia"; and "Combating Anemia with Iron Supplementation: A Double-Edged Sword?".

## *Anemia and Malaria*

Importantly, severe anemia is an important public health problem for areas endemic to *P. falciparum*, as the morbidity and severity of malaria can exacerbate anemia due to other causes, posing especially acute risk to children and pregnant women [79]. In areas of low malaria endemicity, children <5 years old have been shown to be more likely to become anemic than older children [80]. In contrast, in areas with high malaria transmission, all populations, both young and old, tend to have reduced hemoglobin levels. It is thus important to consider the dual role of anemia in malaria infections, as it can be both a contributing factor to the degree of infection susceptibility and severity (both as a risk factor and being associated with protection), and the outcome of infection. It is difficult to identify a single cause of malarial anemia, as its cause seems to be multifactorial.

In severe malarial cases, overlapping syndromes of cerebral malaria, metabolic acidosis, and severe anemia are responsible for the clinical severity of disease [81]. Among African children, severe anemia is associated with 53% of malaria-attributable mortality [82]. Malarial anemia stems from erythrocyte lysis and phagocytosis, sequestration of parasitized RBCs, and an inflammatory process whereby the modulation of iron and hemoglobin levels during the asexual reproductive stages of the *Plasmodium* parasite reduces erythrocyte levels through bone marrow suppression and reduced iron absorption.

Infection from any of the five human *Plasmodium* species can lead to anemia. Recently, there has been renewed appreciation that among *Plasmodium* species, severe anemia is not a hallmark of *P. falciparum* malaria alone [83]. There has been increasing evidence that *P. vivax* infection can lead to severe manifestations of disease [84, 85]. *P. vivax* malaria has a wider geographic distribution than *P. falciparum*, and although *P. vivax* infection has the reputation for being more benign, largely due to lower parasitemia associated with restriction of infection to reticulocytes and a lack of cytoadherence, there is still a risk of severe chronic illness, including anemia. Recent studies have elucidated cases of severe anemia associated with *vivax* malaria as a major cause of morbidity in infancy [86].

Intriguingly, many epidemiological studies have found an association between iron deficiency anemia and protection from malaria caused by *P. falciparum* in pregnant women [87–89] and children [90–92], which may seem counterintuitive. The mechanisms behind this association are related to erythropoiesis to replace the iron-deficient erythrocytes with iron-replete reticulocytes and erythrocytes, which are more susceptible to *Plasmodium* infection due to parasite invasion potential and reticulocyte preference [20].

## Contribution of Anemia to Malaria Severity

Several meta-analyses and systematic reviews have attempted to clarify the complex relationship between malaria and anemia, but a clear answer has been difficult to identify due to the nonspecific and overlapping symptoms, differences in study design and methodology, and confounding factors that contribute to malaria such as coinfections and micronutrient deficiencies [93] (see Box 11.1). Meanwhile, the pathogenic mechanisms of *P. falciparum* can compound the effects of anemia. The destruction of erythrocytes, the sequestration of erythrocytes at the spleen, and dysfunction of erythropoiesis all lead to the loss of function of erythrocytes.

## The Iron-Infection Axis, Hepcidin, and Iron Deficiency Anemia

Iron is a critical nutrient for nearly all living organisms and impacts biological processes such as oxygen transport, cellular respiration, and DNA replication (see Chap. 2) [35]. Iron has a very specific role in host-pathogen interactions with bacteria, viruses, and parasites, and it is a critical nutrient for both the human host and the *Plasmodium* parasite alike. Iron deficiency can be subdivided into three distinct categories: (1) iron deficiency without anemia, (2) iron deficiency with mild anemia, and (3) iron deficiency with severe anemia [20]. Iron deficiency is slow to develop and is often not diagnosed until it is associated with anemia [94]. The WHO estimates that 50% of pregnant women and 40% of young children in low- and middle-income countries are iron deficient [74]. Iron deficiency in pregnancy can cause severe adverse outcomes for both the mother and the child, and iron deficiency in children can result in impaired growth, cognition, brain development, and immune function (see Chap. 2) [35, 95, 96].

Iron is unique in that it is the only micronutrient that has its own regulatory hormone—hepcidin—which can respond and be regulated by both nutrient status and infection status [97]. Hepcidin is a regulatory peptide hormone produced by hepatocytes, the hepcidin antimicrobial peptide (*HAMP*) gene for which is upregulated in the face of high iron stores, inflammation, or elevated erythropoiesis. The body largely regulates iron stores and circulation through intestinal iron absorption and heme recycling from senescent erythrocytes which are ingested by macrophages. To simplify a complex mechanism, hepcidin production results in the degradation of ferroportin molecules, the only known iron exporter, thus reducing iron absorption through ferroportin on the basolateral surface of duodenal enterocyte, increasing macrophage storage of iron, and reducing iron in circulation. This process also affects overall erythropoiesis, causing anemia and microcytosis given the body's iron-restricted state [98]. While iron is an essential nutrient, it can lead to increased oxidative damage and be a growth factor for pathogens if unbound or in excess. Thus, it is evident that biological mechanisms have evolved for careful iron regulation, with hepcidin being a central player [99, 100].

The dynamic between malaria and anemia is complicated and bidirectionally influenced, with hepcidin playing a key role. In explaining the interactions, the extremes on the spectrum of malaria and anemia are more conceptually straightforward. Severe malaria, defined by the WHO as malaria with one or more of a series of clinical or laboratory features [101], can easily lead to significant anemia through direct interactions including RBC loss (hemolysis and phagocytosis of infected RBCs), dysfunction (sequestration of infected erythrocytes and altered integrity of nearby uninfected RBCs), and bone marrow infiltration, as discussed above. By the same token, severe anemia, often accompanied by severe malnutrition, compromises the host immune system and thus increases susceptibility to infection. On a more nuanced level, malaria can also indirectly lead to iron deficiency anemia by impairing or reducing erythropoiesis, even on the level of uncomplicated or asymptomatic infection. This is speculated to be partially linked to malaria infection increasing hepcidin levels and thus in turn reducing iron absorption and altering host iron stores, as well as increasing cytokines such as TNF-$\alpha$ which can also inhibit iron absorption [102–106]. Conversely, mild-moderate anemia itself has been shown to be protective against malaria in both observational epidemiological studies in pregnant women and children [107] and in ex vivo experiments using RBCs from individuals with IDA where microcytic iron-deficient RBCs are shown to be refractory to parasite invasion and growth [20]. Additionally, iron is also known to be a growth factor for *Plasmodium*, as iron chelators have been shown to be cytotoxic to the parasite in in vitro and in vivo experiments, though the precise pathways through which *Plasmodium* acquires and utilizes host iron are unknown [107]. Furthermore, elevated hepcidin has been suggested to impair the initial liver stage of malaria infection in mice, with the intriguing hypothesis that acute malaria infection causes inflammation and hepcidin elevation, thus redistributing iron stores away from hepatocytes and reducing parasite superinfection with other malaria strains [108].

In short, the relationship between malaria, hepcidin, iron, and anemia is complex, with our knowledge still unfolding. Conducting and interpreting population-based studies has not been straightforward, as outlined above. In areas of high malaria transmission, it can be difficult in cross-sectional studies to delineate cause and effect and protection and risk, among people with anemia, nutritional deficiencies, and malaria infection, especially considering that distinguishing iron deficiency anemia from anemia of chronic inflammation (disease) is difficult in areas with high levels of infection and inflammation [105]. Prospective aspects of trials are often confounded by the need to of course provide subjects' extensive antimalarial prevention and treatment resources. Additional confounding factors complicating study interpretation include variable malarial prevalence, seasonality and immunity across regions, and hemoglobinopathies, to name a few. The balance between iron regulatory mechanisms that restrict pathogen access and maintaining availability of iron for the host has often been framed as an evolutionary arms race between the host and pathogen [109]. Certainly, malaria has already solidified its influential role on human genetics with numerous protective erythrocytic mutations appreciated [110], and the scientific literature on this topic continues to evolve.

Recent publications have commented on additional human genetic mutations involving ferroportin. Ferroportin has also been shown to be prevalent in RBC membranes. An initial study speculated that a prevalent ferroportin mutation in sub-Saharan Africa (Q248H), which is relatively resistant to hepcidin-mediated degradation, may have been conserved to protect against malaria [111]. This was based on findings using small human cohort studies looking at differences between carriers and WT individuals in terms of infection rates, parasite density, and disease severity. The authors also observed lower hemoglobin levels among these carriers. In addition, they found ferroportin knockout mice infected with murine *Plasmodium* strains demonstrated increased parasitemia and reduced survival time. Focusing on RBC physiology, they hypothesized that the degradation-resistant ferroportin mutation Q248H allowed for increased iron transport out of RBCs, reducing iron availability to parasites and also protecting RBCs from iron-mediated oxidative stress and hemolysis [111]. However, a follow-up publication using large human cohorts did not corroborate such results, finding instead that the degradation-resistant Q248H ferroportin was mildly protective against anemia but not malaria risk [112]. Interestingly in this follow-up study, parasite growth was also not shown to differ in ex vivo malaria culture in RBCs from wild-type and carrier individuals with the Q248H mutation [112]. These authors suggested the same ferroportin mutation instead allowed for increased intestinal iron absorption and thus overall increased body iron stores, in addition to reduced Fe-mediated hemolysis [112]. These findings demonstrate the complex, multi-organ influence of hepcidin within the human body, and highlight areas of new exploration in relation to malaria.

## *Combating Anemia with Iron Supplementation: A Double-Edged Sword?*

Treatment for both falciparum and non-falciparum malaria includes blood transfusions, antimalarial drug treatment, and in some cases, iron supplementation. While there is the danger that iron supplements may promote pathogen survival and proliferation, metadata have shown that iron supplementation to treat the anemia may aid in hemoglobin recovery during malaria infections as long as regular malaria prevention and treatment services are also provided [113]. The two subpopulations particularly at risk of malaria and with high rates of anemia requiring iron supplementation are children and pregnant women. This is due to their higher physiological requirements, including an increasing need for specific nutrients and vitamins. Iron supplementation in children and in pregnancy is a commonly employed nutritional intervention. However, in the case of iron supplementation, there may be unintended consequences with respect to *Plasmodium* invasion and replication (Fig. 11.2). Iron supplementation has been shown to increase susceptibility to *P. falciparum* infection [66, 68, 114, 115].

Supplementation of children with iron in malaria-endemic areas has been investigated in multiple clinical studies, which results have been reviewed in three meta-analyses [62, 116, 117]. Two large iron supplementation trials in children have also been conducted, in which the relationship between host iron status and malaria infection has been explored: one in Zanzibar in a region with intense malaria transmission [118], and one in Nepal in a region with no malaria transmission [119]. Smaller clinical studies have also been conducted [20]. Despite differences in study design and specific outcome measures, the overarching consensus is that iron deficiency is protective for malaria, and iron supplementation increases malaria risk in the absence of access to adequate health care and malaria management [107, 120–122]. In regions endemic to both malaria and iron deficiency malnutrition, future interventions should consider potential additive effects of treatment on either illness.

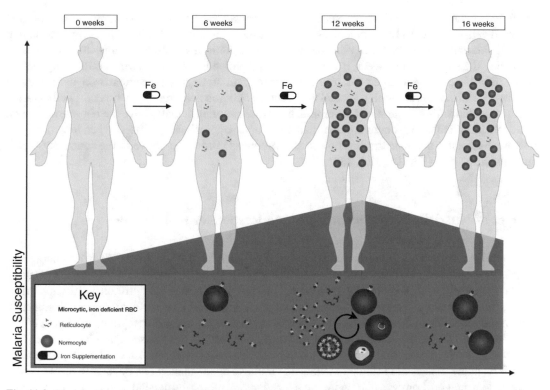

**Fig. 11.2** Model of kinetics of differential susceptibility to malaria with iron supplementation. (Figure adapted from [20]). Kinetics of erythropoiesis and malaria risk with iron supplementation at baseline (0 weeks), 6 weeks, 12 weeks, 16 weeks. At baseline, high levels of iron-deficient erythrocytes are present, which also provides a protective effect for malaria. Iron supplementation results in reticulocytosis and production of iron-replete erythrocytes at 6 weeks. By 12 weeks, most iron-deficient erythrocytes have been cleared, and reticulocyte levels are high—resulting in increased malaria risk. By 16 weeks, iron status has been corrected, and the erythrocyte population has been restored to normal, and as such, malaria risk returns to the individual's standard level

Iron supplementation in pregnancy is also controversial in malaria-endemic regions. The current WHO guidelines recommend 30–60 mg of iron and 0.4 mg folic acid supplemented daily throughout pregnancy to reduce the risk of low birth weight (LBW), preterm birth, maternal iron deficiency, and maternal anemia, and simultaneously recommend intermittent preventative treatment for malaria in areas endemic for malaria [123, 124]. Women of all gravidas are at an increased risk for *P. falciparum* malaria; however, primigravida women are at the highest risk. Some of the reasons behind this increased risk include (1) pregnant women are more attractive to mosquitoes [57]; (2) the higher rates of erythropoiesis and reticulocyte production during pregnancy provide reticulocytes for invasion by *P. falciparum* [107, 125]; and (3) sequestration of var2CSA expressing parasitized cells in the placenta [126] protects the parasite from immune-mediated mechanisms of clearance [127]. Observational studies have indicated that iron deficiency is protective for placental malaria in countries with high malaria transmission [87, 88]. In support of these studies, an observational cohort study conducted in the Gambia measured *P. falciparum* invasion and growth in vitro in erythrocytes from pregnant women during their second and third trimesters. Full hematology panels were performed at time points before and after iron supplementation. The results demonstrated that, similar to the finding in nonpregnant individuals, parasite growth rates and the population of CD71-positive reticulocytes increased with iron supplementation [127]. The caveat to this study was that there was no control cohort of pregnant women not on iron supplementation to specifically address the impact of iron supplementation versus the impact of pregnancy alone. However, in support of these findings, a similar study conducted in children revealed similar associations between iron supplementation and increased parasite growth [128], underscoring WHO's recommendation for both iron supplementation and antimalarials during pregnancy in malaria-endemic countries. Understanding the mechanisms underlying the association between iron deficiency and protection from malaria is critical and essential to inform policy guidelines for iron supplementation strategies to combat iron deficiency in malaria-endemic countries, with a special emphasis on children and pregnant women. As others have speculated, combatting malaria and other infectious diseases may actually have the biggest impact on widespread iron deficiency anemia rather than nutritional supplementation itself when infectious and inflammatory states continue to prevent iron absorption, as introduced above in the context of hepcidin regulation [102, 103, 105, 129, 130]

## Impact of Nutritional Status on Immune Responses to Malaria

Both nutritional status [131] and the gut microbiome [132] in African children may have immunomodulatory effects on human host immunity to malaria, especially in the liver which is the site of sporozoite initiation of infection and additionally drains portal blood [133]. Chronic malnutrition and micronutrient deficiencies (such as zinc, magnesium, iron, selenium, and vitamin A) can result in immune dysfunction of both the innate and adaptive arms of the immune system, by impairing thymic activity, cytokine responses, T cell responses, macrophage activation, and antibody responses (see Chap. 3) [36, 131, 134, 135]. Such immune dysfunction can also result in increased risk of infection. Zinc deficiency, for example, affects many aspects of immune function, and immune dysregulation can be largely reversed with zinc supplementation; however, certain immune functions are more zinc dependent than others, meaning that, depending on the dominant immune mechanism of killing, supplementation may have a stronger protective effect for some pathogens than others (see Chap. 2) [35, 136].

Conflicting data currently exist from studies of the relationship between nutritional status as measured by anthropometry (height-for-age Z (HAZ) scores, weight-for-age Z scores and weight-for-height/length Z scores) and immunity in children with malaria. In a cross-sectional study from young children in Senegal, it was observed that immunoglobulin G (IgG) levels were lower in stunted children (HAZ<−2.0) than controls, irrespective of differences in parasite density [137]). This finding is in contrast to an earlier study in older children in Papua New Guinea in which increased cytokine production was observed in response to antimalarial antigens in stunted and wasted children, and a decrease in antibody response was observed in wasted children [138]. The micronutrient zinc is required for immune function [136], specifically lymphocyte functions implicated in resistance to malaria such as IgG production, interferon-gamma production, TNF-α production, and microbicidal macrophage activity [136, 139]. Zinc supplementation was found to be protective against malaria morbidity in some studies [88, 140, 141], including in a placebo-controlled trial [142], but not in others [143, 144]. The role of other micronutrients in the protection against malaria has also been investigated, such as vitamin C [145], vitamin A [146], and vitamin D [147]. Further studies evaluating the impact of malnutrition on the development of immune responses to malaria are clearly needed to design adequate and appropriate treatment responses that will not exacerbate either condition.

## Adding Hookworm to the Mix

It is important to consider the interaction with hookworms when discussing topics of malaria and malnutrition, as hookworm is also a cause of anemia due to the destruction of the intestinal mucosa and blood loss that ensues [143]. Further, there is often a geographical overlap of malaria, hookworm, and malnutrition, especially in Africa [148]. Children, newborn infants, and pregnant women are impacted more severely by coinfection with malaria and hookworm [149], even though hookworm intensity is typically higher in older children and adults. Data on the direction and magnitude of the effects of coinfection are lacking, and even more so when host nutritional status is also considered. Infections with helminths, such as hookworms, and malaria both modulate the host immune response but often in different directions, although the direction and magnitude of the pathophysiology of coinfections remain unclear (see Chap. 14) [150, 151]. Hookworms, through their complex and long life cycle, modulate host immune responses to escape host defense mechanisms by establishing an anti-inflammatory Th2 and regulatory immune environment [152] that promotes their long-term establishment in the intestine. This anti-inflammatory Th2 response can compromise the pro-inflammatory Th1 immune responses needed to fight malaria infection [153]. The balance of pro- and anti-inflammatory immune modulation is delicate, and subtle shifts can tip the scales in favor of one pathogen or the other. Shifts in nutritional and/or coinfection statuses may change the efficacy or nature of host immune responses to combat the pathogens. The mechanisms of this regulation are not yet well understood and will likely be influenced by the timing and nature of each infection, which was established first, and for how long. Some hypotheses have explored how regulatory T cells can inhibit the pro-inflammatory Th1 cell activity in malaria [154] or how higher nitric oxide concentrations in helminth-infected malaria patients may reduce sequestration of infected erythrocytes [155]. Additionally, the Th2-skewed hookworm response may render the Th1 response required for *Plasmodium* control and elimination ineffective, by producing non-cytophilic antibodies [156]. Regardless, there are many plausible contradicting hypotheses, and results vary depending on the setting, the timing of coinfection, and the specific immune profile of the host.

Meta-analyses have demonstrated a complex malaria-helminth coinfection relationship with variable outcomes on anemia. Pregnant women infected with hookworm had a higher risk of malaria infection compared to those uninfected, and the risk of anemia in malaria-helminth coinfection was increased compared to the association between anemia and malaria infection alone or the association between anemia and hookworm infection alone [157]. In some study sites, no association in clinical outcomes between malaria and hookworms was seen [158]. To further complicate these associations, often hookworm infections occur in the context of other helminth coinfections. These polyparasite infections can either exacerbate the clinical pathology or progression of malaria infections or be protective against further clinical harm [159]. Other environmental or social factors, as well as host immunity and nutritional status, may play a role in this complex relationship (see Chap. 14) [151].

# Drug-Nutrient Interactions in Malaria

## *Impact of Preventative Antimalarials on Nutrition*

In addition to drugs that treat *Plasmodium* infections, several drugs are used prophylactically. The current WHO guidelines for either seasonal malaria chemoprevention (SMC) in children or intermittent preventative treatment for malaria in pregnancy (IPTp) rely on sulfadoxine-pyrimethamine-based (SP) chemoprevention. In the case of SMC, in many countries, amodiaquine has also been included. However, for pregnant women, SP alone remains the safest and standard regimen of choice [160, 161]. Unfortunately, while safe and effective at preventing malaria in pregnancy, the drugs which inhibit folate synthesis in the parasite also inhibit folate synthesis and absorption in the human (see Chap. 13) [162]. Folate is a critical nutrient during pregnancy that decreases the chances of neural tube defects in the developing fetus [163]. However, as with the conundrum of iron supplementation in pregnancy, folate supplementation together with antifolate drugs may decrease the efficacy of the

IPTp and increase the risk of malaria in pregnancy. In humans, there does not seem to be a protective effect of folate deficiency, as seen with iron deficiency, since individuals with megaloblastic anemia (folate deficiency anemia) had greater *Plasmodium* infection rates [164] and pregnant women with high folate diets had low infection rates [165]. In a study of folate supplementation in children in the Gambia, there was no associated risk of malaria [166], similar to the results in pregnant women, even when reticulocyte numbers increased [167], again in striking contrast to what has been observed with iron supplementation [20, 127].

While folic acid is not biologically active, it is converted into dihydrofolate and then tetrahydrofolate (THF) by the dihydrofolate reductase (DHFR) enzyme. While mammalian cells do not synthesize folate de novo, relying instead on scavenging folate from dietary intake, the malaria parasite can both salvage from the host and synthesize it de novo. The inhibition of de novo synthesis alone is enough to kill the malaria parasite—this is the mode of action of SP. In vitro, it has been shown that supplementing with exogenous folic acid or folinic acid and THF decreases the activity of antifolate drugs against the parasite. Likewise, lower folate availability results in greater susceptibility of the parasite to antifolate drugs both in vitro and in vivo [168–176]. Clearly, folate derivative compound concentration plays a role in the activity of antifolate drugs [168]. In a meta-analysis of many in vivo studies, higher concentrations of folic acid impacted SP efficacy; however, at the WHO-recommended doses of 0.4 mg/day of folic acid supplementation in pregnancy, there is no evidence of a decrease in SP efficacy [177].

Taken together, as with iron, it is important to consider the complex interactions between host nutrition and nutritional supplementation, parasite metabolism, and chemoprophylactic treatment in such a way that the balance favors the health of the mother and child. Current WHO-recommended folic acid supplementation should not interfere with the activity of SP for IPTp during pregnancy, but this area should be carefully monitored. As discussed throughout the chapter, there is a multiplicity of host biological and nutritional factors that tie into the risk for infection. Understanding the population profile and implementing multifaceted approaches that synergize (rather than antagonize each other) are important considerations to building an effective and safe malaria prevention program for all.

## *Impact of Nutritional Status on Efficacy on Antimalarial Treatment*

A second active area of research is the impact of nutritional status on first-line antimalarial efficacy, currently with artemisinin-based combination therapies (ACT). There are few studies examining the clinical efficacy of artemisinin combination therapies—the current first-line treatment for malaria—in malnourished children (see Chap. 13) [162, 178–180]; as in general, vulnerable populations such as very young children and malnourished individuals are excluded from studies of antimalarial drug efficacy [181]. In a longitudinal study including over 2000 malaria episodes in a high-transmission setting, the authors found that both artemether lumefantrine and dihydroartemisinin piperaquine were efficacious antimalarial regimens for the treatment of *P. falciparum* malaria in children under 3 years of age, regardless of nutritional status [179]. Yet, in response to the paucity of studies examining the impact of malnutrition on ACT efficacy, the Worldwide Antimalarial Resistance Network has assembled a study group, the ACT Malaria and Malnutrition Study Group, to specifically address this question. As part of baseline data collection, the group has published a systematic literature review on the interactions between malaria and malnutrition. One of the existing knowledge gaps is in the lack of understanding of the pharmacodynamics and pharmacokinetics of ACTs in malnourished children [182]. The objectives of the study group are (1) to measure global malnutrition using anthropometric indicators (weight-for-age (WAZ), height-for-age (HAZ), and weight-for-height (WHZ)) and assess the impact on ACT efficacy for the treatment of uncomplicated malaria in children under 5 years of age, (2) to measure the impact of malnutrition on early parasitological response (first 3 days post ACT

> **Box 11.2 Key Knowledge Gaps to Address in Understanding the Interactions Between Nutrition and Malaria**
> 1. Standardizing definitions of malnutrition and establishing standardized metrics and biomarkers common for both malaria and malnutrition are required for effective surveillance.
> 2. Identifying the nutritional drivers of malaria susceptibility at the level of initial mosquito infection.
> 3. Identifying the aspects of mosquito nutritional status that contribute to enhanced malaria transmission.
> 4. Determining the precise interactions between host iron status, iron deficiency anemia, erythropoiesis, and malaria risk (susceptibility and severity).
> 5. Determining whether iron deficiency and iron supplementation affect *P. falciparum* microvascular adhesion or host endothelial cell activation.
> 6. Determining the effect of nutritional deficiency and supplementation on *P. falciparum* gametocytogenesis and malaria transmission (spread).
> 7. Determining the impact of malnutrition on antimalarial efficacy of ACTs, both early and late parasitological failure.
> 8. Determining the impact of nutritional status on anti-*Plasmodium* immunity.
> 9. Determining the impact of coinfections with malaria and other pathogens (helminths, viruses, bacteria) especially where both organisms modulate nutritional, immunological, and inflammatory responses with potential exacerbation of malaria severity.

treatment), and (3) to measure the impact of malnutrition on late parasitological response post ACT treatment. The results from this study group are highly anticipated and will provide much needed data to answer a key knowledge gap (Box 11.2) in the interaction between nutrition and malaria severity.

## Spread: The Role of Human and Mosquito Nutritional Status on Malaria Transmission

For the *Plasmodium* parasite to be transmitted, an ongoing infection within an infected human host must receive a cue to produce the sexual and transmissible form of the parasite — the gametocyte. In general, sexual conversion or gametocytogenesis is a strategy employed by the parasites in response to adverse conditions in the human host that allows them to be transmitted to another host before the infection is cleared or the host dies [183, 184]. This is referred to as a "terminal investment" [185]. There are many proposed triggers for gametocytogenesis including high parasitemia [186, 187], treatment with antimalarial drugs that are not gametocytocidal [184, 188], low hematocrit [189, 190], lysophosphatidylcholine depletion [191, 192], and increased reticulocytosis [193, 194], to name a few of many [195]. An increase in sexual commitment makes intuitive sense when parasites encounter drugs; however, the situation is less straightforward in the case of reticulocyte production which can be beneficial to asexual parasites, thus a less obvious stress factor [185]. As discussed previously in the section outlining the relationship between malaria, anemia, and erythropoiesis, it is difficult to determine the temporal causality of how malaria parasites either take advantage of enhanced reticulocyte production to promote asexual parasitemia and gametocyte conversion or induce increased reticulocytosis.

While we have considered the nutritional status of the human host in relation to malaria, that of the parasitic vector may also influence transmission of parasites. Many studies have already demonstrated that the environment where larval mosquito development occurs affects adult traits such as size, biting behavior, and vector competency [196]. Food deprivation at larval stages can influence not only the speed of maturation and development of the mosquito [197] but also the development of the parasite within the mosquito resulting from resource deprivation. Studies are inconclusive about the directionality between nutritional stress and the mosquito's ability to acquire, maintain, and transmit pathogens. Some in vitro studies observed that parasite survival in the mosquito can be influenced by nutritional and environmental stress during mosquitoes' larval stages. Deprivation of food and resources, as well as increased temperature, decreases the activity of the mosquito's innate immune response [198], by reducing the mosquito's capability of melanizing (phagocytosis-like mechanism to sequester parasites) parasites [199], thus promoting parasite survival in infected mosquitoes.

The recent interest in the role of the gut microbiota in the ability of insect vectors to carry and transmit parasites has highlighted the potential to develop innovative vector control strategies by altering the vector's gut microbiota to decrease transmission potential [200]. Insects, similar to humans, carry a diverse microbial flora that plays a physiological role in the mosquito's diet and development and can also interact with the microbial pathogens they carry [201]. Microbes in the midgut play an important role in modulating vector physiology and immunology in relation to mosquito pathogens [202]. For example, higher loads of bacteria in the *Anopheles* mosquito digestive tract are associated with lower infection rates with *Plasmodium* [203]. Although the specific mechanisms of parasite-microbiota interactions are yet to be understood, it is suggested that there is a bacteria-mediated antiparasitic effect of the mosquito's innate immune response [204, 205]. Some *Enterobacter* bacteria isolated from the guts of wild mosquito populations in Zambia were found to render the mosquito 99% resistant to *P. falciparum* infection [206]. In the laboratory, both larval diet and the microbiota of the adult mosquitoes have been shown to influence permissiveness of adult mosquitoes to *Plasmodium* [207]. It might be important to consider how these interactions play out in natural populations, as the nutritional status of the mosquito may prove to be important to the transmission of malaria. Interventions that modulate the diet and resulting microbiota of the mosquito may be an innovative way to disrupt the malaria life cycle. Also, if climate change alters mosquito diets, this may have impacts on transmission in the future (see Chap. 15) [208].

# Challenges and Opportunities for Integrated Public Health Interventions

## Challenges

While the goal of this chapter was to explore interactions between nutritional status and malaria susceptibility, severity, and transmission, it is clear that the interactions are far from clearly defined and certainly not unidirectional. Establishing the direction of associations and influence is challenging, and often it is difficult to assign cause or effect (or both). A systems biology approach that considers all the components in the whole biological system is needed. This approach includes considering the human host the malaria parasite, the mosquito vector, and the external environment to explore how nutritional status influences malaria risk (Fig. 11.1). Further, the magnitude of these interactions may differ between different geographical sites and populations based on their specific genetic profile, coexisting infections, and sociocultural factors, and there may be hidden combinatorial effects not yet explored. The complex heterogeneous human life cycle makes it difficult to approach this problem from a single angle, as vulnerable populations including pregnant women, children, and aging adults all present different risk factors that interact differently with malaria infection and/or malnutrition. Heterogeneous and non-standardized biomarkers are being used in research studies involving both malaria and malnutrition, and thus, a more careful definition of appropriate and measurable biomarkers would be required. As there are a multitude of variables to consider, efforts should be made to identify and understand the interaction among these factors. The Biomarkers Reflecting Inflammation and Nutritional Determinants of Anemia is seeking to identify the best biomarkers of nutritional status in the context of inflammation and infection, as one approach to address this question [209, 210]. As a large portion of malaria infections and nutrient deficiencies are asymptomatic, there are obvious limitations in understanding potentially important interactions in asymptomatic individuals. Active and regular surveillance may be required to capture the bulk of those affected by both conditions. Envisioning comprehensive, multifaceted interventions is difficult, but opportunities remain to integrate both surveillance and interventions for malaria and malnutrition.

## *Opportunities*

Because of the clear interactions between malnutrition and malaria, from a public health standpoint, it would be ideal to identify and address them together. One opportunity for synergy is in surveillance. As children and women of childbearing age are at the highest risk for both nutritional deficiencies and malaria, simultaneous surveillance would provide public health practitioners with the information needed to make decisions regarding the appropriate interventions. Current serological tests for malaria biomarkers such as *P. falciparum* histidine-rich protein 2 (PfHRP2) may be inadequate to detect low-intensity infections or infections harboring PfHRP2 deletions that would not be identified by the serologic PfHRP2 test [211–213]. Recently, tools have been developed to allow for simultaneous and multiplexed serological surveillance of biomarkers for iron deficiency, iodine deficiency, vitamin A deficiency, as well as markers of systemic inflammation (which can confuse and confound micronutrient biomarker results), and malaria infection (current or recent) [214]. While there are limitations to this multiplex system, most notably the reliance on PfRHRP2 as the sole marker of *P. falciparum* malaria, it represents an improved approach to simultaneous measurement of biomarkers for each disease state. Further, it offers a platform which could be modified and improved to address other malaria species and other genetic targets. Such a field-deployable, multiplex approach presents the opportunity for integrated surveillance of micronutrient levels, inflammation, and malaria infection in both cross-sectional and longitudinal studies of target populations in endemic countries. Not only would this provide early warning signs of either micronutrient deficiencies or asymptomatic malaria infection, but also it would provide data sets of extreme value for improving our understanding of interactions between malaria and malnutrition.

Next is the opportunity to design interventions that address malnutrition and malaria concurrently. As discussed previously, supplementation of iron or folate may have unintended consequences of increasing malaria risk in *Plasmodium*-endemic areas. The current WHO guidelines emphasize that iron supplementation should be given to pregnant women in these malaria-endemic areas together with malaria prevention and treatment services. Supplementations of other micronutrients, while not discussed in this chapter, have shown mixed results depending on the study site and population, and their safety and usefulness are still being discussed. With appropriate surveillance methods and regular monitoring of at-risk populations, appropriate preventative measures can be designed, and treatments can be delivered. For children, school or community health center-based interventions aimed at reducing malnutrition or malaria could be effectively targeted together, and health workers trained to educate and intervene for one condition could use the opportunity to target both. Such an approach would require coordination between existing governmental and nongovernmental programs to deliver information, nutritional supplements, medications, and prevention tools synergistically. Pregnancy represents another opportunity for addressing both optimal maternal nutrition and malaria prevention. Prenatal care and visits could and should be used as opportunities to monitor and intervene in the overall health of the pregnant mother, including nutritional status and malaria prevention.

## The Way Forward: Addressing Key Knowledge Gaps and Integrating Interventions

To truly make headway in understanding the impact of nutritional status on malaria susceptibility, severity, and spread, a number of key knowledge gaps must be systematically addressed (Box 11.2). Consideration of these gaps provides an opportunity to unravel, in a systematic manner, the complex interactions between nutritional status and malaria susceptibility, severity, and spread.

The WHO recently published a compendium that updated and catalogued its policy recommendations regarding the prevention, diagnosis, treatment, surveillance, and elimination of malaria [215], with a summarized toolkit aimed to guide its global partners. Within a broader context of the Global Technical Strategy for Malaria 2016–2030 [216], the WHO calls for malaria surveillance as a core intervention to eliminate malaria. While these guidelines generally focus on the issue of malaria only, it might be effective for future policies to consider the broader framework of malaria and nutrition when designing interventions or surveillance strategies, as many areas of the world are endemic to both. A more integrative and holistic approach, using collaborative approaches with experts from various fields, will be necessary to realize the goals of eliminating malaria. From a nutritional point of view, scientific organizations such as BRINDA (Biomarkers Reflecting Inflammation and Nutritional Determinants of Anemia) aim to examine relationships between inflammation and nutrition biomarkers and identify key factors associated with anemia [217].

In light of the Sustainable Development Goals set by the United Nations in 2015, the world aims to achieve specific benchmarks by the year 2030, among which are elimination of hunger and poverty and promotion of good health and well-being, under the umbrella of global, multilateral partnership [218]. Much evidence points to the fact that there is significant overlap between malaria and nutrition, and there are potential avenues of reducing the burden of both conditions through research, surveillance, diagnosis, and treatment. The UN acknowledges that a more integrative and holistic approach is necessary to successfully make the sustainable development goals a reality. In this way, perhaps more success will be seen if we work with a holistic framework that encompasses facets of both malaria and malnutrition, with collaborative approaches that can address multitudes of issues simultaneously.

## References

1. Organization WH. World malaria report 2019. Geneva, Switzerland; 2019.
2. Wiser MF. Nutrition and protozoan pathogens of humans – a primer. In: Humphries DL, Scott ME, Vermund SH, editors. Nutrition and infectious diseases: shifting the clinical paradigm. New York: Springer; 2020.
3. Howes RE, Reiner RC Jr, Battle KE, Longbottom J, Mappin B, Ordanovich D, et al. Plasmodium vivax transmission in Africa. PLoS Negl Trop Dis. 2015;9(11):e0004222.
4. Breman JG. The ears of the hippopotamus: manifestations, determinants, and estimates of the malaria burden. Am J Trop Med Hyg. 2001;64(1–2 Suppl):1–11.
5. Grigg MJ, William T, Barber BE, Rajahram GS, Menon J, Schimann E, et al. Age-related clinical spectrum of Plasmodium knowlesi malaria and predictors of severity. Clin Infect Dis. 2018;67(3):350–9.
6. Cox-Singh J, Hiu J, Lucas SB, Divis PC, Zulkarnaen M, Chandran P, et al. Severe malaria – a case of fatal Plasmodium knowlesi infection with post-mortem findings: a case report. Malar J. 2010;9:10.
7. Garnham PC. Immunity against the different stages of malaria parasites. Bull Soc Pathol Exot Filiales. 1966;59(4):549–57.

8. Durocher JR, Payne RC, Conrad ME. Role of sialic acid in erythrocyte survival. Blood. 1975;45(1):11–20.
9. Schroit AJ, Madsen JW, Tanaka Y. In vivo recognition and clearance of red blood cells containing phosphatidyl-serine in their plasma membranes. J Biol Chem. 1985;260(8):5131–8.
10. Waugh RE, Narla M, Jackson CW, Mueller TJ, Suzuki T, Dale GL. Rheologic properties of senescent erythrocytes: loss of surface area and volume with red blood cell age. Blood. 1992;79(5):1351–8.
11. Sim RB, Malhotra V, Ripoche J, Day AJ, Micklem KJ, Sim E. Complement receptors and related complement control proteins. Biochem Soc Symp. 1986;51:83–96.
12. Moldenhauer F, Botto M, Walport MJ. The rate of loss of CR1 from ageing erythrocytes in vivo in normal subjects and SLE patients: no correlation with structural or numerical polymorphisms. Clin Exp Immunol. 1988;72(1):74–8.
13. Kanamaru A, Okuda K, Ueda E, Kitani T, Kinoshita T, Nagai K. Different distribution of decay-accelerating factor on hematopoietic progenitors from normal individuals and patients with paroxysmal nocturnal hemoglobinuria. Blood. 1988;72(2):507–11.
14. Woolley IJ, Hotmire KA, Sramkoski RM, Zimmerman PA, Kazura JW. Differential expression of the duffy antigen receptor for chemokines according to RBC age and FY genotype. Transfusion. 2000;40(8):949–53.
15. Hegner R. Relative frequency of ring-stage plasmodia in reticulocytes and mature erythrocytes in man and mon-key. Am J Epidemiol. 1938;27(3):690–718.
16. Simpson JA, Silamut K, Chotivanich K, Pukrittayakamee S, White NJ. Red cell selectivity in malaria: a study of multiple-infected erythrocytes. Trans R Soc Trop Med Hyg. 1999;93(2):165–8.
17. Pasvol G, Weatherall DJ, Wilson RJ. The increased susceptibility of young red cells to invasion by the malarial parasite Plasmodium falciparum. Br J Haematol. 1980;45(2):285–95.
18. Collins WE, Jeffery GM. Plasmodium malariae: parasite and disease. Clin Microbiol Rev. 2007;20(4):579–92.
19. Koury MJ, Ponka P. New insights into erythropoiesis: the roles of folate, vitamin B12, and iron. Annu Rev Nutr. 2004;24:105–31.
20. Clark MA, Goheen MM, Fulford A, Prentice AM, Elnagheeb MA, Patel J, et al. Host iron status and iron supple-mentation mediate susceptibility to erythrocytic stage Plasmodium falciparum. Nat Commun. 2014;5:4446.
21. Sexton AC, Good RT, Hansen DS, Ombrain MCD, Buckingham L, Simpson K, et al. Transcriptional profiling reveals suppressed erythropoiesis, up-regulated glycolysis, and interferon-associated responses in murine malaria. J Infect Dis. 2004;189(7):1245–56.
22. Xu L, Zheng X, Berzins K, Chaudhuri A. Cytokine dysregulation associated with malarial anemia in Plasmodium yoelii infected mice. Am J Transl Res. 2013;5(2):235–45.
23. Angulo I, Fresno M. Cytokines in the pathogenesis of and protection against malaria. Clin Diagn Lab Immunol. 2002;9(6):1145–52.
24. Oyegue-Liabagui SL, Bouopda-Tuedom AG, Kouna LC, Maghendji-Nzondo S, Nzoughe H, Tchitoula-Makaya N, et al. Pro- and anti-inflammatory cytokines in children with malaria in Franceville, Gabon. Am J Clin Exp Immunol. 2017;6(2):9–20.
25. Joice R, Nilsson SK, Montgomery J, Dankwa S, Egan E, Morahan B, et al. Plasmodium falciparum transmission stages accumulate in the human bone marrow. Sci Transl Med. 2014;6(244):244re5.
26. Sinka ME, Bangs MJ, Manguin S, Rubio-Palis Y, Chareonviriyaphap T, Coetzee M, et al. A global map of domi-nant malaria vectors. Parasit Vectors. 2012;5:69.
27. Sinka ME, Bangs MJ, Manguin S, Coetzee M, Mbogo CM, Hemingway J, et al. The dominant Anopheles vectors of human malaria in Africa, Europe and the Middle East: occurrence data, distribution maps and bionomic precis. Parasit Vectors. 2010;3:117.
28. Gakhar SK, Sharma R, Sharma A. Population genetic structure of malaria vector Anopheles stephensi Liston (Diptera: Culicidae). Indian J Exp Biol. 2013;51(4):273–9.
29. Pimenta PF, Orfano AS, Bahia AC, Duarte AP, Rios-Velasquez CM, Melo FF, et al. An overview of malaria trans-mission from the perspective of Amazon Anopheles vectors. Mem Inst Oswaldo Cruz. 2015;110(1):23–47.
30. Macdonald G. The analysis of equilibrium in malaria. Trop Dis Bull. 1952;49(9):813–29.
31. Macdonald G. The analysis of the sporozoite rate. Trop Dis Bull. 1952;49(6):569–86.
32. Sinden RE. Plasmodium differentiation in the mosquito. Parassitologia. 1999;41(1–3):139–48.
33. Takken W, Smallegange RC, Vigneau AJ, Johnston V, Brown M, Mordue-Luntz AJ, et al. Larval nutrition differen-tially affects adult fitness and Plasmodium development in the malaria vectors Anopheles gambiae and Anopheles stephensi. Parasit Vectors. 2013;6(1):345.
34. Sungvornyothin S, Chareonviriyaphap T, Prabaripai A, Thirakhupt V, Ratanatham S, Bangs MJ. Effects of nutri-tional and physiological status on behavioral avoidance of Anopheles minimus (Diptera: Culicidae) to DDT, del-tamethrin and lambdacyhalothrin. J Vector Ecol. 2001;26(2):202–15.
35. Barffour MA, Humphries DL. Core principles: infectious disease risk in relation to macro and micronutrient status. In: Humphries DL, Scott ME, Vermund SH, editors. Nutrition and infectious disease: shifting the clinical paradigm. New York: Springer, Humana Press; 2020.

36. Stephensen CB. Primer on immune response and interface with malnutrition. In: Humphries DL, Scott ME, Vermund SH, editors. Nutrition and infectious disease: shifting the clinical paradigm. New York: Springer, Humana Press; 2020.
37. Faure E. Malarial pathocoenosis: beneficial and deleterious interactions between malaria and other human diseases. Front Physiol. 2014;5:441.
38. Grantham-McGregor S, Ani C. A review of studies on the effect of iron deficiency on cognitive development in children. J Nutr. 2001;131(2S–2):649S–66S; discussion 666S–8S.
39. Muller O, Traore C, Jahn A, Becher H. Severe anaemia in West African children: malaria or malnutrition? Lancet. 2003;361(9351):86–7.
40. Tusting LS, Bousema T, Smith DL, Drakeley C. Measuring changes in Plasmodium falciparum transmission: precision, accuracy and costs of metrics. Adv Parasitol. 2014;84:151–208.
41. Bhatt S, Weiss DJ, Cameron E, Bisanzio D, Mappin B, Dalrymple U, et al. The effect of malaria control on Plasmodium falciparum in Africa between 2000 and 2015. Nature. 2015;526(7572):207–11.
42. Weiss DJ, Lucas TCD, Nguyen M, Nandi AK, Bisanzio D, Battle KE, et al. Mapping the global prevalence, incidence, and mortality of Plasmodium falciparum, 2000–17: a spatial and temporal modelling study. Lancet. 2019;394(10195):322–31.
43. Gething PW, Casey DC, Weiss DJ, Bisanzio D, Bhatt S, Cameron E, et al. Mapping Plasmodium falciparum mortality in Africa between 1990 and 2015. N Engl J Med. 2016;375(25):2435–45.
44. Gething PW, Kirui VC, Alegana VA, Okiro EA, Noor AM, Snow RW. Estimating the number of paediatric fevers associated with malaria infection presenting to Africa's public health sector in 2007. PLoS Med. 2010;7(7):e1000301.
45. Hay SI, Okiro EA, Gething PW, Patil AP, Tatem AJ, Guerra CA, et al. Estimating the global clinical burden of Plasmodium falciparum Malaria in 2007. PLoS Med. 2010;7(6):e1000290.
46. Korenromp EL, Armstrong-Schellenberg JR, Williams BG, Nahlen BL, Snow RW. Impact of malaria control on childhood anaemia in Africa – a quantitative review. Trop Med Int Health. 2004;9(10):1050–65.
47. Garrett-Jones C. The human blood index of malaria vectors in relation to epidemiological assessment. Bull World Health Organ. 1964;30:241–61.
48. Stanczyk NM, Brugman VA, Austin V, Sanchez-Roman Teran F, Gezan SA, Emery M, et al. Species-specific alterations in Anopheles mosquito olfactory responses caused by Plasmodium infection. Sci Rep. 2019;9(1):3396.
49. Schaber CL, Katta N, Bollinger LB, Mwale M, Mlotha-Mitole R, Trehan I, et al. Breathprinting reveals malaria-associated biomarkers and mosquito attractants. J Infect Dis. 2018;217(10):1553–60.
50. de Boer JG, Robinson A, Powers SJ, Burgers S, Caulfield JC, Birkett MA, et al. Odours of Plasmodium falciparum-infected participants influence mosquito-host interactions. Sci Rep. 2017;7(1):9283.
51. Lacroix R, Mukabana WR, Gouagna LC, Koella JC. Malaria infection increases attractiveness of humans to mosquitoes. PLoS Biol. 2005;3(9):e298.
52. Busula AO, Bousema T, Mweresa CK, Masiga D, Logan JG, Sauerwein RW, et al. Gametocytemia and attractiveness of Plasmodium falciparum-infected Kenyan children to Anopheles gambiae mosquitoes. J Infect Dis. 2017;216(3):291–5.
53. De Moraes CM, Wanjiku C, Stanczyk NM, Pulido H, Sims JW, Betz HS, et al. Volatile biomarkers of symptomatic and asymptomatic malaria infection in humans. Proc Natl Acad Sci U S A. 2018;115(22):5780–5.
54. Robinson A, Busula AO, Voets MA, Beshir KB, Caulfield JC, Powers SJ, et al. Plasmodium-associated changes in human odor attract mosquitoes. Proc Natl Acad Sci U S A. 2018;115(18):E4209–E18.
55. Humphries DL, Scott ME, Vermund SH. Pathways linking nutritional status and infectious disease. In: Humphries D, Scott ME, Vermund SH, editors. Nutrition and infectious disease: shifting the clinical paradigm. New York: Springer, Humana Press; 2020.
56. Weger-Lucarelli J, Auerswald H, Vignuzzi M, Dussart P, Karlsson EA. Taking a bite out of nutrition and arbovirus infection. PLoS Negl Trop Dis. 2018;12(3):e0006247.
57. Ansell J, Hamilton KA, Pinder M, Walraven GE, Lindsay SW. Short-range attractiveness of pregnant women to Anopheles gambiae mosquitoes. Trans R Soc Trop Med Hyg. 2002;96(2):113–6.
58. Mohandas N, An X. Malaria and human red blood cells. Med Microbiol Immunol. 2012;201(4):593–8.
59. Chaudhary K, Darling JA, Fohl LM, Sullivan WJ Jr, Donald RG, Pfefferkorn ER, et al. Purine salvage pathways in the apicomplexan parasite Toxoplasma gondii. J Biol Chem. 2004;279(30):31221–7.
60. Downie MJ, Kirk K, Mamoun CB. Purine salvage pathways in the intraerythrocytic malaria parasite Plasmodium falciparum. Eukaryot Cell. 2008;7(8):1231–7.
61. Wallqvist A, Fang X, Tewari SG, Ye P, Reifman J. Metabolic host responses to malarial infection during the intraerythrocytic developmental cycle. BMC Syst Biol. 2016;10(1):58.
62. Shankar AH. Nutritional modulation of malaria morbidity and mortality. J Infect Dis. 2000;182(Suppl 1):S37–53.
63. Garnham PC. Malaria in the African child. East Afr Med J. 1954;31(4):155–9.

64. Edington GM. Cerebral malaria in the Gold Coast African: four autopsy reports. Ann Trop Med Parasitol. 1954;48(3):300–6.
65. Hendrickse RG, Hasan AH, Olumide LO, Akinkunmi A. Malaria in early childhood. An investigation of five hundred seriously ill children in whom a "clinical" diagnosis of malaria was made on admission to the children's emergency room at University College Hospital, Ibadan. Ann Trop Med Parasitol. 1971;65(1):1–20.
66. Murray MJ, Murray NJ, Murray AB, Murray MB. Refeeding-malaria and hyperferraemia. Lancet. 1975;1(7908):653–4.
67. Murray MJ, Murray AB, Murray MB, Murray CJ. Somali food shelters in the Ogaden famine and their impact on health. Lancet. 1976;1(7972):1283–5.
68. Murray MJ, Murray AB, Murray MB, Murray CJ. The adverse effect of iron repletion on the course of certain infections. Br Med J. 1978;2(6145):1113–5.
69. Murray MJ, Murray AB, Murray NJ, Murray MB. Diet and cerebral malaria: the effect of famine and refeeding. Am J Clin Nutr. 1978;31(1):57–61.
70. Blanc B. Nutritional anemias. Report of a WHO Scientific Group. World Health Organ Tech Rep Ser. 1968;405:1–40.
71. WHO. Haemoglobin concentrations for the diagnosis of anaemia and assessment of severity. Geneva: World Health Organization; 2011. Contract No.: (WHO/NMH/NHD/MNM/11.1).
72. White NJ. Anaemia and malaria. Malar J. 2018;17(1):371.
73. Beutler E, Waalen J. The definition of anemia: what is the lower limit of normal of the blood hemoglobin concentration? Blood. 2006;107(5):1747.
74. Kassebaum NJ, Jasrasaria R, Naghavi M, Wulf SK, Johns N, Lozano R, et al. A systematic analysis of global anemia burden from 1990 to 2010. Blood. 2014;123(5):615–24.
75. Geary TG, Haque M. Human helminth infections. In: Humphries DL, Scott ME, Vermund SH, editors. Nutrition and infectious disease: shifting the clinical paradigm. New York: Springer, Humana Press; 2020.
76. Madu AJ, Ughasoro MD. Anaemia of chronic disease: an in-depth review. Med Princ Pract. 2017;26(1):1–9.
77. Calis JC, Phiri KS, Faragher EB, Brabin BJ, Bates I, Cuevas LE, et al. Severe anemia in Malawian children. N Engl J Med. 2008;358(9):888–99.
78. Fernández-Ballart JD. Iron metabolism during pregnancy. Clin Drug Investig. 2000;19(1):9–19.
79. Ekvall H. Malaria and anemia. Curr Opin Hematol. 2003;10(2):108–14.
80. Price RN, Simpson JA, Nosten F, Luxemburger C, Hkirjaroen L, ter Kuile F, et al. Factors contributing to anemia after uncomplicated falciparum malaria. Am J Trop Med Hyg. 2001;65(5):614–22.
81. Miller LH, Ackerman HC, Su XZ, Wellems TE. Malaria biology and disease pathogenesis: insights for new treatments. Nat Med. 2013;19(2):156–67.
82. Murphy SC, Breman JG. Gaps in the childhood malaria burden in Africa: cerebral malaria, neurological sequelae, anemia, respiratory distress, hypoglycemia, and complications of pregnancy. Am J Trop Med Hyg. 2001;64(1–2 Suppl):57–67.
83. Gosling RD, Hsiang MS. Malaria and severe anemia: thinking beyond Plasmodium falciparum. PLoS Med. 2013;10(12):e1001576.
84. Rodriguez-Morales AJ, Sanchez E, Vargas M, Piccolo C, Colina R, Arria M. Anemia and thrombocytopenia in children with Plasmodium vivax malaria. J Trop Pediatr. 2006;52(1):49–51.
85. Rodriguez-Morales AJ, Sanchez E, Vargas M, Piccolo C, Colina R, Arria M, et al. Is anemia in Plasmodium vivax malaria more frequent and severe than in Plasmodium falciparum? Am J Med. 2006;119(11):e9–10.
86. Poespoprodjo JR, Fobia W, Kenangalem E, Lampah DA, Hasanuddin A, Warikar N, et al. Vivax malaria: a major cause of morbidity in early infancy. Clin Infect Dis. 2009;48(12):1704–12.
87. Kabyemela ER, Fried M, Kurtis JD, Mutabingwa TK, Duffy PE. Decreased susceptibility to Plasmodium falciparum infection in pregnant women with iron deficiency. J Infect Dis. 2008;198(2):163–6.
88. Senga EL, Harper G, Koshy G, Kazembe PN, Brabin BJ. Reduced risk for placental malaria in iron deficient women. Malar J. 2011;10:47.
89. Sangare L, van Eijk AM, Ter Kuile FO, Walson J, Stergachis A. The association between malaria and iron status or supplementation in pregnancy: a systematic review and meta-analysis. PLoS One. 2014;9(2):e87743.
90. Gwamaka M, Kurtis JD, Sorensen BE, Holte S, Morrison R, Mutabingwa TK, et al. Iron deficiency protects against severe Plasmodium falciparum malaria and death in young children. Clin Infect Dis. 2012;54(8):1137–44.
91. Nyakeriga AM, Troye-Blomberg M, Dorfman JR, Alexander ND, Back R, Kortok M, et al. Iron deficiency and malaria among children living on the coast of Kenya. J Infect Dis. 2004;190(3):439–47.
92. Veenemans J, Milligan P, Prentice AM, Schouten LR, Inja N, van der Heijden AC, et al. Effect of supplementation with zinc and other micronutrients on malaria in Tanzanian children: a randomised trial. PLoS Med. 2011;8(11):e1001125.
93. Duffy F, Bernabeu M, Babar PH, Kessler A, Wang CW, Vaz M, et al. Meta-analysis of Plasmodium falciparum var signatures contributing to severe malaria in African children and Indian adults. MBio. 2019;10(2):e00217–9.

94. Stoltzfus RJ. Iron deficiency: global prevalence and consequences. Food Nutr Bull. 2003;24(4 Suppl):S99–103.

95. De-Regil LM, Jefferds ME, Sylvetsky AC, Dowswell T. Intermittent iron supplementation for improving nutrition and development in children under 12 years of age. Cochrane Database Syst Rev. 2011;12:CD009085.

96. De-Regil LM, Suchdev PS, Vist GE, Walleser S, Pena-Rosas JP. Home fortification of foods with multiple micronutrient powders for health and nutrition in children under two years of age (Review). Evid Based Child Health. 2013;8(1):112–201.

97. Drakesmith H, Prentice AM. Hepcidin and the iron-infection axis. Science. 2012;338(6108):768–72.

98. Wallace DF. The regulation of iron absorption and homeostasis. Clin Biochem Rev. 2016;37(2):51–62.

99. Prentice AM. Clinical implications of new insights into hepcidin-mediated regulation of iron absorption and metabolism. Ann Nutr Metab. 2017;71(Suppl 3):40–8.

100. Armitage AE, Eddowes LA, Gileadi U, Cole S, Spottiswoode N, Selvakumar TA, et al. Hepcidin regulation by innate immune and infectious stimuli. Blood. 2011;118(15):4129–39.

101. Severe malaria. Trop Med Int Health. 2014;19 Suppl 1:7–131.

102. Atkinson SH, Uyoga SM, Armitage AE, Khandwala S, Mugyenyi CK, Bejon P, et al. Malaria and age variably but critically control hepcidin throughout childhood in Kenya. EBioMedicine. 2015;2(10):1478–86.

103. Atkinson SH, Armitage AE, Khandwala S, Mwangi TW, Uyoga S, Bejon PA, et al. Combinatorial effects of malaria season, iron deficiency, and inflammation determine plasma hepcidin concentration in African children. Blood. 2014;123(21):3221–9.

104. Mohandas N, Hillyer CD. The iron fist: malaria and hepcidin. Blood. 2014;123(21):3217–8.

105. Muriuki JM, Atkinson SH. How eliminating malaria may also prevent iron deficiency in African children. Pharmaceuticals (Basel). 2018;11(4):96.

106. Spottiswoode N, Duffy PE, Drakesmith H. Iron, anemia and hepcidin in malaria. Front Pharmacol. 2014;5:125.

107. Clark MA, Goheen MM, Cerami C. Influence of host iron status on Plasmodium falciparum infection. Front Pharmacol. 2014;5:84.

108. Portugal S, Carret C, Recker M, Armitage AE, Goncalves LA, Epiphanio S, et al. Host-mediated regulation of superinfection in malaria. Nat Med. 2011;17(6):732–7.

109. Kramer J, Ozkaya O, Kummerli R. Bacterial siderophores in community and host interactions. Nat Rev Microbiol. 2020;18(3):152–63.

110. Lelliott PM, McMorran BJ, Foote SJ, Burgio G. The influence of host genetics on erythrocytes and malaria infection: is there therapeutic potential? Malar J. 2015;14:289.

111. Zhang DL, Wu J, Shah BN, Greutelaers KC, Ghosh MC, Ollivierre H, et al. Erythrocytic ferroportin reduces intracellular iron accumulation, hemolysis, and malaria risk. Science. 2018;359(6383):1520–3.

112. Muriuki JM, Mentzer AJ, Band G, Gilchrist JJ, Carstensen T, Lule SA, et al. The ferroportin Q248H mutation protects from anemia, but not malaria or bacteremia. Sci Adv. 2019;5(9):eaaw0109.

113. Neuberger A, Okebe J, Yahav D, Paul M. Oral iron supplements for children in malaria-endemic areas. Cochrane Database Syst Rev. 2016;2:CD006589.

114. Smith AW, Hendrickse RG, Harrison C, Hayes RJ, Greenwood BM. Iron-deficiency anaemia and its response to oral iron: report of a study in rural Gambian children treated at home by their mothers. Ann Trop Paediatr. 1989;9(1):6–16.

115. Oppenheimer SJ, Gibson FD, Macfarlane SB, Moody JB, Harrison C, Spencer A, et al. Iron supplementation increases prevalence and effects of malaria: report on clinical studies in Papua New Guinea. Trans R Soc Trop Med Hyg. 1986;80(4):603–12.

116. Oppenheimer SJ. Iron and its relation to immunity and infectious disease. J Nutr. 2001;131(2S–2):616S–33S; discussion 33S–35S.

117. Gera T, Sachdev HP. Effect of iron supplementation on incidence of infectious illness in children: systematic review. BMJ. 2002;325(7373):1142.

118. Sazawal S, Black RE, Ramsan M, Chwaya HM, Stoltzfus RJ, Dutta A, et al. Effects of routine prophylactic supplementation with iron and folic acid on admission to hospital and mortality in preschool children in a high malaria transmission setting: community-based, randomised, placebo-controlled trial. Lancet. 2006;367(9505):133–43.

119. Tielsch JM, Khatry SK, Stoltzfus RJ, Katz J, LeClerq SC, Adhikari R, et al. Effect of routine prophylactic supplementation with iron and folic acid on preschool child mortality in Southern Nepal: community-based, cluster-randomised, placebo-controlled trial. Lancet. 2006;367(9505):144–52.

120. Prentice AM, Cox SE. Iron and malaria interactions: research needs from basic science to global policy. Adv Nutr. 2012;3(4):583–91.

121. Spottiswoode N, Fried M, Drakesmith H, Duffy PE. Implications of malaria on iron deficiency control strategies. Adv Nutr. 2012;3(4):570–8.

122. Stoltzfus RJ. Iron and malaria interactions: programmatic ways forward. Adv Nutr. 2012;3(4):579–82.

123. Desai M, ter Kuile FO, Nosten F, McGready R, Asamoa K, Brabin B, et al. Epidemiology and burden of malaria in pregnancy. Lancet Infect Dis. 2007;7(2):93–104.

124. Tuncalp Ö, Pena-Rosas JP, Lawrie T, Bucagu M, Oladapo OT, Portela A, et al. WHO recommendations on antenatal care for a positive pregnancy experience-going beyond survival. BJOG. 2017;124(6):860–2.
125. Lim C, Hansen E, DeSimone TM, Moreno Y, Junker K, Bei A, et al. Expansion of host cellular niche can drive adaptation of a zoonotic malaria parasite to humans. Nat Commun. 2013;4:1638.
126. Duffy PE, Fried M. Plasmodium falciparum adhesion in the placenta. Curr Opin Microbiol. 2003;6(4):371–6.
127. Goheen MM, Bah A, Wegmuller R, Verhoef H, Darboe B, Danso E, et al. Host iron status and erythropoietic response to iron supplementation determines susceptibility to the RBC stage of falciparum malaria during pregnancy. Sci Rep. 2017;7(1):17674.
128. Goheen MM, Wegmuller R, Bah A, Darboe B, Danso E, Affara M, et al. Anemia offers stronger protection than sickle cell trait against the erythrocytic stage of falciparum malaria and this protection is reversed by iron supplementation. EBioMedicine. 2016;14:123–30.
129. Prentice AM, Bah A, Jallow MW, Jallow AT, Sanyang S, Sise EA, et al. Respiratory infections drive hepcidin-mediated blockade of iron absorption leading to iron deficiency anemia in African children. Sci Adv. 2019;5(3):eaav9020.
130. Pasricha SR, Armitage AE, Prentice AM, Drakesmith H. Reducing anaemia in low income countries: control of infection is essential. BMJ. 2018;362:k3165.
131. Schaible UE, Kaufmann SH. Malnutrition and infection: complex mechanisms and global impacts. PLoS Med. 2007;4(5):e115.
132. Molloy MJ, Bouladoux N, Belkaid Y. Intestinal microbiota: shaping local and systemic immune responses. Semin Immunol. 2012;24(1):58–66.
133. Crompton PD, Moebius J, Portugal S, Waisberg M, Hart G, Garver LS, et al. Malaria immunity in man and mosquito: insights into unsolved mysteries of a deadly infectious disease. Annu Rev Immunol. 2014;32:157–87.
134. Cunningham-Rundles S, McNeeley DF, Moon A. Mechanisms of nutrient modulation of the immune response. J Allergy Clin Immunol. 2005;115(6):1119–28; quiz 29.
135. Schlesinger L, Uauy R. Nutrition and neonatal immune function. Semin Perinatol. 1991;15(6):469–77.
136. Shankar AH, Prasad AS. Zinc and immune function: the biological basis of altered resistance to infection. Am J Clin Nutr. 1998;68(2 Suppl):447S–63S.
137. Fillol F, Sarr JB, Boulanger D, Cisse B, Sokhna C, Riveau G, et al. Impact of child malnutrition on the specific anti-Plasmodium falciparum antibody response. Malar J. 2009;8:116.
138. Genton B, Al-Yaman F, Ginny M, Taraika J, Alpers MP. Relation of anthropometry to malaria morbidity and immunity in Papua New Guinean children. Am J Clin Nutr. 1998;68(3):734–41.
139. Good MF, Kaslow DC, Miller LH. Pathways and strategies for developing a malaria blood-stage vaccine. Annu Rev Immunol. 1998;16:57–87.
140. Bates CJ, Evans PH, Dardenne M, Prentice A, Lunn PG, Northrop-Clewes CA, et al. A trial of zinc supplementation in young rural Gambian children. Br J Nutr. 1993;69(1):243–55.
141. Richard SA, Zavaleta N, Caulfield LE, Black RE, Witzig RS, Shankar AH. Zinc and iron supplementation and malaria, diarrhea, and respiratory infections in children in the Peruvian Amazon. Am J Trop Med Hyg. 2006;75(1):126–32.
142. Shankar AH, Genton B, Baisor M, Paino J, Tamja S, Adiguma T, et al. The influence of zinc supplementation on morbidity due to Plasmodium falciparum: a randomized trial in preschool children in Papua New Guinea. Am J Trop Med Hyg. 2000;62(6):663–9.
143. Glinz D, Hurrell RF, Righetti AA, Zeder C, Adiossan LG, Tjalsma H, et al. In Ivorian school-age children, infection with hookworm does not reduce dietary iron absorption or systemic iron utilization, whereas afebrile Plasmodium falciparum infection reduces iron absorption by half. Am J Clin Nutr. 2015;101(3):462–70.
144. Some JW, Abbeddou S, Yakes Jimenez E, Hess SY, Ouedraogo ZP, Guissou RM, et al. Effect of zinc added to a daily small-quantity lipid-based nutrient supplement on diarrhoea, malaria, fever and respiratory infections in young children in rural Burkina Faso: a cluster-randomised trial. BMJ Open. 2015;5(9):e007828.
145. Wintergerst ES, Maggini S, Hornig DH. Immune-enhancing role of vitamin C and zinc and effect on clinical conditions. Ann Nutr Metab. 2006;50(2):85–94.
146. Olofin IO, Spiegelman D, Aboud S, Duggan C, Danaei G, Fawzi WW. Supplementation with multivitamins and vitamin A and incidence of malaria among HIV-infected Tanzanian women. J Acquir Immune Defic Syndr. 2014;67(Suppl 4):S173–8.
147. Cusick SE, Opoka RO, Lund TC, John CC, Polgreen LE. Vitamin D insufficiency is common in Ugandan children and is associated with severe malaria. PLoS One. 2014;9(12):e113185.
148. Brooker S, Clements AC, Hotez PJ, Hay SI, Tatem AJ, Bundy DA, et al. The co-distribution of Plasmodium falciparum and hookworm among African school children. Malar J. 2006;5:99.
149. Menzies SK, Rodriguez A, Chico M, Sandoval C, Broncano N, Guadalupe I, et al. Risk factors for soil-transmitted helminth infections during the first 3 years of life in the tropics; findings from a birth cohort. PLoS Negl Trop Dis. 2014;8(2):e2718.

150. Pullan RL, Smith JL, Jasrasaria R, Brooker SJ. Global numbers of infection and disease burden of soil transmitted helminth infections in 2010. Parasit Vectors. 2014;7:37.

151. Ezenwa VO. Co-infection and nutrition: integrating ecological and epidemiological perspectives. In: Humphries DL, Scott ME, Vermund SH, editors. Nutrition and infectious disease: shifting the clinical paradigm. New York: Springer; 2020.

152. Boef AG, May L, van Bodegom D, van Lieshout L, Verweij JJ, Maier AB, et al. Parasitic infections and immune function: effect of helminth infections in a malaria endemic area. Immunobiology. 2013;218(5):706–11.

153. Hartgers FC, Yazdanbakhsh M. Co-infection of helminths and malaria: modulation of the immune responses to malaria. Parasite Immunol. 2006;28(10):497–506.

154. Hartgers FC, Obeng BB, Kruize YC, Dijkhuis A, McCall M, Sauerwein RW, et al. Responses to malarial antigens are altered in helminth-infected children. J Infect Dis. 2009;199(10):1528–35.

155. Nacher M. Worms and malaria: noisy nuisances and silent benefits. Parasite Immunol. 2002;24(7):391–3.

156. Mwangi TW, Bethony JM, Brooker S. Malaria and helminth interactions in humans: an epidemiological viewpoint. Ann Trop Med Parasitol. 2006;100(7):551–70.

157. Naing C, Whittaker MA, Nyunt-Wai V, Reid SA, Wong SF, Mak JW, et al. Malaria and soil-transmitted intestinal helminth co-infection and its effect on anemia: a meta-analysis. Trans R Soc Trop Med Hyg. 2013;107(11):672–83.

158. Shapiro AE, Tukahebwa EM, Kasten J, Clarke SE, Magnussen P, Olsen A, et al. Epidemiology of helminth infections and their relationship to clinical malaria in Southwest Uganda. Trans R Soc Trop Med Hyg. 2005;99(1):18–24.

159. Abbate JL, Ezenwa VO, Guegan JF, Choisy M, Nacher M, Roche B. Disentangling complex parasite interactions: protection against cerebral malaria by one helminth species is jeopardized by co-infection with another. PLoS Negl Trop Dis. 2018;12(5):e0006483.

160. Bardaji A, Bassat Q, Alonso PL, Menendez C. Intermittent preventive treatment of malaria in pregnant women and infants: making best use of the available evidence. Expert Opin Pharmacother. 2012;13(12):1719–36.

161. van Eijk AM, Hill J, Alegana VA, Kirui V, Gething PW, ter Kuile FO, et al. Coverage of malaria protection in pregnant women in sub-Saharan Africa: a synthesis and analysis of national survey data. Lancet Infect Dis. 2011;11(3):190–207.

162. Boullata JI. Drug-nutrition interactions in infectious diseases. In: Humphries DL, Scott ME, Vermund SH, editors. Nutrition and infectious disease: shifting the clinical paradigm. New York: Springer, Humana Press; 2020.

163. Laurence KM, Campbell H. Trial of folate treatment to prevent recurrence of neural tube defect. Br Med J (Clin Res Ed). 1981;282(6282):2131.

164. Fleming AF, Werblinska B. Anaemia in childhood in the guinea savanna of Nigeria. Ann Trop Paediatr. 1982;2(4):161–73.

165. Hamilton PJ, Gebbie DA, Wilks NE, Lothe F. The role of malaria, folic acid deficiency and haemoglobin AS in pregnancy at Mulago hospital. Trans R Soc Trop Med Hyg. 1972;66(4):594–602.

166. Fuller NJ, Bates CJ, Hayes RJ, Bradley AK, Greenwood AM, Tulloch S, et al. The effects of antimalarials and folate supplements on haematological indices and red cell folate levels in Gambian children. Ann Trop Paediatr. 1988;8(2):61–7.

167. Gail K, Herms V. Influence of pteroylglutamic acid (folic acid) on parasite density (Plasmodium falciparum) in pregnant women in West Africa. Z Tropenmed Parasitol. 1969;20(4):440–50.

168. Metz J. Folic acid metabolism and malaria. Food Nutr Bull. 2007;28(4 Suppl):S540–9.

169. Wang P, Sims PF, Hyde JE. A modified in vitro sulfadoxine susceptibility assay for Plasmodium falciparum suitable for investigating Fansidar resistance. Parasitology. 1997;115(Pt 3):223–30.

170. Watkins WM, Mberu EK, Winstanley PA, Plowe CV. The efficacy of antifolate antimalarial combinations in Africa: a predictive model based on pharmacodynamic and pharmacokinetic analyses. Parasitol Today. 1997;13(12):459–64.

171. Watkins WM, Mberu EK, Winstanley PA, Plowe CV. More on 'the efficacy of antifolate antimalarial combinations in Africa'. Parasitol Today. 1999;15(4):131–2.

172. Salcedo-Sora JE, Ochong E, Beveridge S, Johnson D, Nzila A, Biagini GA, et al. The molecular basis of folate salvage in Plasmodium falciparum: characterization of two folate transporters. J Biol Chem. 2011;286(52):44659–68.

173. Wang P, Wang Q, Sims PF, Hyde JE. Characterisation of exogenous folate transport in Plasmodium falciparum. Mol Biochem Parasitol. 2007;154(1):40–51.

174. Sowunmi A, Fehintola FA, Adedeji AA, Gbotosho GO, Falade CO, Tambo E, et al. Open randomized study of pyrimethamine-sulphadoxine vs. pyrimethamine-sulphadoxine plus probenecid for the treatment of uncomplicated Plasmodium falciparum malaria in children. Trop Med Int Health. 2004;9(5):606–14.

175. Nzila A, Mberu E, Bray P, Kokwaro G, Winstanley P, Marsh K, et al. Chemosensitization of Plasmodium falciparum by probenecid in vitro. Antimicrob Agents Chemother. 2003;47(7):2108–12.

176. Sowunmi A, Adedeji AA, Fateye BA, Fehintola FA. Comparative effects of pyrimethamine-sulfadoxine, with and without probenecid, on Plasmodium falciparum gametocytes in children with acute, uncomplicated malaria. Ann Trop Med Parasitol. 2004;98(8):873–8.

177. Nzila A, Okombo J, Molloy AM. Impact of folate supplementation on the efficacy of sulfadoxine/pyrimethamine in preventing malaria in pregnancy: the potential of 5-methyl-tetrahydrofolate. J Antimicrob Chemother. 2014;69(2):323–30.
178. Hess FI, Nukuro E, Judson L, Rodgers J, Nothdurft HD, Rieckmann KH. Anti-malarial drug resistance, malnutrition and socio-economic status. Trop Med Int Health. 1997;2(8):721–8.
179. Verret WJ, Arinaitwe E, Wanzira H, Bigira V, Kakuru A, Kamya M, et al. Effect of nutritional status on response to treatment with artemisinin-based combination therapy in young Ugandan children with malaria. Antimicrob Agents Chemother. 2011;55(6):2629–35.
180. Mitangala PN, D'Alessandro U, Donnen P, Hennart P, Porignon D, Bisimwa Balaluka G, et al. Malaria infection and nutritional status: results from a cohort survey of children from 6–59 months old in the Kivu province, Democratic Republic of the Congo. Rev Epidemiol Sante Publique. 2013;61(2):111–20.
181. Barnes KI, Lindegardh N, Ogundahunsi O, Olliaro P, Plowe CV, Randrianarivelojosia M, et al. World antimalarial resistance network (WARN) IV: clinical pharmacology. Malar J. 2007;6:122.
182. Das D, Grais RF, Okiro EA, Stepniewska K, Mansoor R, van der Kam S, et al. Complex interactions between malaria and malnutrition: a systematic literature review. BMC Med. 2018;16(1):186.
183. Dixon MW, Thompson J, Gardiner DL, Trenholme KR. Sex in Plasmodium: a sign of commitment. Trends Parasitol. 2008;24(4):168–75.
184. Buckling AG, Taylor LH, Carlton JM, Read AF. Adaptive changes in Plasmodium transmission strategies following chloroquine chemotherapy. Proc Biol Sci. 1997;264(1381):553–9.
185. Carter LM, Kafsack BF, Llinas M, Mideo N, Pollitt LC, Reece SE. Stress and sex in malaria parasites: why does commitment vary? Evol Med Public Health. 2013;2013(1):135–47.
186. Carter R, Miller LH. Evidence for environmental modulation of gametocytogenesis in Plasmodium falciparum in continuous culture. Bull World Health Organ. 1979;57(Suppl 1):37–52.
187. Fivelman QL, McRobert L, Sharp S, Taylor CJ, Saeed M, Swales CA, et al. Improved synchronous production of Plasmodium falciparum gametocytes in vitro. Mol Biochem Parasitol. 2007;154(1):119–23.
188. Buckling A, Ranford-Cartwright LC, Miles A, Read AF. Chloroquine increases Plasmodium falciparum gametocytogenesis in vitro. Parasitology. 1999;118(Pt 4):339–46.
189. Stepniewska K, Price RN, Sutherland CJ, Drakeley CJ, von Seidlein L, Nosten F, et al. Plasmodium falciparum gametocyte dynamics in areas of different malaria endemicity. Malar J. 2008;7:249.
190. Drakeley CJ, Secka I, Correa S, Greenwood BM, Targett GA. Host haematological factors influencing the transmission of Plasmodium falciparum gametocytes to Anopheles gambiae s.s. mosquitoes. Trop Med Int Health. 1999;4(2):131–8.
191. Brancucci NMB, Gerdt JP, Wang C, De Niz M, Philip N, Adapa SR, et al. Lysophosphatidylcholine regulates sexual stage differentiation in the human malaria parasite Plasmodium falciparum. Cell. 2017;171(7):1532–44 e15.
192. Usui M, Prajapati SK, Ayanful-Torgby R, Acquah FK, Cudjoe E, Kakaney C, et al. Plasmodium falciparum sexual differentiation in malaria patients is associated with host factors and GDV1-dependent genes. Nat Commun. 2019;10(1):2140.
193. Trager W, Gill GS, Lawrence C, Nagel RL. Plasmodium falciparum: enhanced gametocyte formation in vitro in reticulocyte-rich blood. Exp Parasitol. 1999;91(2):115–8.
194. Reece SE, Duncan AB, West SA, Read AF. Host cell preference and variable transmission strategies in malaria parasites. Proc Biol Sci. 2005;272(1562):511–7.
195. Baker DA. Malaria gametocytogenesis. Mol Biochem Parasitol. 2010;172(2):57–65.
196. Breaux JA, Schumacher MK, Juliano SA. What does not kill them makes them stronger: larval environment and infectious dose alter mosquito potential to transmit filarial worms. Proc Biol Sci. 2014;281(1786):20140459.
197. Vantaux A, Lefevre T, Cohuet A, Dabire KR, Roche B, Roux O. Larval nutritional stress affects vector life history traits and human malaria transmission. Sci Rep. 2016;6:36778.
198. Suwanchaichinda C, Paskewitz SM. Effects of larval nutrition, adult body size, and adult temperature on the ability of Anopheles gambiae (Diptera: Culicidae) to melanize sephadex beads. J Med Entomol. 1998;35(2):157–61.
199. Christensen BM, Li J, Chen CC, Nappi AJ. Melanization immune responses in mosquito vectors. Trends Parasitol. 2005;21(4):192–9.
200. Cirimotich CM, Ramirez JL, Dimopoulos G. Native microbiota shape insect vector competence for human pathogens. Cell Host Microbe. 2011;10(4):307–10.
201. Kumar A, Srivastava P, Sirisena P, Dubey SK, Kumar R, Shrinet J, et al. Mosquito innate immunity. Insects. 2018;9(3):pii:E95.
202. Gonzalez-Ceron L, Santillan F, Rodriguez MH, Mendez D, Hernandez-Avila JE. Bacteria in midguts of field-collected Anopheles albimanus block Plasmodium vivax sporogonic Development. J Med Entomol. 2003;40(3):371–4.

203. Cirimotich CM, Dong Y, Clayton AM, Sandiford SL, Souza-Neto JA, Mulenga M, et al. Natural microbe-mediated refractoriness to Plasmodium infection in Anopheles gambiae. Science. 2011;332(6031):855–8.
204. Riehle MM, Markianos K, Niare O, Xu J, Li J, Toure AM, et al. Natural malaria infection in Anopheles gambiae is regulated by a single genomic control region. Science. 2006;312(5773):577–9.
205. Dong Y, Manfredini F, Dimopoulos G. Implication of the mosquito midgut microbiota in the defense against malaria parasites. PLoS Pathog. 2009;5(5):e1000423.
206. Telang A, Qayum AA, Parker A, Sacchetta BR, Byrnes GR. Larval nutritional stress affects vector immune traits in adult yellow fever mosquito Aedes aegypti (Stegomyia aegypti). Med Vet Entomol. 2012;26(3):271–81.
207. Linenberg I, Christophides GK, Gendrin M. Larval diet affects mosquito development and permissiveness to Plasmodium infection. Sci Rep. 2016;6:38230.
208. Rocklov J, Ahlm C, Humphries DL. Climate change pathways and potential future risks to nutrition and infection. In: Humphries DL, Scott ME, Vermund SH, editors. Nutrition and infectious disease: shifting the clinical paradigm. New York: Springer, Humana Press; 2020.
209. Namaste SM, Aaron GJ, Varadhan R, Peerson JM, Suchdev PS, Group BW. Methodologic approach for the biomarkers reflecting inflammation and nutritional determinants of anemia (BRINDA) project. Am J Clin Nutr. 2017;106(Suppl 1):333S–47S.
210. Suchdev PS, Namaste SM, Aaron GJ, Raiten DJ, Brown KH, Flores-Ayala R, et al. Overview of the biomarkers reflecting inflammation and nutritional determinants of anemia (BRINDA) project. Adv Nutr. 2016;7(2):349–56.
211. Slater HC, Ross A, Ouedraogo AL, White LJ, Nguon C, Walker PG, et al. Assessing the impact of next-generation rapid diagnostic tests on Plasmodium falciparum malaria elimination strategies. Nature. 2015;528(7580):S94–101.
212. Das S, Jang IK, Barney B, Peck R, Rek JC, Arinaitwe E, et al. Performance of a high-sensitivity rapid diagnostic test for Plasmodium falciparum malaria in asymptomatic individuals from Uganda and Myanmar and Naive human challenge infections. Am J Trop Med Hyg. 2017;97(5):1540–50.
213. Cheng Q, Gatton ML, Barnwell J, Chiodini P, McCarthy J, Bell D, et al. Plasmodium falciparum parasites lacking histidine-rich protein 2 and 3: a review and recommendations for accurate reporting. Malar J. 2014;13:283.
214. Brindle E, Lillis L, Barney R, Hess SY, Wessells KR, Ouedraogo CT, et al. Simultaneous assessment of iodine, iron, vitamin A, malarial antigenemia, and inflammation status biomarkers via a multiplex immunoassay method on a population of pregnant women from Niger. PLoS One. 2017;12(10):e0185868.
215. Organization WH. Compendium of WHO malaria guidance – prevention, diagnosis, treatment, surveillance and elimination. 2019. https://www.who.int/malaria/publications/atoz/compendium/en/. Accessed 20 Feb 2020.
216. Organization WH. Global technical strategy for Malaria 2016–2030. 2015. https://www.who.int/malaria/publications/atoz/9789241564991/en/. Accessed 20 Feb 2020.
217. BRINDA. BRINDA Objectives. https://brinda-nutrition.org/about-us/brinda-objectives/. Accessed 20 Feb 2020.
218. United Nations General Assembly. Transforming our world: the 2030 Agenda for sustainable development. United Nations Population Fund; 2015. https://www.unfpa.org/resources/transforming-our-world-2030-agenda-sustainable-development. Accessed 20 Feb 2020.

# Chapter 12
# Soil-Transmitted Helminths: Does Nutrition Make a Difference?

Marilyn E. Scott and Kristine G. Koski

## Abbreviations

| | |
|---|---|
| APC | Antigen-presenting cell |
| BMI | Body mass index |
| C12–C16 | Carbon 12–carbon 16 |
| CD4 | Immunoglobulin superfamily 4 |
| CRP | C-reactive protein |
| epg | Eggs per gram feces |
| Foxp3 | Forkhead box p3 |
| IFN | Interferon |
| Ig | Immunoglobulin |
| IGF-1 | Insulin-like growth factor-1 |
| IL | Interleukin |
| $L_4$ | Fourth-stage larva |
| M1 macrophages | Classically activated macrophages |
| M2 macrophages | Alternatively activated macrophages |
| MMCP | Mucosal mast cell protease |
| RELM | Resistin-like protein |
| STAT6 | Signal transducer and activator of transcription 6 |
| STH | Soil-transmitted helminth |
| Th | T helper |
| TNF | Tumor necrosis factor |
| Tregs | Regulatory T cells |
| VDR | Vitamin D receptor |

M. E. Scott (✉)
Institute of Parasitology, McGill University (Macdonald Campus), Ste-Anne de Bellevue, QC, Canada
e-mail: marilyn.scott@mcgill.ca

K. G. Koski
School of Human Nutrition, McGill University (Macdonald Campus), Ste-Anne de Bellevue, QC, Canada
e-mail: kris.koski@mcgill.ca

© Springer Nature Switzerland AG 2021
D. L. Humphries et al. (eds.), *Nutrition and Infectious Diseases*, Nutrition and Health,
https://doi.org/10.1007/978-3-030-56913-6_12

**Key Points**
- Food- and agriculture-related risks for exposure to soil-transmitted helminth (STH) infections can be minimized by agricultural interventions and health education, but increasing water scarcity may increase use of wastewater for irrigation and the risk of STH exposure.
- Nutritional status may alter chemical cues that STH larvae use to locate a host and to cross tissue barriers en route to their preferred site in the gastrointestinal tract. Release of a host protein that blocks worm feeding is lowered by high-protein and high-carbohydrate diets. Several deficiencies benefit STH development, survival, and egg production, whereas energy restriction and vitamin D deficiency may reduce STH egg production.
- The Th2 response needed for expulsion of STH infections is impaired by protein, energy, zinc, and selenium deficiencies, and energy and zinc deficiencies also blunt the pro-inflammatory Th1 response. However, protein deficiency increases pro-inflammatory responses in STH-infected rodents.
- STH infections alter host nutritional status by modulating molecular signaling of appetite and taste receptors and by reducing absorption of macronutrients, $\beta$-carotene, and iron, with consequences for growth.
- Low host iron increases pathology associated with hookworm infection, but evidence of other impacts of malnutrition on STH-induced disease severity is limited. On the other hand, STH infections may have beneficial effects. They reduce pathology associated with chronic nutritional diseases including obesity, diabetes, and inflammatory bowel diseases. Also, positive intergenerational benefits include altered pup stomach microbiome with upregulated nutrient biosynthesis pathways, and upregulated expression of pathways needed for synaptogenesis, cognition, and memory in the pup brain.
- There is limited evidence that deworming improves nutritional status, that supplementation reduces STH infection, or that combined interventions are more effective. Benefits are more likely to be detectable if standardized metrics are recorded; if study designs incorporate critical aspects of the STH biology; if a broader set of variables that captures the complex interactions among co-existing infections, co-existing nutrient deficiencies, and the host microbiome is incorporated in epidemiological studies; and if evidence from observational studies and lab experiments is considered.

# Introduction

The interactions between soil-transmitted helminths (STHs) and nutrition have been described as a negative spiral whereby infection may contribute to malnutrition but malnutrition may increase infection [1, 2]. Despite the likely bidirectional nature of this relationship, the common perception is that STH infections are a cause of malnutrition. Less appreciated is the likelihood that STH infections may be affected by host nutritional status. This chapter explores evidence that diet and nutritional status influence STH infections using the conceptual framework provided in Chap. 1 [3] as a guide. An overview of evidence for the inverse that STH infection leads to malnutrition is also included.

The basic biology of those STH infections considered in this chapter has been reviewed in Chap. 7 [4] (Table 12.1). All are directly transmitted nematodes that infect a single host. Eggs released in the feces develop into infective stages (embryonated eggs or third-stage larvae) that either are ingested or penetrate the host skin. Within the host, some nematodes live exclusively in the intestinal lumen, some have direct physical contact with the gut epithelium, and some have an extensive extraintestinal tissue migration phase through the lungs. *Strongyloides* is unique in that it has an autoinfection cycle. For

**Table 12.1** Comparison of key life cycle features of soil-transmitted helminths of humans, livestock, dogs, and rodents referred to in this chapter

| Parasite | Normal host | Infective stage[a] | Mode of transmission | Extraintestinal tissue migration | Intestinal niche |
|---|---|---|---|---|---|
| *Ascaris lumbricoides* | Humans | Egg with $L_2$ | Ingestion | Via lungs | Small intestine, lumen |
| *Trichuris trichiura* | Humans | Egg | Ingestion | None | Large intestine, embedded in epithelium |
| *Necator americanus* | Humans | $L_3$ | Skin penetration | Via lungs | Small intestine, lumen |
| *Ancylostoma duodenale* | Humans | $L_3$ | Skin penetration; ingestion | Via lungs | Small intestine, lumen |
| *Strongyloides stercoralis* | Humans, rats | $L_3$ | Skin penetration; also autoinfection | Via lungs | Small intestine, submucosa; females reproduce parthenogenetically |
| *Enterobius vermicularis* (pinworms) | Humans | Egg | Ingestion | None | Small and large intestine; females attach to mucosa |
| *Ascaris suum* | Pigs | Egg with $L_2$ | Ingestion | Via lungs | Small intestine, lumen |
| *Trichuris suis* | Pigs | Egg | Ingestion | None | Large intestine, embedded in epithelium |
| *Haemonchus contortus* | Sheep and goats | $L_3$ | Ingestion | None | Abomasum submucosa and then lumen |
| *Teladorsagia circumcincta* (*=Ostertagia circumcincta*) | Sheep, goats | $L_3$ | Ingestion | None | Gastric glands, then abomasum |
| *Oesophagostomum bifurcum* | Goats, pigs | $L_3$ | Ingestion | None | Small or large intestine, submucosa and then large intestine, lumen |
| *Cooperia oncophora* | Cattle | $L_3$ | Ingestion | None | Small intestine |
| *Toxocara canis* | Dogs | Egg with $L_2$ | Ingestion | Via lungs | Small intestine |
| *Ascaridia galli* | Chickens | Egg | Ingestion | None | Small intestine submucosa and then lumen |
| *Nippostrongylus brasiliensis* | Rats and mice | $L_3$ | Skin penetration | Via lungs | Small intestine, lumen |
| *Heligmosomoides bakeri* (*=H. polygyrus*) | Mice | $L_3$ | Ingestion | None | Small intestine, submucosa and then lumen |
| *Trichuris muris* | Mice | Egg | Ingestion | None | Cecum and large intestine, epithelium |

[a]$L_2$, second stage larva within egg; $L_3$, infective third-stage larva

conciseness, each nematode will be referred to by genus only, unless clarification of the species is necessary. Hookworm genera will be mentioned only if identified in the study.

STHs are distinct in several important ways from viral, bacterial, and protozoan pathogens. First, the number of individual worms cannot increase within the host in the absence of ongoing transmission, as each adult worm results from a single transmission event. Therefore exposure and transmission are ongoing processes leading to an accumulation of worms in the host. This generates an aggregated distribution within the host population where a small proportion of hosts have a disproportionately high number of worms and most hosts are lightly infected. Second, the severity of disease is normally a function of the number of worms in a host which in turn is a function of the rate of transmission. Third, the T helper (Th) 2 response against STHs induces partial immunity of relatively short

**Table 12.2** Commonly used experimental infection protocols

| Protocol | Description | Benefit |
|---|---|---|
| Primary infection | First exposure of previously uninfected host (naïve host) to a single dose of infective eggs or larvae | Parasite establishment, growth, and development are synchronous; useful for relating immune response to specific time points during a first infection |
| Trickle infection | Controlled exposure of initially uninfected host to repeated doses of infective eggs or larvae | Simulates the normal, ongoing exposure to infective stages in the environment in a controlled manner |
| Challenge infection | Second exposure of host that has already received a primary infection to infective eggs or larvae. For *Heligmosomoides,* this is usually done after drug treatment to terminate the primary infection | Beneficial for distinguishing components of the adaptive immune response |

duration. Fourth, following drug treatment, re-infection occurs rapidly in areas where infection is endemic. These distinctive features underlie many of the relationships between nutrition and STH infection and also account for the experimental approaches used to explore nutrition-infection interactions in livestock and rodent models (Table 12.2).

## Agriculture, Diet, and Nutrient Deficiencies Influence Exposure to STH Eggs and Larvae

Without exposure, STH transmission to the host cannot occur. This section considers how diet and nutritional status may alter the exposure of hosts to STH eggs and larvae.

### *Crop Production and Livestock Practices That Increase Risk of Transmission*

*Irrigation* Among agricultural practices, irrigation is increasingly needed, especially because of the increased frequency and severity of droughts (see Chap. 15, [5]). Well-irrigated soils promote survival of hookworm larvae, and irrigation with wastewater is likely to distribute STH eggs and larvae onto agricultural fields. In Ghana, exposure to irrigation water increased the odds of *Ascaris* and hookworm infection by threefold, but only during the wet season [6]. This seasonal response makes sense as free-living hookworm larvae are susceptible to dessication, whereas *Ascaris* eggs accumulate over time in irrigated soils. In contrast, a cross-sectional survey of Vietnamese farmers working in rice paddies revealed a lower prevalence of *Ascaris* and *Trichuris* if wastewater rather than river water was used for irrigation, even though wastewater had a higher concentration of eggs [7]. The authors attributed the unexpected lower prevalence of STHs to better overall wellbeing (child weight-for-age and household socioeconomic status) that compensated for increased exposure to STH eggs in rice paddies irrigated with wastewater.

*Fertilizers* Farmers who use human feces as a fertilizer benefit from improved soil nutrients and crop production and from reduced cost. However, a meta-analysis revealed a 24% increased risk of becoming infected with STHs in those who applied fresh human feces to their rice paddies [8]. In rural Panama, the risk of infection among preschool children with *Ascaris* and hookworm was higher in children who accompanied their caregivers to distant agricultural plots, presumably because open defecation at the plots increased risk of exposure to STH eggs and larvae where children played [9]. Yet caregivers may not be aware of this risk.

***Livestock***   Raising livestock can put farming communities at risk of STH infection. For example, in Maine, USA, pig farmers were infected with the pig ascarid, *Ascaris suum* [10], and molecular epidemiological studies have demonstrated occasional human infection with *A. suum* in developing countries where infections in pigs are common [11]. Another pig parasite, *Trichuris suis*, is also able to establish patent infections in humans. Evidence of genetic mixing of human and pig *Trichuris* was found in Ecuador [12], and in Uganda it was suggested that cross transmission between pigs and humans occurs [13]. Pigs may also serve as a transport host for hookworms as some hookworm eggs are able to survive passage through the pig gut [14]. In Ghana, hookworm prevalence (predominantly *Necator*) was higher in households that owned a pig [15]. If pigs defecate hookworm eggs after they have eaten human feces, eggs may be more widely dispersed in the environment leading to increased exposure of children to infective hookworm larvae. Therefore, the risk of human infection associated with raising pigs should not be ignored.

## Fruit and Vegetables as a Source of STH Infection

Many surveys report that unwashed fruits and vegetables are contaminated with STH eggs and larvae and that washing reduces the likelihood of infection [16]. In southern Thailand, 35% of vegetable samples were contaminated, most commonly with infective nematode larvae [17]. In Ethiopia, *Ascaris* eggs were the most common pathogen on the 54% of produce from local markets that was contaminated [18], and pregnant women were at higher risk of STH infection (predominately hookworm and *Ascaris*) if they regularly consumed raw or unwashed fruit and vegetables [19]. In Thailand, celery was the most frequently contaminated, perhaps because the structure of celery stalks makes them difficult to clean [17]. An Iranian study showed that leafy vegetables were more likely to be contaminated than root vegetables and that the odds of finding STHs on unwashed vegetables were higher compared with washed vegetables [20]. The importance of leafy greens as a source of STH infection is consistent with leafy greens being a priority concern for microbial safety [21].

Many nutrition interventions in impoverished settings encourage diets that incorporate homegrown or wild fruits and vegetables such as dark green leafy vegetables that are rich in micronutrients including vitamin A and iron. For example, after finding that female Tanzanian small-scale farmers who consumed more dark green leafy vegetables had higher serum retinol and total body iron stores, a diversified agriculture intervention was established that promoted nutrient-sensitive production, growth of dark leafy greens in pocket gardens, and nutritional education [22]. However, achieving nutritional benefits from fruits and vegetables while ensuring that they are not a source of STH transmission requires integrated approaches [16].

Improved water sources are beneficial in reducing transmission of *Ascaris* and *Trichuris*, and improved sanitation reduces transmission of hookworm and *Strongyloides* [23], but training in appropriate methods for washing fruit and vegetables is also needed. This is especially important for *Ascaris* because the eggs are very sticky and resistant to chemicals; soaking vegetables in vinegar for 30 minutes was insufficient to kill *Ascaris* eggs [24]. Use of preventative measures by those who package, transport, store, and sell fresh produce [17] helps to reduce contamination during handling. Interventions also need to consider local perceptions. For example, pregnant women in an urban setting in Ethiopia believe that eating dark green leafy vegetables is a potential source of infection for both the fetus and the mother, and therefore they avoid this food during pregnancy [25], a decision that may reduce risk of STH infection but also may contribute to anemia. If trained to wash produce properly, these women might be convinced to consume these nutrient-rich vegetables. Thus, efforts to reduce open defecation and use of contaminated water for irrigation, and to provide potable water, need to be combined with training in procedures for handling and washing fruits and vegetables [16].

## Geophagia Increases Risk of STH Transmission

Direct ingestion of soil is a potential risk factor for transmission of *Ascaris* and *Trichuris* eggs, as both infections occur when eggs are ingested. Evidence of an association is quite strong for *Ascaris* but less so for *Trichuris*. *Ascaris* infection was associated with geophagia in HIV-infected pregnant women in Tanzania [26]. *Ascaris* was also more common in pregnant and lactating women in western Kenya [27] and school children from KwaZulu-Natal in South Africa [28] if they ingested termite mound soil, but not other forms of soil. Geophagia was also associated with *Ascaris* but not *Trichuris* re-infection in Kenyan school children where the relative risk of *Ascaris* re-infection was higher for children who ingested soil compared to those who did not [29]. A more recent study identified geophagy as a risk behavior directly associated with *Ascaris*, hookworm, *Trichuris*, and to a lesser extent *Strongyloides* infection in pregnant women [30].

Yet not all studies have found a relationship between geophagia and STH transmission [31], and the direction of a causal relationship is not clear [32]. This may be because most studies consider pica (ingestion of unusual items such as chalk, ice or ashes as well as soil) rather than geophagia specifically. Also the stigma associated with geophagia may impede collection of accurate information.

Although the underlying causes of geophagia have yet to be established, micronutrient deficiencies have been suggested as one factor contributing to this craving for soil [33]. Among Hispanic women in the United States, the likelihood of geophagia was inversely related to hemoglobin concentration [34], and geophagia increased the risk of anemia in a longitudinal study in Tanzania [26]. Further information is needed on the risks of geophagia, not only from exposure to STHs but also from exposure to heavy metals and to chelating agents that may interfere with micronutrient absorption [26, 32].

## Low Dietary Intake and Poor Appetite Reduce Risk of STH Infection

Two recent studies have shown that STH prevalence is higher in children whose dietary intakes are below recommendation, likely indicating that lower dietary intake reduces nutritional status and hence increases the likelihood of infection. Above-average intake of animal source foods reduced the odds of *Necator* infection in Ghanaian school children [15]. In school-age children from the Philippines, *Trichuris* prevalence was higher when estimated intakes of energy, iron, thiamine, and riboflavin were below recommendation, and hookworm prevalence was higher in those who did not meet the recommended caloric intake [35].

Many nutritional deficiencies are associated with reduced appetite, and there is clear evidence that improved nutritional status increases appetite. Chao and colleagues [36] demonstrated that zinc supplementation (10 mg/day for 12–24 weeks) improved appetite, especially in children with the lowest serum zinc concentrations at the beginning of the study. Similarly, iron-deficient children responded to iron supplementation with increased concentrations of ghrelin and lower leptin, both of which indicate improved appetite [37].

Children with a poor appetite may have a reduced likelihood of ingesting eggs of STHs on fruit and vegetables, and when the reduced appetite also reduces outdoor activity, exposure to STH larvae may be further reduced. Heitman and colleagues [38] explored the impact of dietary energy restriction on natural transmission of the mouse nematode, *Heligmosomoides,* in small cages where infective larvae were dispersed over the damp peat bedding. Energy restriction reduced grooming and the frequency with which mice dug in the peat, thus reducing contact with infective larvae and subsequent transmission. On the other hand, sheep normally avoid feeding near feces, and this evolved behavior reduces the risk of fecal-oral transmission. However, this advantageous behavior was lost when sheep were nutritionally deprived, as hungry "nutritionally motivated" sheep were more likely to feed near feces than "well-nourished" sheep [39], with potential implications for increased transmission of STHs.

> **Box 12.1 Exposure: Take-Home Messages**
> - Eating unwashed fruits and vegetables increases the risk of exposure particularly to *Ascaris* eggs and especially in regions where wastewater is used for irrigation or human feces is used for fertilizer.
> - Although pigs are an important source of animal protein, they are also a source of zoonotic infection with STHs. Deworming especially of free-range pigs can reduce the risk to farmers and their families.
> - Ingestion of soil and playing in agricultural areas where open defecation occurs increases risk of *Ascaris* transmission.
> - Agricultural interventions and health education can effectively address these risks, although the increasing water scarcity associated with global climate change may lead farmers to increase their use of wastewater for irrigation, increasing the risk of STH infection.

*Take-Home Messages* (Box 12.1)

## Nutritional Status Alters STH Establishment and Passage Across Host Tissue Barriers

STHs, depending on the species, must pass one or more barriers in order to establish an infection (see Chap. 7 [4]). Following ingestion of eggs, *Ascaris* larvae cross the intestinal epithelium to begin their tissue migration to the lungs before returning as adult worms to the intestine. *Trichuris* eggs hatch in the lumen of the colon, and adults burrow into the intestinal mucosa. *Haemonchus* and *Heligmosomoides* larvae are ingested but have an obligate development phase in the gastrointestinal mucosa. In contrast, larvae of human hookworms, *Strongyloides,* and *Nippostrongylus* penetrate the skin barrier and then move through the vascular system to the lower respiratory tract where they cross into the alveolar spaces. Although the skin, lung, and gastrointestinal mucosal membranes are known as important barriers to microbial invasions [40, 41], their role as barriers to STH infections is less appreciated, and the impact of nutritional deficiencies on this barrier function has not been widely explored.

## The Skin Barrier

Infective STH larvae that penetrate skin use a variety of sensory signals to find their host including chemicals, odors, and temperature (see review [42]). In vitro assays have shown that the percentage of hookworm larvae displaying penetration activity was higher when the larvae were exposed to saturated carbon (C)12-C16 fatty acids (lauric, myristic, and palmitic acids) from skin extracts [43] and both hookworms and *Strongyloides* respond to serum components including sodium chloride [42].

*Strongyloides* infective larvae are attracted to urocanic acid [44]. Following enzymatic conversion of histamine in metabolically inactive skin cells, urocanic acid accumulates in the epidermis until it is released in sweat or with skin cells that are sloughed off over the period of a month [45]. Protein-deficient mice were found to have elevated levels of urocanic acid in their skin [46], raising the intriguing possibility that *Strongyloides* larvae may be more attracted to individuals that are protein deficient. Furthermore, as urocanic acid has also been shown to reduce immediate-type hypersensitivity [47], its higher concentration in skin of protein-deficient individuals may minimize the host response to the penetrating larvae.

Vitamins and minerals also affect skin health and function [48, 49] (see also Chap. 3 [50]. Vitamin A carotenoids have a role as antioxidants, whereas retinoids inhibit matrix-degrading enzymes in epidermal keratinocytes and dermal fibroblasts [48, 49]. Vitamin A deficiency is associated with delayed wound healing [51]. Adequate intakes of vitamin C have been associated with collagen formation, increased skin moisture content, and epidermal hydration status, all that are important for skin barrier function [49], and Vitamin C deficiency decreases mature collagen formation [52] and increases focal skin bleeding [53]. Vitamin D is synthesized in skin epithelial cells and is associated with stimulation of antimicrobial host defense pathways and wound healing [54–56]. Vitamin E downregulates oxidative damage induced by ultraviolet A irradiation of keratinocytes [57]. Zinc, copper, and selenium also help in protecting the skin from oxidative damage [49]. Thus, given the importance of vitamins and minerals for skin integrity and moisture, wound healing, repair of antioxidant damage, and antimicrobial defense, it is possible that micronutrient deficiencies may play an unrecognized role in altering penetration of the skin by STH larvae, but we were unable to find any studies that explored this.

## The Lung

The lung architecture provides an important barrier to potentially invasive pathogens [58]. Passage through the lung is an important part of life cycle for *Ascaris*, hookworms, and *Strongyloides* [59], as well as *Nippostrongylus*. Following a primary infection of mice with *Nippostrongylus*, resistin-like protein (RELM)α was evident in interstitial macrophages but not alveolar macrophages. The downregulation of pro-inflammatory processes linked to RELMα-reduced lung damage [60] was consistent with the finding that RELMα exerts beneficial effects both on *Nippostrongylus* by minimizing immune attack of larvae as they move through the lungs and on the host because of less lung pathology [61]. Deficiencies of several nutrients including n-3 long-chain polyunsaturated fatty acid, vitamins A, D, and E and their metabolites, and selenium and zinc impair lung maturation, maintenance of the pulmonary epithelial lining, and normal lung physiology (see reviews [62, 63]). However, the impact of nutrient deficiencies on movement of nematode larvae into the alveolar spaces has not been explored.

## The Stomach

STH eggs and larvae must successfully resist digestion by salivary amylase, pepsin, and hydrochloric acid during the interval between being swallowed and reaching the small intestine. If host nutritional status alters the concentrations of gastric acid or digestive enzymes, survival of infective eggs or migrating larvae might be reduced. Although there are occasional reports of *Strongyloides* causing gastric lesions in immunocompromised hosts [64], and impaired gastric acidity and acid-inhibiting treatments may increase pathology associated with *Strongyloides* in patients [65, 66], there is no epidemiological evidence that presence of stomach ulcers is associated with higher prevalence of any of the STH infections.

## The Intestinal Mucosa

Recent reviews have explored the relationship of intestinal barrier function with STH infections [67] and with intestinal immunity (Chap. 3 [50, 68]). To cross the mucosa, nematode larvae must overcome host mucus production, ion secretion that promotes water efflux and peristalsis, the physical barrier associated with tight junctions and paracellular and transcellular pathways, as well as the multifaceted mucosal immune system that includes immunoglobulin (Ig)A, antimicrobial peptides, and cytokines [67]. Specialized chemosensory epithelial cells detect the invading parasites and release cytokine signals that are transmitted to cells of the innate immune system in the lamina propria that elicit a predominantly Th2 acquired immune response characterized by eosinophils, mast cells, and alternatively activated M2 macrophages. This generalized Th2 response is responsible for several biological processes that disrupt the parasite niche by strengthening the physical barrier of the intestine and promoting tissue repair [68].

Most of our understanding of the impact of specific nutrients on the intestinal barrier function has come from studies done in the absence of STH infections or during intestinal inflammation. From this research, roles for vitamin A [69, 70], vitamin D [71–74], zinc [75], and selenium [76] have been reported. Evidence is emerging that supplementation with specific amino acids, short-chain fatty acids produced by microbiota from undigested polysaccharides, and possibly vitamins A, $D_3$, and C as well as zinc may promote mucosal healing, restoration of tissue structure, and epithelial barrier function following inflammation [77]. Given the importance of the goblet cells in producing mucus, it is of note that protein deficiency did not alter the number of goblet cells either in the proximal or distal duodenum during a challenge infection of mice with *Heligmosomoides* [78].

RELMs contribute to the intestinal barrier function and play an important role in STH infections through regulation of intestinal glucose metabolism and mucus production [68, 79]. Initially identified as a protein secreted by adipocytes that inhibits insulin action and adipose cell differentiation, three homologous RELMs have been identified (RELMα, RELMβ, and RELMγ), and the latter two are secreted mainly by the gut. In uninfected mice, colonic expression of RELMβ mRNA was markedly reduced by high-protein and high-carbohydrate diets [80]. Furthermore, in vitro exposure to a saturated fatty acid (stearic acid), insulin, and TNFα, but not polyunsaturated fatty acids (linoleic acid and oleic acid), increased RELMβ expression in colonic cancer cells, but exposure to glucose downregulated RELMβ expression [80], demonstrating that RELMβ expression was directly influenced by nutrients and hormones [80]. Whether this component of the intestinal barrier plays a role in movement of larvae across the mucosa is not known, although RELMβ is necessary for expulsion of adult *Heligmosomoides* from mice [81].

More recently, researchers have proposed that intestinal eosinophilia itself may be a prehepatic barrier that interferes with movement of STH larvae from the gut lumen to the liver [82, 83]. Eosinophils are involved in several protective responses in the intestine including (1) smooth muscle contraction and increased intestinal motility, (2) stimulation of mucins and immunoglobulin (Ig) A-driven retention of mucus, (3) provision of pro-resolution lipid mediators which inhibit granulocyte infiltration and enhance antigen clearance and prevent bacterial translocation, (4) intestinal uptake and glucose metabolism, (5) differentiation of regulatory T cells (Tregs) and inhibition of Th17 induction which limits intestinal mucosal inflammation, and (6) production of lipid mediators that reduce intestinal pathology and prevent neutrophil infiltration [83]. Lab studies have shown that the eosinophil response associated with intestinal barrier function is more sensitive to protein deficiency during adaptive immunity. Mucosal eosinophilia was reduced by protein deficiency in mice challenged with *Heligmosomoides* but not during a primary infection [84, 85], and high-protein diets increased mucosal eosinophilia in lactating rats that had received a challenge infection with *Nippostrongylus* [86].

## The Intestinal Microbiome

The complexity of STH-microbiome interactions is beginning to be explored. Successful establishment of *Trichuris* in the large intestine of mice was shown to be dependent on microflora as egg hatching required attachment of bacteria including *Salmonella typhimurium*, *Escherichia coli*,

*Pseudomonas aeruginosa,* and *Staphylococcus aureus* to the egg operculum [87]. In contrast, in vitro hatching of *Trichuris suis* from pigs was not affected by presence of *E. coli* or several other bacteria [88]. Interestingly, there is evidence that STHs have their own microbiome, as *Heligmosomoides* infective larvae were shown to bring an entirely distinctive microbiome to the mouse host, but by the time they had developed into adults, their microbiome paralleled that of their host [89].

STH infection can alter the gut microbiome (see review [90]) often distal to the location of the worms and perhaps as a function of the immunomodulatory effect of STHs. Chronic infection of mice with *Trichuris* increased the relative abundance of *Lactobacillus* [91], and the reduced diversity and abundance of *Prevotella* and *Parabacteroides* (phylum *Bacteroidetes*) was no longer evident 50 days after mebendazole treatment [92]. *Heligmosomoides* infection of mice increased the relative abundance of *Lactobacillaceae* in the ileum [89] and of *Gammapro teobacteria/Enterobacteriaceae* in the colon [93]. *Heligmosomoides* infection of lactating mice also led to dysbiosis of the stomach microbiome of the neonates on days 2 and 7 [94]. Furthermore, as explored in more detail in section "STHs Alter Gut Microbiome with Implications for Nutritional Status," STH-induced dysbiosis has been shown to alter microbial metabolic pathways [94–96].

When these recent findings are superimposed on the growing understanding of the complex diet-microbiome-nutrient interactions (see review [97]), the impact of STH-microbiome-nutrient interactions on gut barrier function is unlikely to be fully understood for some time.

## Site Selection in the Intestine

A final step in the migration of STHs through the body is their establishment in a preferred site in the gastrointestinal tract [98]. In *Heligmosomoides* infections, bile acids aid establishment of infective larvae, whereas gastric juices are used as a signal for intestinal site selection of adult worms. When entry of bile into the mouse intestine was surgically reduced, larval establishment was lower [99], and the distribution of adult worms along the intestine shifted in parallel with surgical changes in location of the entry of stomach contents into the intestine [100]. These findings are consistent with the normal location of adults in the upper duodenum but larval penetration more distally.

## Other Barriers

Interestingly, there is evidence in endemic areas of northern India and in some parts of China that vertical transmission of *Ancylostoma* larvae to infants may occur through lactogenic transmission during breastfeeding [101], but in utero exposure has not been reported. As antibodies can cross the placenta, the observation that young children of mothers infected with *Ascaris* and *Trichuris* were at increased risk of postnatal infection with these nematodes raises the possibility that maternal transfer of antiparasite antibodies may induce tolerance not protection [102]. Chronic inflammation of the placenta is accompanied by eosinophilia [103] which is intriguing, given that *Heligmosomoides* infection in pregnant mice increased placental mass [104]. STH infections may contribute to eosinophilia and chronic inflammation of this important barrier.

> **Box 12.2 Barriers: Take-Home Messages**
> - STHs rely on chemical cues to find the skin and select preferred sites in the intestine. They also cross skin, lung, and intestinal barriers to complete their life cycle. Yet remarkably few studies have considered the impact of host nutrition on the ability of STH larvae to cross these barriers.
> - STHs are attracted to fatty acids and urocanic acid in the skin, and urocanic acid concentrations are increased by protein deficiency.
> - The microbiome is critical to STHs. Egg hatching is induced by attachment of microbes to the egg operculum. Worms have their own microbiome that is distinct on arrival in the host and gradually shifts to parallel the host microbiome. Furthermore, STH infections induce dysbiosis of the gut microbiome, and this alters microbial metabolic pathways. How these host-microbiome interactions are influenced by nutrient deficiencies is unexplored.

*Take-Home Messages* (Box 12.2)

## Host Nutrition Affects STH Feeding and Reproduction

Adult STHs live in the gastrointestinal tract where they acquire the nutrients needed to survive and reproduce. However, if nutrients are unavailable or uptake is prevented, this will have a negative impact on their ability to survive and reproduce.

### *Nutrient Absorption and Feeding*

Nematodes acquire nutrients by ingestion or by transport across their cuticle. Using *Heligmosomoides,* it was shown that the RELMβ secreted from intestinal goblet cells interfered with worm feeding, contributing to reduced egg production and a shorter life span in the mouse host [81]. Furthermore, RELMβ was shown to bind to chemosensory organs on *Trichuris muris* and *Strongyloides* and inhibit chemotaxis [105] indicating that goblet cell secretion interferes with the ability of the nematode to find, attach to, and feed on gut epithelial cells. As noted earlier, diets high in protein or fat reduce RELMβ expression [80].

Most research on nutrient uptake was conducted in the 1970s and 1980s using *Ascaris suum* from pigs. The requirement for exogenous pyruvate, amino acids, and vitamins was demonstrated by improved in vitro growth, development, and survival when these elements were included in culture media [106]. Furthermore, it was demonstrated that vitamin $B_{12}$ was absorbed across the worm intestine and that maximal absorption occurred at pH 6.4 [107], a pH similar to the proximal small intestine [108] where adult *Ascaris* live. In contrast to vitamin $B_{12}$, cholesterol is absorbed across the cuticle [109]. Cholesterol is the major sterol in *Ascaris* and other nematodes, and in vitro survival of larval *Ascaris suum* was markedly enhanced by inclusion of cholesterol in culture media [106] since de novo synthesis of cholesterol by nematodes is not possible [106, 110].

In addition to cholesterol, parasitic nematodes, including hookworms, are unable to synthesize long-chain fatty acids and retinol de novo and therefore have evolved means to acquire these nutrients from the host [110, 111]. At least two distinct families of fatty acid-binding proteins have been identified in the parasitic stage of nematodes [112]: the *Ascaris* protein ABA-1, and the fatty acid- and retinol-binding (FAR) proteins that have been found in *Teladorsagia* in sheep, the dog hookworm, as well as the human hookworm *Ancylostoma ceylanicum*. Using a hamster model, the *Ancylostoma* FAR, AceFAR-1, was shown to bind to individual fatty acids in the C12–C22 chain length range including oleic, arachidonic, and eicosapentaenoic acid and was localized in several organs of the adult worms, including the hypodermis that lies just under the cuticle [113]. When hamsters were immunized using recombinant AceFAR-1 together with adjuvant, both worm survival and egg production were reduced, highlighting the importance of this protein to the nematodes. The authors speculated that, by interfering with absorption of essential fatty acids, critical functions such as synthesis and maintenance of the cuticle may have been disrupted [113].

## Macronutrients Alter Egg Reproduction

Energy and fatty acids are critical to nematode egg development. Oocytes in the female uterus of *Ascaris suum* absorb glucose that is converted first to glycogen and then, after fertilization, to chitin in the eggshell [114]. Developing *Heligmosomoides* oocytes accumulate lipoproteins presumably as an energy reserve, given the small amounts of glycogen in mature oocytes [115]. Energy restriction led to lower per capita egg production 3 weeks after a primary *Heligmosomoides* infection [116].

The impact of protein deficiency on *Haemonchus* egg production was explored in pregnant goats given a trickle infection early in pregnancy and fed low- or high-protein diets throughout pregnancy until 6 weeks after delivery. In goats fed high-protein diets, initiation of egg production and net egg production over the course of infection was reduced [117]. In mice, protein deficiency increased per worm egg production following a challenge infection with *Heligmosomoides* [118].

The nature and concentration of dietary fiber included in the formulation of diets affected reproduction of *Heligmosomoides*. In vitro egg production was higher in mice fed pectin (a soluble fiber) than those fed cellulose (an insoluble fiber) [119]. In vivo egg output increased with pectin concentration up to 10% but was very low at 20%, and pectin concentration was positively correlated with villus length, villus/crypt ratio, and mucosal thickness [119].

## Micronutrients Alter Egg Production

***Zinc, Selenium, and Boron*** In the *Heligmosomoides*-mouse model, zinc and selenium deficiencies are favorable for the parasite, whereas boron deficiency is detrimental. During a primary infection (controlling for reduced energy intake), zinc deficiency accelerated worm maturation and increased survival but did not alter zinc concentrations in the worms [116]. During a challenge infection, both zinc deficiency [116] and selenium deficiency [120] prolonged worm survival and increased egg production per worm. In contrast, dietary boron restriction lowered the number of larvae 6 days after a primary infection and enhanced worm expulsion during a challenge infection [121].

***Vitamins A, E, and B₁₂*** Vitamin A deficiency lowered fecal egg production in *Trichuris*-infected pigs at 11 and 12 weeks after infection [122], whereas in vivo egg production was higher following challenge infection with *Heligmosomoides* in mice fed diets restricted in vitamin E [120, 123]. Vitamin $B_{12}$ may be necessary for production of gametes as vitamin $B_{12}$ was found in the reproductive tract of *Ascaris suum* [107, 124].

## Host Hormones Influence STH Development and Reproduction

Several hormones or hormone precursors have been shown to affect nematode reproduction. In vitro exposure to estradiol, testosterone, and cortisone lowered *Heligmosomoides* egg output [125]. Also, two ecdysteroid hormones, best known as molting hormones of insects, were found free within tissues of larvae and young adult *Haemonchus* from sheep [126]. Ecdysteroids were also found within the reproductive tract of adult female *Ascaris suum* and were synthesized within eggs that had been isolated from the uterine tissues, indicating a regulatory role in embryogenesis, cuticular deposition, and gonadogenesis [126].

Finally, prostanoids, derivatives of essential fatty acids including arachidonic and linoleic acid, have been implicated as hormone-like growth regulators [127]. In vitro inhibition of prostanoid synthesis not only inhibited development of *Oesophagostomum* from pigs to the $L_4$ stage but also inhibited larval production and excretion of prostanoid-like compounds during the early phases of development [127]. Given the ability of STHs to respond to host hormonal cues, any nutrient deficiency that interferes with hormonal regulation could impact on STH development and reproduction, but this has been largely unexplored.

## Take-Home Messages (Box 12.3)

## Host Nutrition Influences Immunity Against STHs

The impact of deficiencies on host immunity has been reviewed for zinc [128–130], selenium [131], vitamin A [132], vitamin B [133], vitamin C [134], and vitamin D [135]. Several reviews have been published on the Th2 response induced by STH infections (see Chap. 3 [50] and [68, 79, 136] (see Box 12.4). Evidence that host malnutrition directly influences immune responses to STH infections has also been reviewed [1, 137–142].

---

**Box 12.3 STH Feeding and Reproduction: Take-Home Messages**
- STHs are dependent on the host for a variety of nutrients (pyruvate, amino acids, vitamins, long-chain fatty acids). These nutrients are absorbed across the worm gut (e.g., vitamin $B_{12}$) or transported across the cuticle (e.g., cholesterol), and specialized fatty acid-binding proteins promote uptake of nutrients from the host.
- STH feeding is blocked when RELMβ, secreted by goblet cells, binds to STH chemosensory organs, and expression of RELMβ is downregulated by high-protein and high-carbohydrate diets. STH infections also respond to host hormones, but studies have not considered an impact of nutritional deficiencies.
- Deficiencies of protein, zinc, selenium, and vitamin E increase STH egg production, whereas deficiencies of energy and vitamin D decrease egg production. Soluble fiber also increases egg production compared with insoluble fiber.
- Development and survival of STHs is promoted by zinc and selenium deficiencies.

**Box 12.4 STHs Induce a Distinct Immune Response**
- STH infections induce a Th2 immune response characterized by eosinophilia, mastocytosis, elevated antibody titers (IgG1, IgE), and production of Th2 (interleukin (IL)4, IL5, IL13) and T regulatory (IL10, IL17) cytokines. They also stimulate alternatively activated M2 macrophages and downregulate classical inflammation markers including pro-inflammatory Th1 cytokines.
- Some STHs release immunosuppressive molecules that blunt the effectiveness of immune expulsion. For example, the immunosuppressive molecules released by adult *Heligmosomoides* in mice are sufficiently potent that adults survive in mice for several months following a primary infection. However, during a challenge infection, the adaptive immune response delays larval development and effectively expels worms from the gut lumen. In contrast, *Trichuris* and *Nippostrongylus* are effectively expelled from their rodent host within 2 weeks of a primary infection.

## *Nutritional Deficiencies Alter the Th2 Response*

***Protein and Energy*** In the *Heligmosomoides*-mouse model, both protein deficiency [84, 85] and energy restriction [143] prolonged worm survival and reduced the Th2 response to challenge infection, but there were notable differences in the relative timing of immune responses (Table 12.3). Energy restriction led to an earlier, but transient, lowering of serum Th2 biomarkers [143], whereas protein deficiency led to sustained reduction of serum and intestinal Th2 responses (reduced eosinophilia, mucosal mast cells, and mucosal mast cell protease (MMCP)-1) [85]. Protein deficiency also delayed expression of markers of T and B cell proliferation in *Nippostrongylus*-infected rats [144]. However, protein deficiency increased expression of a wide range of pro-inflammatory cytokines and chemokines including interferon (IFN)γ [78], whereas energy restriction lowered IFNγ [143].

***Vitamins*** There is compelling evidence that vitamin A deficiency triggers expansion of the innate lymphoid cells that produce IL13, increasing the immune response against *Trichuris* and reducing worm numbers in mice [145].

In mouse and livestock studies, vitamin D has been shown to regulate Th2 responses. The vitamin D receptor (VDR) is expressed by all cells of the immune system including T cells and B cells where it participates in the control of IgE class-switching and may be involved in control of IgG1 and IgA classes. *Heligmosomoides*-infected mice that were unable to synthesize the active form of vitamin D (calcitriol) had higher concentrations of total and specific IgE compared with wild-type mice, and the authors concluded that endogenous calcitriol from T cells acts on the VDR in B cells to regulate IgE in vivo and alter migration of specific immune cells [146]. In cattle, the VDR was also involved in the adaptive immune response to *Cooperia oncophora* infection, as gene expression studies of intestinal tissue revealed that VDR activation occurred only during re-infection indicating its importance in immune regulation and the maintenance of mucosal integrity [147]. Together, these results suggest that vitamin D deficiency limits the beneficial effects of endogenous calcitriol regulation of IgE.

The impact of dietary vitamin E was explored by comparing the minimal recommended level with that considered optimal for immune responsiveness in lambs infected with *Haemonchus* 5 weeks after the diet treatments began [148]. There were fewer worms in lambs fed the optimal vitamin E diet, and the number of worms was negatively correlated with eosinophils in the abomasal mucosa, but only in the lambs fed the optimal vitamin E diet [148]. Neither serum IgG nor expression of IL4 or interferon (INF)γ in serum was affected by diet [148].

**Table 12.3** Detailed comparison of impact of dietary protein restriction (3% vs 24%) and energy restriction (75% of control) on worm expulsion and immunological indicators at various times during in a primary (p) or challenge (c) infection of mice with *Heligmosomoides* [84, 85, 143]

| Tissue and outcome variable | Protein restricted Compared to control | | Energy restricted Compared to control [143] | |
|---|---|---|---|---|
| | Primary infection | Challenge infection | Primary infection | Challenge infection |
| Worm expulsion | Delayed [84, 85] | Delayed [84, 85] | Delayed | Delayed |
| *Serum* | | | | |
| IgE | Early elevated (p7) [84] Late lowering (p28) [85] | Unaffected [84] Lower (c3–c28) [85] | Mid-lowering (p18) | Early lowering (c6) |
| Total IgG1 | Lower [84, 85] | Lower [84] | Late lowering (p28) | Early lowering (c6) |
| Parasite-specific IgG1 | Unaffected [84] | Unaffected [84] | | |
| Eosinophilia | Unaffected [84] | Lower [84] | Mid-lowering (p12 & p18) | Early lowering (c6) |
| *Splenic T cells* | | | | |
| Stimulation index | | | Lower (p7 & p18) | Early lowering (c7) |
| In vitro IL4 | Early lowering (p6) [85] | Unaffected [85] | Lower (p7 & p18) | Unaffected |
| In vitro IL5 | | | Unaffected | Early lowering (c7) |
| In vitro IFNγ | Unaffected (p6) [85] | Mid--elevation (c14) [85] | Unaffected | Late lowering (c28) |
| IL4 m-RNA | | Mid-lowering (c14) [85] | | |
| IL10 m-RNA | | Mid-lowering (c14) [85] | | |
| *Mesenteric lymph node T cells* | | | | |
| Stimulation index | | | Lower (p7 and p18) | Unaffected |
| In vitro IL4 | Unaffected (p6) [85] | Early lowering (c3 and c6) [85] | Early lowering (p7) | Unaffected |
| In vitro IL5 | | | Late lowering (p 28) | Unaffected |
| In vitro IFNγ | Unaffected (p6) [85] | Mid-elevation (c14) [85] | Unaffected | Lower (c18 and c28) |
| IL4 mRNA | | Mid-lowering (c14) [85] | | |
| IL10 mRNA | | Mid-lowering (c14) [85] | | |
| *Intestine* | | | | |
| Eosinophilia | Unaffected [85] | Lower (c6–c28) [85] | | |
| MMC/vcu | Unaffected [85] | Lower (c9–c28) [85] | | |
| MMCP-1 | Unaffected [85] | Mid-lower (c6, c14) [85] | | |

***Zinc and Energy***  Zinc deficiency impaired both intestinal and systemic responses to *Heligmosomoides* and worm expulsion (see review [138]). Of particular note, Shi and colleagues [149] were able to distinguish consequences of zinc deficiency from the coincident energy restriction on antigen-presenting cell (APC) and T cell function. Based on in vitro assays that combined APCs and T cells from zinc-deficient, pair-fed, or control mice, zinc deficiency impaired T cell function leading to lower T cell proliferation and IL4 production in response to parasite antigen. On the other hand, energy restriction impaired APC function leading to reduced T cell proliferation and lowered production of both Th2 (IL4 and IL5) and Th1 (IFNγ) cytokines [149]. This finding draws attention to the differential impact of zinc and energy on specific cell populations.

*Selenium*  Selenium deficiency reduced the Th2 response during *Heligmosomoides* challenge infection. Selenium-deficient mice had lower expression of Th2-associated genes, fewer alternatively activated M2 macrophages in cyst tissue surrounding the $L_4$ worms, and reduced production of RELMβ [150]. As a consequence, both worm numbers and egg production per worm were higher in the selenium-deficient mice [120]. Worms from selenium-deficient mice also had higher ATP concentrations indicating higher metabolic activity [150], perhaps because RELMβ has a negative impact on worm ATP production [150].

## Supplementation and Refeeding Restore Components of the Th2 Response

In addition to experimental studies using deficient diets, evidence on the impact of nutrients on STH immunity has been obtained during nutrient intervention studies in humans and in animal refeeding studies where diets are restored to adequate levels.

*Macronutrients*  The impact of protein and energy refeeding on immune response to *Nippostrongylus* was studied in pregnant rats and their pups [86]. Rats infected 14 days prior to pregnancy were fed a diet low in crude protein during the second half of gestation and then fed experimental diets with various concentrations of crude protein and metabolizable energy beginning at parturition. Higher crude protein, but not higher energy, increased worm expulsion following a postpartum challenge, and this coincided with more mucosal mast cells and eosinophils [86]. The combination of high protein and high energy increased total serum IgG, but IL4 and IL13 gene expression in mesenteric lymph nodes was not affected by diet. Of note, the benefit of increased dietary protein was evident within 18 days of refeeding, indicating a relatively rapid response. Similar results have been reported in sheep where supplemental protein counters the periparturient immunosuppression [151], presumably because of the higher protein requirements during periods of reproduction.

Protein refeeding also improved expulsion in the *Heligmosomoides* model. Mice fed a low protein diet beginning 1 week before infection were refed a protein-sufficient diet beginning at various times during a primary and challenge infection, and worm expulsion was compared with mice that remained on either a protein-sufficient or protein-deficient diet. Successful worm expulsion occurred in all refeeding groups, even those that were refed 1 week after the challenge infection. Thus protein deficiency did not interfere with priming of the immune response that occurs during a primary infection [118].

*Micronutrients*  Refeeding with a selenium-sufficient diet during a challenge *Heligmosomoides* infection also had a rapid impact [150]. Egg production increased within 2 days, coincident with restoration of Th2-dependent gene expression in the small intestine. After 4 days of refeeding, parasite-specific IgG1 had returned to normal. After 6 days of refeeding, worm ATP concentrations and worm numbers had declined to control levels [150].

In Mexican infants infected with *Ascaris*, Vitamin A supplementation increased the odds of a Th2 response (fecal IL4) but not a Th1 response (fecal IFNγ) or an inflammatory response (fecal monocyte chemoattractant protein-1) [152, 153]. Though based on a limited set of immunological parameters, this study indicated that improved vitamin A status promoted a Th2 response in a population where 37% of infants had low serum retinol (10–20 μg/dL retinol). Consistent with this, *Ascaris*-infected pigs that received three oral doses (100 µg/kg body weight) of all-trans retinoic acid had a heightened pulmonary Th2 response including higher IL4 and IL13 and more alveolar eosinophils [154].

## Take-Home Messages (Box 12.5)

## Host Nutrition Associated with STH-Induced Pathology

Compared with other infectious diseases, severe disease and mortality are less commonly associated with STH infections, perhaps because both the intensity and the presence of infection determine disease severity and because only a small proportion of the population is heavily infected. Nevertheless, the ability of the host to tolerate STHs is at least in part determined by nutritional status [140]. The majority of studies indicate that nutrient deficiencies exacerbate infection-induced pathologies although there are examples where deficiencies reduce pathology.

## Malnutrition, Immunosuppression, and Strongyloides

*Strongyloides* infection is more likely to develop into an autoinfection cycle (see Box 12.6) and become pathogenic in immunosuppressed individuals [155]. A retrospective study of 27 Taiwanese individuals with disseminated infection found that 74% had low serum albumin [156]. Given the range of nutrient deficiencies that impair protective responses to STH infections (see section "Supplementation and Refeeding Restore Components of the Th2 Response"), it is likely that immunosuppression resulting from malnutrition may increase the risk of disseminated strongyloidiasis.

---

**Box 12.5 STH Immunity: Take-Home Messages**
- The Th2 response to STH infections is impaired by protein, energy, zinc, and selenium deficiencies, resulting in improved worm survival and reproduction.
- The Th1 response is blunted by energy restriction and zinc deficiency, but protein deficiency increases pro-inflammatory responses.
- Priming of the adaptive immune response is not impaired by protein deficiency. Hence adaptive immunity develops rapidly following protein refeeding or supplementation.
- Improvement in dietary intake of protein, selenium, and vitamin A status, but not energy, improves Th2 responses and expulsion of STH infections.

---

**Box 12.6 Autoinfection Cycle of *Strongyloides***
- *Strongyloides* eggs often hatch in the intestine, and the larvae can be prematurely infective leading to autoinfection. This possibility is unique among STH infections and is epidemiologically and clinically relevant.
- The autoinfection cycle allows continuing exposure to larvae without contact with infective stages in the environment.
- If the autoinfection cycle is not properly regulated by host immunity, it can result in a hyperinfection syndrome and disseminated infection to a variety of organs [155].

**Box 12.7 Hookworms Cause Hemorrhaging**
- Adult hookworms feed on blood which they acquire through the physical damage to the gut mucosa by their cutting plates (*Necator*) or teeth (*Ancylostoma*).
- In addition to blood ingested by hookworms, hookworms release anticoagulants that prevent clotting and allow leakage of blood around the site of attachment.
- It is estimated that >1 ml of blood can be lost per day during heavy *Necator* infections [157].

## Iron and Zinc Deficiencies Increase STH-Induced Pathology

Perhaps the best evidence of an impact of malnutrition on disease progression comes from hookworm infections where preexisting anemia or iron deficiency exacerbate the hookworm-induced pathology (see review [157] and Box 12.7). Moderate or severe hookworm infections that cause blood loss may also cause iron deficiency anemia when superimposed on low dietary iron intake, blood loss (e.g., during menstruation), or increased nutritional demands such as during pregnancy [157]. It is important to note that extreme iron restriction can impair hookworm development, resulting in lower worm burdens and less hookworm-induced pathology, as shown in hamsters experimentally infected with *A. ceylanicum* [158]. However, when hamsters were fed a moderately iron-restricted diet that did not impair hookworm development, the combination of iron restriction and hookworm lowered hemoglobin and serum iron, relative to uninfected hamsters, and increased mortality.

In contrast, there is limited direct evidence that the severity of *Ascaris* or *Trichuris* infection is influenced by host micronutrient status. Daily zinc supplementation (with or without vitamin A every 2 months) over a period of a year reduced the frequency of diarrhea reported within 7 days of *Ascaris*-positive stool samples from Mexican children (6–15 months at enrolment) [159] (see also section "Improving Nutritional Status as a Means of Reducing STH Infection").

## Protein Deficiency May Increase or Reduce STH-Induced Pathology

In livestock, a high-protein diet has been shown to reduce STH-associated pathology and improve reproductive outcomes. In comparison with *Haemonchus*-infected goats that were fed a low-protein diet during pregnancy and for 6 weeks following parturition, those fed a high-protein diet were able to sustain serum albumin and globulin levels despite protein loss due to infection [160] and had better maternal and neonatal outcomes (doe weight, birth weight) [117]. A high-protein diet also dampened the periparturient rise in *Teladorsagia* egg counts that accompanies sheep immunosuppression at the time of delivery and paralleled a reduction in mucosal damage as evidenced by lower pepsinogen [161]. Interestingly, these benefits were observed in a strain of sheep considered susceptible to STH infection, but not in a resistant strain, raising the possibility that the response to supplementation is influenced by nutrition-genetic interactions [161]. A possible role of host genetics was also reported for mice infected with *Heligmosomoides*. Protein deficiency increased the intestinal damage as measured by permeability to macromolecules in response to infection in a resistant strain of mouse but not in a susceptible strain [162].

In contrast to the previous examples where protein deficiency exacerbated infection-induced pathology, protein deficiency reduced villus atrophy and fluid leakage into the intestinal lumen despite higher numbers of *Heligmosomoides* 14 days after challenge infection [79], likely because protein deficiency lowered the Th2 response that is responsible for fluid leakage [163]. Protein deficiency also reduced liver pathology induced by trickle *Heligmosomoides* infection in lactating mice, as less infection-induced lobular inflammation was observed in response to co-existing infection and protein deficiency [164]. In the kidney, both infection and protein deficiency independently increased creatinine concentrations, whereas they had antagonistic effects on the percentage of abnormal glomeruli, with infection lowering the pathology induced by protein deficiency [164].

## Vitamin A and E Deficiencies Protect Against STH-Induced Pathology in Mice

During *Heligmosomoides* challenge infection, vitamin E deficiency reversed the infection-induced impairment in glucose absorption, reducing fluid accumulation in the intestine and hypercontractility of intestinal smooth muscles [123]. As noted above (section "Nutritional Deficiencies Alter the Th2 Response" - Vitamins), vitamin A deficiency reduced *Trichuris* intensity in mice [145], a finding that would also be expected to reduce STH-induced pathology. However, as retinoic acid controls the balance of innate lymphoid cell populations in the gut, pathology due to acute bacterial infections was increased [145].

## Lung Pathology Is Increased by Vitamin A Deficiency

All human STHs except *Trichuris* and pinworms have an obligate migration across the epithelium of the lower respiratory tract into the alveolar spaces (see review [59]). As a result of the range of antimicrobial defenses in the upper respiratory tract, the lower respiratory tract is putatively microbe-free and designed to maximize gas exchange by maintaining homeostasis and limiting inflammation. Hence, despite local tissue damage, the pathology associated with movement of coevolved human STH larvae into the alveolar spaces in well-nourished hosts is generally limited to a transient eosinophilic inflammation [59]. The only direct evidence that nutrient deficiencies increase lung pathology due to STH infections comes from zoonotic infections. A history of exposure to zoonotic ascarid infection (*Toxocara*) was shown to reduce forced expiratory volume during analysis of data from the US NHANES III study [165]. Vitamin A deficiency was shown to increase severity of lung inflammation in lactating mice infected with the dog ascarid, *Toxocara canis* [166].

## Take-Home Messages (Box 12.8)

**Box 12.8 STH-Induced Pathology: Take-Home Messages**
- Remarkably few studies explicitly examine the impact of malnutrition on STH pathology.
- Iron deficiency, low iron intake, and blood loss exacerbate hookworm-induced pathology; protein malnutrition may be associated with disseminated *Strongyloides* infection.
- Vitamin A and E deficiencies have been shown to reduce intestinal pathology, but vitamin A deficiency may increase lung inflammation.
- Protein deficiency may exacerbate or reduce infection-induced pathology.

# STHs Cause Host Malnutrition

The premise that STH infections contribute to host malnutrition is not new [167], and two reviews have documented underlying mechanisms [1, 168]. More recently, the role of maternal infection on perinatal growth and development and impacts of STH infections on the host microbiome have been identified as new pathways by which STH infection may lead to host malnutrition.

## *STH Infections Reduce Appetite*

Appetite is reduced not only by nutritional deficiencies (see section "Low Dietary Intake and Poor Appetite Reduce Risk of STH Infection") but also by several STHs that alter mediators of appetite including serum leptin, an appetite suppressant, and neuropeptide Y that is linked to food intake. *Strongyloides*-infected children in Egypt had higher concentrations of leptin [169]. Using the mouse-*Nippostrongylus* model, the reduced food intake that occurred immediately after infection [170] was consistent with a transient increase in serum leptin [171] and dose-dependent expression of neuropeptide Y [172]. Furthermore, the anorexia induced by *Nippostrongylus* in rats and *Trichuris* in mice has been associated with altered expression of taste receptors and/or satiety hormones (see review [173]).

## *STH Infections Reduce Nutrient Absorption*

Despite the perception that STH infections interfere with nutrient absorption, definitive evidence is surprisingly limited (see reviews [139, 174, 175]).

***Macronutrients*** Absorption of nitrogen and fat and retention of nitrogen improved following deworming of school-age boys and the effects were more evident in those who had higher numbers of *Ascaris* prior to treatment [176]. Similarly, carbohydrate absorption was better in Burmese preschool children who had been dewormed every 3 months over 2 years compared with those dewormed only 6 weeks before testing [177]. However, the increase in plasma albumin after deworming of 2–9-year-old Bangladeshi children was not due to improved absorption as intestinal permeability (lactulose/mannitol ratio following a standardized sweet flavored drink) was unaffected [178].

Both *Heligmosomoides* challenge infection and *Nippostrongylus* primary infection are associated with reduced sodium-linked glucose absorption by enterocytes resulting in increased fluid movement into the intestinal lumen and increased mucosal permeability that would facilitate uptake of parasite antigen into circulation and movement of host protective molecules into the intestinal lumen [173, 179]. An earlier study reported that *Heligmosomoides* infection lowered carrier-mediated uptake of labeled glucose (mmol/day/g wet weight) in the small intestine pf lactating mice but that total glucose uptake capacity was unaffected given the infection-induced increase in mucosal mass [180].

***Vitamins*** Deworming of *Ascaris*-infected Bangladeshi preschool children resulted in an increase in serum β-carotene 6 months later indicating that *Ascaris* impaired absorption of β-carotene, but deworming did not improve retinol absorption unless deworming was followed by daily dietary β-carotene supplements [181]. However, plasma retinol concentration was negatively associated with *Ascaris* intensity in Vietnamese school children [182] raising the possibility that *Ascaris* impaired retinol absorption.

There is no evidence that *Ascaris* infection is associated with vitamin $B_{12}$ concentration either in Panamanian preschool children [183] or Guatemalan lactating women [184]. However, despite adequacy of serum $B_{12}$ in Spanish school children (all >200 ng/mL $B_{12}$), serum $B_{12}$ concentrations increased following treatment for pinworms [185]. Pinworms are a common, but understudied, STH in children of developed countries. This raises the possibility that pinworms may impair vitamin $B_{12}$ absorption.

***Minerals and Trace Elements*** A Nigerian study compared *Ascaris*-infected children and pregnant women with age-matched uninfected individuals. *Ascaris*-infected pregnant women had lower serum iron, zinc, and selenium; *Ascaris*-infected preschool children had lower iron, zinc, and vitamin A but higher selenium; and *Ascaris*-infected school-age children had lower zinc and vitamin A but higher selenium [186]. Also, Nigerian school-age children with STH infections had lower zinc and vitamin A but higher transferrin and selenium [187]. Whether infection reduced micronutrient absorption or metabolism is unclear, and it is also possible that micronutrient status altered immunocompetence with consequences for infection.

The presence of *Trichuris* in 3–7-year-old children from urban slums in Bangladesh was negatively associated with serum zinc concentration in a multiple regression model that also included a negative association with C-reactive protein (CRP) and a positive association with maternal education [188]. Furthermore, regression analysis using *Trichuris* egg counts (eggs per gram feces, epg) instead of presence of infection revealed 0.12 µmol/L less serum zinc for each unit increase in $\log_{10}(epg + 1)$, and these findings remained significant when controlling for an acute phase response and stunting. Given that *Trichuris* might have led to lower serum zinc or that low zinc might have been beneficial for *Trichuris,* the authors acknowledged that the direction of causality was unclear, especially as deworming had occurred 3–5 weeks before serum samples were collected [188].

Animal studies have shown that STH infections alter host mineral concentrations (see review [139]) but, as with the human studies, it is not clear if this was due to altered absorption or metabolism. Relative to a primary infection, mice with a challenge *Heligmosomoides* infection had lower concentrations of liver boron, iron, and zinc concentrations but higher liver concentrations of chromium, molybdenum, potassium, sodium, and sulfur [121]. *Heligmosomoides* also reduced spleen calcium, iron, and calcium/zinc ratio as well as serum iron [189].

## Loss of Iron and Protein due to Intestinal Tissue Damage

Among the STH infections, direct damage is most commonly associated with hookworms that directly feed on blood (see Box 12.7) and *Trichuris* adults that insert their anterior end directly into the mucosa (see Chap. 7 [4]). Systematic reviews provide an overview of the evidence that hookworm affects hemoglobin [190–192]. Both light and more severe hookworm infections have been associated with lower hemoglobin in pregnant women [189, 190] and nonpregnant adults [192], but in school-age children, only moderate or heavy infections were associated with lower hemoglobin [192]. Deworming improved various health indicators of women and their children [190, 191]. Deworming with albendazole increased hemoglobin concentrations in nonpregnant populations [192], but there was insufficient evidence to conclude that deworming of pregnant women or children under 5 improved hemoglobin concentrations [190, 191]. However, deworming reduced the prevalence of very low birthweight babies in Peru [193]. During severe hookworm infections, intestinal damage also leads to hypoalbuminemia and hypoproteinemia, which can present as a condition similar to kwashiorkor [157].

*Trichuris*-infected children had lower hemoglobin concentrations and higher odds of anemia [182], and fecal occult blood was found in Thai school children whose *Trichuris* epg was greater than 500, but not in those with lower epgs [194]. Furthermore, during *Trichuris* dysentery syndrome, overt bleeding leads to iron deficiency [195]. *Strongyloides* may also contribute to anemia, given that the odds of anemia were higher in those with *Strongyloides* even when controlling for hookworm in communities in Argentina [196].

## Increased Nutrient Demand

Immunological and inflammatory responses to STH as well as tissue repair are energetically demanding and increase nutritional requirements of the host [197]. In livestock, it is well understood that allocation of nutritional resources to immunity is reduced during periods of rapid host growth or reproduction. As a consequence, dietary interventions are routinely used to minimize the impacts of STH infections on reproductive outcomes in livestock [139, 198, 199]. Nutrient interventions are often used during the perinatal period in human populations where STH infections are endemic [200].

## Consequences of STH Infections on Child Growth and Perinatal Growth and Development

Stunting, normally considered to reflect chronic malnutrition, is now known to have a much wider range of causes including STH infection [201–203]. A meta-analysis of the impact of sanitation interventions concluded that the benefit of reduced STH infections was associated with a marginal reduction in stunting despite the low quality of studies [204]. Also, a 1-year randomized control trial of zinc and/or vitamin A supplementation to infants aged 6–12 months revealed that *Ascaris* infection impaired linear growth benefits of zinc supplementation [205] indicating an impact of STH infection on linear growth. Moderate and heavy intensity of combined *Trichuris* and *Ascaris* infections increased the odds of stunting in Peruvian children in grade 5 [206] and also in preschool children [207]. In general, there is less evidence that STH infections are associated with underweight, although moderate-heavy infection with *Trichuris* increased the odds of underweight in preschool children from Peru [208] and albendazole treatment of Indonesian children reduced the proportion of underweight and severely underweight children [209].

There is some evidence that deworming of hookworm-infected women during pregnancy increases birthweight (see review [210]). Linear growth of infants during the first 6 months was also improved if STH-infected Peruvian mothers were dewormed postpartum [211]. More direct evidence that maternal STH infection affects fetal and neonatal growth and development has been obtained using pregnant and lactating mice that received an ongoing trickle infection with *Heligmosomoides*, with or without concurrent protein deficiency. Of particular relevance here was the impact of maternal infection on the uninfected fetus and neonate. Maternal infection reduced fetal linear growth [104, 212], postpartum length and mass [180, 213], and maternal and fetal serum concentrations of prolactin [104]. Furthermore, maternal infection increased placental mass [104] and altered placental expression of several genes associated with fetal growth, including genes associated with the insulin-like growth factor (IGF)-1 axis [214]. Expression of IGF-1 receptor (*Igf1r*) and prolactin (*Prl*) was increased by maternal infection, but only in protein-deficient dams, whereas expression of a transcription factor that positively regulates osteoblast differentiation was reduced, but only in protein-sufficient dams [214]. Also, the T/B cell ratio of pup spleen cells was lowered by maternal *Heligmosomoides* infection but only if dams were also protein deficient [215].

Remarkably, maternal *Heligmosomoides* infection also altered both fetal [216] and pup [217] brain gene expressions. In the 7-day-old pup brain, pyrimidine and purine metabolic pathways were downregulated, but pathways associated with synaptogenesis, cognition, and memory were upregulated [217]. The possibility that maternal STH infection may influence maturation of other key neonatal organs warrants further study especially considering that an impact of maternal infection on liver and stomach mass of uninfected pups was still evident 2 months after birth [218].

## STHs Alter Gut Microbiome with Implications for Nutritional Status

Evidence that STH infections alter the gut microbial community is emerging (see review [90] and section "The Intestinal Microbiome") with implications for microbial metabolic pathways. The altered composition of the microbiome in the proximal colon of *Trichuris*-infected pigs was linked to a dramatic change in metabolic pathways, including downregulation of 14 protein and carbohydrate metabolism pathways, and the absence of specific metabolites of carbohydrate, lysine, and tryptophan metabolism in the lumen of the colon [95]. In addition, there was evidence that pathways involved in metabolism of vitamins and cofactors were higher in infected pigs [96]. In lactating mice, maternal *Heligmosomoides* infection downregulated carbohydrate, amino acid, and vitamin biosynthesis pathways of the cecal microbial community of the dam. Of particular note, however, was the finding that this maternal infection upregulated microbial pathways in the pup stomach, including those involved with amino acid biosynthesis, energy metabolism and fermentation, short-chain fatty acid synthesis, and vitamin-B biosynthesis [94]. The implications of these metabolic changes have not yet been explored.

## Take-Home Messages (Box 12.9)

## Evidence That STHs Are Protective Against Nutrition-Related Chronic Conditions

One of the fascinating emerging areas of study is the potential therapeutic value of STH infections against a variety of chronic nutrition-related diseases, a finding of particular importance given the rising rates of obesity, diabetes, and inflammatory bowel diseases.

---

**Box 12.9 STHs Cause Malnutrition: Take-Home Messages**
- STH infections alter molecular signals of appetite, leading to reduced food intake.
- Treatment of *Ascaris* improves nitrogen, carbohydrate, and β-carotene absorption and increases plasma albumin concentrations.
- Hookworm, as well as *Trichuris* and *Strongyloides*, are associated with low hemoglobin and iron deficiency. Hookworm also causes loss of protein.
- The resulting lower food intake and nutrient absorption, together with nutrient loss, increase dietary requirements especially during periods of reproduction and rapid growth.
- Evidence that STH infections impair growth is stronger for stunting than for underweight. Moreover, maternal STH infection in mice impairs fetal and neonatal growth, alters neonatal brain gene expression, and alters microbial metabolic pathways with potential implications for the host.

## Why STH Infections May Be Relevant

There is growing evidence that the Th2/Treg response to STH infections may prevent or diminish the symptoms of obesity, diabetes, and inflammatory bowel disease. Obesity and diabetes share a common metabolic profile characterized by insulin resistance and subacute chronic inflammation [219, 220]. Furthermore, adipose tissue is now considered to be an active metabolic tissue with immune properties. In general, adipose tissue from lean individuals is known to secrete anti-inflammatory adipokines and cytokines and has alternatively activated M2 macrophages typical of STH infections, whereas adipose tissue from obese individuals secretes pro-inflammatory cytokines and leptin and classically activated M1 macrophages [221]. Within this context, the ability of low-intensity STH infections to promote Th2 driven responses is relevant (see review [173]).

## Obesity

STHs have been shown to attenuate obesity in mouse models. *Nippostrongylus* infection both prevented and treated obesity and associated metabolic dysfunction [170]. This was, at least in part, attributed to reduced intestinal glucose uptake, to weight loss over and above that expected due to infection-induced reduction in food intake, and to reduced inflammation and fewer M1 macrophages that are often associated with obesity [170], consistent with downregulation of pro-inflammatory responses. Furthermore, infection led to an accumulation of eosinophils associated with IL4 release and stimulation of M2 macrophages expected with an upregulation of Th2/Treg responses [222]. *Nippostrongylus* also altered expression of genes involved in regulation of energy and lipid metabolism, leading to decreased lipogenesis [170]. Similarly, in the *Heligmosomoides* model, it was demonstrated that infection significantly reduced development of obesity in mice fed a high-fat diet, and this was associated with reduced glucose uptake, altered lipid metabolism in adipose tissue, upregulation of a Th2/Treg response, and increased numbers of alternatively activated M2 macrophages in adipose tissue [223].

## Insulin Sensitivity and Diabetes

Several animal studies have shown inhibition of diabetes mellitus due to the ability of STH infections to induce IL10, M2 macrophages, and the Th2-driven IL4/STAT 6 immune axis [224]. Furthermore, IL4 administration alone improved insulin action, lowered insulin, total cholesterol, and triglycerides, and protected against diet-induced obesity in uninfected mice [225]. However, evidence to date in humans is weaker. Wiria and colleagues [226] surveyed Indonesian adults and reported a negative association of STH infection with body mass index (BMI), waist-hip ratio, serum cholesterol, and triglycerides but not with carotid intima thickness, CRP, tumor necrosis factor (TNF), or IL10. A subsequent study found that STH infection modestly improved insulin sensitivity in diabetes mellitus Type 2 subjects when controlling for BMI [227]. Moreover, insulin sensitivity increased with each additional concurrent STH in a study where *Necator* was most the prevalent STH [227].

## *Inflammatory Bowel Disease*

Evidence that STH infections reduce inflammation associated with inflammatory bowel diseases has been accumulating from human volunteers and small-scale trials and from experimental animal models (see reviews [157, 228, 229]). Following the experimental infection of celiac patients with a low dose of *Necator,* patients were able to tolerate gluten and had less mucosal damage [230]. Infection also increased the regulatory responses that dampen inflammation following a gluten challenge, as shown by lower numbers of IFNγ-producing intraepithelial lymphocytes and more CD4+ Foxp3+ T cells within the epithelium [230]. Experimental infection with both *Trichuris trichiura* and *T. suis* has had protective effects in small trials against ulcerative colitis and Crohn's disease [229]. In rodent studies, extracellular vesicles secreted by *Nippostrongylus* were protective against chemical-induced colitis in mice and were associated with lowered Th1 cytokines and an increase in the anti-inflammatory cytokine, IL10 [231]. This raises the possibility that STH products could be used as a therapy instead of live worm infections. Also, microbial production of short-chain fatty acids with an anti-inflammatory effect was increased in a small sample of hookworm-infected celiac patients [232], leading to the suggestion that STH-induced anti-inflammatory response may explain the increased bacterial species richness and shift toward a normal gut microbiome concurrent with reduced inflammatory bowel diseases [233].

## *Take-Home Messages* (Box 12.10)

## Nutrition, Drug Efficacy, and Medicinal Plants

Another potential association between nutrition and STH infection is through dietary components that modulate drug efficacy (see Chap. 13 [234]), or that are toxic to nematodes.

## *Diet and Nutritional Status and Efficacy of Commercially Available Anthelmintic Drugs*

There is limited information on the impact of diet or nutritional status on efficacy of anthelmintic drugs (Chap. 13 [234]). Efficacy against hookworm infection, measured by reduction in fecal egg counts following treatment, was higher in school-age Ghanaian children who had fasted for 6 hours prior to treatment, and, furthermore, the cure rate was higher in children with higher hemoglobin [235].

---

**Box 12.10 STHs and Chronic Diseases: Take-Home Messages**
- By upregulating Th2/Treg responses, STHs reduce several nutrition-related chronic conditions.
- STH infection has been shown to prevent and treat obesity in mice through altered lipid metabolism and increased Th2/Treg responses in adipose tissue.
- Mouse studies and, to some extent, human studies demonstrate that STH infection improves insulin action and sensitivity, indicating potential benefits in diabetes mellitus.
- STH infections reduce intestinal inflammation associated with inflammatory bowel diseases resulting, for example, in improved tolerance to gluten in celiac patients.

## Medicinal Plants

In many cultures, medicinal plants are believed to have anthelmintic properties, and several plants from Africa and the Caribbean have been demonstrated to have in vitro effects on *Ascaris suum* [236]. Traditional healers in Kenya use the roots of *Clausena anisata*, a shrub or small tree with edible fruit, as an anthelmintic, and its ethanolic extracts were shown to inhibit in vitro migration of *Ascaris suum* larvae [236]. Recent reports include a study in Africa where papaya seeds were added to maize flour-based porridge and those children who consumed the snack daily for 2 months had a 63% reduction in *Ascaris* egg counts at the end of the 2 months [237]. Both in vitro and in vivo efficacy of ethanolic extracts from pumpkin seeds were comparable to the commercial anthelmintic, fenbendazole, when used to treat the chicken ascarid, *Ascaridia galli* [238], a finding of considerable interest to producers.

In livestock, hydrolyzed yeast reduced *Haemonchus* fecal egg counts in sheep [239], and protein supplements provided to lambs throughout lactation reduced *Haemonchus* fecal egg counts [240]. Goats of the Mamber breed have been shown to self-medicate by preferentially browsing on shrubs with high-tannin content [241], and sheep have a dietary preference for foods containing tannins and saponins that provide nutritional benefits and also have anthelmintic properties against *Haemonchus* [242]. A high-tannin cultivar of birdsfoot trefoil forage had both preventative and therapeutic effects against *Haemonchus* in free-grazing lambs [243]. The anthelmintic properties of polyphenols, particularly condensed and hydrolyzed tannins, have been extensively investigated (see review [244]), and their mode of action may be associated with binding to proline-rich proteins on the nematode cuticle and the buccal capsule that leads to the intestine. Although efficacy of tannins is less than that of commercially available anthelmintics, they may provide supplementary benefits in worm control [244].

## Toxic Effects of Copper and Boron

Toxicity to STH infections has been documented for copper and boron. The anthelmintic properties of multiple small doses of copper oxide wire particles against STHs in lambs were equivalent to the anthelmintic, levamisole [245], raising the possibility that copper could provide an alternative control strategy in settings of multidrug resistance, especially against *Haemonchus* [246]. Repeated copper oxide administration over 3 months did not result in liver toxicity in treated animals, although the possibility of toxicity needs to be monitored [245]. Furthermore, one study has reported an inverse relationship between boron concentration and in vitro *Heligmosomoides* egg production, indicating possible toxicity of boron to this nematode [247].

## Take-Home Messages (Box 12.11)

> **Box 12.11 Anthelmintic Agents: Take-Home Messages**
> - There is no direct evidence that the efficacy of albendazole, the most widely used anthelmintic for STH infections, is affected by nutrient deficiencies, although it may be improved if taken on any empty stomach.
> - Medicinal plants have anthelmintic properties against STH infections and also provide nutritional benefits. These may provide supplementary benefits to commercially available medications.

## Interventions to Address STH Infections and Malnutrition

Evidence of the effectiveness of deworming STH-infected individuals and of micronutrient supplementation of deficient individuals is well established. Whether deworming also improves nutritional status or supplements reduce STH infection, and whether the combination of deworming and supplements exert synergistic benefits, is less clear, especially at the population level where interventions are typically applied.

### *Reducing STH Infection as a Means of Improving Nutritional Status*

Hall and colleagues [248] in a review of the impact of STHs on nutrition concluded that deworming alone is unlikely to treat nutritional problems that may have been exacerbated by infection and recommended parallel provision of protein, energy, and/or micronutrients. This conclusion has been reiterated by two recent systematic reviews [249, 250] that have identified little or no benefit of mass deworming on child weight and no benefit on height. However, in a global empirical analysis of mass deworming programs (population-based treatment without confirmation that individuals are infected or that treatment clears infection), the odds of stunting were reduced in preschool children whose caregiver recalled that their child had been dewormed within the previous 6 months [251]. This study also showed that deworming reduced anemia within sub-Saharan Africa where hookworm is a very common infection [251]. A distinct feature of this analysis was confirmation (albeit by recall) of individual deworming rather than an assumption that mass deworming reached all children.

### *Improving Nutritional Status as a Means of Reducing STH Infection*

Interventions that improve diet, provide agricultural and nutritional education, and provide supplements with single or multiple nutrients might be expected to reduce STH infection, and this logic has guided some national recommendations. For example, a recent study in Ecuador concluded that nutritional supplementation programs should be prioritized in order to reduce the burden of STH within the Amazon region [252]. In Mexico, when bimonthly vitamin A supplementation and a daily zinc supplement were provided for a year to infants (6–15 months), the duration of *Ascaris* infection (measured as number of months between a positive and a negative stool sample) was reduced, indicating that the immune response to *Ascaris* may have been enhanced by the combination of vitamin A and zinc supplements, but not by vitamin A or zinc alone [159]. Of note, however, is the emerging evidence from *Trichuris*-infected mice that the major metabolite of vitamin A (retinoic acid) induced a pro-inflammatory response [253], raising a caution that vitamin A supplementation may exacerbate acute bacterial infections [145].

Other nutrition interventions, such as shifts in food production, food access, food choices, or improved food security, are likely to have longer-term and more sustainable benefits than nutritional supplements and may also reduce STH transmission. However, the benefits of these interventions are less likely to be detected quickly, and the long-term research needed to detect benefits has not been done.

### *Combined Nutrition and Infection Interventions*

The most common combination interventions that directly target both STH infection and malnutrition are deworming together with either multi-micronutrient or vitamin A supplements. Re-infection rates with *Trichuris* and *Ascaris* were lower in Vietnamese school children who received a multi-micronutrient supplement 5 days/week for 12 weeks following albendazole treatment [254].

Several studies have explored the impact of combined vitamin A and deworming on STH re-infection rates. When deworming occurred prior to a 200,000 IU (60 mg) vitamin A supplement, no impact was seen on *Ascaris, Trichuris*, or hookworm re-infection at 3 or 6 months after deworming in a randomized double-blind placebo controlled trial in Malaysian school children [255]. Similarly, when a single, 60 mg dose of vitamin A was administered together with albendazole to Chinese pre-school children, re-infection rates were unaffected compared with deworming alone, although the combination of albendazole and vitamin A was more effective in reducing anemia and improving hemoglobin [256]. However, when a 60 mg vitamin A supplement preceded deworming by no more than 3 months, supplementation reduced *Ascaris* re-infection epg 3 months after deworming of Panamanian preschool children of normal stature but not stunted preschool children [257]. Although the different results among these studies may be due to the relative timing of supplementation and deworming, it is important to note that serum retinol concentrations were lower in the Panamanian preschool children than in the Chinese preschool children and the Malaysian school children. Both age and preexisting degree of deficiency may modify the potential benefit of the supplement on STH re-infection. Also, if retinol is depleted more rapidly in stunted children [258], the benefit of supplementation on re-infection may be brief.

## Co-existing Infections and Co-existing Nutrient Deficiencies

The challenge of identifying the most appropriate intervention(s) is compounded by co-existing infections not only in the gut but also in other organs and tissues, together with co-existing multiple nutrient deficiencies. A recent multidimensional survey of impoverished indigenous pregnant women in Panama highlights the challenge [259–261]. STH infections were common (hookworm in 57%, *Ascaris* in 32%, *Trichuris* in 12%) and two intestinal protozoa, *Giardia* (11%) and *Entamoeba coli* (2%), were also detected. In addition, clinically determined oral, skin infections and laboratory-diagnosed vaginal and urinary infections were recorded. The number of other infections was staggering. At least one vaginal pathogen was found in 97% of women: bacterial vaginosis was diagnosed in 61% of women, trichomoniasis in 75%, diplococcal infection in 20%, and vaginal yeast in 25%. Also, asymptomatic urinary tract infections were detected in 56% of women, 20% had dental caries, and 17% had scabies [259]. Malaria and HIV were not present in the population, and other blood-borne and viral infections were not measured. Furthermore, serum analysis of vitamins and haemaglobin revealed a high prevalence of deficiencies: vitamin $B_{12}$ (86%), vitamin D (68%), vitamin A (39%), and folic acid (31%) [260] together with anemia (38%) a [261].

Each of these infections and deficiencies may influence others. For example, among the infections, vaginal diplococcal infection was positively associated with *Ascaris* but negatively associated with hookworm, and vaginal *Lactobacillus* increased *Ascaris* epg [259]. Serum C-reactive protein (CRP) concentration was higher in women with hookworm infection and caries but lower in women with *Ascaris* and vaginal bacteria [260]. Also, a complex network of associations emerged between infections and deficiencies with regard to blood pressure indicators [261]. These findings raise concerns that interventions targeted against a specific infection may have unexpected consequences and that clinically relevant biomarkers may be misinterpreted without a more holistic knowledge of co-existing infections and nutrient deficiencies.

This setting in rural Panama is likely unique only in that comparable sets of data have not been collected elsewhere. This arises because of the specialized nature of the research and the limited interaction between nutritionists and infectious disease experts when designing screening and intervention studies. A more detailed consideration of the challenge of co-existing infections and deficiencies is explored in Chap. 14 [262]).

*Take-Home Messages* (Box 12.12)

## Challenges for Future Research and Conclusions

The large number of reported associations between malnutrition and STH infection in human populations would indicate that underlying mechanistic explanations exist. Many such mechanisms have been demonstrated in livestock [141] and in laboratory models especially when animal age parallels developmental periods of greatest concern for human health, when multiple infections or deficiencies are combined, and when natural routes of infection are used [142]. Yet these findings do not provide public health answers to the challenges of malnutrition and STH infection in resource-poor settings. How can we ensure that epidemiological studies are as informative as possible? As summarized below, the answer lies in considering data from observational and experimental studies along with randomized controlled trials (RCTs), in adjusting the design of epidemiological studies to account for unique aspects of STH epidemiology, and in measuring a wider set of variables to account for the complex interactions among co-existing infections and nutrient deficiencies.

First, several recent meta-analyses and systematic reviews of nutrition-STH interactions and interventions have questioned whether sole reliance on RCTs as a means of demonstrating causal relationships is appropriate [174, 191, 251]. Clearly the strength of evidence would be improved if more RCTs were conducted, if all RCTs provided the metrics needed for meta-analyses [203], and if new analytical tools such as agent-based models [203], k-nearest neighbor analysis, k-means analysis, and finite mixture models [263] were used. However, observational studies also advance understanding when associations consistent with causal relationships obtained from experimental studies are repeatedly observed [174, 251].

Second, distinctive aspects of STH infections are often ignored in both RCTs and observational studies, reducing the likelihood of detecting relationships that do exist. (1) Studies need to be conducted in populations where both malnutrition and STH infection are prevalent [191, 248]. Hall and colleagues [248] recommended that >20% should be underweight and >40% should be anemic in order to detect an impact of deworming on these nutritional status indicators and that >70% of a population should be infected with STHs. The recommended prevalence of STHs may seem excessive, but it is important to remember that most infected individuals have only a few worms and that detectable morbidity more often occurs in the few individuals with high numbers of worms. (2) Intensity of STH infection (usually measured through epg), not just presence or absence, needs to be recorded for each participant. Without data on STH intensity, it is impossible to reliably detect associations or to know whether an intervention benefitted those individuals with a moderate- or high-intensity infection, as results from the large proportion of lightly infected individuals would dilute the benefit accrued in more heavily infected individuals [248, 263]. Data on epg would also allow investigators to clarify whether low-intensity STH infections minimize the pro-inflammatory response. (3) The most commonly used anthelmintic to treat STHs (albendazole) has lower efficacy against hookworm and *Trichuris* than against *Ascaris*. Thus, a comparison of fecal epg prior to, and 3 weeks after, deworming is important to confirm that treated individuals are no longer infected [248]. (4) Mass deworming programs provide treatment without prior confirmation that individuals are infected or confirmation that treatment has cleared the infection [251], making it difficult to detect benefits of mass deworming on nutritional status. (5) STH re-infection occurs rapidly following infection, often within 6 months [248], and thus repeated deworming is needed to detect improvements in growth that may not be evident for 1 or 2 years [248].

Third, an expanded range of variables should be measured, given the variety of ways in which host nutritional status and STH infections interact [141]. Child height and weight and maternal BMI are commonly measured, but few studies have considered head circumference. Co-existing nutrient deficiencies and co-existing viral, bacterial, protozoan, helminth, fungal, and ectoparasitic infections may modify relationships, but are rarely recorded. Overwhelming evidence highlights that the microbiome interacts with infections, immunity, inflammation, and nutrition [41], but the composition, structure, and metabolic profile of host microbiomes have been largely ignored. Fortunately, new bioinformatics tools allow researchers to explore vast amounts of data in an unbiased way [142]. Finally, the complex social, economic, and political environment also influences both risk of malnutrition and risk of STH infection and certainly affects the success of interventions programs [203, 250]. Multidisciplinary research teams are most likely to incorporate a broader set of indicators of nutrition, infection, immunology inflammation, and the microbiome, as well as social variables in their study design and to interrogate the results in a broader, and more meaningful, way.

The paradigm that all infections are "bad" needs to be reconsidered. Evolution may have favored a balanced set of low-grade infections and low-grade nutritional deficiencies for optimal health. Evidence now shows that STH infections reduce symptoms of a variety of nutrition-related chronic diseases [173], and STH infections may reduce the risk of other infections [259] and lower concentrations of clinically relevant biomarkers [260, 261]. Hence, attention to the possibility that STH interventions may inadvertently exacerbate disease is needed. This may be of special relevance in remote, impoverished settings and marginalized populations where interactions among the many co-existing mild infections and mild nutrient deficiencies may have coevolved to minimize host disease.

From a public health perspective, a multipronged approach that extends beyond deworming and supplements will be needed to achieve sustainable improvements [142, 201, 264]. Such an approach could include education programs that promote healthy diets, improved sanitation and hygiene, food safety, improved food security, shifts in dietary recommendations to account for energetic costs of infection and immunity, and use of probiotics that together could interrupt the STH life cycle and promote beneficial immune and inflammatory responses. New nutraceuticals and medicinal foods with specific bioactive components that modify the intraluminal environment and enhance skin and intestinal barrier functions may also be helpful.

In conclusion, conceptual frameworks such as those developed in Chap. 1 [3] and by Welch and colleagues [250] expand the list of possible mechanisms by which nutritional status interacts with STH infection beyond the two most obvious (impaired immunity in malnourished hosts increases STH infection, and STHs reduce nutrient absorption). Many of these potential mechanisms have been explored and confirmed in rodent models and livestock. Yet demonstration of causality in epidemiological studies remains elusive, perhaps because each causal interaction is in turn influenced by co-existing infections and nutrient deficiencies and probably by the host microbiome. Through more intentional multidisciplinarity in design of epidemiological studies and intentional integration of experimental findings in interpreting results, evidence that nutritional status influences STH infections is likely to increase, allowing development of more holistic and sustainable public health interventions.

# References

1. Koski KG, Scott ME. Gastrointestinal nematodes, nutrition and immunity: breaking the negative spiral. Annu Rev Nutr. 2001;21:297–321.
2. Geus D, Sifft KC, Habarugira F, Mugisha JC, Mukampunga C, Ndoli J, et al. Co-infections with *Plasmodium, Ascaris* and *Giardia* among Rwandan school children. Trop Med Int Health. 2019;24:409–20.
3. Humphries DL, Scott ME, Vermund SH. Pathways linking nutritional status and infectious disease: a conceptual framework. In: Humphries DL, Scott ME, Vermund SH, editors. Nutrition and infectious diseases: shifting the clinical paradigm. Switzerland: Springer Nature; 2020.
4. Geary TG. Primer on helminth parasites. In: Humphries DL, Scott ME, Vermund SH, editors. Nutrition and infectious diseases: shifting the clinical paradigm. Switzerland: Springer Nature; 2020.
5. Rocklöv J, Ahlm C, Humphries DL. Climate change pathways and potential future risks to nutrition and infection. In: Humphries DL, Scott ME, Vermund SH, editors. Nutrition and infectious diseases: shifting the clinical paradigm. Switzerland: Springer Nature; 2020.
6. Amoah AD, Abubakari A, Stenström TA, Abaidoo RC, Seidu R. Contribution of wastewater irrigation to soil transmitted helminths infection among vegetable farmers in Kumasi, Ghana. PLoS Negl Trop Dis. 2016;10:e0005161.
7. Trang DT, Hoek W, Cam PD, Vinh KT, Hoa NV, Dalsgaard A. Low risk for helminth infection in wastewater-fed rice cultivation in Vietnam. J Water Health. 2006;4:321–31.
8. Tran-Thi N, Lowe RJ, Schurer JM, Vu-Van T, MacDonald LE, Pham-Duc P. Turning poop into profit: cost-effectiveness and soil transmitted helminth infection risk associated with human excreta reuse in Vietnam. PLoS Negl Trop Dis. 2017;11:e0006088.
9. Krause RJ, Koski KG, Pons E, Sinisterra O, Scott ME. *Ascaris* and hookworm transmission in preschool children in rural Panama: role of subsistence agricultural activities. Parasitology. 2016;143:1043–54.
10. Miller LA, Colby K, Manning SE, Hoenig D, McEvoy E, Montgomery S, et al. Ascariasis in humans and pigs on small-scale farms, Maine, USA, 2010–2013. Emerg Infect Dis. 2015;21:332–4.
11. Nejsum P, Betson M, Bendall RP, Thamsborg SM, Stothard JR. Assessing the zoonotic potential of *Ascaris suum* and *Trichuris suis*: looking to the future from an analysis of the past. J Helminthol. 2012;86:148–55.
12. Meekums H, Hawash MBF, Sparks AM, Oviedo Y, Sandoval C, Chico ME, et al. A genetic analysis of *Trichuris trichiura* and *Trichuris suis* from Ecuador. Parasit Vectors. 2015;8:168.
13. Nissen S, Al-Jubury A, Hansen TV, Olsen A, Christensen H, Thamsborg SM, et al. Genetic analysis of *Trichuris suis* and *Trichuris trichiura* recovered from humans and pigs in a sympatric setting in Uganda. Vet Parasitol. 2012;188:68–77.
14. Steenhard NR, Storey PA, Yelifari L, Pit DSS, Nansen P, Polderman AM. The role of pigs as transport hosts of the human helminths *Oesophagostomum bifurcum* and *Necator americanus*. Acta Trop. 2000;76:125–30.
15. Humphries D, Simms BT, Davey D, Otchere J, Quagraine J, Terryah S, et al. Hookworm infection among school age children in Kintampo North Municipality, Ghana: nutritional risk factors and response to albendazole treatment. Am J Trop Med Hyg. 2013;89:540–8.
16. Karshima SN. Parasites of importance for human health on edible fruits and vegetables in Nigeria: a systematic review and meta-analysis of published data. Pathog Glob Health. 2018;112:47–55.
17. Punsawad C, Phasuk N, Thongtup K, Nagavirochana S, Viriyavejakul P. Prevalence of parasitic contamination of raw vegetables in Nakhon Si Thammarat province, Southern Thailand. BMC Public Health. 2019;19:34.
18. Bekele F, Tefera T, Biresaw G, Yohannes T. Parasitic contamination of raw vegetables and fruits collected from selected local markets in Arba Minch town, Southern Ethiopia. Infect Dis Poverty. 2017;6:19.
19. Mengist HM, Zewdie O, Belew A. Intestinal helminthic infection and anemia among pregnant women attending ante-natal care (ANC) in East Wollega, Oromia, Ethiopia. BMC Res Notes. 2017;10:440.
20. Rostami A, Ebrahimi M, Mehravar S, Omrani VF, Fallahi S, Behniafar H. Contamination of commonly consumed raw vegetables with soil transmitted helminth eggs in Mazandaran province, northern Iran. Int J Food Microbiol. 2016;225:54–8.
21. Gil MI, Selma MV, Suslow T, Jacxsens L, Uyttendaele M, Allende A. Pre- and postharvest preventive measures and intervention strategies to control microbial food safety hazards of fresh leafy vegetables. Crit Rev Food Sci Nutr. 2015;55:453–68.
22. Stuetz W, Gowele V, Kinabo J, Bundala N, Mbwana H, Rybak C, et al. Consumption of dark green leafy vegetables predicts Vitamin A and iron intake and status among female small-scale farmers in Tanzania. Nutrients. 2019;11:1025.
23. Echazú A, Bonanno D, Juarez M, Cajal SP, Heredia V, Caropresi S, et al. Effect of poor access to water and sanitation as risk factors for soil-transmitted helminth infection: selectiveness by the infective route. PLoS Negl Trop Dis. 2015;9:e0004111.

24. Beyhan YE, Yilmaz H, Hokelek M. Effects of acetic acid on the viability of *Ascaris lumbricoides* eggs. Is vinegar reliable enough to clean the vegetables? Saudi Med J. 2016;37:288–92.
25. Mohammed SH, Taye H, Larijani B, Esmaillzadeh A. Food taboo among pregnant Ethiopian women: magnitude, drivers, and association with anemia. Nutr J. 2019;18:19.
26. Kawai K, Saathoff E, Antelman G, Msamanga G, Fawzi WW. Geophagy (soil-eating) in relation to anemia and helminth infection among HIV-infected pregnant women in Tanzania. Am J Trop Med Hyg. 2009;80:36–43.
27. Luoba AI, Geissler PW, Estambale B, Ouma JH, Alusala D, Ayah R, et al. Earth-eating and reinfection with intestinal helminths among pregnant and lactating women in western Kenya. Trop Med Int Health. 2005;10:220–7.
28. Saathoff E, Olsen A, Kvalsvig JD, Geissler PW. Geophagy and its association with geohelminth infection in rural school children from northern KwaZulu-Natal, South Africa. Trans R Soc Trop Med Hyg. 2002;96:485–90.
29. Geissler W, Mwaniki D, Thiong F, Friis H. Geophagy as a risk factor for geohelminth infections: a longitudinal study of Kenyan primary school children. Trans R Soc Trop Med Hyg. 1998;92:7–11.
30. Ivoke N, Ikpor N, Ivoke O, Ekeh F, Ezenwaji N, Odo G, et al. Geophagy as risk behaviour for gastrointestinal nematode infections among pregnant women attending antenatal clinics in a humid tropical zone of Nigeria. Afr Health Sci. 2017;17:24–31.
31. Young SL, Goodman D, Farag TH, Ali SM, Khatib MR, Khalfan SS, et al. Association of geophagia with *Ascaris, Trichuris* and hookworm transmission in Zanzibar, Tanzania. Trans R Soc Trop Med Hyg. 2007;101:766–72.
32. Miao D, Young SL, Golden CD. A meta-analysis of pica and micronutrient status. Am J Hum Biol. 2015;27:84–93.
33. Young SL. Craving earth: understanding Pica—the urge to eat clay, starch, ice, and chalk. New York: Columbia University Press; 2012.
34. Roy A, Fuentes-Afflick E, Fernald LCH, Young SL. Pica is prevalent and strongly associated with iron deficiency among Hispanic pregnant women living in the United States. Appetite. 2018;120:163e170.
35. Papier K, Williams GM, Luceres-Catubig R, Ahmed F, Olveda RM, McManus DP, et al. Childhood malnutrition and parasitic helminth interactions. Clin Infect Dis. 2014;59:234–43.
36. Chao H-C, Chang Y-J, Huang W-L. Cut-off serum zinc concentration affecting the appetite, growth, and nutrition status of undernourished children supplemented with zinc. Nutr Clin Pract. 2018;33:701–10.
37. Kucuk N, Orbak Z, Karakelloglu C, Akcay F. The effect of therapy on plasma ghrelin and leptin levels, and appetite in children with iron deficiency anemia. J Pediatr Endocrinol Metab. 2019;32:275–80.
38. Heitman TL, Kosk KG, Scott ME. Energy deficiency alters behaviours involved in transmission of *Heligmosomoides polygyrus* (Nematoda) in mice. Can J Zool. 2003;81:1767–73.
39. Hutchings MR, Kyriazakis I, Papachristou TG, Gordon IJ, Jackson F. The herbivores' dilemma: trade-offs between nutrition and parasitism in foraging decisions. Oecologia. 2000;124:242–51.
40. Moens E, Veldhoen M. Epithelial barrier biology: good fences make good neighbours. Immunology. 2012;135:1–8.
41. Biesalski HK. Nutrition meets the microbiome: micronutrients and the microbiota. Ann N Y Acad Sci. 2016;1372:53–64.
42. Bryant AS, Hallem EA. Terror in the dirt: sensory determinants of host seeking in soil-transmitted mammalian-parasitic nematodes. Int J Parasitol Drugs Drug Resist. 2018;8:496–510.
43. Haas W, Haberl B, Syafruddin, Idris I, Kallert D, Kersten S, et al. Behavioural strategies used by the hookworms *Necator americanus* and *Ancylostoma duodenale* to find, recognize and invade the human host. Parasitol Res. 2005;95:30–9.
44. Safer D, Brenes M, Dunipace S, Schad G. Urocanic acid is a major chemoattractant for the skin-penetrating parasitic nematode *Strongyloides stercoralis*. Proc Natl Acad Sci U S A. 2007;104:1627–30.
45. National Center for Biotechnology Information. PubChem Database. Urocanic acid, CID=736715, https://pubchem.ncbi.nlm.nih.gov/compound/Urocanic-acid. Accessed 15 July 2019.
46. Hug DH, Hunter JK, Dunkerson DD. The potential role for urocanic acid and sunlight in the immune suppression associated with protein malnutrition. J Photochem Photobiol B. 1998;44:117–23.
47. Laihia JK, Taimen P, Kujari H, Leino L. Topical cis-urocanic acid attenuates oedema and erythema in acute and subacute skin inflammation in the mouse. Br J Dermatol. 2012;167:506–13.
48. Richelle M, Sabatier M, Steiling H, Williamson G. Skin bioavailability of dietary vitamin E, carotenoids, polyphenols, vitamin C, zinc and selenium. Br J Nutr. 2006;96:227–38.
49. Park K. Role of micronutrients in skin health and function. Biomol Ther (Seoul). 2015;23:207–17.
50. Stephensen CB. Primer on immune response and interface with malnutrition. In: Humphries DL, Scott ME, Vermund SH, editors. Nutrition and infectious diseases: shifting the clinical paradigm. Switzerland: Springer Nature; 2020.
51. Hunt TK. Vitamin A and wound healing. J Am Acad Dermatol. 1986;15:817–21.
52. Ross R, Benditt EP. Wound healing and collagen formation. IV. Distortion of ribosomal patterns of fibroblasts in scurvy. J Cell Biol. 1964;22:365–89.
53. Hodges RE, Hood J, Canham JE, Sauberlich HE, Baker EM. Clinical manifestations of ascorbic acid deficiency in man. Am J Clin Nutr. 1971;24:432–43.

54. Gombart AF, Luong QT, Koeffler HP. Vitamin D compounds: activity against microbes and cancer. Anticancer Res. 2006;26:2531–42.
55. Gombart AF. The vitamin D-antimicrobial peptide pathway and its role in protection against infection. Future Microbiol. 2009;4:1151–65.
56. Campbell Y, Fantacone ML, Gombart AF. Regulation of antimicrobial peptide gene expression by nutrients and by-products of microbial metabolism. Eur J Nutr. 2012;51:899–907.
57. Wu S, Gao J, Dinh QT, Chen C, Fimmel S. IL-8 production and AP-1 transactivation induced by UVA in human keratinocytes: roles of D-alpha-tocopherol. Mol Immunol. 2008;45:2288–96.
58. Iwasaki A, Foxman EF, Molony RD. Early local immune defences in the respiratory tract. Nat Rev Immunol. 2017;17:7–20.
59. Craig JM, Scott AL. Helminths in the lungs. Parasite Immunol. 2014;36:463–74.
60. Krljanac B, Schubart C, Naumann R, Wirtz S, Culemann S, Krönke G, et al. RELMα-expressing macrophages protect against fatal lung damage and reduce parasite burden during helminth infection. Sci Immunol. 2019;4:pii: eaau3814.
61. Batugedara HM, Li J, Chen G, Lu D, Patel JJ, Jang JC, et al. Hematopoietic cell-derived RELMα regulates hookworm immunity through effects on macrophages. J Leukoc Biol. 2018;104:855–69.
62. Arigliani M, Spinelli AM, Liguoro I, Cogo P. Nutrition and lung growth. Nutrients. 2018;10:919.
63. Timoneda J, Rodríguez-Fernández L, Zaragozá R, Marín MP, Cabezuelo MT, Torres L, et al. Vitamin A deficiency and the lung. Nutrients. 2018;10:1132.
64. Rivasi F, Pampiglione S, Boldorini R, Cardinale L. Histopathology of gastric and duodenal *Strongyloides stercoralis* locations in fifteen immunocompromised subjects. Arch Pathol Lab Med. 2006;130:1792–8.
65. Larner AJ, Hamilton MI. Review article: infective complications of therapeutic gastric acid inhibition. Aliment Pharmacol Ther. 1994;8:579–84.
66. Martinsen TC, Bergh K, Waldum HL. Gastric juice: a barrier against infectious diseases. Basic Clin Pharmacol Toxicol. 2005;96:94–102.
67. McKay DM, Shute A, Lopes F. Helminths and intestinal barrier function. Tissue Barriers. 2017;5:e1283385.
68. Sorobetea D, Svensson-Frej M, Grencis R. Immunity to gastrointestinal nematode infections. Mucosal Immunol. 2018;11:304–15.
69. Moran ET Jr. Nutrients central to maintaining intestinal absorptive efficiency and barrier integrity with fowl. Poult Sci. 2017;96:1348–63.
70. de Medeiros PHQS, Pinto DV, de Almeida JZ, Rêgo JMC, Rodrigues FAP, Lima AÂM, et al. Modulation of intestinal immune and barrier functions by Vitamin A: implications for current understanding of malnutrition and enteric infections in children. Nutrients. 2018;10:pii: E1128.
71. Ruemmele FM, Garnier-Lengliné H. Transforming growth factor and intestinal inflammation: the role of nutrition. Nestle Nutr Inst Workshop Ser. 2013;77:91–8.
72. Ardesia M, Ferlazzo G, Fries W. Vitamin D and inflammatory bowel disease. Biomed Res Int. 2015;2015:470805.
73. Li YC, Chen Y, Du J. Critical roles of intestinal epithelial vitamin D receptor signaling in controlling gut mucosal inflammation. J Steroid Biochem Mol Biol. 2015;148:179–83.
74. Dimitrov V, White JH. Vitamin D signaling in intestinal innate immunity and homeostasis. Mol Cell Endocrinol. 2017;453:68–78.
75. Guthrie GJ, Aydemir TB, Troche C, Martin AB, Chang SM, Cousins RJ. Influence of ZIP14 (slc39A14) on intestinal zinc processing and barrier function. Am J Physiol Gastrointest Liver Physiol. 2015;308:G171–8.
76. Kudva AK, Shay AE, Prabhu KS. Selenium and inflammatory bowel disease. Am J Physiol Gastrointest Liver Physiol. 2015;309:G71–7.
77. Lan A, Blachier F, Benamouzig R, Beaumont M, Barrat C, Coelho D, et al. Mucosal healing in inflammatory bowel diseases: is there a place for nutritional supplementation? Inflamm Bowel Dis. 2015;21:198–207.
78. Tu T, Koski KG, Scott ME. Mechanisms underlying reduced expulsion of a murine nematode infection during protein deficiency. Parasitology. 2008;135:81–93.
79. Reynolds LA, Filbey KJ, Maizels RM. Immunity to the model intestinal helminth parasite *Heligmosomoides polygyrus*. Semin Immunopathol. 2012;34:829–46.
80. Fujio J, Kushiyama A, Sakoda H, Fujishiro M, Ogihara T, Fukushima Y, et al. Regulation of gut-derived resistin-like molecule β expression by nutrients. Diabetes Res Clin Pract. 2008;79:2–10.
81. Herbert DR, Yang JQ, Hogan SP, Groschwitz K, Khodoun M, Munitz A, et al. Intestinal epithelial cell secretion of RELM-β protects against gastrointestinal worm infection. J Exp Med. 2009;206:2947–57.
82. Masure D, Vlaminck J, Wang T, Chiers K, Van den Broeck W, Vercruysse J, Geldhof P. A role for eosinophils in the intestinal immunity against infective *Ascaris suum* larva. PLoS Negl Trop Dis. 2013;7:e2138.
83. Strandmark J, Rausch S, Hartmann S. Eosinophils in homeostasis and their contrasting roles during inflammation and helminth infections. Crit Rev Immunol. 2016;36:193–238.

 84. Boulay M, Scott ME, Conly SL, Stevenson MM, Koski KG. Dietary protein and zinc restrictions independently modify a *Heligmosomoides polygyrus* (Nematoda) infection in mice. Parasitology. 1998;116:449–62.
 85. Ing R, Su Z, Scott ME, Koski KG. Suppressed T helper 2 immunity and prolonged survival of a nematode parasite in protein-malnourished mice. Proc Natl Acad Sci U S A. 2000;97:7078–83.
 86. Jones LA, Houdijk JGM, Sakkas P, Bruce AD, Mitchell M, Knox DP, et al. Dissecting the impact of protein versus energy host nutrition on the expression of immunity to gastrointestinal parasites during lactation. Int J Parasitol. 2011;41:711–9.
 87. Hayes KS, Bancroft AJ, Goldrick M, Portsmouth IS, Grencis RK. Exploitation of the intestinal microflora by the parasitic nematode *Trichuris muris*. Science. 2010;328:139104.
 88. Vejzagić N, Adelfio R, Keiser J, Kringel H, Thamsborg SM, Kapel CM. Bacteria-induced egg hatching differs for *Trichuris muris* and *Trichuris suis*. Parasit Vectors. 2015;8:371.
 89. Walk ST, Blum AM, Ewing SA, Weinstock JV, Young VB. Alteration of the murine gut microbiota during infection with the parasitic helminth *Heligmosomoides polygyrus*. Inflamm Bowel Dis. 2010;16:1841–9.
 90. Zaiss MM, Harris NL. Interactions between the intestinal microbiome and helminth parasites. Parasite Immunol. 2016;38:5–11.
 91. Holm JB, Sorobetea D, Kiilerich P, Ramayo-Caldas Y, Estellé J, Ma T, et al. Chronic *Trichuris muris* infection decreases diversity of the intestinal microbiota and concomitantly increases the abundance of Lactobacilli. PLoS One. 2015;10:e0125495.
 92. Houlden A, Hayes KS, Bancroft AJ, Worthington JJ, Wang P, Grencis RK, et al. Chronic *Trichuris muris* infection in C57BL/6 mice causes significant changes in host microbiota and metabolome: effects reversed by pathogen clearance. PLoS One. 2015;10:e0125945.
 93. Rausch S, Held J, Fischer A, Heimesaat MM, Kühl AA, Bereswill S, et al. Small intestinal nematode infection of mice is associated with increased enterobacterial loads alongside the intestinal tract. PLoS One. 2013;8:1–13.
 94. Haque M. Maternal nematode infection alter neonatal brain gene expression and maternal and neonatal microbiomes. PhD Dissertation. McGill University; 2020, 176 pp.
 95. Li RW, Wu S, Li W, Navarro K, Couch RD, Hill D, et al. Alterations in the colon microbiota induced by the gastrointestinal nematode *Trichuris suis*. Infect Immun. 2012;80:2150–7.
 96. Wu W, Li RW, Li W, Beshah E, Dawson HD, Urban JF Jr. Worm burden-dependent disruption of the porcine colon microbiota by *Trichuris suis* infection. PLoS One. 2012;7:e35470.
 97. Valdes AM, Walter J, Segal E, Spector TD. Role of the gut microbiota in nutrition and health. BMJ. 2018;361:k2179.
 98. Sukhdeo MV, Bansemir AD. Critical resources that influence habitat selection decisions by gastrointestinal helminth parasites. Int J Parasitol. 1996;26:483–98.
 99. Sukhdeo MVK, Croll NA. The location of parasites within their hosts: bile and the site selection behaviour of *Nematospiroides dubius*. Int J Parasitol. 1981;11:157–62.
100. Sukhdeo MV, Mettrick DF. Site selection by *Heligmosomoides polygyrus* (Nematoda): effects of surgical alteration of the gastrointestinal tract. Int J Parasitol. 1983;13:355–8.
101. Yu SH, Jiang ZX, Xu LQ. Infantile hookworm disease in China. A review. Acta Trop. 1995;59:265–70.
102. Menzies SK, Rodriguez A, Chico M, Sandoval C, Broncano N, Guadalupe I, et al. Risk factors for soil-transmitted helminth infections during the first 3 years of life in the tropics; findings from a birth cohort. PLoS Negl Trop Dis. 2014;8:e2718.
103. Katzman PJ. Chronic inflammatory lesions of the placenta. Semin Perinatol. 2015;39:20–6.
104. Starr LM, Scott ME, Koski KG. Protein deficiency and intestinal nematode infection in pregnant mice differentially impact fetal growth through specific stress hormones, growth factors, and cytokines. J Nutr. 2015;145:41–50.
105. Artis D, Wang ML, Keilbaugh SA, He W, Brenes M, Swain GP, et al. RELMβ/FIZZ2 is a goblet cell-specific immune-effector molecule in the gastrointestinal tract. Proc Natl Acad Sci U S A. 2004;101:13596–600.
106. Urban JF, Douvres FW, Xu S. Culture requirements of *Ascaris suum* larvae using a stationary multi-well system: increased survival, development and growth with cholesterol. Vet Parasitol. 1984;14:33–42.
107. Zam SG, Martin WE, Thomas LJ Jr. In vitro uptake of $Co^{60}$-vitamin $B_{12}$ by *Ascaris suum*. J Parasitol. 1963;49:190–6.
108. Evans DF, Pye G, Bramley R, Clark AG, Dyson TJ, Hardcastle JD. Measurement of gastrointestinal pH profiles in normal ambulant human subjects. Gut. 1988;29:1035–41.
109. Fleming MW, Fetterer RH. *Ascaris suum*: continuous perfusion of the pseudocoelom and nutrient absorption. Exp Parasitol. 1984;57:142–8.
110. Harder A. The biochemistry of *Haemonchus contortus* and other parasitic nematodes. Adv Parasitol. 2016;93:69–94.
111. Behm CA. Metabolism. In: Lee DL, editor. The biology of nematodes. London: Taylor & Francis; 2002. p. 261–90.
112. Kennedy MW. The polyprotein lipid binding proteins of nematodes. Biochim Biophys Acta. 2000;1476:149–64.
113. Fairfax KC, Vermeire JJ, Harrison LM, Bungiro RD, Grant W, Husain SZ, et al. Characterization of a fatty acid and retinol binding protein orthologue from the hookworm *Ancylostoma ceylanicum*. Int J Parasitol. 2009;39:1561–71.
114. Dubinský P, Rybos M, Turceková L, Ossikovski E. Chitin synthesis in zygotes of *Ascaris suum*. J Helminthol. 1986;60:187–92.

115. MacKinnon BM. An ultrastructural and histochemical study of oogenesis in the trichostrongylid nematode *Heligmosomoides polygyrus*. J Parasitol. 1987;73:390–9.

116. Shi HN, Scott ME, Koski KG, Boulay M, Stevenson MM. Energy restriction and severe zinc deficiency influence development, survival and reproduction of *Heligmosomoides polygyrus* (Nematoda) during primary and challenge infections in mice. Parasitology. 1995;110:599–609.

117. Nnadi PA, Kamalu TN, Onah DH. The effect of dietary protein on the productivity of West African Dwarf (WAD) goats infected with *Haemonchus contortus*. Vet Parasitol. 2009;161:232–8.

118. Tu T, Koski KG, Wykes LJ, Scott ME. Refeeding rapidly restores protection against *Heligmosomoides bakeri* (Nematoda) in protein-deficient mice. Parasitology. 2007;134:899–909.

119. Sun Y, Koski KG, Wykes LJ, Scott ME. Dietary pectin, but not cellulose, influences *Heligmosomoides polygyrus* (Nematoda) reproduction and intestinal morphology in the mouse. Parasitology. 2002;124:447–55.

120. Smith A, Madden KB, Yeung KJ, Zhao A, Elfrey J, Finkelman F, et al. Deficiencies in selenium and/or vitamin E lower the resistance of mice to *Heligmosomoides polygyrus* infections. J Nutr. 2005;135:830–6.

121. Bourgeois A-C, Scott ME, Sabally K, Koski KG. Low dietary boron reduces parasite (Nematoda) survival and alters cytokine profiles but the infection modifies liver minerals in mice. J Nutr. 2007;137:2080–6.

122. Pedersen S, Saeed I, Jensen SK, Michaelsen KF, Friis H. Marginal vitamin A deficiency in pigs experimentally infected with *Trichuris suis*: a model for vitamin A inadequacy in children. Trans R Soc Trop Med Hyg. 2001;95:557–65.

123. Au Yeung K, Smith A, Zhao A, Madden K, Elfrey J, Sullivan C, et al. Impact of vitamin E or selenium deficiency on nematode-induced alterations in murine intestinal function. Exp Parasitol. 2005;109:201–8.

124. Weinstein PP, Jaffe JJ. Cobalamin and folate metabolism in helminths. Blood Rev. 1987;1:245–53.

125. Richardson TL, Mackinnon BM. *Heligmosomoides polygyrus*: effect of exogenous steroid hormones on egg output in vitro. J Helminthol. 1990;64:123–32.

126. Fleming MW. Ecdysteroids during development in the ovine parasitic nematode, *Haemonchus contortus*. Comp Biochem Physiol B. 1993;104:653–5.

127. Daugschies A. *Oesophagostomum dentatum*: population dynamics and synthesis of prostanoids by histotropic stages cultured in vitro. Exp Parasitol. 1995;81:574–83.

128. Maares M, Haase H. Zinc and immunity: an essential interrelation. Arch Biochem Biophys. 2016;611:58–65.

129. Gammoh NZ, Rink L. Zinc in infection and inflammation. Nutrients. 2017;9:624.

130. Wessels I, Maywald M, Rink L. Zinc as a gatekeeper of immune function. Nutrients. 2017;9:1286.

131. Avery JC, Hoffmann PR. Selenium, selenoproteins, and immunity. Nutrients. 2018;10:1203.

132. Bono MR, Tejon G, Flores-Santibañez F, Fernandez D, Rosemblatt M, Sauma D. Retinoic acid as a modulator of T cell immunity. Nutrients. 2016;8:349.

133. Spinas E, Saggini A, Kritas SK, Cerulli G, Caraffa A, Antinolfi P, et al. Crosstalk between vitamin B and immunity. J Biol Regul Homeost Agents. 2015;29:283–8.

134. Carr AC, Maggini S. Vitamin C and immune function. Nutrients. 2017;9:1211.

135. Lang PO, Aspinall R. Vitamin D status and the host resistance to infections: what it is currently (not) understood. Clin Ther. 2017;39:930–45.

136. Grencis RK. Immunity to helminths: resistance, regulation, and susceptibility to gastrointestinal nematodes. Annu Rev Immunol. 2015;33:201–25.

137. Scrimshaw NS, SanGiovanni JP. Synergism of nutrition, infection, and immunity: an overview. Am J Clin Nutr. 1997;66:464S–77S.

138. Scott ME, Koski KG. Zinc deficiency impairs immune responses against parasitic nematode infections at intestinal and systemic sites. J Nutr. 2000;130:1412S–20S.

139. Koski KG, Scott ME. Gastrointestinal nematodes, trace elements and immunity. J Trace Elem Exp Med. 2003;16:237–51.

140. Athanasiadou S. Nutritional deficiencies and parasitic disease: lessons and advancements from rodent models. Vet Parasitol. 2012;189:97–103.

141. Hoste H, Torres-Acosta JF, Quijada J, Chan-Perez I, Dakheel MM, Kommuru DS, et al. Interactions between nutrition and infections with *Haemonchus contortus* and related gastrointestinal nematodes in small ruminants. Adv Parasitol. 2016;93:239–351.

142. Ibrahim MK, Zambruni M, Melby CL, Melby PC. Impact of childhood malnutrition on host defense and infection. Clin Microbiol Rev. 2017;30:919–71.

143. Koski KG, Su Z, Scott ME. Energy deficits suppress both systemic and gut immunity during infection. Biochem Biophys Res Commun. 1999;264:796–801.

144. Athanasiadou S, Jones LA, Burgess STG, Pemberton A, Kyriazakis I, Huntley JF, et al. Genome-wide transcriptomic analysis of intestinal tissue to assess the impact of nutrition and a secondary nematode challenge in lactating rats. PLoS One. 2011;6:e20771.

145. Spencer SP, Wilhelm C, Yang Q, Hall JA, Bouladoux N, Boyd A, et al. Adaptation of innate lymphoid cells to a micronutrient deficiency promotes Type 2 barrier immunity. Science. 2014;343:432–7.

146. Lindner J, Rausch S, Treptow S, Geldmeyer-Hilt K, Krause T, St-Arnaud R, et al. Endogenous calcitriol synthesis controls the humoral IgE response in mice. J Immunol. 2017;199:3952–8.

147. Li RW, Li C, Gasbarre LC. The vitamin D receptor and inducible nitric oxide synthase associated pathways in acquired resistance to *Cooperia oncophora* infection in cattle. Vet Res. 2011;42:48.

148. de Wolf BM, Zajac AM, Hoffer KA, Sartini BL, Bowdridge S, LaRoith T, et al. The effect of vitamin E supplementation on an experimental *Haemonchus contortus* infection in lambs. Vet Parasitol. 2014;205:140–9.

149. Shi HN, Scott ME, Stevenson MM, Koski KG. Energy restriction and zinc deficiency impair the functions of murine T cells and antigen-presenting cells during gastrointestinal nematode infection. J Nutr. 1998;128:20–7.

150. Smith AD, Cheung L, Beshah E, Shea-Donohue T, Urban JF Jr. Selenium status alters the immune response and expulsion of adult *Heligmosomoides bakeri* worms in mice. Infect Immun. 2013;81:2546–53.

151. Kyriazakis I, Houdijk J. Immunonutrition: nutritional control of parasites. Small Rumin Res. 2006;62:79–82.

152. Long KZ, Estrada-Garcia T, Rosado JL, Santos JI, Haas M, Firestone M, et al. The effect of vitamin A supplementation on the intestinal immune response in Mexican children is modified by pathogen infections and diarrhea. J Nutr. 2006;136:1365–70.

153. Long KZ, Santos JI, Garcia TE, Haas M, Firestone M, Bhagwat J, et al. Vitamin A supplementation reduces the monocyte chemoattractant protein-1 intestinal immune response of Mexican children. J Nutr. 2006;136:2600–5.

154. Dawson H, Solano-Aguilar G, Beal M, Beshah E, Vangimalla V, Jones E, et al. Localized Th1-, Th2-, T regulatory cell-, and inflammation-associated hepatic and pulmonary immune responses in *Ascaris suum*-infected swine are increased by retinoic acid. Infect Immun. 2009;77:2576–87.

155. Nutman TB. Human infection with *Strongyloides stercoralis* and other related *Strongyloides* species. Parasitology. 2017;144:263–73.

156. Tsai HC, Lee SS, Liu YC, Lin WR, Huang CK, Chen YS, et al. Clinical manifestations of strongyloidiasis in southern Taiwan. J Microbiol Immunol Infect. 2002;35:29–36.

157. Loukas A, Hotez PJ, Diemert D, Yazdanbakhsh M, McCarthy JS, Correa-Oliveira R, et al. Hookworm infection. Nat Rev Dis Primers. 2016;2:16088.

158. Held MR, Bungiro RD, Harrison LM, Hamza I, Cappello M. Dietary iron content mediates hookworm pathogenesis in vivo. Infect Immun. 2006;74(1):289–95.

159. Long KZ, Rosado JL, Montoya Y, Solano ML, Hertzmark E, DuPont HL, et al. Effect of vitamin A and zinc supplementation on gastrointestinal parasitic infections among Mexican children. Pediatrics. 2007;120:e846.

160. Nnadi PA, Kamalu TN, Onah DN. The effect of dietary protein supplementation on the pathophysiology of *Haemonchus contortus* infection in West African Dwarf goats. Vet Parasitol. 2007;148:256–61.

161. Zaralis K, Tolkamp BJ, Houdijk JGM, Wylie ARG, Kyriazakis I. Consequences of protein supplementation for anorexia, expression of immunity and plasma leptin concentrations in parasitized ewes of two breeds. Br J Nutr. 2009;101:499–509.

162. Clough D, Prykhodko O, Råberg L. Effects of protein malnutrition on tolerance to helminth infection. Biol Lett. 2016;12:20160189.

163. Sun R, Urban JF Jr, Notari L, Vanuytsel T, Madden KB, Bohl JA, et al. Interleukin-13 receptor α1-dependent responses in the intestine are critical to parasite clearance. Infect Immun. 2016;84:1032–44.

164. Starr LM, Odiere MR, Koski KG, Scott ME. Protein deficiency alters impact of intestinal nematode infection on intestinal, visceral and lymphoid organ histopathology in lactating mice. Parasitology. 2014;141:801–13.

165. Walsh MG. *Toxocara* infection and diminished lung function in a nationally representative sample from the United States population. Int J Parasitol. 2011;41:243–7.

166. Moreira DS, Rocha GM. *Toxocara canis*: impact of preweaning nutritional deprivation on the pathogenesis of pneumonia in the mouse. Exp Parasitol. 2005;110:349–52.

167. Scrimshaw NS, Taylor CE, Gordon JE. Interactions of nutrition and infection. Am J Med Sci. 1959;237:367–403.

168. Stephenson LS, Latham MC, Ottesen EA. Malnutrition and parasitic helminth infections. Parasitology. 2000;121:S23–38.

169. Yahya RS, Awad SI, Kizilbash N, El-Baz HA, Atia G. Enteric parasites can disturb leptin and adiponectin levels in children. Arch Med Sci. 2018;14:101–6.

170. Yang Z, Grinchuk V, Smith A, Qin B, Bohl JA, Sun R, et al. Parasitic nematode-induced modulation of body weight and associated metabolic dysfunction in mouse models of obesity. Infect Immun. 2013;81:1905–14.

171. Roberts HC, Hardie LJ, Chappell LH, Mercer JG. Parasite-induced anorexia: leptin, insulin and corticosterone responses to infection with the nematode, *Nippostrongylus brasiliensis*. Parasitology. 1999;118:117–23.

172. Horbury SR, Mercer JG, Chappell LH. Anorexia induced by the parasitic nematode, *Nippostrongylus brasiliensis*: effects on NPY and CRF gene expression in the rat hypothalamus. J Neuroendocrinol. 1995;7:867–73.

173. Shea-Donohue T, Qin B, Smith A. Parasites, nutrition, immune responses, and biology of metabolic tissues. Parasite Immunol. 2017;39:e12422.

174. de Gier B, Ponce MC, van de Bor M, Doak CM, Polman K. Helminth infections and micronutrients in school-age children: a systematic review and meta-analysis. Am J Clin Nutr. 2014;99:1499–509.
175. Strunz EC, Suchdev PS, Addiss DG. Soil-transmitted helminthiasis and vitamin a deficiency: two problems, one policy. Trends Parasitol. 2016;32:10–7.
176. Brown KH, Gilman RH, Khatun M, Ahmed MG. Absorption of macronutrients from a rice-vegetable diet before and after treatment of ascariasis in children. Am J Clin Nutr. 1980;33:1975–82.
177. Linklater JM, Khin-Maung-U, Bolin TD, Thane-Toe, Pereira SP, Myo-Khin, et al. Absorption of carbohydrate from rice in Ascaris lumbricoides infected Burmese village children. J Trop Pediatr. 1992;38:323–6.
178. Northrop CA, Lunn PG, Wainwright M, Evans J. Plasma albumin concentrations and intestinal permeability in Bangladeshi children infected with *Ascaris lumbricoides*. Trans R Soc Trop Med Hyg. 1987;81:811–5.
179. Madden KB, Yeung KA, Zhao A, Gause WC, Finkelman FD, Katona IM, et al. Enteric nematodes induce stereotypic STAT6-dependent alterations in intestinal epithelial cell function. J Immunol. 2004;172:5616–21.
180. Kristan DM. Effects of intestinal nematodes during lactation: consequences for host morphology, physiology and offspring mass. J Exp Biol. 2002;205:3955–65.
181. Haque R, Ahmed T, Wahed MA, Mondal D, Rahman ASMH, Albert MJ. Low-dose β-carotene supplementation and deworming improve serum vitamin A and β-carotene concentrations in preschool children of Bangladesh. J Health Popul Nutr. 2010;28:230–7.
182. de Gier B, Nga TT, Winichagoon P, Dijkhuizen MA, Khan NC, van de Bor M. Species-specific associations between soil-transmitted helminths and micronutrients in Vietnamese school children. Am J Trop Med Hyg. 2016;95:77–82.
183. Scatliff CE, Koski KG, Scott ME. Diarrhea and novel dietary factors emerge as predictors of serum $B_{12}$ in Panamanian children. Food Nutr Bull. 2011;32:54–9.
184. Casterline JE, Allen LH, Ruel MT. Vitamin B-12 deficiency is very prevalent in lactating Guatemalan women and their infants at three months postpartum. J Nutr. 1997;127:1966–72.
185. Olivares JL, Fernández R, Fleta J, Ruiz MY, Clavel A. Vitamin B12 and folic acid in children with intestinal parasitic infection. J Am Coll Nutr. 2002;21:109–13.
186. Arinola GO, Morenikeji OA, Akinwande KS, Alade AO, Olateru-Olagbegi O, Alabi PE, et al. Serum micronutrients in helminth-infected pregnant women and children: suggestions for differential supplementation during anti-helminthic treatment. Ann Glob Health. 2015;81:705–10.
187. Akinwande KS, Morenikeji OA, Arinola OG. Anthropometric indices and serum micronutrient status of helminth – infected school children from semi-urban communities in Southwestern Nigeria. Niger J Physiol Sci. 2017;32:195–200.
188. Kongsbak K, Wahed MA, Friis H, Thilsted SH. Acute phase protein levels, *T. trichiura*, and maternal education are predictors of serum zinc in a cross-sectional study in Bangladeshi children. J Nutr. 2006;136:2262–8.
189. Tu T, Scott ME, Sabally K, Koski KG. Tissue mineral distributions are differentially modified by dietary protein deficiency and a murine nematode infection. Biol Trace Elem Res. 2009;127:234–44.
190. Brooker S, Hotez PJ, Bundy DA. Hookworm-related anaemia among pregnant women: a systematic review. PLoS Negl Trop Dis. 2008;2:e291.
191. Thayer WM, Clermont A, Walker N. Effects of deworming on child and maternal health: a literature review and meta-analysis. BMC Public Health. 2017;17(S4):830.
192. Smith JL, Brooker S. Impact of hookworm infection and deworming on anaemia in non-pregnant populations: a systematic review. Trop Med Int Health. 2010;15:776–95.
193. Larocque R, Casapia M, Gotuzzo E, MacLean JD, Soto JC, Rahme E, et al. A double-blind randomized controlled trial of antenatal mebendazole to reduce low birthweight in a hookworm-endemic area of Peru. Trop Med Int Health. 2006;11:1485–95.
194. Wanachiwanawin D, Wongkamchai S, Loymek S, Suvuttho S, Monkon N, Chinabutra P, et al. Determination of fecal occult blood in primary schoolchildren infected with *Trichuris trichiura*. Southeast Asian J Trop Med Public Health. 2005;36:1110–3.
195. Khuroo MS, Khuroo MS, Khuroo NS. *Trichuris* dysentery syndrome: a common cause of chronic iron deficiency anemia in adults in an endemic area (with videos). Gastrointest Endosc. 2010;71:200–4.
196. Echazú A, Juarez M, Vargas PA, Cajal SP, Cimino RO, Heredia V, Caropresi S, et al. Albendazole and ivermectin for the control of soil-transmitted helminths in an area with high prevalence of *Strongyloides stercoralis* and hookworm in northwestern Argentina: a community-based pragmatic study. PLoS Negl Trop Dis. 2017;11:e0006003.
197. Piwoz E, Sundberg S, Rooke J. Promoting healthy growth: what are the priorities for research and action? Adv Nutr. 2012;3:234–41.
198. Coop RL, Kyriazakis I. Nutrition–parasite interaction. Vet Parasitol. 1999;84:187–204.
199. Coop RL, Kyriazakis I. Influence of host nutrition on the development and consequences of nematode parasitism in ruminants. Trends Parasitol. 2001;17:325–30.

200. Vaivada T, Gaffey MF, Das JK, Bhutta ZA. Evidence-based interventions for improvement of maternal and child nutrition in low-income settings: what's new? Curr Opin Clin Nutr Metab Care. 2017;20:204–10.
201. Prendergast AJ, Humphrey JH. The stunting syndrome in developing countries. Paediatr Int Child Health. 2014;34:250–65.
202. de Onis M, Branca F. Childhood stunting: a global perspective. Matern Child Nutr. 2016;12(S1):12–26.
203. Mosites E, Dawson-Hahn E, Walson J, Rowhani-Rahbar A, Neuhouser ML. Piecing together the stunting puzzle: a framework for attributable factors of child stunting. Paediatr Int Child Health. 2017;37:158–65.
204. Weatherhead JE, Hotez PJ. Worm infections in children. Pediatr Rev. 2015;36:341–52.
205. Rosado JL, Caamaño MC, Montoya YA, Solano ML, Santos JI, Long KZ. Interaction of zinc or vitamin A supplementation and specific parasite infections on Mexican infants' growth: a randomized clinical trial. Eur J Clin Nutr. 2009;63:1176–84.
206. Casapía M, Joseph SA, Núñez C, Rahme E, Gyorkos TW. Parasite risk factors for stunting in grade 5 students in a community of extreme poverty in Peru. Int J Parasitol. 2006;36:741–7.
207. Gyorkos TW, Maheu-Giroux M, Casapía M, Joseph SA, Creed-Kanashiro H. Stunting and helminth infection in early preschool-age children in a resource-poor community in the Amazon lowlands of Peru. Trans R Soc Trop Med Hyg. 2011;105:204–8.
208. Casapía M, Joseph SA, Núñez C, Rahme E, Gyorkos TW. Parasite and maternal risk factors for malnutrition in preschool-age children in Belen, Peru using the new WHO Child Growth Standards. Br J Nutr. 2007;98:1259–66.
209. Sungkar S, Ridwan AS, Kusumowidagdo G. The effect of deworming using triple-dose albendazole on nutritional status of children in Perobatang Village, Southwest Sumba, Indonesia. J Parasitol Res. 2017;5476739
210. Larocque R, Gyorkos TW. Should deworming be included in antenatal packages in hookworm-endemic areas of developing countries? Can J Public Health. 2006;97:222–4.
211. Mofid LS, Casapía M, Aguilar E, Silva H, Montresor A, Rahme E, et al. A double-blind randomized controlled trial of maternal postpartum deworming to improve infant weight gain in the Peruvian Amazon. PLoS Negl Trop Dis. 2017;11:e0005098.
212. Odiere MR, Koski KG, Weiler HA, Scott ME. Concurrent nematode infection and pregnancy induce physiological responses that impair linear growth in the murine foetus. Parasitology. 2010;137:991–1002.
213. Odiere MR, Scott ME, Weiler HA, Koski KG. Protein deficiency and nematode infection during pregnancy and lactation reduce maternal bone mineralization and neonatal linear growth in mice. J Nutr. 2010;140:1638–45.
214. Starr LM, Koski KG, Scott ME. Expression of growth-related genes in the mouse placenta is influenced by interactions between intestinal nematode (Heligmosomoides bakeri) infection and dietary protein deficiency. Int J Parasitol. 2016;46:97–104.
215. Odiere MR, Scott ME, Leroux L-P, Dzierszinski FS, Koski KG. Maternal protein deficiency during a gastrointestinal nematode infection alters developmental profile of lymphocyte populations and selected cytokines in neonatal mice. J Nutr. 2013;143:100–7.
216. Haque M, Starr LM, Koski KG, Scott ME. Differential expression of genes in fetal brain as a consequence of maternal protein deficiency and nematode infection. Int J Parasitol. 2018;48:51–8.
217. Haque M, Koski KG, Scott ME. Maternal gastrointestinal nematode infection up-regulates expression of genes associated with long-term potentiation in perinatal brains of uninfected developing pups. Sci Rep. 2019;9:4165.
218. Kristan DM. Maternal and direct effects of the intestinal nematode Heligmosomoides polygyrus on offspring growth and susceptibility to infection. J Exp Biol. 2002;205:3967–77.
219. Hotamisligil GS, Shargill NS, Spiegelman BM. Adipose expression of tumor necrosis factor-alpha: direct role in obesity-linked insulin resistance. Science. 1993;259:87–91.
220. Hotamisligil GS. Inflammation and metabolic disorders. Nature. 2006;444:860–7.
221. Ouchi N, Parker JL, Lugus JJ, Walsh K. Adipokines in inflammation and metabolic disease. Nat Rev Immunol. 2011;11:85–97.
222. Wu D, Molofsky AB, Liang HE, Ricardo-Gonzalez RR, Jouihan HA, Bando JK, et al. Eosinophils sustain adipose alternatively activated macrophages associated with glucose homeostasis. Science. 2011;332:243–7.
223. Su CW, Chen C-Y, Li Y, Long SR, Massey W, Kumar DV, et al. Helminth infection protects against high fat diet-induced obesity via induction of alternatively activated macrophages. Sci Rep. 2018;8:4607.
224. Wiria AE, Djuardi Y, Supali T, Sartono E, Yazdanbakhsh M. Helminth infection in populations undergoing epidemiological transition: a friend or foe? Semin Immunopathol. 2012;34:889–901.
225. Ricardo-Gonzalez RR, Eagle AR, Odegaard JI, Jouihan H, Morel CR, Heredia JE, et al. IL-4/STAT6 immune axis regulates peripheral nutrient metabolism and insulin sensitivity. Proc Natl Acad Sci U S A. 2010;107:22617–22.
226. Wiria AE, Wammes LJ, Hamid F, Dekkers OM, Prasetyani MA, May L, et al. Relationship between carotid intima media thickness and helminth infections on Flores Island, Indonesia. PLoS One. 2013;8:e54855.
227. Wiria AE, Hamid F, Wammes LJ, Prasetyani MA, Dekkers OM, May L, et al. Infection with soil-transmitted helminths is associated with increased insulin sensitivity. PLoS One. 2015;10:e0127746.

228. Smallwood TB, Giacomin PR, Loukas A, Mulvenna JP, Clark RJ, Miles JJ. Helminth immunomodulation in auto-immune disease. Front Immunol. 2017;8:453.
229. Varyani F, Fleming JO, Maizels RM. Helminths in the gastrointestinal tract as modulators of immunity and pathology. Am J Physiol Gastrointest Liver Physiol. 2017;312:G537–49.
230. Croese J, Giacomin P, Navarro S, Clouston A, McCann L, Dougall A, et al. Experimental hookworm infection and gluten microchallenge promote tolerance in celiac disease. J Allergy Clin Immunol. 2015;135:508–16.
231. Eichenberger RM, Ryan S, Jones L, Buitrago G, Polster R, Montes de Oca M, et al. Hookworm secreted extracellular vesicles interact with host cells and prevent inducible colitis in mice. Front Immunol. 2018;9:850.
232. Zaiss MM, Rapin A, Lebon L, Dubey LK, Mosconi I, Sarter K, et al. The intestinal microbiota contributes to the ability of helminths to modulate allergic inflammation. Immunity. 2015;43:998–1010.
233. Giacomin P, Croese J, Krause L, Loukas A, Cantacessi C. Suppression of inflammation by helminths: a role for the gut microbiota? Philos Trans R Soc Lond B Biol Sci. 2015;370:20140296.
234. Boullata JI. Drug-nutrition interactions in infectious diseases. In: Humphries DL, Scott ME, Vermund SH, editors. Nutrition and infectious diseases: shifting the clinical paradigm. Switzerland: Springer Nature; 2020.
235. Humphries D, Nguyen S, Kumar S, Quagraine JE, Otchere J, Harrison LM. Effectiveness of albendazole for hookworm varies widely by community and correlates with nutritional factors: a cross-sectional study of school-age children in Ghana. Am J Trop Med Hyg. 2017;96:347–54.
236. Williams AR, Soelberg J, Jäger AK. Anthelmintic properties of traditional African and Caribbean medicinal plants: identification of extracts with potent activity against *Ascaris suum* in vitro. Parasite. 2016;23:24.
237. Kugo M, Keter L, Maiyo A, Kinyua J, Ndemwa P, Maina G, et al. Fortification of *Carica papaya* fruit seeds to school meal snacks may aid Africa mass deworming programs: a preliminary survey. BMC Complement Altern Med. 2018;18:327.
238. Abdel Aziz AR, AbouLaila MR, Aziz M, Omar MA, Sultan K. In vitro and in vivo anthelmintic activity of pumpkin seeds and pomegranate peels extracts against *Ascaridia galli*. Beni Suef Univ J Basic Appl Sci. 2018;7:231–4.
239. Silva NCS, Lima AS, Silva CR, Brito DRB, Cutrim-Junior JAA, Milhomem MN, et al. In vitro and in vivo activity of hydrolyzed *Saccharomyces cerevisiae* against goat nematodes. Vet Parasitol. 2018;254:6–9.
240. de Melo GKA, Ítavo CCBF, Monteiro KLS, da Silva JA, da Silva PCG, Ítavo LCV, et al. Effect of creep-fed supplement on the susceptibility of pasture-grazed suckling lambs to gastrointestinal helminths. Vet Parasitol. 2017;239:26–30.
241. Amit M, Cohen I, Marcovics A, Muklada H, Glasser TA, Ungar ED, et al. Self-medication with tannin-rich browse in goats infected with gastro-intestinal nematodes. Vet Parasitol. 2013;198:305–11.
242. Copani G, Hall JO, Miller J, Priolo A, Villalba JJ. Plant secondary compounds as complementary resources: are they always complementary? Oecologia. 2013;172:1041–9.
243. Mata-Padrino DJ, Belesky DP, Crawford CD, Walsh B, MacAdam JW, Bowdridge SA. Effects of grazing birdsfoot trefoil-enriched pasture on managing *Haemonchus contortus* infection in Suffolk crossbred lambs. J Anim Sci. 2019;97:172–83.
244. Spiegler V, Liebau E, Hensel A. Medicinal plant extracts and plant-derived polyphenols with anthelmintic activity against intestinal nematodes. Nat Prod Rep. 2017;34:627–43.
245. Burke JM, Miller JE. Evaluation of multiple low doses of copper oxide wire particles compared with levamisole for control of *Haemonchus contortus* in lambs. Vet Parasitol. 2006;139:145–9.
246. Burke JM, Miller JE, Terrill TH, Smyth E, Acharya M. Examination of commercially available copper oxide wire particles in combination with albendazole for control of gastrointestinal nematodes in lambs. Vet Parasitol. 2016;215:1–4.
247. Bourgeois AC, Koski KG, Scott ME. Comparative sensitivity of feeding and non-feeding stages of *Heligmosomoides bakeri* (Nematoda) to boron. Comp Parasitol. 2007;74:319–26.
248. Hall A, Hewitt G, Tuffrey V, de Silva N. A review and meta-analysis of the impact of intestinal worms on child growth and nutrition. Matern Child Nutr. 2008;4(Suppl 1):118–236.
249. Taylor-Robinson DC, Maayan N, Soares-Weiser K, Donegan S, Garner P. Deworming drugs for soil-transmitted intestinal worms in children: effects on nutritional indicators, haemoglobin, and school performance. Cochrane Database Syst Rev. 2015;2015:CD000371.
250. Welch VA, Ghogomu E, Hossain A, Awasthi S, Bhutta ZA, Cumberbatch C, et al. Mass deworming to improve developmental health and wellbeing of children in low-income and middle-income countries: a systematic review and network meta-analysis. Lancet Glob Health. 2017;5:e40–50.
251. Lo NC, Snyder J, Addiss DG, Heft-Neal S, Andrews JR, Bendavid E. Deworming in pre-school age children: a global empirical analysis of health outcomes. PLoS Negl Trop Dis. 2018;12:e0006500.
252. Moncayo AL, Lovato R, Cooper PJ. Soil-transmitted helminth infections and nutritional status in Ecuador: findings from a national survey and implications for control strategies. BMJ Open. 2018;8:e021319.
253. Hurst RJM, Caul AD, Little MC, Kagechika H, Else KJ. The retinoic acid receptor agonist Am80 increases mucosal inflammation in an IL-6 dependent manner during *Trichuris muris* infection. J Clin Immunol. 2013;33:1386–94.

254. Nga TT, Winichagoon P, Dijkhuizen MA, Khan NC, Wasantwisut E, Furr H, et al. Multi-micronutrient-fortified biscuits decreased prevalence of anemia and improved micronutrient status and effectiveness of deworming in rural Vietnamese school children. J Nutr. 2009;139:1013–21.

255. Al-Mekhlafi HM, Anuar TS, Al-Zabedi EM, Al-Maktari MT, Mahdy MAK, Ahmed A, et al. Does vitamin A supplementation protect schoolchildren from acquiring soil-transmitted helminthiasis? A randomized controlled trial. Parasit Vectors. 2014;7:367.

256. Chen K, Xie HM, Tian W, Zheng X, Jiang AC. Effect of single-dose albendazole and vitamin A supplementation on the iron status of pre-school children in Sichuan, China. Br J Nutr. 2016;115:1415–23.

257. Payne LG, Koski KG, Ortega-Barria E, Scott ME. Benefit of vitamin A supplementation on *Ascaris* reinfection is less evident in stunted children. J Nutr. 2007;137:1455–9.

258. Pedro MR, Madriaga JR, Barba CV, Habito RC, Gana AE, Deitchler M, et al. The national vitamin A supplementation program and subclinical vitamin A deficiency among preschool children in the Philippines. Food Nutr Bull. 2004;25:319–29.

259. González-Fernández D, Koski KG, Sinisterra OT, Del Carmen PE, Murillo E, Scott ME. Interactions among urogenital, intestinal, skin, and oral infections in pregnant and lactating Panamanian Ngäbe women: a neglected public health challenge. Am J Trop Med Hyg. 2015;92:1100–10.

260. González-Fernández D, Pons EDC, Rueda D, Sinisterra OT, Murillo E, Scott ME, et al. C-reactive protein is differentially modulated by co-existing infections, vitamin deficiencies and maternal factors in pregnant and lactating indigenous Panamanian women. Infect Dis Poverty. 2017;6:94.

261. González-Fernández D, Pons EC, Rueda D, Sinisterra OT, Murillo E, Scott ME, Koski KG. Identification of high-risk pregnancies in a remote setting using ambulatory blood pressure: the MINDI cohort. Front Public Health 8:86.

262. Ezwena V. Nutrition and co-infections. In: Humphries DL, Scott ME, Vermund SH, editors. Nutrition and infectious diseases: shifting the clinical paradigm. Switzerland: Springer Nature; 2020.

263. de Silva N, Ahmed B-N, Casapia M, de Silva H, Gyapong J, Malecela M, et al. Cochrane reviews on deworming and the right to a healthy, worm-free life. PLoS Negl Trop Dis. 2015;9:e0004203.

264. Yap P, Utzinger J, Hattendorf J, Steinmann P. Influence of nutrition on infection and re-infection with soil-transmitted helminths: a systematic review. Parasit Vectors. 2014;7:229.

# Part IV
# Integration of Cross-Cutting Issues in Nutrition/Infection Interactions

# Chapter 13
# Drug-Nutrition Interactions in Infectious Diseases

Joseph I. Boullata

## Abbreviations

| | |
|---|---|
| ALT | Alanine aminotransferase |
| AUC | Area under the concentration-time curve |
| BCRP | Breast cancer-related protein |
| BMI | Body mass index |
| cf | Correction factor |
| Cl | Clearance |
| CNT | Concentrative nucleoside transporter |
| CYP | Cytochrome $P_{450}$ |
| HIV | Human immunodeficiency virus |
| MIC | Minimum inhibitory concentration |
| OATP | Organic anion-transporting polypeptide |
| PEM | Protein-energy malnutrition |
| PEPT | Peptide transporter |
| RUTF | Ready-to-use therapeutic food |
| Vd | Volume of distribution |

**Key Points**
- Interactions between antimicrobial agents (antibacterial, antiviral, antifungal, antiparasitic) and nutrition (i.e., drug-nutrition interaction) occur and are superimposed on the already complex relationship between pathogen and host.
- A meal, specific food, food component (including a nutrient), or nutritional status may influence the physiologic disposition of an antimicrobial agent.
- If a drug-nutrition interaction is not recognized and addressed, an altered drug concentration may adversely influence clinical progress and outcome including the risk for drug resistance.
- An antimicrobial regimen may influence whole body nutritional status, metabolic status, or the concentration of individual nutrients requiring close monitoring and management as needed.

J. I. Boullata (✉)
Clinical Nutrition Support Services, Hospital of the University of Pennsylvania, Philadelphia, PA, USA
e-mail: joseph.boullata@pennmedicine.upenn.edu

© Springer Nature Switzerland AG 2021
D. L. Humphries et al. (eds.), *Nutrition and Infectious Diseases*, Nutrition and Health,
https://doi.org/10.1007/978-3-030-56913-6_13

# Introduction

There are numerous relationships between nutrition and infectious diseases, well described in the many valuable chapters in this volume. Added into that complex mix are the potential interactions between nutrition and antimicrobial agents (Fig. 13.1). These agents include those used to manage bacterial, viral, fungal, and parasitic infections, whether systemic or isolated to the gastrointestinal tract. The valuable therapeutic interactions between these medications and infecting organisms in support of the host's inflammatory response to the infection as coordinated by the immune system are well documented [1]. By targeting the pathogen, antimicrobials may be seen as tipping the balance in favor of the host.

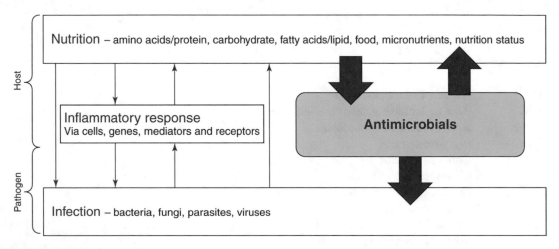

**Fig. 13.1** Interaction of antimicrobials superimposed on the interactions between nutrition, inflammatory response, and infectious disease domains in a patient (host)

## *Nutrition and Infection*

Interactions between host and pathogen necessarily involve nutrition through both specific nutrients and broader nutritional status. For example, one area of "metabolic cross talk" between host and pathogen may occur with amino acids, as the host and pathogen compete for proteins in general, and specific amino acids [2]. The effects of such competitions likely influence the outcome of an infection. The interacting influence of poor diet and infection on growth and development at various life stages (e.g., infancy, childhood, pregnancy) is well-described [3]. The synergistic effects between nutrition and the inflammatory response are particularly important in the face of malnutrition and infection when biomarker assessments become challenging [4]. Malnutrition is also a significant predictor of healthcare-associated infections in hospitalized patients [5]. Hence, interactions between antimicrobials and nutrition have the potential to be favorable or unfavorable to the host, sometimes depending upon the specific microbes.

## *Nutrition and the Microbiota*

With respect to the gut microbiota, the influence of nutrition (diet) is known to be critical [6–8]. Malnutrition also impacts the abundance and diversity of the gut microbiota, increasing the risk for gut pathogens to access both local and systemic tissues [9]. Although interactions involving this domain are beyond the scope of this chapter, the influence of antimicrobials on the microbiota has also been well described in recent years to include roles in resistance patterns as well as altering functional gene diversity [10]. Regimens as short as 7 days may have lasting impacts on reduced microbial diversity and gene functionality [11]. The effects will vary by drug. For example, anthelminthic regimens may alter (e.g., ivermectin) or have no influence (e.g., albendazole) on the gut microbiota in the days following therapy [12].

## Antimicrobials and Nutrition

Tipping the balance in favor of the host does not mean that antimicrobials are without an adverse effect on the host. The oral bioavailability and the clinical effect of these valuable drugs are influenced by a variety of factors including interactions. Although drug-drug interactions are commonly recognized by clinicians, drug-nutrition interactions are less familiar but are no less important. This chapter will define drug-nutrition interactions and then describe the various types of drug-nutrition interactions using a variety of antimicrobials as examples. Table 13.1 provides a list, by class, of select antimicrobials mentioned in the chapter. Additional information on these drugs (Tables 13.2, 13.3, 13.4, and 13.5) provides further clinical context.

**Table 13.1**  Selected antimicrobials used for infectious diseases

| Target organisms | Drug class | Examples |
|---|---|---|
| Antibacterials | Aminoglycosides | Gentamicin |
| | Antituberculars | Ethambutol, isoniazid, pyrazinamide, rifampin |
| | Beta-lactams | Meropenem, cefdinir, penicillins |
| | Ketolides or macrolides | Azithromycin, clarithromycin |
| | Lipopeptides or glycopeptides | Daptomycin, vancomycin |
| | Quinolones | Ciprofloxacin |
| | Tetracyclines | Doxycycline |
| | Others | Chloramphenicol, clindamycin, cotrimoxazole, linezolid |
| Antifungals | Azoles | Fluconazole, itraconazole, posaconazole, voriconazole |
| | Classic | Amphotericin, flucytosine, griseofulvin |
| | Echinocandins | Caspofungin, micafungin |
| Antivirals | Antiretroviral reverse transcriptase inhibitors | Abacavir, efavirenz, lamivudine, nevirapine, tenofovir |
| | Antiretroviral protease inhibitors | Atazanavir, darunavir, saquinavir |
| | Antiretroviral integrase inhibitors | Dolutegravir, elvitegravir |
| | Others | Acyclovir, adefovir, entecavir, oseltamivir, ribavirin, sofosbuvir |
| Antiparasitics | Anthelmintics | Albendazole, ivermectin, praziquantel |
| | Antimalarials | Artesunate, chloroquine, lumefantrine, mefloquine, sulfadiazine |
| | Antiprotozoals | Metronidazole, pyrimethamine |

Functionally, antimicrobials can be classified into one of three groups by the method that best describes how drug exposure leads to killing activity. They may be described as (1) time-dependent killing (serum drug concentrations remain above the minimum inhibitory concentration [MIC] of the pathogen for a minimum period of time [e.g., penicillins, cephalosporins]); (2) concentration-dependent killing (maximum serum drug concentrations [i.e., "peak"] well above the MIC [e.g., ami-

**Table 13.2** Antibacterial agents

| Antimicrobial common name | Antimicrobial trade name (USA) | Therapeutic action or class | Routinely susceptible organisms[a] | Predominant clinical infection | Taken with food?[b] |
|---|---|---|---|---|---|
| Amoxicillin | Amoxil, others | Cell wall synthesis inhibitor | *Streptococcus* spp., *Enterococcus* spp. | Otitis media, sinusitis, pharyngitis, endocarditis, respiratory tract, urinary tract infection | Y |
| Ampicillin | Various | Cell wall synthesis inhibitor | *Streptococcus* spp., *Enterococcus* spp. | Otitis media, sinusitis, pharyngitis, endocarditis, respiratory tract, urinary tract infection | N |
| Azithromycin | Zithromax, others | Protein synthesis inhibitor | *Streptococcus* spp., *Staphylococcus* spp., *Neisseria* spp., *Haemophilus influenzae*, *Moraxella catarrhalis*, *Escherichia coli*, *Shigella* spp., *Salmonella* spp., *Chlamydia* spp., *Legionella* spp., *Toxoplasma gondii* | Upper respiratory tract, lower respiratory tract, pertussis, skin and skin structure, gastrointestinal infections | Y (tablet) N (capsule) |
| Cefdinir | Various | Cell wall synthesis inhibitor | *Staphylococcus* spp., *Streptococcus* spp., *Neisseria* spp., *Haemophilus influenzae*, *Moraxella catarrhalis*, *Escherichia coli*, *Klebsiella* spp., *Salmonella* spp., *Shigella* spp., *Proteus* spp. | Respiratory tract infection, tonsillitis, skin infection | N |
| Cefoxitin | Mefoxin, others | Cell wall synthesis inhibitor | *Staphylococcus* spp., *Streptococcus* spp., *Escherichia coli*, *Klebsiella* spp., *Proteus mirabilis*, *Bacteroides fragilis* | Intra-abdominal infection | IV |
| Cefpodoxime | Various | Cell wall synthesis inhibitor | *Staphylococcus* spp., *Streptococcus* spp., *Neisseria* spp., *Haemophilus influenzae*, *Moraxella catarrhalis*, *Escherichia coli*, *Klebsiella* spp., *Salmonella* spp., *Shigella* spp., *Proteus* spp. | Respiratory tract infection, tonsillitis, skin infection | Y |

**Table 13.2** (continued)

| Antimicrobial common name | Antimicrobial trade name (USA) | Therapeutic action or class | Routinely susceptible organisms[a] | Predominant clinical infection | Taken with food?[b] |
|---|---|---|---|---|---|
| Chloramphenicol | Various | Protein synthesis inhibitor | *Staphylococcus* spp., *Streptococcus* spp., *Enterococcus* spp., *Neisseria* spp., *Clostridium* spp., *Bacteroides* spp. | (An alternative agent) | Y/N |
| Ciprofloxacin | Cipro, others | DNA synthesis inhibitor | *Escherichia coli, Klebsiella* spp., *Enterobacter* spp., *Proteus* spp., *Morganella* spp., *Citrobacter* spp., *Serratia* spp., *Legionella* spp., *Haemophilus influenzae, Vibrio* spp., *Salmonella* spp., *Shigella* spp. | Urinary tract infection, prostatitis, gastroenteritis, intra-abdominal, peritonitis, osteomyelitis, skin and soft tissue infections | Y (if no dairy or calcium-fortified food) |
| Clarithromycin | Biaxin, others | Protein synthesis inhibitor | *Streptococcus* spp., *Staphylococcus* spp., *Neisseria* spp., *Haemophilus influenzae, Moraxella catarrhalis, Escherichia coli, Shigella* spp., *Salmonella* spp., *Helicobacter pylori, Mycobacterium avium* complex, *Chlamydia* spp., *Legionella* spp. | Upper respiratory tract, lower respiratory tract, pertussis, pulmonary and disseminated *Mycobacterium avium* complex, skin and skin structure, gastrointestinal infections including *H. pylori*-associated gastritis | Y/N |
| Clindamycin | Cleocin, others | Protein synthesis inhibitor | *Staphylococcus aureus,* coagulase-negative *Staphylococcus* spp., *Streptococcus* spp., *Corynebacterium diphtheria, Bacteroides fragilis, Clostridium tetani, Clostridium perfringens* | Skin and connective tissue infection, necrotizing fasciitis, bite wound, respiratory tract, diphtheria, endocarditis, osteomyelitis | Y/N |
| Cotrimoxazole[c] | Bactrim, Septra, others | Folic acid antagonist | *Staphylococcus* spp., *Streptococcus* spp., *Corynebacterium* spp., *Enterobacteriaceae, Pneumocystis jirovecii* | Urinary tract infection, bacterial pneumonia, others | Y/N |
| Daptomycin | Cubicin, others | Cell membrane depolarization | *Staphylococcus* spp., *Streptococcus* spp., *Enterococcus* spp. | Skin and skin structure infection, Staph bacteremia and endocarditis, osteomyelitis | IV |

(continued)

**Table 13.2** (continued)

| Antimicrobial common name | Antimicrobial trade name (USA) | Therapeutic action or class | Routinely susceptible organisms[a] | Predominant clinical infection | Taken with food?[b] |
|---|---|---|---|---|---|
| Doxycycline | Vibramycin, others | Protein synthesis inhibitor | *Streptococcus pneumonia, Bacillus anthracis, Enterobacteriaceae, Listeria monocytogenes, Chlamydia* spp., *Yersinia pestis* | Respiratory tract infection, gastrointestinal infection, sexually transmitted infection, others | N |
| Ethambutol | Myambutol, others | Arabinosyl transferase inhibitor | *Mycobacterium* spp. | Tuberculosis, *Mycobacterium avium* complex | Y/N |
| Gentamicin | Various | Protein synthesis inhibitor | Enterobacteriaceae | Bacteremia, urinary tract infection | IV |
| Isoniazid | Various | Mycolic acid synthesis inhibitor | *Mycobacterium tuberculosis* | Pulmonary and extrapulmonary tuberculosis | N |
| Linezolid | Zyvox, others | Protein synthesis inhibitor | *Staphylococcus* spp., *Enterococcus* spp., *Streptococcus* spp. | Bacteremia, respiratory tract infection, endocarditis, skin/ structure infection | Y/N |
| Meropenem | Merrem, others | Cell wall synthesis inhibitor | *Staphylococcus* spp., *Streptococcus* spp., *Enterococcus* spp., *Enterobacteriaceae, Haemophilus influenzae, Neisseria meningitides* | Skin/structure infection, intra-abdominal infection, bacterial meningitis | IV |
| Norfloxacin | Various | DNA synthesis inhibitor | *Staphylococcus* spp., *Enterobacteriaceae* | Urinary tract infection, prostatitis, bacterial diarrhea | N |
| Omadacycline | Nuzyra | Protein synthesis inhibitor | *Staphylococcus* spp., *Enterococcus faecalis, Streptococcus* spp., *Haemophilus* spp., *Klebsiella pneumonia, Legionella pneumonia, Mycoplasma pneumonia* | Community-acquired pneumonia, skin and skin structure infection | N |
| Penicillin | Various | Cell wall synthesis inhibitor | *Staphylococcus* spp., *Streptococcus* spp., *Neisseria* spp. | Strep throat, cellulitis, otitis, sinusitis | N |
| Pyrazinamide | Various | Antitubercular | *Mycobacterium tuberculosis* | Tuberculosis | N |
| Rifampin | Various | RNA polymerase inhibitor | *Mycobacterium* spp., *Staphylococcus* spp., *Legionella pneumonia, Neisseria meningitides, Listeria monocytogenes* | Tuberculosis, *Mycobacterium avium* complex, staph bacteremia | Y/N |

**Table 13.2** (continued)

| Antimicrobial common name | Antimicrobial trade name (USA) | Therapeutic action or class | Routinely susceptible organisms[a] | Predominant clinical infection | Taken with food?[b] |
|---|---|---|---|---|---|
| Tigecycline | Tygacil, others | Protein synthesis inhibitor | *Staphylococcus* spp., *Streptococcus* spp., *Enterococcus faecalis*, *Bacteroides* spp., *Enterobacter cloacae*, *Escherichia coli*, *Haemophilus influenzae*, *Klebsiella pneumonia*, *Legionella pneumonia* | Intra-abdominal infection, skin and skin structure infection, community-acquired infection | IV |
| Vancomycin | Various | Cell wall synthesis inhibitor | *Staphylococcus* spp., *Streptococcus* spp., *Enterococcus faecalis* | Bacteremia, endocarditis, peritonitis, *Clostridium difficile*-associated colitis | IV |

[a]Local susceptibility patterns vary by organism (genus and species)
[b]Y = yes; N = No; Y/N = either; IV = only available intravenously
[c]Cotrimoxazole = sulfamethoxazole + trimethoprim

**Table 13.3** Antifungal agents

| Antimicrobial common name | Antimicrobial trade name (USA) | Therapeutic action or class | Routinely susceptible organisms[a] | Predominant clinical infection | Taken with food?[b] |
|---|---|---|---|---|---|
| Amphotericin | Various | Cell membrane disruptor | *Cryptococcus neoformans, Candida* spp. | Cryptococcosis, candidemia, candidiasis | IV |
| Caspofungin | Cancidas, others | β-glucan synthesis inhibitor | *Candida* spp., *Aspergillus* spp. | Candidiasis, aspergillosis | IV |
| Fluconazole | Diflucan, others | Fungal cytochrome P450 inhibitor | *Candida* spp., *Cryptococcus neoformans* | Candidemia, candidiasis, cryptococcosis | Y/N |
| Flucytosine | Ancobon, others | Protein synthesis inhibitor | *Candida* spp., *Cryptococcus neoformans* | Candidemia, candidiasis, cryptococcosis | Y/N |
| Griseofulvin | Various | Microtubule disruptor | *Trichophyton* spp., *Epidermophyton* spp., *Microsporum* spp. | Dermatophyte infections | Y |
| Itraconazole | Sporanox, others | Fungal cytochrome P450 inhibitor | *Candida* spp., *Cryptococcus neoformans, Blastomyces* spp., *Histoplasma* spp., *Aspergillus* spp. | Candidemia, candidiasis, cryptococcosis, blastomycosis, histoplasmosis, aspergillosis, others | Y |
| Micafungin | Mycamine, others | β-glucan synthesis inhibitor | *Candida* spp. | Candidemia, candidiasis | IV |
| Posaconazole | Noxafil, others | Fungal cytochrome P450 inhibitor | *Aspergillus* spp., *Candida* spp. | Aspergillosis, mucosal candidiasis | Y |
| Voriconazole | Vfend, others | Fungal cytochrome P450 inhibitor | *Aspergillus* spp., *Candida* spp., *Fusarium* spp. | Aspergillosis, candidemia, invasive candidiasis | N |

[a]Local susceptibility patterns vary by organism (genus and species)
[b]Y = yes; N = No; Y/N = either; IV = only available intravenously

**Table 13.4** Antiviral agents

| Antimicrobial common name | Antimicrobial trade name (USA) | Therapeutic action or class | Routinely susceptible organisms[a] | Predominant clinical infection | Taken with food?[b] |
|---|---|---|---|---|---|
| Abacavir | Ziagen, others | Nucleoside reverse transcriptase inhibitor | Human immunodeficiency virus-1, Human immunodeficiency virus-2 | HIV infection | N |
| Acyclovir | Zovirax, others | DNA polymerase inhibitor | Herpes simplex virus-1, Herpes simplex virus-2, Varicella-zoster virus | Genital herpes, herpes labialis, HSV encephalitis, disseminated herpes, varicella, zoster | Y/N |
| Adefovir | Hepsera, others | Nucleotide reverse transcriptase inhibitor | Hepatitis B virus, Varicella-zoster virus, Cytomegalovirus | Chronic hepatitis B infection | Y/N |
| Atazanavir | Reyataz, others | Protease inhibitor | Human immunodeficiency virus-1 | HIV infection | Y |
| Cobicistat | Tybost[c] | CYP3A inhibitor | (to increase antiretroviral availability) | HIV infection | Y/N |
| Daclatasvir | Daklinza | NS5A inhibitor | Hepatitis C virus | Hepatitis C infection | N |
| Darunavir | Prezista, others | Protease inhibitor | Human immunodeficiency virus-1 | HIV infection | Y |
| Dolutegravir | Tivicay, others | Integrase inhibitor | Human immunodeficiency virus-1 | HIV infection | Y |
| Doravirine | Pifeltro | Non-nucleoside reverse transcriptase inhibitor | Human immunodeficiency virus-1 | HIV infection | Y/N |
| Efavirenz | Sustiva, others | Non-nucleoside reverse transcriptase inhibitor | Human immunodeficiency virus-1 | HIV infection | Y |
| Elvitegravir | Vitekta | Integrase inhibitor | Human immunodeficiency virus-1 | HIV infection | Y |
| Emtricitabine | Emtriva, others | Nucleoside reverse transcriptase inhibitor | Human immunodeficiency virus-1 | HIV infection | Y/N |
| Entecavir | Baraclude, others | Nucleoside reverse transcriptase inhibitor | Hepatitis B virus | Chronic hepatitis B infection | N |
| Faldaprevir | [BI-201335] | Protease inhibitor | Hepatitis C virus | Hepatitis C infection | Y/N |
| Lamivudine | Epivir, others | Nucleoside reverse transcriptase inhibitor | Human immunodeficiency virus-1 | HIV infection | Y/N |
| Lopinavir | Kaletra[d], others[d] | Protease inhibitor | Human immunodeficiency virus-1 | HIV infection | Y |

**Table 13.4**   (continued)

| Antimicrobial common name | Antimicrobial trade name (USA) | Therapeutic action or class | Routinely susceptible organisms[a] | Predominant clinical infection | Taken with food?[b] |
|---|---|---|---|---|---|
| Nevirapine | Viramune, others | Non-nucleoside reverse transcriptase inhibitor | Human immunodeficiency virus-1 | HIV infection | Y/N |
| Oseltamivir | Tamiflu, others | Neuroaminidase inhibitor | Influenza A virus, Influenza B virus | Influenza A and B infections, avian H5N1 infection | Y/N |
| Ribavirin | Rebetol, others | Nucleoside RNA polymerase inhibitor | Hepatitis C virus, respiratory syncytial virus | Chronic hepatitis C infection | Y |
| Saquinavir | Invirase | Protease inhibitor | Human immunodeficiency virus-1 | HIV infection | Y |
| Sofosbuvir | Sovaldi | Nucleotide polymerase inhibitor | Hepatitis C virus | Chronic hepatitis C infection | Y > N |
| Tenofovir | Viread, others | Nucleotide reverse transcriptase inhibitor | Human immunodeficiency virus-1, Hepatitis B virus | HIV infection, chronic hepatitis B infection | Y > N |

[a]Local susceptibility patterns vary by virus
[b]Y = yes; N = No; Y/N = either; Y > N = either but food preferred, IV = only available intravenously
[c]Cobicistat most commonly used in combination with products with other retroviral agents
[d]Lopinavir only available in combination products with ritonavir

**Table 13.5**   Antiparasitic agents

| Antimicrobial common name | Antimicrobial trade name (USA) | Therapeutic action or class | Routinely susceptible organisms[a] | Predominant clinical infection | Taken with food?[b] |
|---|---|---|---|---|---|
| Albendazole | Albenza, others | Tubulin polymerization inhibitor | *Ancylostoma* spp., *Necator* spp., Soil-transmitted helminths:Necator., *Enterobius* spp., *Trichuris* spp., *Ascaris* spp., *Strongyloides* spp., *Giardia duodenalis* | Hookworm, whipworm, pinworm, ascariasis, strongyloidiasis, giardiasis, microsporidiosis | Y/N |
| Artemisinin (Quinhaosu) | n/a | Reactive metabolite damage to organelles and/or interference with calcium homeostasis | *Plasmodium falciparum, Plasmodium vivax, Schistosoma* spp., *Leishmania* spp. | Malaria | Y > N |
| Artesunate | n/a | Reactive metabolite damage to organelles and/or interference with calcium homeostasis | *Plasmodium falciparum, Plasmodium vivax, Schistosoma* spp., *Leishmania* spp. | Schistosomiasis, leishmaniasis, malaria | Y > N |

(continued)

**Table 13.5** (continued)

| Antimicrobial common name | Antimicrobial trade name (USA) | Therapeutic action or class | Routinely susceptible organisms[a] | Predominant clinical infection | Taken with food?[b] |
|---|---|---|---|---|---|
| Chloroquine | Aralen, others | Increases ferrprotoporphyrin IX (heme) induced cell lysis | *Plasmodium vivax, Plasmodium ovale, Entamoeba histolytica, Giardia duodenalis* | Schistosomiasis, leishmaniasis, malaria (erythrocytic stages) | N |
| Ivermectin | Stromectol, others | Selective muscle paralysis | *Ascaris lumbricoides, Enterobius vermicularis, Strongyloides stercoralis, Onchocerca volvulus* | Ascariasis, pinworm, strongyloidiasis, onchocerciasis | Y |
| Lumefantrine | Coartem[c] | Increases ferrprotoporphyrin IX (heme) induced cell lysis | *Plasmodium falciparum, Plasmodium vivax* | Malaria (erythrocytic stages) | Y |
| Mefloquine | Various | Efflux pump inhibitor | *Plasmodium falciparum, Plasmodium vivax* | Malaria | Y > N |
| Metronidazole | Flagyl, others | DNA synthesis inhibitor | *Bacteroides fragilis, Clostridium* spp., *Peptostreptococcus* spp., *Trichomonas vaginalis, Giardia duodenalis, Entamoeba histolytica* | Intra-abdominal infection, genital infection, bacterial vaginosis, osteomyelitis, trichomoniasis, giardiasis, amebiasis | N |
| Praziquantel | Biltricide, others | Calcium-channel binding associated tetany | *Schistosoma* spp., *Opistorchis viverrini, Clonorchis sinensis* | Schistosomiasis, opisthorchiasis, clonorchiasis | Y |
| Pyrimethamine | Daraprim | Folic acid antagonist | *Plasmodium falciparum, Toxoplasma gondii, Pneumocystis jirovecii, Cystoisospora belli* | Malaria, toxoplasmosis, pneumocystis pneumonia, cystoisosporiasis | Y/N |
| Sulfadiazine | Various | Folic acid antagonist | *Staphylococcus* spp., *Streptococcus* spp., Enterobacteriaceae, *Toxoplasma gondii, Plasmodium falciparum* | Urinary tract infection, respiratory tract infection, toxoplasmosis, malaria | Y/N |

*n/a* not available
[a]Local susceptibility patterns vary by organism (genus and species)
[b]Y = yes; N = No; Y/N = either; Y > N = either but food preferred, IV = only available intravenously
[c]Lumefantrine only available in combination products with artemether

noglycosides, lipopeptides]); or (3) concentration-dependent killing with time dependency (area under the drug concentration-time curve [AUC] above the MIC or above an AUC:MIC cut-off value for the organism [e.g., macrolides, fluoroquinolones, glycopeptides, azole antifungals]). The clinical effect of drug-nutrition interactions may have the potential to alter this pharmacologic activity.

## Definitions and Clinical Relevance

In a distinctly broad definition, the term drug-nutrition interaction reflects a physical, chemical, physiological, or pathophysiological relationship between a medication and one or more nutrients, food in general, specific foods or food components, nutritional status, or metabolic status [13–15]. One part of the relationship is considered the *precipitating* factor, while the other component is the *object* of the interaction (Table 13.6). The precipitating element may be any one of the listed components (i.e., drug, nutrient, food, or nutritional status), with any other component serving as the object of the interaction. As a result, several subtypes of drug-nutrition interaction exist which can be described by their precipitating factor and object as "food-drug" interactions or "drug-nutrient" interactions, among others. The systematic approach to identifying, recognizing, and understanding the many interactions, when classified into subtypes, is more inclusive and allows evolving interactions to be classified as new data become available [14, 15].

**Table 13.6** Classes of drug-nutrition interactions

| Precipitating factor (The perpetrator) | Object (The victim) |
| --- | --- |
| Food | Drug |
| Specific food component / Nutrient | Drug |
| Nutritional status | Drug |
| Drug | Nutritional status |
| Drug | Metabolic status |
| Drug | Nutrient |

For a drug-nutrition interaction to be considered clinically significant, there is an expectation that nutritional status is compromised and/or therapeutic drug response is modified. The alteration may be represented by a 20% or greater change in biomarkers, physiologic indicators, or kinetic parameters from a baseline value or an anticipated effect. The time frame over which the change occurs will vary with the precipitating factor and object. The severity of consequences may vary, with some individuals at higher risk based on their age, genetic variants, organ function, or disease state. As a result, the clinical significance or severity of a drug-nutrition interaction may be difficult to predict. The management of an interaction may only require close clinical monitoring in some instances but may require significant changes in eating patterns or pharmacotherapeutic regimens in others. For clinicians to recognize or predict drug-nutrition interactions, assess their clinical relevance, and manage them requires keen awareness, a basic understanding of pharmacology, and an appreciation for the mechanisms of interactions.

Although electronic medical record systems often have basic built-in alerts to help prescribers and pharmacists identify drug-nutrition interactions in healthcare settings, the content and capability remain quite limited and do not address much of what is described in this chapter. As of mid-2019, there are no stand-alone software tools that address drug-nutrition interactions. Clinicians continue to rely on summaries of the primary literature in review articles and reference texts.

# Mechanisms of Interaction

## *General*

Generally, drug-nutrition interactions occur because of two fundamental reasons: (1) the inherent physicochemical properties of drugs, nutrients, and the food matrix and (2) similarities in their physiologic disposition (i.e., absorption, distribution, metabolism, excretion) and effect. The physical chemistry that is operational for each substance governs their interactions when combined. Physiologically, absorption, distribution, and excretion require transporters; metabolism requires one or more enzyme systems; and therapeutic effect requires molecular targets. These transporters, enzymes, and targets are proteins coded for by genes. The expression of the genes themselves comes under the influence of compounds – be they nutrients or drugs. Additionally, the proteins nearly always require micronutrients for optimal function. Although reference here is to medication, the obvious parallels with the disposition of nutrients are unmistakable.

## Pharmaceutical

The current model of drug-nutrition interactions links an interaction with its physiologic effect and clinical outcome, through differentiating mechanisms [14]. Some interactions are based on physico-chemical reactions that take place in the lumen of the gastrointestinal tract or ex vivo in a nutrition support delivery device. These interactions, referred to as pharmaceutical interactions, have the distinct potential to alter the bioavailability of one or more substances (nutrient or drug). For example, alben-dazole must be taken with food in order to create adequate dissolution to support drug absorption and achieve therapeutic blood concentrations [16]. However, if the intent of therapy is for local gut action on helminths, then administration on an empty stomach may enhance that local effectiveness [17].

## Pharmacokinetic

Other associations exist beyond the physical and chemical interactions. These are the result of actions at the level of cell membrane transporters or metabolizing enzymes, referred to as pharmacokinetic interactions. The potential consequences of these interactions are altered bioavailability, distribution, and clearance (through metabolism and/or excretion). These may occur by competition for the same cellular target or indirectly by the influence of nutritional status on kinetic parameters. For example, dietary exposure to compounds in grapefruit inhibits a critical metabolizing enzyme within entero-cytes, leading to reduced clearance of enzyme-susceptible drugs at the intestinal barrier, thereby increasing systemic bioavailability of the drug (e.g., saquinavir, an antiretroviral) [18]. In the case of nutritional status, drug exposure and toxicity may be increased in protein-energy malnutrition (PEM) as the result of altered drug distribution or clearance (e.g., clarithromycin, an antibiotic) [19].

## Pharmacodynamic

Still other interactions may take place at target receptors that influence cell signaling, referred to as pharmacodynamic interactions, which yield an effect on physiologic function. Because most antimi-crobials target the pathogen primarily, it is the off-target effects of the drug on the host that are evalu-ated. The potential consequences are altered cellular response(s) that may translate to a biomarker change, or clinical effect of the drug or nutrient, or a change in physiologic function that affects food intake or disposition. For example, azole antifungal agents may be associated with fatigue, arthralgia, myalgia, tremor, and gastrointestinal complaints (e.g., dry mouth, anorexia, nausea, vomiting, diar-rhea, abdominal pain), with potential to decrease food intake and body weight when present together in an individual. Whenever an interaction is sufficient to alter food intake, drug or nutrient disposition, or their clinical effects, it can be clinically significant. The remainder of the chapter will provide a closer look at each type of interaction as listed in Table 13.6.

## Limitations

It should be noted that mechanisms are difficult to tease out in some instances when discussing infec-tious diseases. For example, chronic exposure to poor sanitation and hygiene can result in an environ-mentally induced enteric dysfunction (even in the absence of diarrhea) with potential malabsorption, among other consequences [20]. The degree to which this will influence the bioavailability of systemic antimicrobials is not well described, but the expected pro-inflammatory profile has the potential, through gene expression, to alter drug transporter and enzyme function. Additionally, consider the difficulty in interpreting the strong association between dietary intake of ω-3 fatty acids and cholesterol and the poor success rate of the antimicrobial regimen that otherwise results in successful eradication rate of *Helicobacter pylori* [21]. It is unclear whether this is related to altered drug disposition (i.e., a "nutrient-drug" interaction) or to increased virulence, accelerated antibiotic resistance, immune modulation, or merely an interesting association without currently ascertainable cause and effect.

## Food-Antimicrobial Interactions

### Mechanism

Food is well established for influencing oral drug absorption and bioavailability [22, 23]. The impact of food on the absorption of a medication is a potential interaction that all new drug applications to the US Food and Drug Administration (FDA) are required to describe. This type of interaction can occur for a variety of physicochemical and physiologic reasons. The latter include alterations to gastric emptying rate, proximal intestinal pH, bile flow, splanchnic blood flow, and enterocyte permeability, transport, and metabolism. The so-called meal effect occurs because the presence of a meal changes the conditions within the gut lumen into which a drug is administered. Depending on the drug, altered conditions in the gut may influence the *rate* of drug absorption or the *extent* of drug absorption (i.e., bioavailability). Bioavailability is more clinically relevant than absorption rate and is evaluated by examining the area under the serum drug AUC in the fed state compared to the fasted state.

### Meal Conditions

Well-designed food-effect studies are useful in recognizing food-drug interactions and designing management strategies. Although not always used in trials, the FDA recommends a "test meal" of ~800–1000 kcal containing ~50% of energy from fat. Clinical significance is noted if the $AUC_{fed}$-to-$AUC_{fasted}$ ratio is <0.8 or >1.25. Generally, drugs with low solubility but high permeability/metabolism, which account for a good proportion of oral medications, are expected to have an increased bioavailability in the presence of food [24]. Although the bioavailability of a specific drug may be increased (positive effect) or decreased (negative effect) in the presence of food, some drugs exhibit no significant meal effect and can therefore be administered without regard to a meal. To make an informed practice recommendation, it is important to note what test meal conditions have been used in a study.

A meal may increase (e.g., cefpodoxime) or decrease (e.g., ampicillin, penicillin, norfloxacin) the extent of drug absorption [25–28]. For the latter agents, administering the antimicrobial at least 1 hour before or 2 hours after food is recommended to improve bioavailability. In other cases, oral bioavailability may be significantly reduced by a concurrent meal or when administered 2 hours following a meal (e.g., omadacycline), compared with the fasting state [29]. Of note, not taking into account the reduced drug bioavailability with a meal may lead to subtherapeutic drug concentrations, risking therapeutic failure and drug resistance.

The meal effect may have different outcomes even on agents within the same drug class. For example, the antifungal posaconazole should be administered with food, while voriconazole needs to be administered on an empty stomach to optimize oral bioavailability [30, 31]. The bioavailability of posaconazole increases about threefold with a meal, regardless of caloric density, compared with administration in the fasted state [32]. Mixed findings are also reported for agents to treat tuberculosis where food may reduce the oral bioavailability of isoniazid and pyrazinamide, but not likely of rifampin [33]. Hence, administration of antituberculosis medicines in the fasted state is suggested.

Antiviral agents also differ in their need to be administered with food (e.g., atazanavir, darunavir, dolutegravir, elvitegravir, sofosbuvir, tenofovir) to support absorption or on an empty stomach (e.g., daclatasvir, entecavir) because of a negative meal effect [34–37]. In other cases, the meal effect may be positive (e.g., faldaprevir) but without clinical relevance [38]. For still others there is no clinical effect at all (e.g., doravirine), and such drugs can therefore be administered without regard to food [39]. The administration of a four-component (elvitegravir, cobicistat, emtricitabine, tenofovir) fixed-dose antiviral tablet to healthy subjects in crossover studies under both fed and fasted states revealed drug-specific effects [40, 41]. Although bioavailability of cobicistat, emtricitabine, and tenofovir from this product were similar in the fasted, standard breakfast fed and enteral nutrition formula fed states, the bioavailability of elvitegravir was significantly greater in the fed state regardless of nutrient content. Consequently, this combination antiviral product is best administered with a meal. One can appreciate the complexities in clinical care management for clinicians, patients, and caretakers.

Ready-to-use therapeutic foods (RUTFs) as public health interventions in communities with malnutrition have not been specifically studied with respect to a meal effect. Lipid-based nutrition supplements used to support patients in HIV programs may reduce systemic exposure to nevirapine but not to efavirenz compared to those not receiving the supplements [42].

Sometimes the formulation of a drug may make a difference. For example, azithromycin capsules and tablets are considered bioequivalent in the fasted state; however, there is a significant meal effect seen only with the capsules resulting in decreased bioavailability compared with the tablets [43]. A further point to consider is that a drug may be administered with a meal not only to improve bioavailability but also to minimize adverse gastrointestinal effects (e.g., mefloquine) [44]. In some cases, the type of meal (i.e., macronutrient content) makes a difference on the food effect.

## Fat Content

The fat component (percent energy) of a meal may have significant influence on oral bioavailability of a drug. For the classic example of the antifungal drug griseofulvin, the oral bioavailability increases between 35% and 120% with a meal depending specifically on fat content, compared to its administration in the fasted state [45]. Bioavailability of the anthelminthic ivermectin increased ~2.5-fold when administered with a meal, especially with a high-fat meal [46, 47]. Based on an animal study, this may be related to altered post-absorptive distribution as well as improved gut dissolution/absorption following a high-fat meal [48]. However, administration of ivermectin with a grain-based meal did not alter bioavailability from that in the fasted state [49].

## Other Meal Components

Other meal components may influence bioavailability. Dietary garlic intake at up to 15 cloves per week may reduce protease inhibitor (e.g., darunavir) concentrations enough that HIV plasma viral load increases [50]. This is most likely associated with the garlic-induced increase in expression of the

P-glycoprotein efflux transporter in enterocytes, thereby significantly reducing drug bioavailability. A high purine-containing (>190 mg) meal competes with a dose of ribavirin for the absorption transporter (CNT2) in the gut, reducing drug bioavailability compared to a low-purine (<10 mg) meal [51]. Administration of oseltamivir, the influenza treatment, with milk reduces initial drug bioavailability by 35% compared to administration with water, possibly the result of competition at the PEPT1 transporter for absorption [52]. The influence of dairy products in reducing the bioavailability of some fluoroquinolones (e.g., ciprofloxacin) by at least 30% is the result of chelation with calcium in the intestinal lumen [53]. While there is occasionally an interest in mixing powdered medication directly in with food to facilitate administration in patients unable to swallow intact pills, this too needs to be considered. For example, when ciprofloxacin is crushed and mixed in water, it is much more chemically stable compared with mixing it with any of several common foods and beverages or with enteral nutrition formula [54, 55].

## Enteral Feeding

For hospitalized patients requiring enteral nutrition through a feeding tube, the administration of medication is not a simple matter and may be confounded by altered bioavailability, among other complications [56]. For example, the administration of an appropriately weight-based fixed-dose four-drug antitubercular product (rifampin, isoniazid, pyrazinamide, ethambutol) by crushing and suspending in water before administration through a feeding tube resulted in subtherapeutic responses for rifampin in six of ten patients and for isoniazid in two of the ten patients [57].

Despite available data on optimal administration with respect to meals, many patients do not adhere to directions resulting in subtherapeutic drug concentrations as was recently described in a cohort of adults receiving antiretroviral therapy [58]. The risk for the emergence of drug-resistant pathogens co-exists with the diminished clinical efficacy.

## Specific Food Component or Nutrient-Antimicrobial Interactions

Individual components of a meal or food (i.e., nutrients or other bioactive substances) or those specific ingredients consumed independently as dietary supplement products may influence drug disposition and clinical effect. For example, a number of beverages, containing a wide variety of polyphenols, are known to influence drug bioavailability. Grapefruit juice is a commonly recognized example that with typical use can influence a number of drug-metabolizing enzymes and drug transporters to increase bioavailability of some drugs and reduce the bioavailability of others [59]. An individual's susceptibility will in part depend on the transporter and enzyme genotype.

## Grapefruit

Grapefruit contains furanocoumarins which are metabolized by CYP3A4 in gut enterocytes. The metabolites then bind to and irreversibly inactivate the enzyme making it unavailable to metabolize medication. This has an effect of increasing bioavailability and serum concentrations for HIV drugs such as saquinavir and efavirenz, but has no influence on abacavir because the latter drug is not a substrate for CYP3A4 [18]. The clinical risk for subsequent adverse effects due to the greater bioavailability varies with the patient. Grapefruit juice contents (furanocoumarins, flavanones, polymethoxyflavones) can also inhibit transporter function – more so with uptake (e.g., OATP) than efflux transporters – at the intestinal mucosa [60]. For example, sulfasalazine is susceptible to grapefruit juice as a substrate for OATP2B1 resulting in reduced drug absorption [61]. Similar interactions also occur with other fruit juices to varying degrees depending on bioactive contents by altering the bioavailability of vulnerable drugs [62]. For example, clementine and mandarin juices inhibit transporters (i.e., BCRP, OATP) to a similar extent as grapefruit juice, but grapefruit is more potent an inhibitor of CYP3A4 and CYP1A2 than are the other two citrus juices [63].

## Nutrition Supplements

In a group of adults co-infected with HIV and receiving intensive phase treatment for tuberculosis, supplementation of a high-energy micronutrient-enriched biscuit slightly improved rifampin bioavailability from a multi-component product [64]. Adding multi-micronutrient supplementation (as a fortified biscuit) to an anthelmintic regimen (albendazole) resulted in a lower parasite load at 4 months compared with drug alone in high-risk children [65].

## Dietary Supplements

The widespread use of dietary supplement (also known as "natural health") products has been associated with adverse effects including drug interactions [66]. A classic interaction with garlic supplements resulted in significant reduction (~50%) of saquinavir bioavailability in healthy volunteers [67]. Other isolated bioactive food substances found in dietary supplements can influence drug disposition, due to the effect on metabolizing enzymes and transporters. These ingredients are found at higher concentrations in dietary supplement products and may be more of a concern in some circumstances than food sources with regard to interactions [68]. Supplement products may include compounds isolated from a variety of foods including fruits and spices [69–71].

Traditional supplements containing macro- and micronutrients are also important. The effects (positive or negative) of these supplements on pharmacologic interventions used to manage the infection have received limited attention. Protein supplements, possibly with source-specific effects, can increase drug metabolism through an influence on transporters and metabolizing enzymes [72, 73]. Several nutrients (e.g., amino acids, vitamin A, vitamin D, iodine, zinc) are used in supplementation studies individually or as part of multiple-micronutrient products in patients with or at high risk for infection.

### Vitamin Supplements

The use of high-dose retinol (60 mg) at the time of albendazole deworming may reduce *Ascaris lumbricoides* or *A. suum* re-infection in at-risk children, but with an effect that is less enduring in those who are stunted compared to normal height [74]. This same dose of retinol, when combined with albendazole, significantly improved iron status as well as vitamin A status [75]. Conversely, response of hookworm infection to albendazole does not seem to be related to nutrition status [76].

Interesting in vitro data suggest a benefit of nicotinamide alone or in combination with artemisinin, chloroquine, and pyrimethamine against circulating stages of malaria (*Plasmodium falciparum*), possibly related to the vitamin's effect on sirtuins which are proteins that affect aging via cellular regulation [77]. In the management of chronic hepatitis B infection, adding carnitine along with entecavir resulted in higher normalization rates for ALT concentrations than entecavir alone [78]. As a natural inhibitor of hepatitis C viral replication, the supplementation of vitamin $B_{12}$ by injection along with an interferon-ribavirin regimen significantly improved viral response compared to those receiving the drug regimen alone including those with higher viral loads [79].

The potential benefit of vitamin B complex as an adjuvant intervention to fluconazole therapy has been described including identified reductions in drug MIC for *Candida* [80]. At pharmacologic concentrations studied in vitro, vitamin C enhanced the killing of *Candida albicans*, but when combined with fluconazole the activity of the antifungal was significantly reduced [81, 82]. High-dose ascorbic acid may reduce aminoglycoside nephrotoxicity as described in an animal model [83]. Including ascorbic acid (250 mg) in an *H. pylori* triple-therapy (omeprazole, amoxicillin, clarithromycin) eradication regimen allows similar success rates despite using half the clarithromycin dose compared with the control group [84]. In another randomized trial, adding vitamin C (500 mg) and vitamin E (200 IU) to triple-therapy (lansoprazole, amoxicillin, clarithromycin) at standard doses significantly improved eradication rates [85]. Another randomized trial added vitamin C (250 mg) and vitamin E (200 mg) to a different triple-therapy regimen (lansoprazole, amoxicillin, metronidazole) and found no difference in *H. pylori* eradication rates [86]. The regimen with the vitamins was actually associated with a reduced eradication rate when metronidazole-susceptible strains were evaluated independently [86]. This again reinforces the need to know what specific supplements and drug regimen a patient is receiving to best anticipate potential interaction. In an animal model of methicillin-resistant *Staphylococcus aureus* wound infection, the addition of vitamin E treatment to an antibacterial (daptomycin, tigecycline) modulated immune function, reduced bacterial counts, and improved tissue repair [87, 88].

Nutrient status plays an important role in modulating the inflammatory response to tuberculosis [89]. A number of randomized controlled trials have administered vitamin D at varying pharmacologic doses as adjunctive treatment of pulmonary tuberculosis. Based on individual participant data from 1850 patients across 8 studies, the vitamin D intervention accelerated sputum culture conversion in those with multidrug-resistant disease [90]. It is difficult to separate a synergistic effect on the medication regimen from a direct effect of the nutrient. Including a pharmacological dose of cholecalciferol along with metronidazole did not reduce recurrence of bacterial vaginosis in a randomized controlled trial despite some improvements in vitamin D status in the treatment group [91]. In some infections, such as leishmaniasis, no data are available on the influence of nutrition intervention on therapy or outcomes (i.e., cure, treatment completion, nutrition status, or drug disposition) [92].

## Mineral Supplements

Micronutrient mineral supplements are often applied to underserved or vulnerable populations to support health especially for children and women. This strategy should take into account any potential interaction with antimicrobials. At therapeutic doses, multivalent mineral supplements can interfere with antimicrobial (ciprofloxacin, levofloxacin, minocycline) absorption due to chelation [93, 94]. Co-administration of mineral supplements (e.g., calcium, iron, magnesium, or zinc) also significantly reduces the bioavailability of the antiretroviral drug dolutegravir, unless taken concurrently with a fat-containing meal [95]. This may complicate decision-making for the HIV-infected patient requiring mineral supplements but not tolerating meals.

Albendazole or zinc (20 mg/days × 14 days) treatment reduced potential malabsorption associated with the subclinical condition "environmental enteropathy" seen in rural African children compared with placebo, although the combination of albendazole with zinc was not evaluated [96]. Combining an iron-folic acid supplement with albendazole in women of childbearing age significantly reduced the prevalence of anemia as well as hookworm infection [97].

Although typically appropriate from a nutrition perspective, the plans to include any nutrient or other dietary supplement product in a patient receiving an antimicrobial regimen should be considered in the context of potential interactions that may influence the bioavailability or clinical efficacy of the drug.

## Nutritional Status-Antimicrobial Interactions

### Infection Risk with Nutritional Status

Both PEM and obesity affect morbidity and mortality, nowhere truer than with the relationship to infectious diseases. The prevalence of overweight and obesity is well recognized in developed nations. Concern over the nutrition transition in low- and middle-income countries reveals the presence of both forms of malnutrition. Although the burden of malnutrition in developing countries is well appreciated, malnutrition is now commonly observed in pediatric and adult patients within the healthcare systems of developed countries as well, often related to the underlying disease condition itself with consequent malabsorption or limited food intake.

PEM is associated with immunosuppression, and obesity is associated with chronic inflammation, with both leading to impaired host protection against pathogens [98]. As a result, the risk for morbidity and mortality from infection is elevated in both undernourished and obese individuals [99, 100]. It turns out that both forms of malnutrition also can influence drug disposition and effect. So potential changes in antimicrobial pharmacokinetics need to be taken into account when managing an undernourished or obese patient. The influence of malnutrition on antimicrobial effect can be confounded by malnutrition's impact on host defense and the resultant infection requiring treatment (see Chap. 3) [101, 102].

### Antimicrobial Prophylaxis in Malnutrition

In children with uncomplicated severe acute malnutrition, an oral antimicrobial regimen is considered along with a nutritional intervention (e.g., RUTFs) [103]. Antibiotics (e.g., amoxicillin, cefdinir) have been used prophylactically in this setting to reduce the risk for infection [104]. For those with complicated malnutrition, inpatient care using parenteral antimicrobials is recommended. The value of antibiotic treatment, especially in the community setting where most uncomplicated malnutrition is found, remains controversial given the available evidence [105–110]. An antimicrobial intervention in severe acute malnutrition may not necessarily improve nutritional recovery and may depend on the presence of additional risk factors [108]. Whether poor adaptation of antimicrobial dosing regimens to malnutrition influenced negative studies with higher morbidity and mortality is not clear [111, 112].

Although beyond the scope of this chapter, there is a need to strike a balance between treating covert infection and reducing inflammation-associated nutrient loss with the risk for unnecessary adverse effects and potential antimicrobial resistance. The selection of the most appropriate antimicrobial based on common pathogens and local susceptibility patterns should be paired with a dosing regimen that is appropriate for the type and degree of malnutrition. The rest of this section will describe information on antimicrobials in altered nutrition states and implications for dosing adjustments.

## *Approach to Dosing*

An individual's nutrition status (i.e., PEM, micronutrient deficits, obesity) can be a determining factor in drug disposition and effect [113, 114]. A drug product developer seldom evaluates a drug's profile with respect to nutritional status, so the influence of PEM or obesity on a drug's disposition is rarely described for most drugs [115]. There is currently no regulatory requirement to do so. Despite increasing attention paid specifically to the potential impact of malnutrition (whether undernutrition or overweight/obesity) on antimicrobials, there is a dearth of adequate pharmacokinetic and pharmacodynamics studies [105, 114, 116–118]. Given the widespread prevalence of malnutrition and obesity globally, it remains troubling that so little data are available on the effect of nutrition status on drug disposition to guide clinical decision-making. Applying some principles around dosing may be helpful in the meantime. The approach to understanding the implications of nutritional status on antimicrobial dosing regimens starts with two issues: dose format and body composition.

### Dose Format

Dose formats for antimicrobials may be either a fixed dose (mg) or weight-based (mg/kg). The fixed dose is based on the expected beneficial effects in patients of otherwise healthy weight. The set value for adults often differs for children. Weight-based dosing most often uses total body weight. For drugs prescribed using weight-based dosing, it can be particularly challenging in a patient with elevated body mass index (BMI) [114, 119]. Neither body surface area nor an "ideal" body weight relative to height is considered appropriate in these circumstances [114]. The dosing weight to use depends on drug-specific characteristics in obese patients. The total body weight may be appropriate for some drugs; the lean body weight for others. A validated predictive equation for lean weight (i.e., the Duffull-Green equation), which considers body composition, may be suitable for weight-based dosing to account for the altered distribution of a drug [120, 121]. For other drugs an adjusted body weight may be more fitting. This value falls between total and lean weight (= lean body weight + [cf] [total body weight – lean body weight]), where the correction factor (cf), when known, represents the fraction of excess weight that normalizes the volume of distribution for that drug in the obese to that in a non-obese patient. This is where body composition comes into play.

### Body Composition

The change in body composition that accompanies PEM and obesity can influence a drug's pharmacokinetics [122, 123]. The two important kinetic parameters to examine for each drug are the volume of distribution (Vd) and the clearance (Cl); the former governs the drug loading dose, while the latter shapes the maintenance dose and/or dosing interval. Assuming a uniform body composition, using the two-compartment framework, in patients of an otherwise healthy weight or BMI, lean mass and fat mass transform as lower and upper extremes of BMI are approached. A drug's Vd correlates with both anatomic compartments, while its Cl correlates predominantly with lean body mass.

So altered body composition can modify the Vd and Cl which in turn will yield unexpected drug concentrations following a "usual" dose. Optimal drug dosing is required to achieve therapeutic serum concentrations and pathogen control while limiting adverse effects associated with supratherapeutic concentrations or resistance with suboptimal exposures. Aside from the absorption step required of oral doses, the Vd (L/kg) and Cl (L/min) of antimicrobials determine the serum and tissue concentrations available for killing microorganisms. So any influence of altered nutrition status on these two parameters will be important to recognize as it may have clinical implications for pathogen eradication.

Generally, the initial (loading) dose is adjusted to account for drug distribution into existing lean and fat mass, and dosing interval is adjusted to account for altered hepatic (or renal) clearance. The mistake is to evaluate absolute value of Vd in liters rather than indexed to total body mass (L/kg). The latter will give an indication of the modified distribution in the individual with altered body composition and help determine the appropriate initial dosing.

## Protein-Energy Malnutrition

The limited human data on antimicrobials in PEM come from case reports and cohort studies for the most part, so general recommendations are based on these findings combined with the approach described above. For orally administered drugs, any impact of malnutrition on the extent of absorption is valuable to appreciate. Oral bioavailability of chloramphenicol, chloroquine, penicillin, and rifampin is often decreased in malnutrition compared with controls [28, 124–126]. The bioavailability of metronidazole is not significantly affected, while sulfadiazine and cotrimoxazole may be significantly increased in malnourished children relative to controls [127–129]. Despite reduced absorption, the elevated serum concentrations of chloramphenicol with repeated dosing are a result of reduced drug Cl [130–132].

### Volume of Distribution (Vd)

The Vd for the aminoglycosides has variably been reported to increase or decrease, likely based on the degree of edema accompanying the malnutrition as these agents distribute into the extracellular fluid space [133–135]. In small series of malnourished children, gentamicin exhibited increased Vd and/or reduced Cl suggesting that larger doses administered less frequently might be appropriate as confirmed in a prospective study [136]. Individualized drug monitoring is recommended. Drug concentrations of sulfadiazine increase in PEM because of reduced Vd [137], and Vd is also reduced for quinine and chloroquine [138, 139]. The Vd may also be unchanged for other agents (e.g., cotrimoxazole) in malnutrition [129]. The oral bioavailability, Vd, and Cl of ciprofloxacin vary widely in children with severe malnutrition [140]. However, the generally greater Vd suggests larger doses (mg/kg) to achieve adequate AUC:MIC for the infecting organism.

### Clearance (Cl)

For drugs cleared primarily by renal excretion, some (e.g., cefoxitin, penicillin) are significantly reduced by malnutrition, whereas others (e.g., the aminoglycosides, cotrimoxazole) are insignificantly affected [28, 129, 133, 141, 142]. PEM is associated with increased chloramphenicol concentrations despite increases in renal Cl because of a concurrent decrease in hepatic metabolism due to reduced enzyme activity [143, 144].

Hepatically cleared drugs will be influenced by any malnutrition-associated alterations in the enzymes of the phase 1 or phase 2 enzyme systems for metabolism and elimination of xenobiotics. Rarely there may be a reported increase in drug metabolic Cl (e.g., chloroquine, quinine), but more often overall metabolic Cl is reduced (e.g., chloramphenicol, isoniazid, metronidazole, quinine) [124, 127, 132, 145–148]. Although inter-individual variability in the small sample was too great to identify statistical significance in chloroquine kinetics, mildly malnourished children had smaller Vd and slower drug Cl than normally nourished children resulting in potentially greater exposure – and associated adverse effects – of parent drug and metabolite [139]. Quinine Vd and Cl are both significantly reduced in malnourished children resulting in higher drug exposure, but this may be no different than the influence of malarial infection itself [138]. Close monitoring is recommended for chloramphenicol, given the wide variability in absorption and Cl of chloramphenicol in malnourished children with the impact on treatment outcome and toxicity risk.

As would be expected, modeling the pharmacokinetics based on data from malnourished patients better predicts serum concentrations than a model derived in non-malnourished individuals [149]. The reduced Cl led to lower total daily dose recommendations for malnourished children (e.g., metronidazole) [150]. Keep in mind that following nutritional rehabilitation, the pharmacokinetics may return towards expected values as seen for chloramphenicol and penicillin [131, 141].

## Antituberculars

The metabolism (acetylation) of isoniazid was decreased in children with PEM which over time increases the risk for hepatotoxicity [151, 152]. A similar synergism between malnutrition and rifampin toxicity was reported in adults despite reduced drug bioavailability [125]. The systemic exposure to oral rifampin is no different in malnourished adults than those not malnourished using a fixed daily dose [153]. Malnutrition also increases the systemic exposure of clarithromycin and itraconazole compared with controls due to reduced drug Cl [19, 154]. Tuberculosis is treated over many months, making these nutritional influences on drug levels and toxicities especially critical to consider and manage.

## Antivirals

Severe acute malnutrition in HIV-infected children influenced lopinavir pharmacokinetics including poor bioavailability and increased drug Cl [155]. Conversely, saquinavir absorption may be increased in PEM [156]. Systemic exposure to both efavirenz and lopinavir was reduced in malnourished HIV-infected children, while nevirapine exposure was increased, relative to values in children from environments with less malnutrition [157]. Previous study of nevirapine pharmacokinetics noted no significant differences between malnourished and well-nourished children [158]. The different findings may be related to varying degrees of malnutrition, change in body composition, and their influence on drug Vd and Cl. Many viral diseases are not cured with antiviral medications, as with some herpesviruses and HIV. Hence, the chronic use of antiviral agents requires careful management of nutritional side effects and drug level alterations.

## Antimalarials

Although pharmacokinetic data are not available for artemisinin-based antimalarial therapies in malnutrition, the clinical response is considered adequate for most children except those with height-for-age $z$-scores less than $-1$ who were at higher risk for recurrent parasitemia [159]. An artemisinin-based therapy with lumefantrine was studied in combination with RUTFs in severely malnourished children and those without severe acute malnutrition in terms of clinical and microbiologic response [160]. Although therapeutic efficacy was comparable, there was a higher re-infection rate in malnourished children combined with lower lumefantrine concentrations despite receiving higher weight-based doses [161]. Artesunate-containing regimens in a clinical trial resulted in similar treatment efficacy, adequate clinical and parasitological response, regardless of weight status by $z$-score, although rate of re-infection was higher in the overweight children [162].

## *Micronutrient Deficits*

Micronutrient deficits can also influence drug disposition based in part on their roles in the function or stability of enzyme systems involved in drug metabolism [113]. Data available from animal models suggest that malnutrition increases aminoglycoside-induced hearing loss compared with control [163]. Magnesium and zinc deficits compound this ototoxicity making it potentially irreversible [164]. Isoniazid-induced loss of glutathione activity is exacerbated in the presence of malnutrition which increases the risk for hepatotoxicity from this drug [165]. When the opportunity to analyze pharmacokinetics is taken in those with severe malnutrition receiving antimicrobials, a subsequent rational dosing approach can then be prospectively evaluated and validated [166].

## *Obese and Overweight*

Product labeling rarely includes specific dosing guidance for antimicrobial administration in persons with higher BMI [167]. This translates into a lack of available guidelines for the local clinical setting where drugs are administered as a fixed dose by age or a weight-based dose using total body weight [168]. The limited human data again come predominantly from case reports and cohort studies. A critical caveat that emerges from clinical reports is that body composition – which can vary significantly at any specific BMI – is rarely evaluated. The variability in proportions of lean-to-fat mass in obesity from what is expected in the non-obese patient can impact drug dosing regimens based on any significant change in Vd or Cl. This appears most obvious at high BMI but may be operative at any degree of overweight and obesity. So general recommendations take this limitation and the approach described previously into account.

### Antibacterials

Beta-Lactam Antibiotics

Beta-lactam antibacterials (e.g., penicillins, cephalosporins) are relatively hydrophilic as a class, distributing into lean mass which, on average, is increased in absolute terms in obesity. These agents are associated with time-dependent killing activity (i.e., duration above MIC). The expected greater Vd, even when weight-normalized (L/kg) compared with non-obese values, suggests total body weight would be an appropriate dosing metric. Therefore, use of fixed doses at the upper limit of the usual range or weight-based dosing using total body weight is suggested, with similar or more frequent dose intervals. Using a standard preoperative prophylactic dose of a cephalosporin in obesity resulted in serum concentrations below the MIC for potential pathogens [169]. Adjusting fixed doses to the upper limit significantly reduced postoperative surgical site infection rates [169].

Aminoglycosides

For concentration-dependent antimicrobial killing activity (e.g., the aminoglycosides), the loading dose will depend on the expected alteration in drug distribution. The aminoglycosides do not fully distribute into the excess body weight (only ~40%) given their degree of hydrophilicity. The weight-normalized Vd is modestly lower than in the non-obese suggesting use of an adjusted body weight. The weight-normalized volume of distribution is also reduced in obese children [170]. When using actual body weight in obese children, despite a lower initial total dose, the resultant gentamicin serum trough concentrations associated with toxicity risk were significantly higher than healthy weight patients as reported in a case-control study [170]. However, given that the aminoglycosides distribute into fat-free mass, dosing based on an estimated lean body mass (Duffull-Green equation) may simplify regimens from malnourished to obese adult patients [171]. Similar findings were seen in obese children using a pediatric-specific equation for fat-free mass [172]. Drug Cl may be increased in obesity, but dosing intervals will best be determined by evaluating serum drug trough concentrations and renal function.

## Glycopeptides

Daptomycin serves as an interesting example as it has been administered to obese patients using either fixed or weight-based dosing; the latter has used either actual body weight or an adjusted body weight [173–175]. When using weight-based doses, there was no significant difference in clinical failure rate, 90-day mortality, when using actual or an adjusted body weight, from a single center retrospective study of 101 obese patients (BMI 30–69 kg/m$^2$) [175]. However, a 90-day readmission was more likely in the group dosed based on actual body weight, and dose-related adverse effects were more common in the adjusted body weight group. Interestingly, over 80% of patients in the actual body weight group received no more than 6 mg/kg, while in the adjusted weight group, nearly 80% received over 6–8 mg/kg. At doses of 4 mg/kg total body weight, the Vd (L/kg) was significantly lower in obese than in non-obese adults, without significant increases in total body Cl, with increased body exposure suggesting that dosing should be based on an adjusted body weight with a correction factor of about 0.3 [114, 176, 177]. Excessive drug exposure increases the risk for creatinine phosphokinase elevations requiring close monitoring with high-dose regimens [173, 178, 179].

Vancomycin Vd correlates with total body weight, so for vancomycin weight-based dosing, the actual body weight can be used for children and adults [180, 181]. Monitoring of vancomycin exposure in obesity, where variability in Vd occurs, benefits from obtaining both trough and peak drug concentrations to guide therapy and limit toxicity [181–183]. The Cl of the drug, to identify maintenance doses, may be best estimated by an adjusted body weight [184]. With standard intermittent maintenance doses, the extremely obese (BMI ≥ 40 kg/m$^2$) required less drug (mg/kg) than the obese to achieve similar target serum concentrations [185]. Although not a common practice, the administration of vancomycin by continuous infusion, following a similar weight-based loading dose, revealed that obese patients required less drug (mg/kg) than non-obese patients to achieve the same therapeutic endpoint [186].

## Others

An adjusted body weight with a cf of ~0.3, comes closest to representing the characteristic behavior of linezolid in obese patients based on available case reports and could be empirically dosed at 10 mg/kg twice daily [187–189]. Otherwise the usual fixed dosing range is considered acceptable for linezolid in obese patients as long as it achieves adequate serum concentrations relative to the MIC.

Fluoroquinolones exhibit larger Vd in obesity but do not adequately distribute into excess adipose tissue but only the excess lean, so an adjusted body weight or otherwise standard doses are considered acceptable. Dosing for clindamycin does not need to be adjusted in obesity so that either a standard dose at the higher end of normal range or a weight-based dose using actual body weight is acceptable [190]. Rifampin, and possibly other antituberculosis agents, could be dosed using a lean body weight; however weight-based dosing using total body weight may be necessary in obesity to avoid subtherapeutic rifampin concentrations [191].

Overweight and obesity influences both the Vd and Cl of cotrimoxazole based on analysis in adults of BMI 16.2–59.1 kg/m$^2$, i.e., ranging from very slim to morbidly obese [192]. Neither "ideal" nor lean body weight is appropriate to use for cotrimoxazole, rather favoring an adjusted or total body weight, although body composition was not taken into account to help refine further. The upper dose limit for cotrimoxazole (trimethoprim-sulfamethoxazole 20 mg–100 mg/kg) is based on total body weight assuming linearity in drug distribution and Cl at a wide BMI range from underweight through obese patients.

## Antifungals

Adequate AUC:MIC values are achievable in obese patients treated with fluconazole when a lean body weight is used for loading and maintenance doses, although some suggest using actual body weight to target pathogens with higher MICs while avoiding fixed dose regimens altogether [193, 194]. The dose of fluconazole should be increased to account for the increased Cl seen in obesity [195]. Voriconazole is more lipophilic, so that a fixed dose is acceptable in obesity, but if weight-based dosing is applied, the lean (or an adjusted) weight could be relied on. Using total body weight for voriconazole dosing may yield excessive drug exposure and increase the risk for toxicity [196–198]. Even the use of an adjusted body weight, if in a patient with CYP2C19 poor metabolizer phenotype, has resulted in excessive voriconazole concentrations [199]. Itraconazole and posaconazole are very lipophilic, and drug is lost from systemic exposure based on lower AUC in obesity.

Echinocandins can be dosed using standard doses or higher as they have good safety profiles. Using standard doses of caspofungin in adults appears to be similarly effective in various fungal infections regardless of obesity category despite lower systemic exposure in some patients [200, 201]. The AUC:MIC was achieved for caspofungin with clinical resolution in an obese patient when using a fixed dose 30% higher than the usual dose [202]. Micafungin requires higher standard dosing in obesity to achieve adequate AUC:MIC cut-off values for specific fungal organisms [203]. Further improvements at higher BMI may require weight-based dosing for echinocandins and azole antifungals to improve outcomes for invasive candidiasis [195, 202].

Amphotericin Vd is higher in obesity so total body weight is most commonly used for weight-based dosing. Flucytosine should use lean body weight due to the decreased weight-normalized Vd and the reduced Cl in obesity [204].

## Antivirals and Antiretrovirals

Several cases reported on obese patients receiving usual doses (weight-based) of acyclovir who developed the drug-induced adverse effect of renal failure [205–207]. Administration of a low dose based on an "ideal" body weight yielded insufficient systemic drug exposure in obese patients compared with non-obese patients receiving the dose based on total body weight in a prospective study [208]. In the management of HIV infection, obesity is associated with lower exposures to efavirenz, lopinavir, and tenofovir over time compared to exposure in normal-weight patients, but no significant differences were seen for abacavir, atazanavir, darunavir, emtricitabine, lamivudine, nevirapine, or raltegravir [209]. Efavirenz exposure using a standard dose is subtherapeutic in obesity requiring a much higher dose to achieve therapeutic concentrations [210]. No dose adjustment is expected to be required for the administration of oseltamivir in obese patients [211–213].

As becomes evident from the inadequate and sometimes inconsistent information, generalizations cannot be made with confidence in the place of drug-specific data. Such data are needed for many commonly used antimicrobials in undernourished, overweight, and obese individuals of all ages. Increased regulatory attention is needed to ensure that clinicians have the critical information for nutritional status-drug dosing interactions and their proper management.

## Antimicrobial-Nutrition Status Interactions

### Subset of Adverse Drug Effects

In addition to any therapeutic benefit, medication use is associated with potential adverse effects. Among the adverse effects are those that can influence metabolic biomarkers, nutrition status in general, or the status of specific nutrients, all of which are important to consider during patient care [214]. A variety of mechanisms can lead to altered metabolism (e.g., dysglycemia, dyslipidemia), overall nutritional status (i.e., body weight, volume status), or individual nutrient stores (e.g., hypokalemia, iron deficiency). Common general effects of a drug on metabolic or nutritional parameters are often available from clinical trials and in the FDA's product labeling [215]. Many of these are summarized in this section and grouped together by their adverse effect rather than their antimicrobial class. More specific, nutrient biomarkers of interest are rarely available until post-marketing case studies are reported. The adverse effects of antimicrobials include not only the host as a target but the microbiota as well. For example, the influence on weight gain or weight loss may be indirect through a change in the gut microbiota [216, 217].

An individual drug may cause several adverse effects that together influence nutrition status – fatigue, loss of appetite, and disturbances of gastrointestinal function – that together can lead to reduced dietary intake and decreased body weight. The effect on intake may occur through the central nervous system, more local gut mechanisms, or both. The impairment of the ability to gather, prepare, and ingest food may even occur following drug-induced cognitive, visual, movement, or gait disturbances. Changes in body weight, body mass index, or extracellular fluid volume over time are easier to recognize. The effects can be additive if multiple drugs are being used.

### Overall Nutritional Status

Reduced appetite has been reported for several unrelated antimicrobials (e.g., aminoglycosides, fluconazole, posaconazole, voriconazole, lamivudine, tenofovir), which with other factors may contribute to weight loss. Occasionally a drug (e.g., amphotericin, clindamycin) may result in reduced appetite in the absence of any other influences. An effect on appetite or body weight is especially important to recognize for antimicrobials used chronically. Weight gain including body fat accumulation (central, dorsocervical) or redistribution with peripheral wasting may occur with several antiretroviral agents (e.g., abacavir, atazanavir, dolutegravir, efavirenz, lamivudine, nevirapine, saquinavir, tenofovir).

In developing countries, persons with HIV infection and low BMI have reported increased appetites once they are placed on antiretroviral therapy, perhaps due to increased metabolic demands of the partial immune reconstitution occurring with declining viral load and pathogenicity. In this case, food supplements may be needed to ensure adherence to antiretroviral therapy since patients may not take a drug that makes them hungry in the absence of available food [218–221].

## Nervous and Musculoskeletal Systems

Central nervous system effects that may contribute to reductions in food gathering, preparation, and intake can include severe headache (e.g., acyclovir, amphotericin, antiretrovirals, azole antifungals, caspofungin, cephalosporins, cotrimoxazole, daptomycin, macrolides, metronidazole, rifampin), dizziness (e.g., cephalosporins, daptomycin, efavirenz, macrolides), fatigue (e.g., abacavir, azole antifungals, cotrimoxazole, dolutegravir, efavirenz, lamivudine, macrolides, nevirapine, rifampin, saquinavir, sofosbuvir, tenofovir), ataxia (e.g., acyclovir, cotrimoxazole, efavirenz, flucytosine, metronidazole, rifampin), and/or tremor (e.g., amphotericin, azole antifungals). Visual disturbances (e.g., rifampin) and optic neuritis (e.g., chloramphenicol) may also influence food gathering, preparation, and intake.

Peripheral neuropathy (e.g., abacavir, atazanavir, aminoglycosides, amphotericin, efavirenz, daptomycin, fluoroquinolones, flucytosine, isoniazid, lamivudine, metronidazole) and even myositis, myalgia, and/or arthralgia (e.g., acyclovir, atazanavir, azole antifungals, cephalosporins, cotrimoxazole, dolutegravir, efavirenz, fluoroquinolones, lamivudine, nevirapine, saquinavir) may influence food gathering, preparation, and intake. These adverse effects can negatively impact nutritional status over time.

## Gastrointestinal System

Dry mouth and altered taste (e.g., amphotericin, azole antifungals, flucytosine, fluoroquinolones, macrolides, metronidazole) as well as glossitis (e.g., cephalosporins, chloramphenicol, cotrimoxazole, metronidazole, penicillins, tetracyclines) or stomatitis (e.g., abacavir, aminoglycosides, amphotericin, tetracyclines, chloramphenicol, cotrimoxazole, metronidazole, nevirapine, penicillins) can also interfere with food intake. Furthermore, common gastrointestinal disturbances (i.e., anorexia, nausea, vomiting, abdominal pain, liver function abnormalities, and diarrhea or constipation) are found with most oral medication. Less commonly occurring are dysphagia (e.g., saquinavir, tetracyclines), hepatitis (e.g., dolutegravir, efavirenz, nevirapine, saquinavir and the macrolides), and pancreatitis (e.g., abacavir, cotrimoxazole, lamivudine, macrolides, metronidazole, saquinavir).

## Metabolic Effects

Metabolic changes can include hyperglycemia as seen with several antiretrovirals (e.g., abacavir, atazanavir, dolutegravir, lamivudine, saquinavir) and other antimicrobials (e.g., posaconazole), as well as hypoglycemia (e.g., fluoroquinolones, flucytosine). Hypertriglyceridemia and hypercholesterolemia have been reported with some agents (e.g., clindamycin, dolutegravir, efavirenz) [222]. Therapy with meropenem in an infant was reported to cause significantly elevated serum triglycerides (966 mg/dL) and total cholesterol (258 mg/dL) concentrations that were reversible with discontinuation of the antibacterial [223].

## Electrolyte Status

Electrolyte abnormalities are also associated with a number of antimicrobials. This includes hyponatremia (e.g., cotrimoxazole), hypokalemia (e.g., aminoglycosides, amphotericin, caspofungin, flucytosine, posaconazole), hypomagnesemia (e.g., aminoglycosides, amphotericin, posaconazole, caspofungin), and hypocalcemia (e.g., aminoglycosides, amphotericin, posaconazole). Hyperkalemia (e.g., cotrimoxazole, macrolides) and hyperphosphatemia (e.g., macrolides) may also occur. Cotrimoxazole is associated with reversible hyperkalemia likely due to inhibition of renal potassium secretion attributed to the trimethoprim fraction of the combination product [224].

Although rarely administered orally, the aminoglycosides can cause gut damage leading to malabsorption of several vitamins, minerals, and electrolytes. In the absence of pseudomembranous colitis associated with *Clostridium difficile*, clindamycin-induced diarrhea may be related to drug-induced malabsorption of bicarbonate-stimulated water and electrolyte absorption in the jejunum [225].

## Antimicrobial-Nutrient Interactions

The classic term "drug-nutrient interaction" has been used as an all-encompassing term, but in its stricter sense only refers to the subtype in which a medication alters the disposition of an individual nutrient. For example, the classic influence that isoniazid has on pyridoxine metabolism has been well described for decades in the treatment of tuberculosis [226, 227]. The resultant influence of pyridoxine deficits on niacin status has also been reported [228–230]. To prevent associated peripheral neuropathy or seizures, or to manage the presenting adverse effect, pyridoxine is administered along with the isoniazid regimen [231, 232]. In the presence of tuberculosis-HIV co-infection, the risk for peripheral neuropathy appears greater and may be multifactorial despite modest pyridoxine supplementation [233, 234]. Adequate pyridoxine supplementation is required in patients being treated for this co-infection [235]. Of note, although the co-administration of high-dose pyridoxine with isoniazid may reduce intestinal drug absorption, based on an in situ model, the overall bioavailability is not significantly affected [236].

Given that vitamin D deficiency is associated with a higher risk for acquiring tuberculosis, it is interesting to note that isoniazid and rifampin may themselves decrease 25-OH vitamin D concentrations by inhibiting 25-hydroxylation and by accelerating 24,25-hydroxylation respectively [237]. This was not, however, identified in a cohort in Africa treated with these agents, where vitamin D status was good to begin with and actually improved somewhat over the course of the first 2 months [238]. Knowing a patient's vitamin D status may help determine whether supplementation is required as part of their antitubercular regimen.

Despite low 25-OH-vitamin D concentrations often found at baseline in HIV infection, efavirenz as part of an antiretroviral regimen is associated with significant vitamin D deficits, increased bone turnover, and risk for osteomalacia [239–241]. This may occur as a result of drug-induced interference with vitamin D metabolism and regulation in osteoblasts [242]. Vitamin D supplementation not only increased serum 25-OH-vitamin D concentrations in patients receiving efavirenz but also significantly improved biomarkers of bone metabolism [243]. Another antiviral, tenofovir, is also associated with vitamin D deficits, hypophosphatemia, increased bone turnover, and osteomalacia [239, 244–246]. Multiple mechanisms may be responsible for the functional deficiency seen with tenofovir including decreased FGF-23 concentrations with elevated vitamin D binding protein [247]. Supplementation with vitamin D increases FGF-23 and unbound $1,25(OH)_2$ vitamin D [248]. Chronic adefovir treatment for viral hepatitis is also associated with renal tubular dysfunction, hypophosphatemia, and osteomalacia [249]. The periostitis reported with long-term use of voriconazole is accompanied by significantly elevated serum fluoride concentrations seen in patients receiving this agent [250, 251].

The use of highly active antiretroviral therapy was associated with lower folate and vitamin $B_{12}$ concentrations and higher soluble transferrin receptors in postpartum HIV-infected women [252]. Lipid-based nutrient supplements corrected most of the low B-vitamin concentrations found in the breast milk of HIV-infected women receiving antiretroviral therapy [253]. In the absence of B-vitamin deficits at baseline, the mechanisms for the poor status of these micronutrients is unclear, but drug-induced changes in gut integrity may play a role as might B-vitamin distribution into breast milk. Highly active antiretroviral therapy is also associated with reduced α-tocopherol concentrations in nearly 20% of patients with long-standing HIV, especially using the combination of nucleoside reverse transcriptase inhibitors with other classes [254]. Carnitine deficits have also been suspected as an adverse effect of antiretroviral therapy [255].

Elevated partial thromboplastin time (PTT) and international normalized ratio (INR) without bleeding were reported in a child receiving chronic azithromycin that was attributed to vitamin K deficits when corrected with a parenteral dose of phytonadione [256]. A possible vitamin K deficiency (elevated prothrombin time, PTT, INR) with gastrointestinal bleeding was reported in a patient who had been receiving cotrimoxazole prophylactically for several months, with a marginal dietary intake despite no history of malabsorption, that responded to oral vitamin K supplementation [257].

Based on in vitro and in vivo studies, it has been suggested that aminoglycosides may interfere with host selenium (Se-cys) incorporation into proteins (selenoprotein P being most sensitive) requiring further examination [258]. Whether this is additive to the decline in circulating selenium concentrations seen with infection will need to be explored. Plasma selenium and selenoprotein P can serve as valuable biomarkers in such studies [259].

# Drug-Nutrition Interactions from the CoVid-19 Experience

## Overview of the CoVid-19 Experience

Of the thousands of coronaviruses (CoV) that exist in nature, only seven are recognized human pathogens [260]. Several seasonal CoV are endemic causing upper respiratory infections (i.e., "common cold") but may cause pneumonia and sepsis in at-risk individuals. CoV include the β-coronaviruses responsible for previous human infectious outbreaks such as severe acute respiratory syndrome (SARS) and Middle East respiratory syndrome (MERS) and the novel SARS-CoV-2 [261]. The latter is a large, single-strand, non-segmented, positive-sense RNA virus responsible for the recent CoVid-19 pandemic. Risk factors associated with developing CoVid-19 can include advanced age, poor nutrition status, and certain comorbidities (e.g., cardiovascular, pulmonary, endocrine). Similar characteristics (i.e., older patients with comorbidities) were noted in critically ill patients who succumbed to CoVid-19 [262]. The approach to management has included prophylaxis and treatment, including nutritional interventions, with varying success.

### Approach to Management

Many infected individuals are asymptomatic, while others develop upper respiratory illness (cough, fever/chills, shortness of breath, fatigue) that recover with mild supportive care. These latter patients may receive therapy, but more severe cases require hospitalization with a significant proportion requiring intensive care to manage pneumonia, acute respiratory distress syndrome, systemic inflammation, and organ dysfunction. The imbalance between insufficient innate natural defenses and excessive cytokine expression is most pronounced in those developing critical illness with CoVid-19 [263].

The management of CoVid-19 caused by the novel SARS-CoV-2 has included a number of potential therapeutic drug interventions. In the absence of drugs approved for management of CoVid-19, approaches have been based on earlier experience with SARS and MERS or repurposing available agents with theoretical benefit extrapolated from previous experiences. There have been general treatments (e.g., micronutrients, immunoenhancers) and CoV-specific treatments (e.g., antiretrovirals [lopinavir, nelfinavir], spike-protein blockers [chloroquine, hydroxychloroquine], others [ribavirin, remdesivir]) [261]. Given the limited evidence available at the time of writing, additional data based on randomized controlled trials are still needed to determine safety, efficacy, and relative clinical value for prophylactic and treatment interventions for CoVid-19. Many clinical trials of therapeutic agents are currently underway across the globe [264]. Other medications used in acutely ill patients target end organ consequences of the infection (e.g., analgesics [fentanyl], sedatives [propofol], vasopressors [norepinephrine], paralytics [cisatracurium], anti-thromboembolics [enoxaparin]) but will not be addressed here with the exception of propofol.

## Prophylactic Measures

Aside from isolating newly infected symptomatic patients, protecting those at risk by wearing masks, limiting dense social gatherings, and practicing standard health hygiene, there has been a surge of interest in prophylactic therapy. Among the interventions considered are those aimed at improving or maintaining good nutrition status (see section "Role of Nutrition Status and Interventions").

Given the difficulty and time required to design and develop a vaccine, along with the concerns following previous CoV vaccine attempts, and the reticence for moving into gene therapy using RNA- or DNA-based vaccines, it is unlikely that a safe and effective vaccine will be available for wide adoption in the short term [265–267]. In the meantime, some antimalarial drugs (e.g., chloroquine, hydroxychloroquine), which have long been recognized as immunomodulatory agents (i.e., used to manage immune activation diseases), have been considered for post-exposure prophylaxis. But given the low rates of conversion to infection, a study would have to enroll a large number of participants to determine any benefit.

## Treatment Measures

Although considered an antimalarial, chloroquine also has activity against some bacteria, fungi, and viruses. Its hydroxyl analog (hydroxychloroquine) has similar properties and activity with lower toxicity [1]. Both agents have antiretroviral clinical effects. At clinically achievable concentrations of ~9–10 μmol/L, chloroquine inhibited SARS-CoV replication and spread even when added to a primate cell culture up to 5 hours' post-infection [268, 269]. In vitro studies support activity against SARS-CoV by impairing activation of the cell receptor for CoV (angiotensin-converting enzyme-II [ACE-II]), thereby interfering with virus binding to cells [267, 268]. The same has now been identified for SARS-CoV-2 [270]. Clinical use of chloroquine/hydroxychloroquine alone or in combination with azithromycin has been reported effective, but is not a consistent finding and will await further clinical trials [271–273]. Both hydroxychloroquine and azithromycin are weak bases that accumulate in acidic cell organelles including endosomes and lysosomes, which could interfere with pH-dependent steps in viral replication [274]. Additionally, in the case of macrophages, these agents may polarize them to the M2 (anti-inflammatory) phenotype [260].

Remdesivir, an adenosine analog pro-drug, was developed for Ebola virus but has in vitro activity against MERS and SARS to inhibit RNA-dependent RNA polymerase. It has now been used with limited success and awaits results of trials as does favipiravir [275, 276]. Lopinavir with ribavirin has been used effectively in SARS but awaits results for use in CoVid-19. Other antivirals being considered besides lopinavir and ribavirin include sofosbuvir and tenofovir (all discussed earlier in the chapter).

Non-selective angiotensin-converting enzyme inhibition may be counterproductive compared with selective ACE-II blockade. Even so, excess selective blockade with accumulation of its substrate (angiotensin-II) may increase pulmonary and gut pathology, but this needs to be evaluated. A recombinant soluble ACE-II is being evaluated as are type 1 interferons. Other biologic agents have been proposed to target the cytokine response in CoVid-19 infection [277]. For example, tocilizumab, an IL-6-receptor monoclonal antibody, to try to neutralize increased circulating IL-6 associated with the cytokine storm has been used [278–280]. Cytokine storm targeted therapy may also include PPAR-γ as a focus [281]. This includes agonist drugs (e.g., the glitazones) as well as nutrient ligands (e.g., curcumin, eicosapentaenoic acid [EPA], and docosahexaenoic acid [DHA]).

As presented in this book, nutrition is critical for maintaining immune function and preventing viral infections. Relevant general recommendations have been provided to prevent or manage CoVid-19 [282]. As discussed earlier in the chapter, poor nutrition status may in turn have implications for the effectiveness of medication.

## Role of Nutrition Status and Interventions

Susceptibility to developing infection following exposure and the ability to fight the infection when present are both influenced by nutrition status. The western diet, including high content of saturated fatty acids, can alter the balance between arms of the immune system in favor of chronic activation of innate immunity with subsequent risk for viral infection [283]. As was noted in previous influenza epidemics, malnutrition (both undernutrition and obesity) is associated with worse prognosis, with prolonged viral shedding in obesity [284]. For CoVid-19 there appear to be implications for the obese as well as undernourished patient. Poor nutrition status is a known virulence factor to be considered and may increase the risk of developing a more severe presentation of CoVid-19 [261, 285]. Whether comorbid disease-related or not, malnutrition impairs immune cell activation allowing viral persistence and increased systemic inflammation [286]. The presence of anosmia and ageusia in CoVid-19 infection may alter dietary intake. Of older adults developing CoVid-19, the majority of inpatients were at risk for or already had malnutrition, which predicted weight loss, disease severity, and length of stay [287, 288]. Malnutrition was also well represented among fatalities but not survivors of CoVid-19 based on early reports [289].

As described elsewhere in this volume, cell-mediated non-specific immunity is most influenced by single micronutrient deficits (e.g., vitamins A, D, E, C, pyridoxine, folate, and vitamin $B_{12}$, copper, iron, selenium, and zinc). Addressing micronutrient deficits (e.g., vitamin D, zinc) may improve immune function, but supplementation in the absence of deficits remains a question mark.

Vitamin D drives endogenous production of antimicrobial peptides that include activity against viruses as part of innate immunity and limits the production of $T_H1$ cytokines that have excessive response to infection while promoting $T_H2$ and $T_{REG}$ responses [290]. Additionally, in a murine model, low vitamin D status activates the renin-angiotensin system detrimental for cardiopulmonary function [291]. Given the apparent decreasing North-South gradient for the CoVid-19 outbreak, patients with vitamin D deficits may benefit from supplementation as a prophylactic measure [292–294]. Vitamin D supplements have been considered to maintain 25-OH vitamin D concentrations above 100 nmol/L for its immunomodulatory, anti-inflammatory, and antiviral properties [295]. In a cohort of patients with symptoms of acute airway disease, significantly lower 25-OH vitamin D concentrations were observed in those testing positive for SARS-CoV-2 compared to those testing negative [296].

Zinc's role in antiviral immunity, particularly for the elderly, is recognized even if not yet fully understood [297–299]. Given that moderate zinc deficits are associated with increased severity of pneumonia, there could be a role for zinc therapy [298]. Zinc has been suggested as a preventative therapy for CoVid-19 as it may reduce ACE-II activity, upregulate interferon-α production, and modulate NF-κB signaling [300]. Keeping in mind zinc's narrow therapeutic index for immunomodulation, excess dosing in sufficient individuals may carry its own risk, which may include attenuating beneficial effects of other micronutrients. Alternative viewpoints dissuade the use of nutrition supplements in favor of exclusive drug interventions recommended by authorities despite inconclusive data for all [301].

Micronutrients are not alone in prophylactic or treatment roles. High cell turnover with systemic inflammation also consumes amino acids. The obese patient will need adequate amino acids available to support the inflammatory response and limit worsening sarcopenia [286]. The protective effect on illness severity by an upregulation of the gene ACE-II has been postulated to benefit from high resveratrol intake and low-fat intake via modulation of gene expression [302]. Nutritional interventions are also considered vital therapy for patients with SARS-CoV-2 infection to support the immune system and disease recovery [303–306]. But they have come up against the issue of tolerance in CoVid-19, given gut dysfunction and metabolic limits (i.e., hyperglycemia, hypertriglyceridemia). Oral nutrition supplements, enteral nutrition, and parenteral nutrition each have a role based on the patient and their ability to tolerate oral intake as assessed by the clinical nutrition team.

Of the CoVid-19 patients ill enough to be admitted to hospital, many have experienced rapid onset of organ dysfunction requiring intensive care management. These patients are extremely hypermetabolic and catabolic requiring nutrition support therapy while intubated and mechanically ventilated. Energy and protein debt are to be avoided while balancing against overfeeding in the face of the risk for hyperglycemia and hypertriglyceridemia in CoVid-19 patients. At the same time the critically ill patient exhibits significant gut dysfunction and fluid-volume sensitivity. Whenever gut function permitted, gastric access for enteral nutrition was preferred to avoid any aerosol generation that violates airborne isolation and healthcare provider exposure that may come with attempting to place a post-pyloric tube using endoscopy or fluoroscopy. Rarely, parenteral nutrition would need to be used to support the patient's metabolic condition. But a low threshold exists for starting parenteral nutrition if unable to meet needs because of gut intolerance or limitations of other interventions (e.g., prone ventilation).

Enteral or parenteral nutrition products containing MCT and omega-9 fatty acids with their neutral profile in the inflammatory response and omega-3 fatty acids which serve as precursors to less inflammatory and pro-resolving mediators are preferred over the pro-inflammatory omega-6 long-chain triglycerides. Incidentally, in the USA, the widely used sedative propofol is formulated in a soybean oil vehicle in which the pro-inflammatory omega-6 fatty acids predominate. Given the considerable energy load from propofol administration (110 kcal/dL), limitation is placed on providing more appropriate fatty acids from enteral or parenteral nutrition sources. The inclusion of EPA and DHA has the benefit of yielding pro-resolving mediators (e.g., the protectins) and reducing inflammatory consequences of viral illness [307, 308]. In critically ill patients, the question of the utility of high-dose intravenous ascorbic acid is being addressed by an ongoing trial (NCT04264533) [309].

Outside the intensive care unit, early nutrition supplementation is also important given severe inflammation and poor oral intake in most hospitalized patients. Given the overwhelming numbers of patients at some hospitals, a pragmatic and general approach has been taken when individualized intervention is not practical [303]. This includes high-energy diets/snacks of varying textures and consistencies that are easily digestible. The availability of high-energy high-protein oral nutrition supplements, especially those that incorporate whey protein, has been suggested. For the patient requiring enteral nutrition, peptide-based formulations and continuous feeding regimens may improve tolerance. Enteral nutrition can be used cautiously when non-invasive ventilation methods are in use but with a low threshold to convert to parenteral nutrition when nutrient needs remain unmet by gut feeding [303]. Patients managed at home require adequate hydration with recommendations to include fluids containing macro- and micronutrients [306]. A high-energy/high-protein diet with oral nutrition supplements throughout the day is also recommended.

## Drug-Nutrition Interactions

With that overview of the evolving management of CoVid-19, this section will describe observations on potential drug-nutrition interactions of agents being used. Interactions associated with some antiviral agents were discussed earlier in the chapter.

Several agents are administered parenterally (e.g., interferons, remdesivir, sarilumab, tocilizumab) and will not be susceptible to food effects. However, in hospitalized patients who require enteral nutrition, oral agents may be administered via enteral feeding tube which remains an incompletely appreciated issue [56]. For example, the azithromycin suspension requires further dilution with purified water just prior to administration by feeding tube to aid the delivery of the full dose through the enteral device to the patient. Additionally, close proximity of azithromycin to enteral nutrition may improve gut tolerance (abdominal discomfort) to the drug, so no need to hold the feed beyond the time taken to flush the tube, administer the drug, and flush again. Lopinavir drug absorption is limited if delivered into the small bowel but remains successful via gastrostomy tube, although the liquid formulation may adsorb to small-bore feeding tubes [56]. Based on data with meals, the presence of fat-containing enteral nutrition may improve lopinavir bioavailability. Chloroquine tablets are to be dispersed in purified water and administered in close proximity to enteral feeds to reduce gut irritation. Keep in mind that chloroquine bioavailability may be decreased in malnutrition [125].

A number of the drugs can cause alterations to gut function besides azithromycin and chloroquine. Dexamethasone, hydroxychloroquine, interferons, and lopinavir are also known to cause nausea, vomiting, abdominal pain, and diarrhea, with possible loss in appetite and body weight over time. The study drug remdesivir may also cause nausea and diarrhea. Liver function tests can become elevated with several agents (e.g., dexamethasone, remdesivir, sarilumab, tocilizumab). Tocilizumab may cause stomatitis, oral mucositis, and gastric ulcer. Sarilumab and tocilizumab may increase the risk for intestinal perforation.

Chloroquine/hydroxychloroquine may also cause vertigo and myopathy including proximal muscle weakness that may limit the ability to prepare meals for patients managed at home. Similarly, dexamethasone and interferons may influence nutrition status indirectly secondary to headache, dizziness, and fatigue. Some drugs are associated with edema (e.g., dexamethasone) that may increase body weight or interfere with the ability to note loss of body mass over time. Dexamethasone is also associated with protein catabolism and a negative nitrogen balance, along with loss of muscle mass and weakness.

Additionally, several of the drugs used in CoVid-19 can cause more specific metabolic and nutrition effects. Some agents cause hyperglycemia (e.g., dexamethasone, interferons, lopinavir), while others may cause hypoglycemia (e.g., chloroquine, hydroxychloroquine). Hypertriglyceridemia (e.g., interferons, lopinavir, sarilumab, tocilizumab) and hypercholesterolemia (e.g., lopinavir, sarilumab, tocilizumab) can also occur. Remdesivir has been reported to cause altered serum potassium concentrations. Dexamethasone can cause hypokalemia by increasing potassium excretion, while azithromycin may cause hyperkalemia and hyperphosphatemia. Favipiravir is associated with reductions in renal phosphate and uric acid excretion with subsequent increases in serum values.

Chloroquine/hydroxychloroquine inhibits a transporter (OATP1A2) responsible for all-*trans*-retinol uptake critical to the visual cycle, thereby contributing to the retinopathy associated with treatment [310]. Weight-based dosing of these agents in the obese patient is better based on a lean body weight to lower the retinopathy risk [311]. The drugs additionally can inhibit thiamin transport with a potential risk for thiamin deficits including central nervous system manifestations [312].

Taking into account overall nutrition status, drug effect in obese patients may differ from the non-obese. Based on findings using fixed standard doses in chronic hepatitis C, the bioavailability of ribavirin and interferon was reduced in obese patients which adversely impacted clinical outcome [313]. Aside from exhibiting altered pharmacokinetics in obesity, dexamethasone sensitivity increases in obesity suggesting that dosing based on a lean or adjusted body weight may be most appropriate [314].

As for positive interactions of nutrients on drug therapy, there are some ongoing trials that involve combinations (e.g., hydroxychloroquine + azithromycin + vitamin C + vitamin D) [264]. Potential benefits will await forthcoming results. The suggestion of adding zinc (oral or intravenous) to a regimen of chloroquine or hydroxychloroquine has been suggested [274, 315]. This is based on the ability of zinc to inhibit viral RNA-dependent RNA polymerase and downstream cell signal transduction [316]. Although these antimalarials are zinc ionophores, it remains unclear whether supplemental zinc would benefit a patient with adequate pre-morbid zinc status in the midst of a systemic inflammatory response.

# Conclusions

The wide variety of antimicrobials indicated for a diverse set of infectious diseases remains a vital therapeutic intervention for people every day across the globe. Appropriate drug regimens and clinical monitoring assures safety and effectiveness in the face of factors that may influence outcomes. Interactions between drug and nutrition can play an important role and need to be taken into account. This includes the influence of diet patterns, meals, supplements, or nutrition status on the disposition and clinical effect of the drug, as well as the potential effect of each drug on the status of global nutrition or the status of individual nutrients.

# References

1. Grayson ML, editor-in-chief. Kucers' the use of antibiotics. 6th ed. London: Hodder Arnold; 2010.
2. Ren W, Rajendran R, Zhao Y, et al. Amino acids as mediators of metabolic cross talk between host and pathogen. Front Immunol. 2018;9:319.
3. Millward DJ. Nutrition, infection and stunting: the roles of deficiencies of individual nutrients and foods, and of inflammation, as determinants of reduced linear growth of children. Nutr Res Rev. 2017;30:50–72.
4. Bresnahan KA, Tanumihardjo SA. Undernutrition, the acute phase response to infection, and its effects on micronutrient status indicators. Adv Nutr. 2014;5:702–11.
5. Fitzpatrick F, Skally M, O'Hanlon C, et al. Food for thought: malnutrition risk associated with increased risk of healthcare-associated infection. J Hosp Infect. 2019;101:300–4.
6. Graf D, DiCagno R, Fak F, et al. Contribution of diet to the composition of the human gut microbiota. Microb Ecol Health Dis. 2015;26:26164.
7. Singh RK, Chang HW, Yan D, et al. Influence of diet on the gut microbiome and implications for human health. J Transl Med. 2017;15:73.
8. Partula V, Mondot S, Torres MJ, et al. Association between usual diet and gut microbiota composition: results from the *Milieu Intérieur* cross-sectional study. Am J Clin Nutr. 2019;109:1472–83.
9. Million M, Diallo A, Raoult D. Gut microbiota and malnutrition. Microb Pathog. 2017;106:127–38.
10. Nogueira T, David PHC, Pothier J. Antibiotics as both friends and foes of the human gut microbiome: the microbial community approach. Drug Dev Res. 2018:1–12.
11. Reijnders D, Goossens GH, Hermes GDA, et al. Effects of gut microbiota manipulation by antibiotics on host metabolism in obese humans: a randomized double-blind placebo-controlled trial. Cell Metab. 2016;24:63–74.
12. Schneeberger PHH, Coulibaly JT, Gueuning M, et al. Off-target effects of tribendimidine, tribendimidine plus ivermectin, tribendimidine plus oxantel-pamoate, and albendazole plus oxantel-pamoate on the human gut microbiota. Int J Parasitol Drugs Drug Resist. 2018;8:372–8.
13. Santos CA, Boullata JI. An approach to evaluating drug-nutrient interactions. Pharmacotherapy. 2005;25:1789–800.
14. Boullata JI, Hudson LM. Drug-nutrient interactions: a broad view with implications for practice. J Acad Nutr Diet. 2012;112:506–17.
15. Boullata JI. Drug and nutrition interactions: not just food for thought. J Clin Pharm Ther. 2013;38:269–71.

16. Lange H, Eggers R, Bircher J. Increased systemic availability of albendazole when taken with a fatty meal. Eur J Clin Pharmacol. 1988;34:315–7.
17. Humphries D, Nguyen S, Kumar S, et al. Effectiveness of albendazole for hookworm varies widely by community and correlates with nutritional factors: a cross-sectional study of school-age children in Ghana. Am J Trop Med Hyg. 2017;96:347–54.
18. Kupferschmidt HH, Fattinger KE, Ha HR, Follath F, Krahenbuhl S. Grapefruit juice enhances the bioavailability of the HI protease inhibitor saquinavir in man. Br J Clin Pharmacol. 1998;45:355–9.
19. Ahn CY, Kim EJ, Kwon JW, et al. Effects of cysteine on the pharmacokinetics of intravenous clarithromycin in rats with protein-calorie malnutrition. Life Sci. 2003;73:1783–94.
20. Humphrey JH. Child undernutrition, tropical enteropathy, toilets, and handwashing. Lancet. 2009;374:1032–5.
21. Ikezaki H, Furusyo N, Jacques PF, et al. Higher dietary cholesterol and ω-3 fatty acid intakes are associated with a lower success rate of *Helicobacter pylori* eradication therapy in Japan. Am J Clin Nutr. 2017;106:581–8.
22. Fleisher D, Sweet BV, Parekh A, Boullata JI. Drug absorption with food. In: Boullata JI, Armenti VT, editors. Handbook of drug-nutrient interactions. 2nd ed. New York: Humana Press; 2010. p. 209–41.
23. Deng J, Zhu X, Chen Z, et al. A review of food-drug interactions on oral drug absorption. Drugs. 2017;77:1833–55.
24. Benet LZ. The role of BCS (Biopharmaceutics Classification System) and BDDCS (Biopharmaceutics Drug Disposition Classification System) in drug development. J Pharm Sci. 2013;102:34–42.
25. Hughes GS, Heald DL, Barker KB, et al. The effects of gastric pH and food on the pharmacokinetics of a new oral cephalosporin, cefpodoxime proxetil. Clin Pharmacol Ther. 1989;46:674–85.
26. Eshelman FN, Spyker DA. Pharmacokinetics of amoxicillin and ampicillin: crossover study of the effect of food. Antimicrob Agents Chemother. 1978;14:539–43.
27. Minami R, Inotsume N, Nakano M, et al. Effect of milk on absorption of norfloxacin in healthy volunteers. J Clin Pharmacol. 1993;33:1238–40.
28. Bolme P, Eriksson M, Paalzow L, et al. Malnutrition and pharmacokinetics of penicillin in Ethiopian children. Pharmacol Toxicol. 1995;76:259–62.
29. Tzanis E, Manley A, Villano S, et al. Effect of food on the bioavailability of omadacycline in healthy participants. J Clin Pharmacol. 2017;57:321–7.
30. Courtney R, Wexler D, Radwanski E, Lim J, Laughlin M. Effect of food on the relative bioavailability of two oral formulations of posaconazole in healthy adults. Br J Clin Pharmacol. 2004;57:218–2.
31. Purkins L, Wood N, Kleinermans D, Greenhalgh K, Nichols D. Effect of food on the pharmacokinetics of multiple-dose oral voriconazole. Br J Clin Pharmacol. 2003;56(Suppl 1):17–23.
32. Lin T-Y, Yang M-H, Chang F-Y. A randomized, phase I, 3-way crossover study to examine the effects of food on the pharmacokinetics of single doses of 400 mg posaconazole oral suspension in healthy male Taiwanese subjects. Ther Drug Monit. 2013;35:223–7.
33. Kumar AKH, Chandrasekaran V, Kumar AK, et al. Food significantly reduces plasma concentrations of first-line anti-tuberculosis drugs. Indian J Med Res. 2017;145:530–5.
34. Busti AJ, Hall RG, Margolis DM. Atazanavir for the treatment of human immunodeficiency virus infection. Pharmacotherapy. 2004;24:1732–47.
35. Sekar V, Kestens D, Spinosa-Guzman S, et al. The effect of different meal types on the pharmacokinetics of darunavir (TMC114)/ritonavir in HIV-negative healthy volunteers. J Clin Pharmacol. 2007;47:479–84.
36. Zhang QH, Yang J, He Y, Liu F, Wang JP, Davey AK. Food effect on the pharmacokinetics of entecavir from dispersible tablets following oral administration in healthy Chinese volunteers. Arzneimittelforschung. 2010;60:640–4.
37. O'Shea JP, Holm R, O'Driscoll CM, Griffin BT. Food for thought: formulating away the food effect – a PEARRL review. J Pharm Pharmacol. 2019;71:510–35.
38. Wu J, Gießmann T, Lang B, Elgadi M, Huang F. Investigation of the effect of food and omeprazole on the relative bioavailability of a single oral dose of 240 mg faldaprevir, a selective inhibitor of HCV NS3/4 protease, in an open-label, randomized, three-way cross-over trial in healthy participants. J Pharm Pharmacol. 2016;68:459–66.
39. Behm MO, Yee KL, Liu R, et al. The effect of food on doravirine bioavailability: results from two pharmacokinetic studies in healthy subjects. Clin Drug Investig. 2017;37:571–9.
40. Shiomi M, Matsuki S, Ikeda A, et al. Effects of a protein-rich drink or a standard meal on the pharmacokinetics of elvitegravir, cobicistat, emtricitabine and tenofovir in healthy Japanese male subjects: a randomized, three-way crossover study. J Clin Pharmacol. 2014;54:640–8.
41. Yamada H, Ikushima I, Nemoto T, et al. Effects of a nutritional protein-rich drink on the pharmacokinetics of elvitegravir, cobicistat, emtricitabine, tenofovir alafenamide, and tenofovir compared with a standard meal in healthy Japanese male subjects. Clin Pharmacol Drug Dev. 2018;7:132–42.
42. Abdissa A, Olsen MF, Yilma D, et al. Lipid-based nutrient supplements do not affect efavirenz but lower plasma nevirapine concentrations in Ethiopian adult HIV patients. HIV Med. 2015;16:403–11.
43. Curatolo W, Liu P, Johnson BA, et al. Effects of food on a gastrically degraded drug: azithromycin fast-dissolving gelatin capsules and HPMC capsules. Pharm Res. 2011;28:1531–9.

44. Crevoisier C, Handschin J, Barre J, Roumenov D, Kleinbloesem C. Food increases the bioavailability of mefloquine. Eur J Clin Pharmacol. 1997;53:135–9.
45. Ogunbona FA, Smith IF, Olawoye OS. Fat contents of meals and bioavailability of griseofulvin in man. J Pharm Pharmacol. 1985;37:283–4.
46. Guzzo CA, Furtek CI, Porras AG, et al. Safety, tolerability, and pharmacokinetics of escalating high doses of ivermectin in healthy adults subjects. J Clin Pharmacol. 2002;42:1122–33.
47. Raman S, Polli JE. Prediction of positive food effect: bioavailability enhancement of BCS class II drugs. Int J Pharm. 2016;506:110–5.
48. Miyajima A, Yamamoto Y, Hirota T. Effect of high fat intake on the pharmacokinetic profile of ivermectin in rabbits. Drug Metab Pharmacokinet. 2015;30:253–6.
49. Homeida MM, Malcolm SB, ElTayeb AZ, et al. The lack of influence of food and local alcoholic brew on the blood level of Mectizan® (ivermectin). Acta Trop. 2013;127:97–100.
50. Cloarec N, Solas C, Ladaique A, et al. Sub-therapeutic darunavir concentration and garlic consumption; a "Mediterranean" drug-food interaction, about 2 cases. Eur J Clin Pharmacol. 2017;73:1331–3.
51. Li L, Koo SH, Limenta LMG, et al. Effect of dietary purines on the pharmacokinetics of orally administered ribavirin. J Clin Pharmacol. 2009;49:661–7.
52. Morimoto K, Kishimura K, Nagami T, et al. Effect of milk on the pharmacokinetics of oseltamivir in healthy volunteers. J Pharm Sci. 2011;100:3854–61.
53. Neuvonen PJ, Kivistö KT, Lehto P. Interference of dairy products with the absorption of ciprofloxacin. Clin Pharmacol Ther. 1991;50(5 Pt 1):498–502.
54. Sadrieh N, Brower J, Yu L, et al. Stability, dose uniformity, and palatability of three counterterrorism drugs: human subject and electronic tongue studies. Pharm Res. 2005;22:1747–56.
55. Wright DH, Pietz SL, Konstatinides FN, Rotschafer JC. Decreased in vitro fluoroquinolone concentrations after admixture with an enteral feeding formulation. JPEN J Parenter Enteral Nutr. 2000;24:42–8.
56. Boullata JI. Drug preparation & administration, with a user guide to the monographs. In: Boullata JI, editor. Guidebook on enteral medication administration. Silver Spring: American Society for Parenteral and Enteral Nutrition; 2019. p. 94–117.
57. Koegelenberg CFN, Nortje A, Lalla U, et al. The pharmacokinetics of enteral antituberculosis drugs in patients requiring intensive care. S Afr Med J. 2013;103:394–8.
58. Cattaneo D, Baldelli S, Minisci D, et al. When food can make the difference: the case of elvitegravir-based co-formulation. Int J Pharm. 2016;512:301–4.
59. Bailey DG. Grapefruit and other fruit juices interactions with medicines. In: Boullata JI, Armenti VT, editors. Handbook of drug-nutrient interactions. 2nd ed. New York: Humana Press; 2010. p. 267–302.
60. Johnson EJ, Won CS, Köck K, Paine MF. Prioritizing pharmacokinetic drug interaction precipitants in natural products: application to OATP inhibitors in grapefruit juice. Biopharm Drug Dispos. 2017;38:251–9.
61. Kashihara Y, Ieiri I, Yoshikado T, et al. Small-dosing clinical study: pharmacokinetic, pharmacogenomics (SLCO2B1 and ABCG2), and interaction (atorvastatin and grapefruit juice) profiles of 5 probes for OATP2B1 and BCRP. J Pharm Sci. 2017;106:2688–94.
62. Chen M, Zhou S-Y, Fabriaga E, Zhang P-H, Zhou Q. Food-drug interactions precipitated by fruit juices other than grapefruit juice: an update review. J Food Drug Anal. 2018;26:S61–71.
63. Theile D, Hohmann N, Kiemel D, et al. Clementine juice has the potential for drug interactions: in vitro comparison with grapefruit and mandarin juice. Eur J Pharm Sci. 2017;97:247–56.
64. Jeremiah K, Denti P, Chigutsa E, et al. Nutritional supplementation increases rifampin exposure among tuberculosis patients coinfected with HIV. Antimicrob Agents Chemother. 2014;58:3468–74.
65. Nga TT, Winichagoon P, Dijkhuizen MA, et al. Decreased parasite load and improved cognitive outcomes caused by deworming and consumption of multi-micronutrient fortified biscuits in rural Vietnamese schoolchildren. Am J Trop Med Hyg. 2011;85:333–40.
66. Ronis MJJ, Pedersen KB, Watt J. Adverse effects of nutraceuticals and dietary supplements. Annu Rev Pharmacol. 2018;58:583–601.
67. Piscitelli SC, Burstein AH, Welden N, Gallicano KD, Falloon J. The effect of garlic supplements on the pharmacokinetics of saquinavir. Clin Infect Dis. 2002;34:234–8.
68. Egert S, Rimbach G. Which sources of flavonoids: complex diets or dietary supplements? Adv Nutr. 2011;2:8–14.
69. Dreiseitel A, Oosterhuis B, Vukman KV, Schreier P, Oehme A, Locher S, et al. Berry anthocyanins and anthocyanidins exhibit distinct affinities for the efflux transporters BCRP and MDR1. Br J Pharmacol. 2009;158:1942–50.
70. Sand PG, Dreiseitel A, Stang M, Schreier P, Oehme A, Locher S, et al. Cytochrome P450 2C19 inhibitory activity of common berry constituents. Phytother Res. 2010;24:304–7.
71. Bahramsoltani R, Rahimi R, Farzaei MH. Pharmacokinetic interactions of curcuminoids with conventional drugs: a review. J Ethnopharmacol. 2017;209:1–12.

72. Anderson KE. Effects of specific foods and dietary components on drug metabolism. In: Boullata JI, Armenti VT, editors. Handbook of drug-nutrient interactions. 2nd ed. New York: Humana Press; 2010. p. 243–65.

73. Ronis MJJ, Chen Y, Liu X, et al. Enhanced expression and glucocorticoid-inducibility of hepatic cytochrome P450 3A involve recruitment of the pregnane-X-receptor promoter elements in rats fed soy protein isolate. J Nutr. 2011;141:10–6.

74. Payne LG, Koski KG, Ortega-Barria E, Scott ME. Benefit of vitamin A supplementation on Ascaris reinfection is less evident in stunted children. J Nutr. 2007;137:1455–9.

75. Chen K, Xie HM, Tian W, Zheng X, Jiang AC. Effect of single-dose albendazole and vitamin A supplementation on the iron status of pre-school children in Sichuan, China. Br J Nutr. 2016;115:1415–23.

76. Humphries D, Simms BT, Davey D, et al. Hookworm infection among school age children in Kintampo North Municipality, Ghana: nutritional risk factors and response to albendazole treatment. Am J Trop Med Hyg. 2013;89:540–8.

77. Tcherniuk SO, Chesnokova O, Oleinikov IV, Oleinikov AV. Nicotinamide inhibits the growth of *P. falciparum* and enhances the antimalarial effect of artemisinin, chloroquine and pyrimethamine. Mol Biochem Parasitol. 2017;216:14–20.

78. Jun DW, Kim BI, Cho YK, et al. Efficacy and safety of entecavir plus carnitine complex (GODEX) compared to entecavir monotherapy in patient with ALT elevated chronic hepatitis B: randomized, multicenter open-label trials. Clin Mol Hepatol. 2013;19:165–72.

79. Rocco A, Compare D, Coccoli P, et al. Vitamin $B_{12}$ supplementation improves rates of sustained viral response in patients chronically infected with hepatitis C virus. Gut. 2013;62:766–73.

80. Sun M-G, Huang Y, Xu Y-H, Cao Y-X. Efficacy of vitamin B complex as an adjuvant therapy for the treatment of complicated vulvovaginal candidiasis: an in vivo and in vitro study. Biomed Pharmacother. 2017;88:770–7.

81. Avci P, Freire F, Banvolgyi A, et al. Sodium ascorbate kills *Candida albicans* in vitro via iron-catalyzed Fenton reaction: importance of oxygenation and metabolism. Future Microbiol. 2016;11:1535–47.

82. Wang Y, Jia XM, Jia JH, et al. Ascorbic acid decreases the antifungal effect of fluconazole in the treatment of candidiasis. Clin Exp Pharmacol Physiol. 2009;36:e40–6.

83. Moreira MA, Nascimento MA, Bozzo TA, et al. Ascorbic acid reduces gentamicin-induced nephrotoxicity in rats through the control of reactive oxygen species. Clin Nutr. 2014;33:296–301.

84. Kaboli SA, Zojaji H, Mirsattari D, et al. Effect of addition of vitamin C to clarithromycin-amoxicillin-omeprazole triple regimen on *Helicobacter pylori* eradication. Acta Gastroenterol Belg. 2009;72:222–4.

85. Sezikli M, Çetinkaya ZA, Güzelbulut F, et al. Supplementing vitamins C and E to standard triple therapy for the eradication of *Helicobacter pylori*. J Clin Pharm Ther. 2012;37:282–5.

86. Chuang C-H, Sheu B-S, Huang A-H, Yang H-B, Wu J-J. Vitamin C and E supplements to lansoprazole-amoxicillin-metronidazole triple therapy may reduce the eradication rate of metronidazole-susceptible *Helicobacter pylori* infection. Helicobacter. 2002;7:310–6.

87. Pierpaoli E, Cirioni O, Barucca A, et al. Vitamin E supplementation in old mice induces antimicrobial activity and improves the efficacy of daptomycin in an animal model of wounds infected with methicillin-resistant *Staphylococcus aureus*. J Antimicrob Chemother. 2011;66:2184–5.

88. Provinciali M, Cirioni O, Orlando F, et al. Vitamin E improves the in vivo efficacy of tigecycline and daptomycin in an animal model of wounds infected with methicillin-resistant *Staphylococcus aureus*. J Med Microbiol. 2011;60:1806–12.

89. Chandrasekaran P, Saravanan N, Bethunaickan R, Tripathy S. Malnutrition: modulator of immune responses in tuberculosis. Front Immunol. 2017;8:1316.

90. Jolliffe DA, Ganmaa D, Wejse C, et al. Adjunctive vitamin D in tuberculosis treatment: meta-analysis of individual participant data. Eur Respir J. 2019;53:1802003.

91. Turner AN, Carr Reese P, Fields K. A blinded, randomized controlled trial of high-dose vitamin D supplementation to reduce recurrence of bacterial vaginosis. Am J Obstet Gynecol. 2014;11:479.

92. Custodio E, López-Alcalde J, Herrero M, et al. Nutritional supplements for patients being treated for active visceral leishmaniasis. Cochrane Database Syst Rev. 2018;3:CD012261.

93. Lomaestro BM, Bailie GR. Quinolone-cation interaction: a review. Ann Pharmacother. 1991;25:1249–58.

94. Pai MP, Allen SE, Amsden GW. Altered steady state pharmacokinetics of levofloxacin in adult cystic fibrosis patients receiving calcium carbonate. J Cyst Fibros. 2006;5:153–7.

95. Song I, Borland J, Arya N, Wynne B, Piscitelli S. Pharmacokinetics of dolutegravir when administered with mineral supplements in healthy adult subjects. J Clin Pharmacol. 2015;55:490–6.

96. Ryan KN, Stephenson KB, Trehan I, et al. Zinc or albendazole attenuates the progression of environmental enteropathy: a randomized controlled trial. Clin Gastroenterol Hepatol. 2014;12:1507–13.

97. Casey GJ, Tinh TT, Tien NT, et al. Sustained effectiveness of weekly iron-flic acid supplementation and regular deworming over 6 years in women in rural Vietnam. PLoS Negl Trop Dis. 2017;11:e0005446.

98. Alwarawrah Y, Kiernan K, MacIver NJ. Changes in nutritional status impact immune cell metabolism and function. Front Immunol. 2018;9:1055.
99. Falagas ME, Kompoti M. Obesity and infection. Lancet Infect Dis. 2006;6:438–46.
100. Black RE, Allen LH, Bhutta ZA, et al. Maternal and child undernutrition: global and regional exposures and health consequences. Lancet. 2008;371:243–60.
101. Ibrahim MK, Zambruni M, Melby CL, Melby PC. Impact of childhood malnutrition on host defense and infection. Clin Microbiol Rev. 2017;30:919–71.
102. Stephenson CB. Primer on immune response and interface with malnutrition. In: Humphries DL, Scott ME, Vermund SH, editors. Nutrition and infectious disease: shifting the clinical paradigm. Springer Nature Switzerland AG, 2021.
103. World Health Organization. Updates on the management of severe acute malnutrition in infants and children. Geneva: WHO; 2013.
104. Trehan I, Goldbach HS, LaGrone LN, et al. Antibiotics as part of the management of severe acute malnutrition. N Engl J Med. 2013;368:425–35.
105. Lazzerini M, Tickell D. Antibiotics in severely malnourished children: systematic review of efficacy, safety and pharmacokinetics. Bull World Health Organ. 2011;89:593–606.
106. Alcoba G, Kerac M, Breysse S, et al. Do children with uncomplicated severe acute malnutrition need antibiotics? A systematic review and meta-analysis. PLoS One. 2013;8:e53184.
107. Trehan I, Maleta KM, Manary MJ. Antibiotics for uncomplicated severe malnutrition. N Engl J Med. 2013;368:2436–7.
108. Isanaka S, Langendorf C, Berthé F, et al. Routine amoxicillin for uncomplicated severe acute malnutrition in children. N Engl J Med. 2016;374:444–53.
109. Berkley JA, Ngari M, Thitiri J, et al. Daily co-trimoxazole prophylaxis to prevent mortality in children with complicated severe acute malnutrition: a multicentre, double-blind, randomized placebo-controlled trial. Lancet Glob Health. 2016;4:e464–73.
110. Williams PCM, Berkley JA. Guidelines for the treatment of severe acute malnutrition: a systematic review of the evidence for antimicrobial therapy. Paediatr Int Child Health. 2018;38:S32–49.
111. Chisti MJ, Salam MA, Bardhan PK, et al. Treatment failure and mortality amongst children with severe acute malnutrition presenting with cough or respiratory difficulty and radiological pneumonia. PLoS One. 2015;10:e0140327.
112. Maitland K, Berkley JA, Shebbe M, Peshul N, English M, Newon CR. Children with severe malnutrition: can those at highest risk of death be identified with the WHO protocol? PLoS Med. 2006;3:2431–9.
113. Walter-Sack I, Klotz U. Influence of diet and nutritional status on drug metabolism. Clin Pharmacokinet. 1996;31:47–64.
114. Boullata JI. Drug disposition in obesity and protein-energy malnutrition. Proc Nutr Soc. 2010;69:543–50.
115. Jacques KA, Erstad BL. Availability of information for dosing injectable medications in underweight or obese patients. Am J Health Syst Pharm. 2010;67:1948–50.
116. Oshikoya KA, Sammons HM, Choonara I. A systematic review of pharmacokinetics studies in children with protein-energy malnutrition. Eur J Clin Pharmacol. 2010;66:1025–35.
117. Polso AK, Lassiter JL, Nagel JL. Impact of hospital guideline for weight-based antimicrobial dosing in morbidly obese adults and comprehensive literature review. J Clin Pharm Ther. 2014;39:584–608.
118. Natale S, Bradley J, Nguyen WH, et al. Pediatric obesity: pharmacokinetic alterations and effects on antimicrobial dosing. Pharmacotherapy. 2017;37:361–78.
119. Pai MP. Drug dosing based on weight and body surface area: mathematical assumptions and limitations in obese adults. Pharmacotherapy. 2012;32:856–68.
120. Janmahasatian S, Duffull SB, Ash S, et al. Quantification of lean body-weight. Clin Pharmacokinet. 2005;44:1051–65.
121. Beckman LM, Boullata JI, Fisher PL, Compher CW, Earthman CP. Evaluation of lean body weight equation by dual-energy X-ray absorptiometry measures. JPEN J Parenter Enteral Nutr. 2017;41:392–7.
122. Compher CW, Boullata JI. Influence of protein-calorie malnutrition on medication. In: Boullata JI, Armenti VT, editors. Handbook of drug-nutrient interactions. 2nd ed. New York: Humana Press; 2010. p. 137–65.
123. Boullata JI. Influence of overweight and obesity on medication. In: Boullata JI, Armenti VT, editors. Handbook of drug-nutrient interactions. 2nd ed. New York: Humana Press; 2010. p. 167–205.
124. Eriksson M, Paalzow L, Bolme P, Mariam TW. Chloramphenicol pharmacokinetics in Ethiopian children of differing nutritional status. Eur J Clin Pharmacol. 1983;24:819–23.
125. Polasa K, Murthy KJR, Krishnaswamy K. Rifampicin kinetics in undernutrition. Br J Clin Pharmacol. 1984;17:481–4.
126. Walker O, Dawodu AH, Salako LA, Alvan G, Johnson AOK. Single disposition of chloroquine in kwashiorkor and normal children: evidence for decreased absorption in kwashiorkor. Br J Clin Pharmacol. 1987;23:467–2.

127. Lares-Asseff I, Cravioto J, Santiago P, Perez-Ortiz B. Pharmacokinetics of metronidazole in severely malnourished and nutritionally rehabilitated children. Clin Pharmacol Ther. 1992;51:42–50.

128. Mehta S, Nain CK, Sharma B, Mathur VS. Metabolism of sulfadiazine in children with protein calorie malnutrition. Pharmacology. 1980;21:369–74.

129. Bravo IG, Bravo ME, Plate G, Merlez J, Arancibia A. The pharmacokinetics of cotrimoxazole sulphonamide in malnourished (marasmic) infants. Pediatr Pharmacol. 1984;4:167–76.

130. Mehta S, Nain CK, Sharma B, Mathur VS. Steady state of chloramphenicol in malnourished children. Indian J Med Res. 1981;73:538–42.

131. Mehta S, Nain CK, Kalsi HK, Mathur VS. Bioavailability and pharmacokinetics of chloramphenicol palmitate in malnourished children. Indian J Med Res. 1981;74:244–50.

132. Ashton M, Bolme P, Alemayehu E, Eriksson M, Paalzow L. Decreased chloramphenicol clearance in malnourished Ethiopian children. Eur J Clin Pharmacol. 1993;45:181–6.

133. Bravo ME, Arancibia A, Jarpa S, Carpentier PM, Jahn AN. Pharmacokinetics of gentamicin in malnourished infants. Eur J Clin Pharmacol. 1982;21:499–504.

134. Seaton C, Ignas J, Muchohi S, et al. Population pharmacokinetics of a single daily intramuscular dose of gentamicin in children with severe malnutrition. J Antimicrob Chemother. 2007;59:681–9.

135. Buchanan N, Davis MD, Eyberg C. Gentamicin pharmacokinetics in kwashiorkor. Br J Clin Pharmacol. 1979;8:451–3.

136. Khan AM, Ahmed T, Alam NH, Chowdhury AK, Fuchs GJ. Extended-interval gentamicin administration in malnourished children. J Trop Pediatr. 2006;52:179–84.

137. Nehru B, Mehta S, Nain CK, Mathur VS. Disposition of sulphadiazine in young rhesus monkeys with protein calorie malnutrition. Int J Clin Pharmacol Ther Toxicol. 1988;26:509–12.

138. Pussard E, Barennes H, Daouda H, et al. Quinine disposition in globally malnourished children with cerebral malaria. Clin Pharmacol Ther. 1999;65:500–10.

139. Kadam PP, Gogtay NJ, Karande S, Shah V, Thatte UM. Evaluation of pharmacokinetics of single-dose chloroquine in malnourished children with malaria: a comparative study with normally nourished children. Indian J Pharmacol. 2016;48:498–502.

140. Thuo N, Ungphakorn W, Karisa J, et al. Dosing regimens of oral ciprofloxacin for children with severe malnutrition: a population pharmacokinetic study with Monte Carlo simulation. J Antmicrob Chemother. 2011;66:2336–45.

141. Buchanan N, Robinson P, Koornhof HJ, Eyberg C. Penicillin pharmacokinetics in kwashiorkor. Am J Clin Nutr. 1979;32:2233–6.

142. Buchanan N, Mithal Y, Witcomb M. Cefoxitin: intravenous pharmacokinetics and intramuscular bioavailability in kwashiorkor. Br J Clin Pharmacol. 1980;9:623–7.

143. Kohli K, Aggarwal KK, Bhatt IN. The pharmacokinetic profile of chloramphenicol in protein-malnourished rats. Indian J Med Res. 1981;73:208–17.

144. Smith JA, Butler TC, Poole DT. Effect of protein depletion in guinea-pigs on glucoronate conjugation of chloramphenicol by liver microsomes. Biochem Pharmacol. 1973;22:981–3.

145. Tulupule A, Krishnaswamy K. Chloroquine kinetics in the undernourished. Eur J Clin Pharmacol. 1984;24:273–6.

146. Roy V, Gupta D, Gupta P, Sethi GR, Mishra TK. Pharmacokinetics of isoniazid in moderately malnourished children with tuberculosis. Int J Tuberc Lung Dis. 2010;14:374–6.

147. Treluyer JM, Roux A, Mugnier C, Largadere B. Metabolism of quinine in children with global malnutrition. Pediatr Res. 1996;40:558–63.

148. Salako LA, Sowunmi A, Akinbami FO. Pharmacokinetics of quinine in African children suffering from kwashiorkor. Br J Clin Pharmacol. 1989;28:197–201.

149. Lares-Asseff I, Lugo-Goytia G, Pérez-Guillé MG, et al. Bayesian prediction of chloramphenicol blood levels in children with sepsis and malnutrition. Rev Investig Clin. 1999;51:159–65.

150. Lares-Asseff I, Cravioto J, Santiago P, Pérez-Ortíz B. A new dosing regimen for metronidazole in malnourished children. Scand J Infect Dis. 1993;25:115–21.

151. Mehta S. Malnutrition and drugs: clinical implications. Dev Pharmacol Ther. 1990;15:159–65.

152. Eriksson M, Bolme P, Habte D, Paalzow L. INH and streptomycin in Ethiopian children with tuberculosis and different nutritional status. Acta Paediatr Scand. 1988;77:890–4.

153. te Brake LHM, Ruslami R, Later-Nijland H, et al. Exposure to total and protein-unbound rifampin is not affected by malnutrition in Indonesian tuberculosis patients. Antimicrob Agents Chemother. 2015;59:3233–9.

154. Lee AEK, Ahn CY, Kim EJ, et al. Effects of cysteine on the pharmacokinetics of itraconazole in rats with protein-calorie malnutrition. Biopharm Drug Disp. 2003;24:63–70.

155. Archary M, McIlleron H, Bobat R, et al. Population pharmacokinetics of lopinavir in severely malnourished HIV-infected children and the effect on treatment outcome. Pediatr Infect Dis J. 2018;37:349–55.

156. Catalán-Latorre A, Nácher A, Merino V, Jiménez-Torres NV, Merino-Sanjuán M. In situ study of the effect of naringin, talinolol and protein-energy undernutrition on intestinal absorption of saquinavir in rats. Basic Clin Pharmacol Toxicol. 2011;109:245–52.
157. Bartelink IH, Savic RM, Dorsey G, et al. The effect of malnutrition on the pharmacokinetics and virologic outcomes of lopinavir, efavirenz and nevirapine in food insecure HIV-infected children in Tororo, Uganda. Pediatr Infect Dis J. 2015;34:e63–70.
158. Pollock L, Else L, Poerksen G, et al. Pharmacokinetics of nevirapine in HIV-infected children with and without malnutrition receiving divided adult fixed-dose combination tablets. J Antimicrob Chemother. 2009;64:1251–9.
159. Verret WJ, Arinaitwe E, Wanzira H, et al. Effect of nutritional status on response to treatment with artemisinin-based combination therapy in young Ugandan children with malaria. Antimicrob Agents Chemother. 2011;55:2629–35.
160. Denoeud-Ndam L, Dicko A, Baudin E, et al. A multi-center, open-label trial to compare the efficacy and pharmacokinetics of artemether-lumefantrine in children with severe acute malnutrition versus children without severe acute malnutrition: study protocol for the MAL-NUT study. BMC Infect Dis. 2015;15:228.
161. Denoeud-Ndam L, Dicko A, Baudin E, et al. Efficacy of artemether-lumefantrine in relation to drug exposure in children with and without severe acute malnutrition: an open comparative intervention study in Mali and Niger. BMC Med. 2016;14:167.
162. Djimde M, Samouda H, Jacobs J, et al. Relationship between weight status and anti-malarial drug efficacy and safety in children in Mali. Malar J. 2019;18:40.
163. Lautermann J, Schacht J. Reduced nutritional status enhances ototoxicity. Laryngoscope. 1995;74:724–7.
164. Gunther T, Rebentisch E, Vormann J, Konig M, Ising H. Enhanced ototoxicity of gentamicin and salicylate caused by Mg deficiency and Zn deficiency. Biol Trace Elem Res. 1988;16:43–50.
165. Sodhi CP, Rana SF, Attri S, Mehta S, Yaiphei K, Mehta SK. Oxidative-hepatic injury of isoniazid-rifampicin in young rats subjected to protein and energy malnutrition. Drug Chem Toxicol. 1998;21:305–17.
166. Lares-Asseff I, Pérz-Guillé MG, Camacho Vieyra GA, et al. Population pharmacokinetics of gentamicin in Mexican children with severe malnutrition. Pediatr Infect Dis J. 2016;35:872–8.
167. Boyd SE, Charani E, Lyons T, Frost G, Holmes AH. Information provision for antibacterial dosing in the obese patient: a sizeable absence? J Antimicrob Chemother. 2016;71:3588–92.
168. Gade C, Christensen HR, Dalhoff KP, Holm JC, Holst H. Inconsistencies in dosage practice in children with overweight or obesity: a retrospective cohort study. Pharmacol Res Perspect. 2018;2:e00398.
169. Forse RA, Karam B, MacLean LD, Christ NV. Antibiotic prophylaxis for surgery in morbidly obese patients. Surgery. 1989;106:750–7.
170. Choi JJ, Moffett BS, McDade EJ, Palazzi DL. Altered gentamicin serum concentrations in obese pediatric patients. Pediatr Infect Dis J. 2011;30:347–9.
171. Pai MP, Nafziger AN, Bertino JS. Simplified estimation of aminoglycoside pharmacokinetics in underweight and obese adult patients. Antimicrob Agents Chemother. 2011;55:4006–11.
172. Moffett BS, Kam C, Galati M, et al. The "ideal" body weight for pediatric gentamicin dosing in the era of obesity: a population pharmacokinetic analysis. Ther Drug Monit. 2018;40:322–9.
173. Bookstaver PB, Bland CM, Qureshi ZP, et al. Safety and effectiveness of daptomycin across a hospitalized obese population: results of a multicenter investigation in the southeastern United States. Pharmacotherapy. 2013;33:1322–30.
174. Butterfield-Cowper JM, Lodise TP, Pai MP. A fixed versus weight-based dosing strategy of daptomycin may improve safety in obese adults. Pharmacotherapy. 2018;38:981–5.
175. Fox AN, Smith WJ, Kupiec KE, et al. Daptomycin dosing in obese patients: analysis of the use of adjusted body weight versus actual body weight. Ther Adv Infect Dis. 2019;6:1–10.
176. Dvorchik BH, Damphousse D. The pharmacokinetics of daptomycin in moderately obese, morbidly obese, and matched nonobese subjects. J Clin Pharmacol. 2005;45:48–56.
177. Pai MP, Norenberg JP, Anderson T, et al. Influence of morbid obesity on the single-dose pharmacokinetics of daptomycin. Antimicrob Agents Chemother. 2007;51:2741–7.
178. Bhavnani SM, Rubino CM, Ambrose PG, Drusano GL. Daptomycin exposure and the probability of elevations in the creatine phosphokinase level: data from a randomized trial of patients with bacteremia and endocarditis. Clin Infect Dis. 2010;50:1568–74.
179. Pea F, Cojutti P, Sbrojavacca R, et al. TDM-guided therapy with daptomycin and meropenem in a morbidly obese, critically ill patient. Ann Pharmacother. 2011;45:e37.
180. Miller M, Miller JL, Hagemann TM, et al. Vancomycin dosage in overweight and obese children. Am J Health Syst Pharm. 2011;68:2062–8.
181. Reynolds DC, Waite LH, Alexander DP, DeRyke CA. Performance of a vancomycin dosage regimen developed for obese patients. Am J Health Syst Pharm. 2012;69:944–50.
182. Pai MP, Hong J, Krop L. Peak measurement for vancomycin AUC estimation in obese adults improves precision and lowers bias. Antimicrob Agents Chemother. 2017;61:e02490–16.

183. Choi YC, Saw S, Soliman D, et al. Intravenous vancomycin associated with the development of nephrotoxicity in patients with class III obesity. Ann Pharmacother. 2017;51:937–44.

184. Leong JVB, Boro MS, Winter ME. Determining vancomycin clearance in an overweight and obese population. Am J Health Syst Pharm. 2011;68:599–603.

185. Morrill HJ, Caffrey AR, Noh E, LaPlante KL. Vancomycin dosing considerations in a real-world cohort of obese and extremely obese patients. Pharmacotherapy. 2015;35:869–75.

186. Lin H, Yeh DD, Levine AR. Daily vancomycin dose requirements as a continuous infusion in obese versus non-obese SICU patients. Crit Care. 2016;20:205.

187. Mersfelder TL, Smith CL. Linezolid pharmacokinetics in an obese patient. Am J Health Syst Pharm. 2005;62:464–7.

188. Tsuji Y, Hiraki Y, Matsumoto K. Evaluation of the pharmacokinetics of linezolid in an obese Japanese patient. Scand J Infect Dis. 2012;44:626–9.

189. Muzevich KM, Lee KB. Subtherapeutic linezolid concentrations in a patient with morbid obesity and methicillin-resistant *Staphylococcus aureus* pneumonia: case report and review of the literature. Ann Pharmacother. 2013;47:e25.

190. Smith MJ, Gonzalez D, Goldman JL, et al. Pharmacokinetics of clindamycin in obese and nonobese children. Antimicrob Agents Chemother. 2017;61:e02014–6.

191. Hall RG. Evolving larger: dosing anti-tuberculosis (TB) drugs in an obese world. Curr Pharm Des. 2015;21:4748–51.

192. Hall RG, Pasipanodya JG, Meek C, et al. Fractal geometry-based decrease in trimethoprim-sulfamethoxazole concentrations in overweight and obese people. CPT Pharmacometrics Syst Pharmacol. 2016;5:674–81.

193. Lopez ND, Phillips KM. Fluconazole pharmacokinetics in a morbidly obese, critically ill patient receiving continuous venovenous hemofiltration. Pharmacotherapy. 2014;34:e162–8.

194. Alobaid AS, Wallis SC, Jarrett P, et al. Effect of obesity on the population pharmacokinetics of fluconazole in critically ill patients. Antimicrob Agents Chemother. 2016;60:6550–7.

195. Payne KD, Hall RG. Dosing of antifungal agents in obese people. Expert Rev Anti-Infect Ther. 2016;14:257–67.

196. Pai MP, Lodise TP. Steady-state plasma pharmacokinetics of oral voriconazole in obese adults. Antimicrob Agents Chemother. 2011;55:2601–5.

197. Koselke E, Kraft S, Smith J, Nagel J. Evaluation of the effect of obesity on voriconazole serum concentrations. J Antimicrob Chemother. 2012;67:2957–62.

198. Davies-Vorbrodt S, Ito JI, Tegtmeier BR, Dadwal SS, Kriengkauykiat J. Voriconazole serum concentrations in obese and overweight immunocompromised patients: a retrospective review. Pharmacotherapy. 2013;33:22–30.

199. Moriyama B, Jarosinski PF, Figg WD, et al. Pharmacokinetics of intravenous voriconazole in obese patients: implications of CYP2C19 homozygous poor metabolizer genotype. Pharmacotherapy. 2013;33:e19–22.

200. Ryan DM, Lupinacci RJ, Kartsonis NA. Efficacy and safety of caspofungin in obese patients. Med Mycol. 2011;49:748–54.

201. Hall RG, Swancutt MA, Meek C, Leff R, Gumbo T. Weight drives caspofungin pharmacokinetic variability in overweight and obese people: fractal power signatures beyond two-thirds or three-fourths. Antimicrob Agents Chemother. 2013;57:2259–64.

202. Ferriols-Lisart R, Aguilar G, Pérez-Pitarch A, et al. Plasma concentrations of caspofungin in a critically ill patient with morbid obesity. Crit Care. 2017;21:200.

203. Maseda E, Grau S, Luque S, et al. Population pharmacokinetics/pharmacodynamics of micafungin against *Candida* species in obese, critically ill, and morbidly obese critically ill patients. Crit Care. 2018;22:94.

204. Gillum JG, Johnson M, Lavoie S, Venitz J. Flucytosine dosing in an obese patient with extrameningeal cryptococcal infection. Pharmacotherapy. 1995;15:251–3.

205. Hernandez JO, Norstrom J, Wysock G. Acyclovir-induced renal failure in an obese patient. Am J Health Syst Pharm. 2009;66:1288–91.

206. Seedat A, Winnett G. Acyclovir-induced acute renal failure and the importance of an expanding waist line. BMJ Case rep. 2012; pii:bcr2012006264.

207. Smith TC, Kim JH, Gast CM, Benefield RJ. Pharmacokinetics of acyclovir in a morbidly obese patient with renal impairment. Int J Antimicrob Agents. 2016;47:340–1.

208. Turner RB, Cumpston A, Sweet M, et al. Prospective, controlled study of acyclovir pharmacokinetics in obese patients. Antimicrob Agents Chemother. 2016;60:1830–3.

209. Madelain V, Le MP, Champenois K, et al. Impact of obesity on antiretroviral pharmacokinetics and immunovirological response in HIV-infected patients: a case-control study. J Antimicrob Chemother. 2017;72:1137–46.

210. de Roche M, Siccardi M, Stoeckle M, et al. Efavirenz in an obese HIV-infected patient: a report and an in vitro-in vivo extrapolation model indicate risk of underdosing. Antivir Ther. 2012;17:1381–4.

211. Pai MP, Lodise TP. Oseltamivir and oseltamivir carboxylate pharmacokinetics in obese adults: dose modification for weight is not necessary. Antimicrob Agents Chemother. 2011;55:5640–5.

212. Jittamala P, Pukrittayakamee S, Tarning J, et al. Pharmacokinetics of orally administered oseltamivir in healthy obese and nonobese Thai subjects. Antimicrob Agents Chemother. 2014;58:1615–21.

213. Chairat K, Jittamala P, Hanpithakpong W, et al. Population pharmacokinetics of oseltamivir and oseltamivir carboxylate in obese and non-obese volunteers. Br J Clin Pharmacol. 2016;81:1103–12.
214. Piccolo KM, Boullata JI. The influence of polypharmacy on nutrition. In: Bendich A, Deckelbaum RJ, editors. Preventive nutrition. 5th ed. New York: Humana Press; 2016. p. 83–113.
215. U.S. Food and Drug Administration. Drug databases: FDA approved drug products. https://www.accessdata.fda.gov/scripts/cder/daf/. Accessed 29 July 2019.
216. Angelakis E, Merhej V, Raoult D. Related actions of probiotics and antibiotics on gut microbiota and weight modification. Lancet Infect Dis. 2013;13:889–99.
217. Raoult D. Microbiota, obesity and malnutrition. Microb Pathog. 2017;106:1–2.
218. Chop E, Duggaraju A, Malley A, Burke V, Caldas S, Yeh PT, et al. Food insecurity, sexual risk behavior, and adherence to antiretroviral therapy among women living with HIV: a systematic review. Health Care Women Int. 2017;38(9):927–44.
219. Cousins T. Antiretroviral therapy and nutrition in Southern Africa: citizenship and the grammar of hunger. Med Anthropol. 2016;35(5):433–46.
220. Koethe JR, Blevins M, Bosire C, Nyirenda C, Kabagambe EK, Mwango A, et al. Self-reported dietary intake and appetite predict early treatment outcome among low-BMI adults initiating HIV treatment in sub-Saharan Africa. Public Health Nutr. 2013;16(3):549–58.
221. Sunguya BF, Poudel KC, Otsuka K, Yasuoka J, Mlunde LB, Urassa DP, et al. Undernutrition among HIV-positive children in Dar es Salaam, Tanzania: antiretroviral therapy alone is not enough. BMC Public Health. 2011;11:869.
222. D'Amico AV, Stanford J. Probiotic use and clindamycin-induced hypercholesterolemia. J Altern Complement Med. 2009;15:470–1.
223. Esposito S, Pinzani R, Raffaeli G, et al. A young infant with transient severe hypertriglyceridemia temporarily associated with meropenem administration. Medicine. 2016;95(38):e4872.
224. Marinella MA. Case report: reversible hyperkalemia associated with trimethoprim-sulfamethoxazole. Am J Med Sci. 1995;310:115–7.
225. Spiller RC, Higgins BE, Frost PG, Silk DB. Inhibition of jejunal water and electrolyte absorption by therapeutic doses of clindamycin in man. Clin Sci. 1984;67:117–20.
226. Biehl JP, Vilter RW. Effects of isoniazid on pyridoxine metabolism. JAMA. 1954;156:1549–52.
227. Clark F. Drugs and vitamin deficiency. Adv Drug React Bull. 1976;57:196–9.
228. McConnell RB, Cheetham HD. Acute pellagra during isoniazid therapy. Lancet. 1952;2:959–60.
229. Okan G, Yaylaci S, Alzafer S. Pellagra: will we see it more frequently? J Eur Acad Dermatol Venereol. 2009;23:365–6.
230. Post FA. Pellagra: a rare complication of isoniazid therapy. Int J Tuberc Lung Dis. 2016;20:1136.
231. Minns AB, Ghafouri N, Clark RF. Isoniazid-induced status epilepticus in a pediatric patient after inadequate pyridoxine therapy. Pediatr Emerg Care. 2010;26:380–1.
232. Aiwale AS, Patel UA, Barvaliya MJ, Jha PR, Tripathi C. Isoniazid induced convulsions at therapeutic dose in an alcoholic and smoker patient. Curr Drug Saf. 2015;10:94–5.
233. van der Watt JJ, Harrison TB, Benatar M, Heckmann JM. Polyneuropathy, anti-tuberculosis treatment and the role of pyridoxine in the HIV/AIDS era: a systematic review. Int J Tuberc Lung Dis. 2011;15:722–8.
234. Centner CM, Carrara H, Harrison TB, Benatar M, Heckmann JM. Sensory polyneuropathy in human immunodeficiency virus-infected patients receiving tuberculosis treatment. Int J Tuberc Lung Dis. 2014;18:27–33.
235. van der Watt JJ, Benatar M, Harrison TB, Carrara H, Heckmann JM. Isoniazid exposure and pyridoxine levels in human immunodeficiency virus associated distal sensory neuropathy. Int J Tuberc Lung Dis. 2015;19:1312–9.
236. Zhou Y, Jiao Y, Yu-Hui W, et al. Effects of pyridoxine on the intestinal absorption and pharmacokinetics of isoniazid in rats. Eur J Drug Metab Pharmacokinet. 2013;38:5–13.
237. Brodie MJ, Boobis AR, Hillyard CJ, et al. Effect of rifampicin and isoniazid on vitamin D metabolism. Clin Pharmacol Ther. 1982;32:525–30.
238. Tostmann A, Wielders JPM, Kibiki GS, et al. Serum 25-hydroxy-vitamin D3 concentrations increase during tuberculosis treatment in Tanzania. Int J Tuberc Lung Dis. 2010;14:1147–52.
239. Welz T, Childs K, Ibrahim F, et al. Efavirenz is associated with severe vitamin D deficiency and increased alkaline phosphatase. AIDS. 2010;24:1923–8.
240. Orkin C, Wohl DA, Williams A, Deckx H. Vitamin D deficiency in HIV: a shadow on long-term management? AIDS Rev. 2014;16:59–74.
241. Nylen H, Habtewold A, Makonnen E, et al. Prevalence and risk factors for efavirenz-based antiretroviral treatment-associated severe vitamin D deficiency: a prospective cohort study. Medicine. 2016;95(34):e4631.
242. Wegler C, Wikvall K, Norlin M. Effects of osteoporosis-inducing dugs on vitamin D-related gene transcription and mineralization in MG-63 and Saos-2 cells. Basic Clin Pharmacol Toxicol. 2016;119:436–42.

243. Etminani-Esfahani M, Khalili H, Jafari S, Abdollahi A, Dashti-Khavidaki S. Effects of vitamin D supplementation on the bone specific biomarkers in HIV infected individuals under treatment with efavirenz. BMC Res Notes. 2012;5:204.

244. Kumar N, Bower M, Nelson M. Severe vitamin D deficiency in a patient treated for hepatitis B with tenofovir. Int J STD AIDS. 2012;23:59–60.

245. Mateo L, Holgado S, Mariñosa ML, et al. Hypophosphatemic osteomalacia induced by tenofovir in HIV-infected patients. Clin Rheumatol. 2016;35:1271–9.

246. Hajek J, Ouma S, Hemmett J, Starko R, Apiyo P. Chest deformity and disability due to tenofovir-induced hypophosphatemia osteomalacia: case report and call for improved global access to laboratory testing. J Int Assoc Provid AIDS Care. 2017;16:430–2.

247. Havens PL, Kiser JJ, Stephensen CB, et al. Association of higher plasma vitamin D binding protein and lower free calcitriol levels with tenofovir disoproxil fumarate use and plasma and intracellular tenofovir pharmacokinetics: cause of a functional vitamin D deficiency? Antimicrob Agents Chemother. 2013;57:5619–28.

248. Havens PL, Hazra R, Stephensen CB, et al. Vitamin D3 supplementation increases fibroblast growth factor-23 in HIV-infected youth treated with tenofovir disoproxil fumarate. Antivir Ther. 2014;19:613–8.

249. Chen N, Zhang J-B, Zhang Q, et al. Adefovir dipivoxil induced hypophosphatemic osteomalacia in chronic hepatitis B: a comparative study of Chinese and foreign case series. BMC Pharmacol Toxicol. 2018;19:23.

250. Gerber B, Guggenberger R, Fasler D, et al. Reversible skeletal disease and high fluoride serum levels in hematologic patients receiving voriconazole. Blood. 2012;120:2390–4.

251. Moon WJ, Scheller EL, Sunej A, et al. Plasma fluoride level as a predictor of voriconazole-induced periostitis in patients with skeletal pain. Clin Infect Dis. 2014;59:1237–45.

252. Flax VL, Adair LS, Allen LH, et al. Plasma micronutrient concentrations are altered by antiretroviral therapy and lipid-based nutrient supplements in lactating HIV-infected Malawian women. J Nutr. 2015;145:1950–7.

253. Allen LH, Hampel D, Shahab-Ferdows S, et al. Antiretroviral therapy provided to HIV-infected Malawian women in a randomized trial diminishes the positive effects of lipid-based nutrient supplements on breast-milk B vitamins. Am J Clin Nutr. 2015;102:1468–74.

254. Kaio DJI, Rondó PHC, Luzia LA, et al. Vitamin E concentrations in adults with HIV/AIDS on highly active antiretroviral therapy. Nutrients. 2014;6:3641–52.

255. Mintz M. Carnitine in human immunodeficiency virus type 1 infection/acquired immune deficiency syndrome. J Child Neurol. 1995;10(Suppl):2S40–4.

256. Stork CM, Marraffa JM, Ragosta K, Wojcik SM, Angelino KL. Elevated international normalized ratio associated with long-term azithromycin therapy in a child with cerebral palsy. Am J Health Syst Pharm. 2011;68:1012–4.

257. Fotouhie A, Desai H, King S, Parsa NA. Gastrointestinal bleeding secondary to trimethoprim-sulfamethoxazole-induced vitamin K deficiency. BMJ Case Rep. 2016. https://doi.org/10.1136/bcr-2016-214437.

258. Renko K, Martitz J, Hybsier S, et al. Aminoglycoside-driven biosynthesis of selenium-deficient selenoprotein P. Sci Rep. 2017;7:4391.

259. Wiehe L, Cremer M, Wisniewska M, et al. Selenium status in neonates with connatal infection. Br J Nutr. 2016;116:504–13.

260. Felsenstein S, Herbert JA, McNamara PS, Hedrich CM. COVID-19: immunology and treatment options. Clin Immunol. 2020;215:108448.

261. Zhang L, Liu Y. Potential interventions for novel coronavirus in China: a systemic review. J Med Virol. 2020;92:479–90.

262. Li X, Wang L, Yan S, et al. Clinical characteristics of 25 death cases with COVID-19: a retrospective review of medical records in a single medical center, Wuhan, China. Int J Infect Dis. 2020;94:128–32.

263. Blanco-Melo D, Nilsson-Payant BE, Liu WC, et al. Imbalanced host response to SARS-CoV-2 drives development of COVID-19. Cell. 2020;181:1036–45.

264. Esposito S, Noviello S, Pagliano P. Update on treatment of COVID-19: ongoing studies between promising and disappointing results. Infez Med. 2020;2:198–211.

265. Wang D, Lu J. Glycan arrays lead to the discovery of autoimmunogenic activity of SARS-CoV. Physiol Genomics. 2004;18:245–8.

266. Marshall E, Enserink M. Caution urged on SARS vaccines. Science. 2004;303:944–6.

267. Bolles M, Deming D, Long K, et al. A double-inactivated severe acute respiratory syndrome coronavirus vaccine provides incomplete protection in mice and induces increased eosinophilic proinflammatory pulmonary response upon challenge. J Virol. 2011;85:12201–15.

268. Keyaerts E, Vijgen L, Maes P, Neyts J, Van Ranst M. In vitro inhibition of severe acute respiratory syndrome coronavirus by chloroquine. Biochem Biophys Res Commun. 2004;323:264–8.

269. Vincent MJ, Bergeron E, Benjannet S, et al. Chloroquine is a potent inhibitor of SARS coronavirus infection and spread. Virol J. 2005;2:69.

270. Wang M, Cao R, Zhang L, et al. Remdesivir and chloroquine effectively inhibit the recently emerged novel coronavirus (2019-nCoV) in vitro. Cell Res. 2020;30:269–71.
271. Gao J, Tian Z, Yang X. Breakthrough: chloroquine phosphate has shown apparent efficacy in treatment of COVID-19 associated pneumonia in clinical studies. Biosci Trends. 2020;14:72–3.
272. Gautret P, Lagier JC, Parola P, et al. Hydroxychloroquine and azithromycin as a treatment of COVID-19: results of an open-label non-randomized clinical trial. Int J Anticmicrob Agents. 2020. https://doi.org/10.1016/j.ijantimicag.2020.105949.
273. Molina JM, Delaugerre C, Le Goff J, et al. No evidence of rapid antiviral clearance or clinical benefit with the combination of hydroxychloroquine and azithromycin in patients with severe COVID-19 infection [letter]. Med Mal Infect. 2020;50:384.
274. Derwand R, Scholz M. Does zinc supplementation enhance the clinical efficacy of chloroquine/hydroxychloroquine to win today's battle against COVID-19? Med Hypotheses. 2020;142:109815.
275. Holshue ML, DeBolt C, Lindquist S, et al. First case of 2019 novel coronavirus in the United States. N Engl J Med. 2020;382:929–36.
276. Grein J, Ohmagari N, Shin D, et al. Compassionate use of remdesivir for patients with severe Covid-19. N Engl J Med. 2020;382:2327–36.
277. Zabetakis I, Lordan R, Norton C, Tsoupras A. COVID-19: the inflammation link and the role of nutrition in potential mitigation. Nutrients. 2020;12:1466.
278. Zhang X, Song K, Tong F, et al. First case of covid-19 in a patient with multiple myeloma successfully treated with tocilizumab. Blood Adv. 2020;4:1307–10.
279. Mihai C, Dobrota R, Schröder M, et al. COVID-19 in a patient with systemic sclerosis treated with tocilizumab for SSc-ILD. Ann Rheum Dis. 2020;79:668–9.
280. Luo P, Liu Y, Qiu L, et al. Tocilizumab treatment in COVID-19: a single center experience. J Med Virol. 2020;92:814–8.
281. Ciavarella C, Motta I, Valente S, Pasquinelli G. Pharmacological (or synthetic) and nutritional agonists of PPAR-g as candidates for cytokine storm modulation in COVID-19 disease. Molecules. 2020;25:2076.
282. Jayawardena R, Sooriyaarachchi P, Chourdakis M, Jeewandara C, Ranasinghe P. Enhancing immunity in viral infections, with special emphasis on COVID-19: a review. Diabetes Metab Syndr Clin Res Rev. 2020;14:367–82.
283. Butler MJ, Barrientos RM. The impact of nutrition on COVID-19 susceptibility and long-term consequences. Brain Behav Immun. 2020. https://doi.org/10.1016/j.bbi.2020.04.040.
284. Luzi L, Radaelli MG. Influenza and obesity: its odd relationship and the lessons for COVID-19 pandemic. Acta Diabetol. 2020;57:759–64.
285. Beck MA, Handy J, Levander OA. Host nutritional status: the neglected virulence factor. Trends Microbiol. 2004;12:417–23.
286. Briguglio M, Pregliasco FE, Lombardi G, Perazzo P, Banfi G. The malnutritional status of the host as a virulence factor for new coronavirus SARS-CoV-2. Front Med. 2020;7:146.
287. Liu G, Zhang S, Mao Z, Wang W, Hu H. Clinical significance of nutritional risk screening for older adult patients with COVID-19. Eur J Clin Nutr. 2020;74:876–83.
288. Li T, Zhang Y, Gong C, et al. Prevalence of malnutrition and analysis of related factors in elderly patients with COVID-19 in Wuhan, China. Eur J Clin Nutr. 2020;74:871–5.
289. Yang X, Yu Y, Xu J, et al. Clinical course and outcomes of critically ill patients with SARS-CoV-2 pneumonia in Wuhan, China: a single-centered, retrospective, observational study. Lancet Respir Med. 2020;8:475–81.
290. Grant WB, Lahore H, McDonnell SL, et al. Evidence that vitamin D supplementation could reduce risk of influenza and COVID-19 infections and deaths. Nutrients. 2020;12:988.
291. Shi Y, Liu T, Yao LI, et al. Chronic vitamin D deficiency induces lung fibrosis through activation of the renin-angiotensin system. Sci Rep. 2017;7:3312.
292. Panareses A, Shahini E. Covid-19, and vitamin D [letter]. Aliment Pharmacol Ther. 2020;51:993–5.
293. Jakovac H. COVID-19 and vitamin D: is there a link and an opportunity for intervention? Am J Physiol Endocrinol Metab. 2020;318:E589.
294. Facchiano A, Facchiano A, Bartoli M, Ricci A, Facchiano F. Reply to Jakovac: about COVID-19 and vitamin D. Am J Physiol Endocrinol Metab. 2020;318:E838.
295. Teymoori-Rad M, Shokri F, Salimi V, Marashi SM. The interplay between vitamin D and viral infections. Rev Med Virol. 2019;29:e2032.
296. D'Avolio A, Avataneo V, Manca A, et al. 25-Hydroxyvitamin D concentrations are lower in patients with positive PCR for SARS-CoV-2. Nutrients. 2020;12:1359.
297. Bogden JD. Influence of zinc on immunity in the elderly. J Nutr Health Aging. 2004;8:48–54.
298. Barnett JB, Hamer DH, Meydani SN. Low zinc status: a new risk factor for pneumonia in the elderly? Nutr Rev. 2009;68:30–7.
299. Read SA. The role of zinc in antiviral immunity. Adv Nutr. 2019;10:696–710.

300. Skalny A, Rink L, Ajsuvakova OP, et al. Zinc and respiratory tract infections: perspectives for COVID-19. Int J Mol Med. 2020;46:17–26.
301. Adams KK, Baker WL, Sobieraj DM. Myth busters: dietary supplements and COVID-19. Ann Pharmacother. 2020. https://doi.org/10.1177/10600280209280.
302. Horne JR, Vohl M-C. Biological plausibility for interactions between dietary fat, resveratrol, ACE2, and SARS-CoV illness severity. Am J Physiol Endocrinol Metab. 2020;318:E830–3.
303. Caccialanza R, Laviano A, Lobascio F, et al. Early nutritional supplementation in non-critically ill patients hospitalized for the 2019 novel coronavirus disease (COVID-19): rationale and feasibility of a shared pragmatic protocol. Nutrition. 2020;74:110835.
304. Barazzoni R, Bischoff SC, Krznaric Z, et al. ESPEN expert statements and practice guidance for nutritional management of individuals with SARS-CoV-2 infection. Clin Nutr. 2020;39:1631–8.
305. Romano L, Bilotta F, Dauri M, et al. Short report: medical nutrition therapy for critically ill patients with COVID-19. Eur Rev Med Pharmacol Sci. 2020;24:4035–9.
306. American Society for Parenteral & Enteral Nutrition. Resources for clinicians caring for patients with coronavirus (12 June 2020). Available at: https://www.nutritioncare.org/ResourcesCOVID19/
307. Morita M, Kuba K, Ichikawa A, et al. The lipid mediator protectin D1 inhibits influenza virus replication and improves severe influenza. Cell. 2013;153:112–25.
308. Russell CD, Schwarze J. The role of pro-resolution lipid mediators in infectious disease. Immunology. 2013;141:166–73.
309. Cheng RZ. Can early and high intravenous dose of vitamin C prevent and treat coronavirus disease 2019 (COVID-19)? Med Drug Discov. 2020;5:100028.
310. Xu C, Zhu L, Chan T, et al. Chloroquine and hydroxychloroquine are novel inhibitors of human organic anion transporting polypeptide 1A2. J Pharm Sci. 2016;105:P884–90.
311. Browning DJ, Easterbrook M, Lee C. The 2016 American Academy of Ophthalmology hydroxychloroquine dosing guidelines for short, obese patients. Ophthalmol Retina. 2019;3:809–13.
312. Liang X, Chien H-C, Yee SW, et al. Metformin is a substrate and inhibitor of the human thiamine transporter, THTR-2 (SLC19A3). Mol Pharm. 2015;12:4301–10.
313. Alsiö Å, Rembeck K, Askarieli G, et al. Impact of obesity on the bioavailability of peginterferon-α2a and ribavirin and treatment outcome for chronic hepatitis C genotype 2 or 3. PLoS One. 2012;7:e37521.
314. Delaleu J, Destere A, Hachon L, Declèves X, Lloret-Linares C. Glucocorticoids dosing in obese subjects: a systematic review. Therapie. 2019;74:451–8.
315. Shittu MO, Afolami OI. Improving the efficacy of chloroquine and hydroxchloroquine against SARS-CoV-2 may require zinc additives: a better synergy for future COVID-19 clinical trials. Infez Med. 2020;2:192–7.
316. te Velthuis AJW, van den Worm SHE, Sims AC, et al. $Zn^{2+}$ inhibits coronavirus and arterivirus RNA polymerase activity in vitro and zinc ionophores block the replication of these viruses in cell culture. PLoS Pathog. 2010;6:e1001176.

# Chapter 14
# Co-infection and Nutrition: Integrating Ecological and Epidemiological Perspectives

Vanessa O. Ezenwa

## Abbreviations

| | |
|---|---|
| IL | Interleukin |
| STH | Soil-transmitted helminth |
| HIV | Human immunodeficiency virus |
| IFN | Interferon |
| pABA | Para-aminobenzoic acid |
| TB | Tuberculosis |
| Th | T helper |

**Key Points**

- Most hosts, including humans, livestock, and wild animals, are infected by more than one parasite species simultaneously.
- Like co-infection, the co-occurrence of multiple nutritional deficiencies is common, and both phenomena frequently affect the same populations.
- Ecological approaches that construct and analyze feeding relationships between species can shed light on complex co-infection-nutrition interactions.
- A feeding relationship (or "trophic") approach suggests at least two key pathways by which constraints on the availability of nutrients to a host might influence interactions between parasites: resource competition and immune-mediated interactions.
- Combining a trophic approach with epidemiological data has practical clinical applications for developing a better understanding of how changes in nutritional status influence disease severity during co-infection and predicting how disease control strategies (e.g., drug treatment, vaccination) might impact nutritional status.
- For example, simultaneous resource- and immune-mediated interactions between hookworm and *Plasmodium falciparum* during co-infection may explain a counterintuitive protective effect of co-infection on anemia.

V. O. Ezenwa (✉)
Odum School of Ecology & Department of Infectious Diseases, College of Veterinary Medicine, University of Georgia, Athens, GA, USA
e-mail: vezenwa@uga.edu

© Springer Nature Switzerland AG 2021
D. L. Humphries et al. (eds.), *Nutrition and Infectious Diseases*, Nutrition and Health, https://doi.org/10.1007/978-3-030-56913-6_14

- Likewise, accounting for the interrelationships among host nutrient availability, parasite resource use, and host immune function suggests that protein deficiency may affect the outcome of helminth-tuberculosis co-infection.

## Introduction

Heterogeneities in both nutrition and infection pose ongoing challenges to global health. A common phenomenon that contributes to these heterogeneities is concurrent infection, or co-infection. Most hosts, including humans, livestock, and wild animals, are infected by more than one parasite species simultaneously [1, 2], and co-infection is the norm rather than the exception in real-world populations. For example, a survey of 500 residents of a single village in Côte d'Ivoire aged 5 days to 91 years revealed that 75% of the population carried three or more parasite infections simultaneously [3]. The study only considered a subset of helminth and protozoan parasites, so it is likely that true co-infection rates were even higher than reported. A similar study, focused on a broader set of parasites, including bacteria, protozoa, helminths, and arthropods, showed that among pregnant and lactating women in rural Panama, co-infections between multiple pairs of parasite species were common [4]. For example, 80% of pregnant women were co-infected by *Bacteroides/Gardnerella* and *Mobiluncus* bacteria, while nearly 50% were co-infected by the bacteria *Lactobacillus* and the protozoa *Trichomonas* [4]. These anecdotes illustrate the magnitude of the co-infection problem. Yet despite the fact that co-infection is so common, its range of consequences are still poorly understood.

One consequence of co-infection that warrants particular attention is the link between co-infection and nutrition. Like co-infection, the co-occurrence of multiple nutritional deficiencies is extremely common, and both phenomena frequently affect the same populations. Indeed, nearly 50% of women in the Panamanian study cohort where frequent co-infection was described [4] also had two or more vitamin deficiencies [5]. For single parasite infections, interactions between infection and nutrition, including effects of infection on nutrition and effects of nutrition on infection, have been the subject of considerable study (see Chap. 1 [6]). Synergistic interactions between nutrition and infection have also been considered, where undernutrition increases susceptibility to infection and resulting increases in infection further magnify undernutrition [7, 8]. Applying the same level of scrutiny to the bidirectional linkages between co-infection and nutrition, including the potential for "vicious circles" to operate, remains a critical frontier in nutrition-infection research.

A small but growing number of studies on nutrition and infection are now considering co-infection. For example, in one of the first studies of its kind, Ezeamama and colleagues [9] showed that, among children in the Philippines, concurrent infection with multiple helminth species increased the odds of anemia five- to eight-fold, including for low-intensity infections previously thought to have very little impact on child morbidity. Given that iron deficiency anemia is a major driver of nutritional deficiency worldwide [10], this study highlighted the disproportionately strong effects co-infection could have on nutritional outcomes when compared to single infection. More generally, over the past 25 years, studies focused specifically on co-infection and malnutrition have gone from less than 1% of papers published on the topic of infection and malnutrition in 1995–1999 to over 4% in 2014–2018 (Fig. 14.1). The central focus of this emerging body of co-infection-malnutrition research has been on a few key infections including human immunodeficiency virus (HIV), tuberculosis (TB), helminths, malaria, and various intestinal pathogens (e.g., enteroinvasive *Escherichia coli*, *Giardia*, *Helicobacter pylori*). HIV-TB co-infection is by far the single most common co-infection studied (see Chap. 9 [11]), followed by co-infections between gastrointestinal intestinal parasites (including helminths) and helminth-malaria co-infection. While the majority of this work has focused on humans, recent studies are also expanding the suite of animal models used to investigate co-infection-malnutrition phenomenon to laboratory

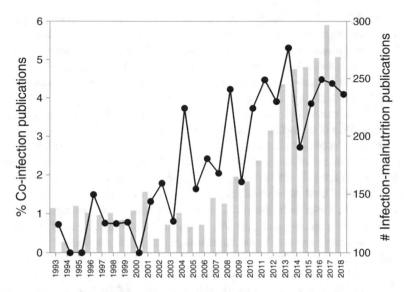

**Fig. 14.1** Annual percent of papers published on the topic of malnutrition and co-infection between 1993 and 2018 (primary axis) as compared to the total number of papers published on nutrition and any type of infection (secondary axis). Data are from a PubMed search performed on 29 May 2019. Search terms were: Title/Abstract = ((co-infection* OR coinfection* OR polyparasitism*) AND (malnutrition OR undernutrition)) for determining the number of papers focused on co-infection and Title/Abstract = ((infection* OR parasitism*) AND (malnutrition OR undernutrition) NOT (co-infection* OR coinfection* OR polyparasitism*)) for determining the number of papers focused on single infections. Counts from the two searches were summed to estimate the total number of papers published on any type of infection (plotted on secondary axis)

animals (e.g., mice: [12]) and non-model species (e.g., *Daphnia*: [13]). Overall, this body of work provides an important starting point for understanding the clinical consequences of nutrition-co-infection interactions and identifying the mechanisms that underlie these outcomes.

The goal of this chapter is to explore our current understanding of co-infection-nutrition interactions by integrating ideas and data from the ecological and epidemiological literature. To do this, I begin by describing an ecological framework for studying species interactions that can be applied to co-infection and nutrition. Second, with this framework in mind, I use two common co-infections as case studies to examine what we know about how co-infection affects nutrition (helminths and malaria) and, reciprocally, how nutrition affects co-infection (helminths and TB). Co-infection and nutrition are complex problems in their own right, and the body of literature on their interactions is still relatively small (see Chap. 9 for a detailed discussion of HIV-TB-nutrition interactions [11]). As such, the ultimate objective of this exercise is not to provide an exhaustive summary of the current state of knowledge on co-infection-nutrition interactions but rather to draw insights from a melding of ecological ideas with epidemiological data that may help guide future research. I conclude with a discussion of the practicalities of merging ecological and epidemiological approaches to study co-infection and nutrition and an outlook on the future.

## An Ecological Framework for Integrating Co-infection and Nutrition

Ecological communities are characterized by complex networks of interactions among species [14]. These interactions can be direct, occurring between two species, or indirect, with the relationship between two species mediated by a third species or the environmental context [15]. Importantly, species interactions differ in both direction and strength: some species affect other species negatively, such as a predator that consumes its prey, whereas some species have positive effects on other species, such as a pollinator that disperses the pollen of its host plant. These interactions can be strong, having relatively large impacts on individuals within the community, or weak [16]. Furthermore, interactions between species are often context dependent, where the outcome changes depending on the context in which it is embedded [17]. Theory and approaches from community ecology provide tools for characterizing and quantifying interactions and dealing with context dependency, and many of these ideas are applicable to communities of parasites residing within individual hosts [18].

One tool for studying species interactions is the food web (Fig. 14.2a). Feeding (or "trophic") relationships between species are often conceptualized as food webs in which primary producers (e.g., plants) comprise the first level; the second level consists of species that consume the primary producers (e.g., herbivores); the third level consists of species that consume the herbivores (e.g., carnivores); and so forth [19]. In this way, a trophic framework is used to understand how energy flows between different compartments of a community and how these flows translate into changes in individual species abundances and community structure. Trophic frameworks are readily applicable to parasite communities residing within hosts (Fig. 14.2b). For parasites, the first level of the food web consists of host resources, represented by specific host tissues on which parasites depend for food or habitat [20]. The second level consists of the parasites, and the third level consists of the host immune system, which is akin to a predator that consumes the parasites [20]. Unique to within-host parasite communities, the first and third levels of the food web are connected because host resources and immune function are

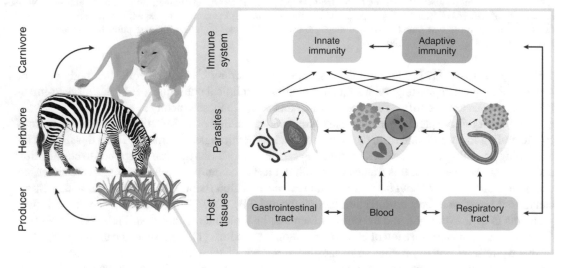

**Fig. 14.2** (a) A classical ecological food web showing feeding or "trophic" relationships between a primary producer (grass), an herbivore (zebra), and a carnivore (lion). (b) A hypothetical within-host food web for a zebra host with an analogous three levels. In this case, the first level of the food web is represented by host tissues in which parasites live and acquire resources (e.g., gastrointestinal tract, blood, respiratory tract). Each of these compartments is connected via a single host energy pool. The second level is occupied by the parasites which reside in different tissue compartments (e.g., gastrointestinal tract, Cyathostomins, *Eimeria*, *Oxyuris*; blood, African horse sickness virus, *Babesia*, *Theileria*; respiratory tract, *Dictyocaulus*, Equine herpesvirus). Strong direct interactions, such as resource competition, can occur between parasites within the same compartment. The third level is comprised of components of the host immune system, which attack parasites from the different compartments. Immune responses triggered by individual parasites can cause indirect, immune-mediated, interactions between parasites within or between tissue compartments. Finally, unlike the classical ecological food web, the top (immune system) and bottom (host tissues) levels of the within-host food web are connected because they both depend on the same pool of host energy

inextricably linked [20]. With this framework in mind, for any given parasite community, trophic relationships can be constructed that link co-infecting species in a manner that facilitates the formulation and testing of hypotheses about which types of parasites are most likely to interact, the mechanisms that drive the interactions, and how these interactions might be shaped by variation in host nutrition. This *trophic approach* is particularly useful for understanding interactions between co-infection and nutrition because the basal layers of within-host food webs (i.e., host tissues) rely on various micro- and macronutrients for growth and maintenance. Consequently, trophic links help identify suites of parasites that are most likely to interact and specific nutrient deficiencies most likely to affect these interactions. For example, red blood cell production is iron dependent, so deficiencies in this micronutrient should most strongly affect interactions between parasites that depend on red blood cells. More broadly, by considering the availability of host nutritional resources, resource use by parasites, host immune defenses, and the interconnections among these processes simultaneously (Fig. 14.2b), a trophic approach can help unravel the myriad complexities associated with co-infection-nutrition interactions. For example, scrutiny of the hypothetical parasite food web in Figure 14.2b reveals at least two key pathways by which constraints on the availability of nutrients to a host might influence interactions between parasites.

First, because multiple parasites often rely on a common pool of host resources, *resource competition* should be a major force shaping interactions between species. Importantly, depletion of the host resource pool due to changes in nutritional status should affect the direction or magnitude of these resource-mediated interactions. Evidence of resource competition between parasite species infecting various animal species is widespread [21]. Recently, the relevance of resource-mediated interactions between human parasites has also gained attention [22]. For example, a longitudinal study of helminth-malaria co-infection showed that blood-sucking hookworms (*Necator americanus* and *Ancylostoma duodenale*) and *Plasmodium* species, all of which rely on red blood cells, interact via this shared resource [23]. This interaction was revealed by a negative effect of hookworm infection on the density of concurrent *P. vivax* (a malaria species which specializes on young RBCs), which was reversed in response to anthelmintic treatment. Interestingly, hookworm had no effect on the density of *P. falciparum*, which unlike *P. vivax* is a red blood cell generalist and thus is potentially less likely to suffer the consequences of resource limitation imposed by hookworms. However, *P. falciparum* co-infection was associated with reduced *Necator* intensity which is likely a manifestation of *P. falciparum*'s superior competitive ability, an idea borne out by the dominant negative effect of *P. falciparum* on host red blood cells [23]. Indeed, the outcome of competitive interactions between parasites is frequently asymmetrical with one species (the weaker competitor) showing large declines in numbers and the other showing little to no change [21]. Identifying and understanding these asymmetries may help with interpreting clinical outcomes of co-infection-nutrition interactions. Importantly, the outcome of competitive interactions between parasites can also depend on the availability of shared resources, as revealed by a study of mouse malaria (*P. chabaudi*) showing strong nutrient-driven changes in the intensity of competitive interactions between two parasite strains [24]. While this observation suggests that in many circumstances host nutrition should be a key mediator of both resource competition between parasites and clinical consequences for the host, few studies have tested this idea empirically (but see [24, 25]).

Second, because parasite species commonly share a "predator," i.e., components of the host immune system, *immune-mediated* interactions should also be a key mechanism shaping interactions between parasites. Furthermore, because host nutrition is critical to the functioning of the immune system, variation in host nutrition should strongly affect the outcome of immune-mediated interactions between parasites. As with resource-mediated interactions, interactions between parasites driven by the host immune system also occur [26, 27]. Interactions between helminths and microparasites (including viruses, bacteria, and protozoa), where helminth infections may facilitate infections such as HIV, malaria, and TB, have captured particular attention in the literature [28]. One mechanistic explanation for this interaction is the mutually inhibitory immune defense pathways triggered by helminths vs. intracellular microparasites. Specifically, helminths trigger T helper (Th) 2 type immune responses, characterized by the production of cytokines such as interleukin (IL)4, which downregulate Th1 type cytokines such as interferon gamma (IFN)$\gamma$ and IL12 which are involved in defense against many intracellular pathogens [29, 30]. As one example, a challenge of laboratory mice with either of the helminths *Heligmosomoides*[1] or *Schistosoma mansoni* induced reactivation of murine $\gamma$-herpesvirus 68, a virus that typically establishes lifelong latency in its host [32]. This reactivation effect was due to the upregulation of IL4 in helminth-infected mice, which promoted virus replication and blocked the antiviral effects of IFN$\gamma$, demonstrating a clear immune-mediated interaction. IL4 treatment had similar effects on human Kaposi's sarcoma-associated herpesvirus in human cells [32].

Finally, it is important to note that resource-mediated interactions are not always competitive and immune-mediated interactions are not always facilitative. For example, parasites that share the same habitat within a host may facilitate one another, rather than compete, if one species modifies the habitat for the other in a way that promotes its colonization or growth [33]. Likewise, closely related parasite species often inhibit, rather than facilitate, one another as a result of cross-protective immune responses mounted by the host [34]. Furthermore, resource- and immune-mediated interactions can also occur in tandem. Indeed, many parasites both share a common resource within a host and are subject to the same or mutually inhibitory immune responses, setting the stage for multiple modes of interaction to occur. The beauty of the trophic approach is that it allows for an entire network of possible interactions to be considered simultaneously (Fig. 14.2b). This approach thus provides an excellent starting point for understanding how complex interactions between parasite species shape and are, in turn, shaped by variation in host nutrition. The rest of this chapter uses a trophic perspective to explore these questions, focusing on two prominent examples of helminth co-infections.

# Effects of Co-infection on Nutrition: Helminths and Malaria as a Case Study

The geographic extent and potentially profound clinical consequences of co-infection between helminths and falciparum malaria make it an ideal case study for exploring how co-infection affects nutrition. In Africa, geographic overlap between *Plasmodium falciparum* and the soil-transmitted helminths (STH: *Ascaris lumbricoides*, *Trichuris trichiura*, and hookworms) is extensive, and 17–32 million children in sub-Saharan Africa are estimated to be at risk of coincident STH-*P. falciparum* infection [35]. Hookworm-*P. falciparum* co-infection is particularly interesting because both parasites independently cause anemia. Hookworms cause iron deficiency anemia by inducing intestinal blood loss [36], while *P. falciparum* causes anemia via a number of mechanisms including destruction and removal of red blood cells, reduced erythrocyte production in the bone marrow, and cytokine-mediated dyserythropoiesis [37]. Thus, whether the dual effects of hookworm and *P. falciparum* exacerbate anemia is a topic of emerging interest, with great relevance for managing clinical outcomes of malaria infection.

In the past decade, a number of studies have examined the impact of helminth-malaria co-infection on anemia with mixed results. A large proportion of these studies focused on impacts on children, and the outcomes have been variable (Fig. 14.3). The presence of anemia, defined as a deficiency of red blood cells or hemoglobin, is typically assessed using hemoglobin concentrations. In children, anemia is defined according to WHO guidelines as hemoglobin concentrations below 12 g/dL with severity increasing as hemoglobin concentrations decline [41]. Some studies show

---

[1] *Heligmosomoides bakeri* is synonymous with *Nematospiroides dubius*, *Heligmosomoides polygyrus*, and *Heligmosomoides polygyrus bakeri* [31].

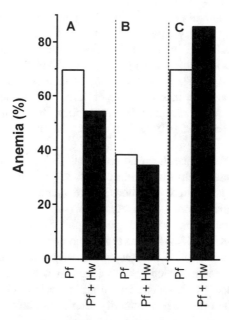

**Fig. 14.3** Examples of variable outcomes from studies comparing anemia prevalence in children infected with malaria (*Plasmodium falciparum*, Pf) only compared to those co-infected with Pf and hookworms (Hw). (**a**) Anemia prevalence was higher in Pf single infection compared to Pf + Hw co-infection for 6–15-year-old children in Ghana (data from [38]). (**b**) The protective effect of Pf + Hw co-infection was similar but weaker for preschool and school-age children in Tanzania (data from [39]). (**c**) However, this pattern was reversed in another study of school-age children in Tanzania, with anemia prevalence increasing by >15% in Pf + Hw co-infected children (data from [40]). Intriguingly, Hw infection intensity was classified as "light" in **a–b**, but "heavy" in **c**

that co-infection tends to worsen anemia. For example, Brooker et al. [42] found that for both preschool and school-age children in Kenya, mean hemoglobin concentrations were lower among hookworm-*P. falciparum* co-infected individuals compared to those infected with hookworm or *P. falciparum* alone. Although this relationship was significant only for preschool children, co-infected school-age children had an average hemoglobin concentration 4.2 g/dL lower than their single-infected counterparts [42]. A study of school-age children in Tanzania reported similar patterns; in this case, the prevalence of anemia increased by >15% among co-infected children compared to those infected with hookworm or *P. falciparum* alone [40]. In direct contrast, other studies found that co-infection had a moderating effect on anemia, particularly when compared to the effects of *P. falciparum* alone. For example, Humphries et al. [38] showed that *P. falciparum* infection significantly increased anemia risk in Ghanaian children aged 6–15, whereas hookworm-*P. falciparum* co-infection did not, suggesting a protective effective of co-infection. Studies of school-age children in Côte d'Ivoire and Tanzania found similar patterns. In Côte d'Ivoire, Righetti et al. [43] reported that for 6–8-year-old children, hookworm-*P. falciparum* co-infection significantly increased hemoglobin concentrations compared to *P. falciparum* infection alone. Likewise, a national school-based survey of children in Côte d'Ivoire found that *P. falciparum* single infection was a significant risk factor for anemia, whereas hookworm-*P. falciparum* co-infection was not [44]. In the Tanzania study, mean hemoglobin concentration was higher in hookworm-*P. falciparum* co-infected preschool and school-age children, and anemia prevalence was correspondingly lower, although these effects were not significant [39]. Overall then, empirical studies either found that hookworm-*P. falciparum* co-infection exacerbates anemia by reducing hemoglobin concentrations or that co-infection improves anemia outcomes relative to single *P. falciparum* infection. Echoing this discordance in the literature, two recent meta-analyses examining the implications of

STH-malaria co-infection for anemia also came to different conclusions. Both analyses were based on a small number (n = 3) of primary studies, two of which were the same and only one of which included hookworm as a focal STH infection. The first of these analyses, Naing et al. [45], concluded that hemoglobin levels in single malaria infected vs. STH-*P. falciparum* co-infected children are comparable. More recently, Degarege et al. [46] concluded that compared to *P. falciparum* infection alone, the odds of anemia in school-age children tend to decrease during STH-*P. falciparum* co-infection. Clearly, more research on the implications of hookworm-*P. falciparum* co-infection for anemia is required to clarify the underlying factors accounting for different patterns observed across studies.

A qualitative analysis of the research on hookworm-*P. falciparum* co-infection and anemia in children reveals trends that may help guide future studies. Crucially, studies where hookworm-*P. falciparum* co-infection was associated with more severe anemia reported that a majority of hookworm-infected children suffered from heavy infections (shedding >2000 parasite eggs per gram feces (epg; [40, 42])). In contrast, studies showing the opposite effect reported that most children had light hookworm infections [38, 39, 43, 44]. This type of context-dependency is a common feature of parasite interactions, with factors such as the density/intensity or virulence of the species involved in the interaction [47], or the order in which species establish within the host [48], determining the outcome of the interaction (Box 14.1). Thus, accounting for variation in hookworm intensity may be key to explaining the opposite outcomes commonly seen in hookworm-*P. falciparum* co-infection studies.

**Box 14.1 Virulence Affects the Outcome of Parasite Co-infection**

Competition between strains of the vector-borne protozoan parasite, *Trypanosoma brucei*, provides an illustrative example of how parasite virulence can alter the outcome of competition during co-infection. *T. brucei* is the causative agent of human trypanosomiasis or African sleeping sickness, a disease of significant public health concern in sub-Saharan Africa. The parasite is transmitted between mammal hosts by the tsetse fly and proliferates in the bloodstream of the host (see Chap. 6). Balmer and colleagues [47] examined the outcome of *T. brucei* strain competition on host survival and condition when competing parasite strains were of equal compared to variable virulence. The researchers created variable and equal virulence treatments by manipulating the virulence of one competing strain (low-virulence "green" strain) but not the other (high-virulence "red" strain). Next, the effects of strain competition on lab mouse hosts were quantified during single and mixed infections under both variable and equal virulence conditions. In the variable virulence experiments (VVE), mixed infection significantly improved mouse survival compared to single infection with the high-virulence "red" strain (Fig. 14.4a). However, in the equal virulence experiments (EVE), survival during mixed infection and single high-virulence infection did not differ (Fig. 14.4a). In terms of host condition, levels of anemia and thrombocytopenia were higher for single high-virulence infections compared to mixed infections in variable virulence conditions, whereas mixed infections caused higher anemia and equivalent thrombocytopenia levels compared to single high-virulence infections in equal virulence conditions (Fig. 14.4b, c). Intriguingly, the outcomes of anemia described under the different *T. brucei* competition scenarios recapitulate exactly the patterns observed in hookworm-*P. falciparum* co-infection for light versus heavy hookworm infections. This similarity in observed patterns suggests there may be a set of general principles that help explain what at first appears to be disparate outcomes of interactions between the same pairs of parasites.

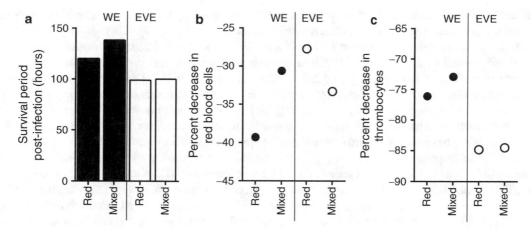

**Fig. 14.4** (**a**) Mean number of hours mice survived after infection with a single high-virulence *Trypanosoma brucei* strain (red) compared to a mixed infection comprised of either the high-virulence red strain and a low-virulence green strain (= variable virulence experiment [VVE]) or the high-virulence red strain and a high-virulence green strain (= equal virulence experiment [EVE]). (**b**) Percent decrease in red blood cells among mice infected with the single high-virulence red strain compared to mixed infections comprised of the high-virulence red strain and the low-virulence green strain (VVE) or the high-virulence red strain and the high-virulence green strain (EVE). (**c**) Percent decrease in thrombocytes among mice infected with the single high-virulence red strain compared to mixed infections comprised of the high-virulence red strain and the low-virulence green strain (VVE) or the high-virulence red strain and the high-virulence green strain (EVE). (Data are from [47])

Similar to the outcome of co-infection between *T. brucei* strains (Box 14.1), the changing nature of the interaction between hookworm and *P. falciparum* in response to variability in the degree to which one parasite negatively affects the host (i.e., virulence) may help explain divergent outcomes of co-infection on anemia. *P. falciparum* tends to be a strong resource extractor nearly always exerting strong virulence effects on its host [49], while the damaging effects of hookworm on hosts are more variable, depending on the intensity of infection [50]. Thus, the presence of light vs. heavy hookworm burdens during co-infection with *P. falciparum* is somewhat analogous to the presence of the low- vs. high-virulence phenotype during *T. brucei* strain co-infection. Interestingly, when hookworm and *P. falciparum* co-occur under light hookworm infection intensity (analogous to the variable virulence experiment described in Box 14.1), the net outcome for the host is a moderation of the negative effect of *P. falciparum*. This is reflected by reduced levels of anemia in light hookworm-*P. falciparum* co-infection compared to single *P. falciparum* infection, a result that qualitatively matches the lower anemia and higher survival rates of mice infected with mixed high- and low-virulence *T. brucei* strains compared to single high-virulence infections (Box 14.1; Fig. 14.4a, b). Thus, a reduction in the severity of infection outcomes may be a general phenomenon arising from co-infection between high- and low-virulence parasites that compete for a shared resource. For hookworm-*P. falciparum* competition specifically, an obvious question is: what are the mechanisms underlying such an effect?

The combined effects of resource-mediated and immune-mediated interactions may explain the reduction in anemia during light hookworm-*P. falciparum* co-infection. At first glance, resource-mediated interactions alone could drive anemia reduction if hookworm has a net suppressive effect on *P. falciparum* density that is not compensated for by direct negative effects of hookworm itself. Mechanistically, this can happen if hookworm imposes resource competition on *P. falciparum* by depleting shared red blood cell resources, thereby reducing *P. falciparum* density. However, this explanation seems unlikely because there is only weak support for strong negative effects of hookworm on *P. falciparum* density in the literature (e.g., [23] but see [51]). Moreover, an alternative hypothesis on immune-mediated interactions suggests that hookworm may facilitate *P. falciparum*, increasing its density by upregulating Th2 cytokines that suppress Th1 responses [52]. Such an effect would increase rather than decrease anemia, but this explanation also seems unlikely because the evidence for positive associations between hookworm and *P. falciparum* density is also weak [46]. It is plausible though that both mechanisms operate in tandem such that negative (resource-mediated) and positive (immune-mediated) effects of hookworm on *P. falciparum* density tend to cancel each other out—this could explain the mixed results regarding correlations between hookworm and *P. falciparum* density during co-infection [46, 53]. In this scenario, there would be no net effect of hookworm on *P. falciparum* density, and since hookworm intensity is light, very little change in anemia would be expected due to effects of hookworm itself. How then does the reduction in anemia come about? A reduction in anemia might plausibly be caused by a third mechanism: the upregulation of anti-inflammatory cytokines (e.g., IL4, IL10) in response to hookworm [52] and concomitant suppression of inflammation-associated anemia [43, 46, 54]. Reductions in anemia during light hookworm-*P. falciparum* co-infection may thus be a direct result of an anti-inflammatory response induced by hookworm. A similar mechanistic explanation has been proposed for why some STH infections are associated with a reduced risk of cerebral malaria [55]. Ultimately then, anemia reduction could be the product of hookworm-associated changes in the inflammatory response occurring in the absence of (i) changes in the density of *P. falciparum* (due to the counterbalanced effects of resource-mediated and immune-mediated interactions between hookworm and *P. falciparum*) and (ii) direct negative effects of hookworm (due to the low intensity of infection). If so, the protective effects of co-infection on anemia emerge from multiple and simultaneous interactions between the two parasites and the immune and resource compartments of the parasite food web (Fig. 14.5). Importantly, because these interactions are identifiable and quantifiable when the

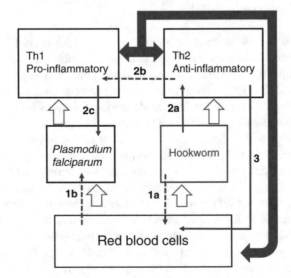

**Fig. 14.5** A full suite of known feeding relationships connecting hookworm and *Plasmodium falciparum* infection that potentially explain the protective effect of light hookworm-*P. falciparum* co-infection on anemia. Open block arrows represent feeding links: both *P. falciparum* and hookworm depend on the same host resource (red blood cells), but different components of the host immune response (Th1 vs. Th2) prey on the two parasites. Solid block arrows show the intrinsic links between different host compartments (immunity [Th1, Th2, pro-inflammatory, anti-inflammatory] and resources [red blood cells]). Red arrows indicate the positive (solid arrows) and negative (dashed arrows) direct and indirect effects of light hookworm infection on *P. falciparum* and consequences for red blood cell numbers. First, hookworm might negatively affect *P. falciparum* by depleting red blood cells (1a) and imposing competitive pressure on *P. falciparum* (1b). Simultaneously, hookworm might positively affect *P. falciparum* by causing the upregulation of the host Th2 response (2a) which downregulates the Th1 response (2b), thereby facilitating *P. falciparum* (2c). These concurrent negative (1b) and positive (2c) indirect effects of hookworm on *P. falciparum* might cancel each other out such that there is no change in the net effect of *P. falciparum* on red blood cell numbers compared to *P. falciparum* single infection. However, because hookworm promotes an anti-inflammatory immune response in the host (2a) which improves red blood cell production (3), but light hookworm infection may not cause substantial red blood cell loss (1a), the net outcome for anemia is positive in this scenario

entire suite of trophic links between hookworm and *P. falciparum* are considered, a trophic approach is a practical tool for making predictions about the clinical outcomes of co-infection (e.g., anemia presence or severity) and how these outcomes should differ by context.

The pattern of increased anemia severity under heavy hookworm-*P. falciparum* co-infection is more intuitive than the anemia reduction observed under light hookworm-*P. falciparum* co-infection—both parasites independently consume host red blood cells inducing more severe anemia. However, the precise mechanisms accounting for this effect still require clarification. For example, under heavy hookworm infection, as with light infection, negative (resource competition) and positive (immune facilitation) effects of hookworm on *P. falciparum* density might still cancel each other out resulting in no net change in *P. falciparum* density and no density-mediated effect on anemia. In addition, inflammation-associated suppression of anemia (via immune effects induced by hookworm) might be counterbalanced by high levels of resource (red blood cell) destruction resulting from heavy hookworm infection, thereby eliminating any protective effect of co-infection. Together these two sets of opposing forces might enable an additive effect of hookworm and *P. falciparum* on anemia. Thus, the combined effects of resource- and immune-mediated interactions might still be in play for heavy hookworm-*P. falciparum* co-infection as is likely for light hookworm co-infection. Even when the clinical outcomes of co-infection are intuitive, understanding the mechanistic basis of these outcomes may help in designing effective intervention strategies.

Overall, the hypothesized web of interactions between hookworm and *P. falciparum* relies on the simultaneous operation of both resource- and immune-mediated mechanisms to explain divergent outcomes of co-infection on anemia. Importantly, this hypothesized suite of interactions is readily tested in the field by integrating the measurement of immunity and inflammation markers into studies that track changes in parasite intensities (both helminths and malaria) and host nutrition/condition (e.g., red blood cell density, hemoglobin concentration). Once these data are in hand, ecological approaches commonly applied to food webs can be used to draw inferences about which hypothetical interactions are most likely to be occurring, the relative strengths of these different interactions, and the effect of context (e.g., parasite traits [intensity, virulence, establishment order]) on clinical outcomes for the host.

## Effects of Nutrition on Co-infection: Helminths and TB as a Case Study

As with helminths and malaria, geographic overlap between helminths and TB (caused by *Mycobacterium tuberculosis*) is substantial. Approximately one third of the world's population is infected with TB [56], while over 1 billion people are infected with helminths [57]. Endemic regions for TB and helminths also correspond to regions where malnutrition is common, and malnutrition is a risk factor for both TB and helminth infection. For *M. tuberculosis*, deficiencies in protein and energy as well as micronutrients can accelerate progression from latent to active infection [58]. Likewise, macro- and micronutrient deficiencies can promote the establishment and survival of various helminth species [59, 60]. These consequences are due, in large part, to the potent effects of malnutrition on the immune response [7, 61] (see Chaps. 2 and 3). However, because immune responses to TB and helminths are distinct, mutually inhibitory (Th1 vs. Th2 [29]), and respond differently to distinct forms of nutrient deficiency [59, 62], understanding how malnutrition affects disease outcomes under helminth-TB co-infection is a fascinating topic of considerable importance.

Macro- and micronutrient deficiencies have differential effects on T-cell development and differentiation [62]. As such, the magnitude and direction of immune-mediated interactions between helminths and TB may depend critically on the nutritional context of the host. In laboratory mouse models, for example, deficits in protein led to suppressed Th2 responses and increased Th1 responses [63], while energy deficits suppressed both Th1 and Th2 responses [64]. In terms of micronutrients, zinc deficiency suppressed Th2 but not Th1 responses in mouse models [65], while in humans, Th1 but not Th2 responses were suppressed in response to zinc deficiency [66]. Finally, while the predominant effect of vitamin A deficiency on immunity is suppression of Th2 responses, upregulation of Th1 responses can also occur [67]. Overall, one interesting consequence of these complicated effects of nutrient deficiency on immune function is that nutrient restriction might suppress immune function and also affect the magnitude of Th1-Th2 cross-regulation. In support, among wild buffalo co-infected with gastrointestinal helminths and bovine TB (*M. bovis*), circulating levels of the Th1 cytokine, IFNγ, were not only lower during the dry season when protein and energy intake is restricted [68], but the expected trade-off between Th1 and Th2 responses was only detectable during the resource-restricted time period [69].

Despite accumulating evidence that helminths dampen host immune responses to TB [28, 70], clinical field studies on the impact of helminths on TB disease progression show mixed results [71–73]. Yet, in a mouse helminth (*Nippostrongylus brasiliensis*)-*M. tuberculosis* co-infection model, helminth-associated changes in the immune response impaired resistance to *Mycobacterium* [74]. In lab animal studies, subjects typically receive ad libitum food, and there is little to no variation in the nutritional status of hosts. This is certainly not the case in field studies, where many hosts suffer from nutrient deficiencies and often differ from one another in the extent or type of deficiencies experienced (e.g., [5]). Thus, accounting for underlying variation in nutritional status in study populations may provide new insight, and a trophic approach in which host nutritional resources, parasite resource use, as well as host immune defenses are considered simultaneously (Fig. 14.2b) may be useful for conceptualizing how variation in host nutrition (i.e., macro- and micronutrients) can shape helminth-TB interactions.

In a rare test of how nutrient deficiency affects interactions between parasite species, Budischak et al. [75] used a trophic approach to investigate the effects of protein limitation on interactions between two helminths (*Heligmosomoides* and *Nippostrongylus*) and *M. tuberculosis* in a mouse model. Mice were fed either a standard (21%) or low (14%)-protein diet, infected with one or both helminths, and subsequently challenged with *Mycobacterium*. The study design mimics a common infection sequence in the real world where infection with multiple helminths often precedes exposure to TB. Crucially, all three parasites have the potential to interact via the host immune system. *Nippostrongylus* triggers a Th2 response, and *Mycobacterium* triggers a Th1 response, so mutual inhibition could drive an interaction between these two parasites. *Heligmosomoides* triggers a regulatory T-cell (Treg) response that can suppress both Th1 and Th2 responses, providing a mechanism by which *Heligmosomoides* might interact with both *Nippostrongylus* and *Mycobacterium*. The two helminths could also interact via shared resources. Two key findings emerged from the study. First, immune-mediated interactions were more important than resource-mediated interactions in driving variation in parasite numbers. Second, resource limitation altered the strength and direction of immune-mediated interactions. Two specific results illustrate the second point: (i) *Heligmosomoides* facilitated *Nippostrongylus* during co-infection via suppression of Th2 responses, but this effect was weaker under low-protein conditions; and (ii) *Mycobacterium* facilitated *Nippostrongylus*, also via Th2 suppression, but facilitation only occurred under low-protein conditions. The pattern of immune-mediated facilitation of *Nippostrongylus* by *Mycobacterium* under protein limitation aligns with evidence showing that protein deficiency suppresses Th2 responses and promotes Th1 responses [63]. More generally, the explicit trophic approach to studying nutrition effects on co-infection, characterized by identifying interrelationships among host nutrient availability, parasite resource use, and host immune function, revealed profound effects of nutrient limitation on co-infection outcomes and identified key mechanisms (i.e., resource-associated changes in immune-interactions) accounting for the observed effects.

Protein limitation is a common cause of human malnutrition particularly in regions with coincident helminth and TB infections. The study by Budischak and colleagues [75] suggests protein deficiency can shift the outcome of co-infection, magnifying TB facilitation of helminths. Since the study did not quantify Th1 cytokines or evaluate the severity of *Mycobacterium* infection, the specific consequences of this stronger interaction for TB are not clear. However, hosts gained less weight during periods of high helminth egg production, and co-infection with helminths and *Mycobacterium* also affected weight gain [75]. This pattern suggests that nutrition-associated shifts in parasite interactions during co-infection can further worsen host nutrition and condition, contributing to vicious nutrition-co-infection cycles that are analogous to those described for single infections. Given the current paucity of information on the implications of nutrition for co-infection outcomes, this is a critical area for future work. As a first step, incorporating the measurement of nutrients into immune-focused studies of helminth-TB (and other) co-infections and accounting for variability among hosts in their nutritional status may help with identifying new patterns. Importantly, incorporating a trophic perspective can help with this goal.

## Applying a Trophic Approach to Co-infection-nutrition Interactions in Practice

Food webs are networks of the feeding (or "trophic") relationships in a community used to understand the underlying structure, function, and stability of communities [76]. In the context of an ecological community, a practical use of a trophic framework could be identifying the cascading effects of the removal of one species (e.g., via extinction) on other species (e.g., [77]). In terms of nutrition and co-infection, trophic approaches could be used, for example, to investigate the effects of perturbations such as targeted treatment of one parasite, or nutrient manipulation of the host, on co-occurring parasite species. A recent application of such an ecological framework to the problem of antimicrobial drug resistance [25] highlights how understanding trophic interactions can have practical clinical value. In this study, Wale and colleagues [25] tested whether the proliferation of drug-resistant parasites can be managed by limiting the availability of a within-host resource required by the parasite. Specifically, because mouse malaria parasites (*Plasmodium chabaudi*) resistant to the drug pyrimethamine require more para-aminobenzoic acid (pABA: a nutrient used by malaria parasites to synthesize folate) than do drug-susceptible parasites, the authors hypothesized that depleting pABA from the host environment would intensify competition with co-occurring susceptible parasites allowing the susceptible parasites to suppress the emergence of resistant parasites during drug treatment. This hypothesis was strongly supported by an experiment comparing how frequently drug resistance emerged in mice that did or did not receive supplementary pABA in their diets [25]. pABA limitation completely prevented the emergence of drug-resistant parasites (Fig. 14.6), suggesting that resource-mediated ecological interactions between parasites can be harnessed to manage some of the most challenging clinical problems.

The two case studies described earlier in this chapter provide concrete illustrations of the importance of both resource- and immune-mediated interactions for understanding co-infection-nutrition interactions. Current evidence also suggests that both types of interactions frequently operate in tandem to determine host outcomes, but our understanding of the relative contributions of these distinct forms of interaction is still very poor. Yet, information on these relative contributions is crucial for public health, since only then will it be possible to manage these interactions (e.g., via drug treatment, vaccination, nutrient manipulation) in ways that improve individual and population health outcomes [22, 25]. Quantifying interaction strengths is an active area of interest in community ecology [16], and a number of the methodological approaches used for achieving this task in free-living animal or plant communities can be applied to within-host parasite communities (Table 14.1). Ultimately, the ability to apply trophic frameworks to co-infection-nutrition problems relies on assembling the underlying data required for constructing food webs. Interestingly, most lab- and field-based studies of co-infection typically collect data on at least two of the three trophic levels (see Fig. 14.2b: resource level, parasite level, immunity level) required for constructing a food web. Other studies already collect all the necessary data (e.g., [80]). As such, incorporating an explicitly trophic approach seems highly feasible for many studies. Furthermore, the methodological approaches applied to food webs (e.g., Table 14.1) are compatible with common longitudinal, experimental (e.g., clinical trial), and cross-sectional designs of co-infection and nutrition studies.

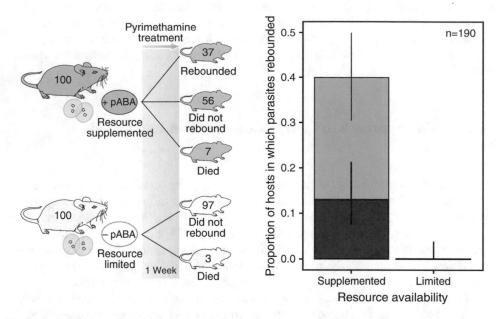

**Fig. 14.6** (**a**) Number of pABA-supplemented vs. pABA-limited mice in which *Plasmodium chabaudi* parasite populations rebounded after drug treatment. (**b**) Proportion of mice in which parasites rebounded (light red bar) that harbored drug-resistant parasites (dark red bar). Error bars are 95% confidence intervals, *n* = number of mice. (Reprinted from Wale et al. 2017 [25] under terms of Creative Commons License https://creativecommons.org/licenses/by-nc-nd/4.0/)

**Table 14.1** A sampling of methods available for quantifying within-host parasite interactions

| Method | Description | Example reference |
|---|---|---|
| Structural equation modeling | A modeling framework used for testing hypotheses about the causal relationships occurring in a system. Provides a powerful way to test the relative strength and direction of different hypothesized interactions in a food web, especially when coupled with directed experiments. | Scherber et al. 2010 [78] |
| Network analysis | A method for visualizing and characterizing the components of a system and the interactions that connect these components. System components are represented as interconnected nodes (e.g., species) and edges (e.g., feeding links between species), allowing the attributes of the system, such as the structure and stability of the network or the strength of interactions between components, to be quantified. | Griffiths et al. 2014 [22] |
| Random decision forests | A machine learning method for classifying observations based on the creation of an ensemble of decision trees that are pooled together to improve predictive power. When sufficient data on known interactions between species are available, this approach can be used to make inferences about missing links to identify new interactions. | DiMucci et al. 2018 [79] |

## Conclusion

Most research on interactions between nutrition and infection focuses on single infections (Fig. 14.1). However, co-infection is ubiquitous. Moreover, the regions of the world where co-infection is most common are also the areas where malnutrition is a pervasive threat [7]. For this reason, there is a compelling need for more research on co-infection-nutrition interactions. Approaches from community ecology, which construct and analyze the feeding relationships that link species, may be particularly well suited to addressing questions about co-infection and nutrition. Indeed, applying this framework to two common helminth co-infections suggests that multiple modes of interaction (resource- and immune-mediated) determine infection and nutritional outcomes, and this perspective could help interpret the mixed outcomes of field studies. In this way, the integration of ecological theory and epidemiological data may provide new insight for tackling the clinical consequences of coincident co-infection and malnutrition. Practical applications include developing a better understanding of how changes in nutritional status influence disease severity during co-infection, predicting how disease control strategies (e.g., drug treatment, vaccination) might impact nutritional status, and anticipating the consequences of nutritional interventions (e.g., nutrient supplementation or restriction). Crucially, as our understanding of the multi-faceted associations between infection and nutrition continues to expand, the trophic approach provides a flexible framework for layering on additional complexity. A key example would be the addition of host-associated microbes, which play a critical role in both host resource acquisition and immune function, into within-host co-infection food webs. More generally, given the rising interest in co-infection-nutrition interactions, a merging of perspectives across disciplines may help spur real progress.

**Acknowledgments**  This chapter was inspired by work supported by the National Science Foundation (NSF DEB-1102493) and National Institutes of Health (NIH R01GM131319) as part of the joint NSF/NIH/USDA Ecology of Infectious Diseases Grant Program. I thank Nina Wale for providing Fig. 14.6, Kate Sabey for drawing Fig. 14.2, and D. Humphries, M. Scott, and M. Seguel for helpful comments on the manuscript.

# References

1. Petney TN, Andrews RH. Multiparasite communities in animals and humans: frequency, structure and pathogenic significance. Int J Parasitol. 1998;28(3):377–93.
2. Brogden KA, Guthmiller JM, Taylor CE. Human polymicrobial infections. Lancet. 2005;365(9455):253–5.
3. Raso G, Luginbuhl A, Adjoua CA, Tian-Bi NT, Silue KD, Matthys B, et al. Multiple parasite infections and their relationship to self-reported morbidity in a community of rural Cote d'Ivoire. Int J Epidemiol. 2004;33(5):1092–102.
4. González-Fernández D, Koski KG, Sinisterra OT, Pons EDC, Murillo E, Scott ME. Interactions among urogenital, intestinal, skin, and oral infections in pregnant and lactating Panamanian Ngäbe women: a neglected public health challenge. Am J Trop Med Hyg. 2015;92(6):1100–10.
5. Gonzalez-Fernández D, Pons EDC, Rueda D, Sinisterra OT, Murillo E, Scott ME, et al. C-reactive protein is differentially modulated by co-existing infections, vitamin deficiencies and maternal factors in pregnant and lactating indigenous Panamanian women. Infect Dis Poverty. 2017;6(1):94.
6. Humphries DL, Scott ME, Vermund SH. Pathways linking nutritional status and infectious disease: a conceptual framework. In: Humphries DL, Scott ME, Vermund SH, editors. Nutrition and infectious diseases: shifting the clinical paradigm. Cham: Springer Nature; 2020.
7. Schaible UE, Kaufmann SH. Malnutrition and infection: complex mechanisms and global impacts. PLoS Med. 2007;4(5):e115.
8. Beldomenico PM, Telfer S, Gebert S, Lukomski L, Bennett M, Begon M. Poor condition and infection: a vicious circle in natural populations. Proc Roy Soc Biol Sci. 2008;275(1644):1753–9.
9. Ezeamama AE, Friedman JF, Olveda RM, Acosta LP, Kurtis JD, Mor V, et al. Functional significance of low-intensity polyparasite helminth infections in anemia. J Infect Dis. 2005;192(12):2160–70.
10. Stoltzfus RJ. Iron-deficiency anemia: reexamining the nature and magnitude of the public health problem. Summary: implications for research and programs. J Nutr. 2001;131(2S-2):697S–700S.
11. Wanke C. Nutrition in HIV and TB. In: Humphries DL, Scott ME, Vermund SH, editors. Nutrition and infectious diseases: shifting the clinical paradigm. Cham: Springer Nature; 2020.
12. Bartelt LA, Bolick DT, Mayneris-Perxachs J, Kolling GL, Medlock GL, Zaenker EI, et al. Cross-modulation of pathogen-specific pathways enhances malnutrition during enteric co-infection with *Giardia lamblia* and enteroaggregative *Escherichia coli*. PLoS Path. 2017;13(7):e1006471.
13. Lange B, Reuter M, Ebert D, Muylaert K, Decaestecker E. Diet quality determines interspecific parasite interactions in host populations. Ecol Evol. 2014;4(15):3093–102.

14. Williams RJ, Berlow EL, Dunne JA, Barabasi AL, Martinez ND. Two degrees of separation in complex food webs. Proc Natl Acad Sci U S A. 2002;99(20):12913–6.
15. Wootton JT. Predicting direct and indirect effects: an integrated approach using experiments and path analysis. Ecology. 1994;75(1):151–65.
16. Wootton JT, Emmerson M. Measurement of interaction strength in nature. Ann Rev of Ecol Evol Syst. 2005;36(1):419–44.
17. Agrawal AA, Ackerly DD, Adler F, Arnold AE, Cáceres C, Doak DF, et al. Filling key gaps in population and community ecology. Front Ecol Env. 2007;5(3):145–52.
18. Johnson PT, de Roode JC, Fenton A. Why infectious disease research needs community ecology. Science. 2015;349(6252):1259504.
19. Pimm SL. Food webs. Netherlands: Springer; 1982.
20. Pedersen AB, Fenton A. Emphasizing the ecology in parasite community ecology. Trends Ecol Evol. 2007;22(3):133–9.
21. Poulin R. Evolutionary ecology of parasites. Princeton: Princeton University Press; 2011.
22. Griffiths EC, Pedersen AB, Fenton A, Petchey OL. Analysis of a summary network of co-infection in humans reveals that parasites interact most via shared resources. Proc Roy Soc Biol Sci. 2014;281(1782):20132286.
23. Budischak SA, Wiria AE, Hamid F, Wammes LJ, Kaisar MMM, van Lieshout L, et al. Competing for blood: the ecology of parasite resource competition in human malaria-helminth co-infections. Ecol Lett. 2018;21(4):536–45.
24. Wale N, Sim DG, Read AF. A nutrient mediates intraspecific competition between rodent malaria parasites in vivo. Proc Roy Soc Biol Sci. 2017;284(1859):20171067.
25. Wale N, Sim DG, Jones MJ, Salathe R, Day T, Read AF. Resource limitation prevents the emergence of drug resistance by intensifying within-host competition. Proc Natl Acad Sci U S A. 2017;114(52):13774–19.
26. Graham AL. Ecological rules governing helminth-microparasite coinfection. Proc Natl Acad Sci U S A. 2008;105(2):566–70.
27. Ezenwa VO, Jolles AE. From host immunity to pathogen invasion: the effects of helminth coinfection on the dynamics of microparasites. Integr Comp Biol. 2011;51(4):540–51.
28. Salgame P, Yap GS, Gause WC. Effect of helminth-induced immunity on infections with microbial pathogens. Nat Immunol. 2013;14(11):1118–26.
29. Mosmann TR, Sad S. The expanding universe of T-cell subsets: Th1, Th2 and more. Immunol Today. 1996;17(3):138–46.
30. Stephensen C. Immunology primer. In: Humphries DL, Scott ME, Vermund SH, editors. Nutrition and infectious diseases: shifting the clinical paradigm. Cham: Springer Nature; 2020.
31. Cable J, Harris PD, Lewis JW, Behnke JM. Molecular evidence that *Heligmosomoides polygyrus* from laboratory mice and wood mice are separate species. Parasitology. 2006;133(Pt 1):111–22.
32. Reese TA, Wakeman BS, Choi HS, Hufford MM, Huang SC, Zhang X, et al. Coinfection. Helminth infection reactivates latent gamma-herpesvirus via cytokine competition at a viral promoter. Science. 2014;345(6196):573–7.
33. Xu DH, Pridgeon JW, Klesius PH, Shoemaker CA. Parasitism by *Ichthyophthirius multifiliis* enhanced invasion of *Aeromonas hydrophila* in tissues of channel catfish. Vet Parasitol. 2012;184(2–4):101–7.
34. Romano A, Doria NA, Mendez J, Sacks DL, Peters NC. Cutaneous infection with *Leishmania major* mediates heterologous protection against visceral infection with *Leishmania infantum*. J Immunol. 2015;195(8):3816–27.
35. Brooker S, Clements AC, Hotez PJ, Hay SI, Tatem AJ, Bundy DA, et al. The co-distribution of *Plasmodium falciparum* and hookworm among African schoolchildren. Malar J. 2006;5:99.
36. Hotez PJ, Brooker S, Bethony JM, Bottazzi ME, Loukas A, Xiao S. Hookworm infection. N Engl J Med. 2004;351(8):799–807.
37. Castelli F, Sulis G, Caligaris S. The relationship between anaemia and malaria: apparently simple, yet controversial. Trans R Soc Trop Med Hyg. 2014;108(4):181–2.
38. Humphries D, Mosites E, Otchere J, Twum WA, Woo L, Jones-Sanpei H, et al. Epidemiology of hookworm infection in Kintampo North Municipality, Ghana: patterns of malaria coinfection, anemia, and albendazole treatment failure. Am J Trop Med Hyg. 2011;84(5):792–800.
39. Kinung'hi SM, Magnussen P, Kaatano GM, Kishamawe C, Vennervald BJ. Malaria and helminth co-infections in school and preschool children: a cross-sectional study in Magu district, north-western Tanzania. PLoS One. 2014;9(1):e86510.
40. Mboera LE, Senkoro KP, Rumisha SF, Mayala BK, Shayo EH, Mlozi MR. *Plasmodium falciparum* and helminth coinfections among schoolchildren in relation to agro-ecosystems in Mvomero District, Tanzania. Acta Trop. 2011;120(1–2):95–102.
41. WHO. Haemoglobin concentrations for the diagnosis of anaemia and assessment of severity. In: Vitamin and mineral nutrition information system. Geneva: World Health Organization; 2011. (WHO/NMH/NHD/MNM/11.1). http://www.who.int/vmnis/indicators/haemoglobin. Accessed 30 July 2019.
42. Brooker S, Akhwale W, Pullan R, Estambale B, Clarke SE, Snow RW, et al. Epidemiology of *Plasmodium*-helminth co-infection in Africa: populations at risk, potential impact on anemia, and prospects for combining control. Am J Trop Med Hyg. 2007;77(6 Suppl):88–98.

43. Righetti AA, Glinz D, Adiossan LG, Koua AY, Niamke S, Hurrell RF, et al. Interactions and potential implications of *Plasmodium falciparum*-hookworm coinfection in different age groups in south-central Cote d'Ivoire. PLoS Negl Trop Dis. 2012;6(11):e1889.
44. Hurlimann E, Houngbedji CA, Yapi RB, N'Dri PB, Silue KD, Ouattara M, et al. Antagonistic effects of Plasmodium-helminth co-infections on malaria pathology in different population groups in Cote d'Ivoire. PLoS Negl Trop Dis. 2019;13(1):e0007086.
45. Naing C, Whittaker MA, Nyunt-Wai V, Reid SA, Wong SF, Mak JW, et al. Malaria and soil-transmitted intestinal helminth co-infection and its effect on anemia: a meta-analysis. Trans R Soc Trop Med Hyg. 2013;107(11):672–83.
46. Degarege A, Veledar E, Degarege D, Erko B, Nacher M, Madhivanan P. *Plasmodium falciparum* and soil-transmitted helminth co-infections among children in sub-Saharan Africa: a systematic review and meta-analysis. Parasit Vect. 2016;9(1):344.
47. Balmer O, Stearns SC, Schotzau A, Brun R. Intraspecific competition between co-infecting parasite strains enhances host survival in African trypanosomes. Ecology. 2009;90(12):3367–78.
48. Hoverman JT, Hoye BJ, Johnson PT. Does timing matter? How priority effects influence the outcome of parasite interactions within hosts. Oecologia. 2013;173(4):1471–80.
49. Menendez C, Fleming AF, Alonso PL. Malaria-related anaemia. Parasitol Today. 2000;16(11):469–76.
50. Stoltzfus RJ, Chwaya HM, Tielsch JM, Schulze KJ, Albonico M, Savioli L. Epidemiology of iron deficiency anemia in Zanzibari schoolchildren: the importance of hookworms. Am J Clin Nutr. 1997;65(1):153–9.
51. Njua-Yafi C, Achidi EA, Anchang-Kimbi JK, Apinjoh TO, Mugri RN, Chi HF, et al. Malaria, helminths, co-infection and anaemia in a cohort of children from Mutengene, south western Cameroon. Malar J. 2016;15:69.
52. Gaze S, McSorley HJ, Daveson J, Jones D, Bethony JM, Oliveira LM, et al. Characterising the mucosal and systemic immune responses to experimental human hookworm infection. PLoS Path. 2012;8(2):e1002520.
53. Degarege A, Erko B. Epidemiology of *Plasmodium* and helminth coinfection and possible reasons for heterogeneity. Biomed Res Int. 2016;2016:3083568.
54. Ganz T, Nemeth E. Iron sequestration and anemia of inflammation. Semin Hematol. 2009;46(4):387–93.
55. Hartgers FC, Yazdanbakhsh M. Co-infection of helminths and malaria: modulation of the immune responses to malaria. Parasite Immunol. 2006;28(10):497–506.
56. Li XX, Zhou XN. Co-infection of tuberculosis and parasitic diseases in humans: a systematic review. Parasit Vect. 2013;6:79.
57. Pullan RL, Smith JL, Jasrasaria R, Brooker SJ. Global numbers of infection and disease burden of soil transmitted helminth infections in 2010. Parasit Vect. 2014;7:37.
58. Cegielski JP, McMurray DN. The relationship between malnutrition and tuberculosis: evidence from studies in humans and experimental animals. Int J Tuberc Lung Dis. 2004;8(3):286–98.
59. Koski KG, Scott ME. Gastrointestinal nematodes, nutrition and immunity: breaking the negative spiral. Annu Rev Nutr. 2001;21:297–321.
60. Scott ME, Koski KG. Soil-transmitted helminths – does nutrition make a difference? In: Humphries DL, Scott ME, Vermund SH, editors. Nutrition and infectious diseases: shifting the clinical paradigm. Cham: Springer Nature; 2020.
61. Chandra RK. Nutrition, immunity and infection: from basic knowledge of dietary manipulation of immune responses to practical application of ameliorating suffering and improving survival. Proc Natl Acad Sci U S A. 1996;93(25):14304–7.
62. Long KZ, Nanthakumar N. Energetic and nutritional regulation of the adaptive immune response and trade-offs in ecological immunology. Am J Hum Biol. 2004;16(5):499–507.
63. Ing R, Su Z, Scott ME, Koski KG. Suppressed T helper 2 immunity and prolonged survival of a nematode parasite in protein-malnourished mice. Proc Natl Acad Sci U S A. 2000;97(13):7078–83.
64. Koski KG, Su Z, Scott ME. Energy deficits suppress both systemic and gut immunity during infection. Biochem Biophys Res Commun. 1999;264(3):796–801.
65. Scott ME, Koski KG. Zinc deficiency impairs immune responses against parasitic nematode infections at intestinal and systemic sites. J Nutr. 2000;130(5S Suppl):1412S–20S.
66. Prasad AS. Effects of zinc deficiency on Th1 and Th2 cytokine shifts. J Infect Dis. 2000;182(Suppl 1):S62–8.
67. Stephensen CB. Vitamin A, infection, and immune function. Annu Rev Nutr. 2001;21:167–92.
68. Ezenwa VO, Etienne RS, Luikart G, Beja-Pereira A, Jolles AE. Hidden consequences of living in a wormy world: nematode-induced immune suppression facilitates tuberculosis invasion in African Buffalo. Am Nat. 2010;176(5):613–24.
69. Jolles AE, Ezenwa VO, Etienne RS, Turner WC, Olff H. Interactions between macroparasites and microparasites drive infection patterns in free-ranging African buffalo. Ecology. 2008;89(8):2239–50.
70. Chatterjee S, Nutman TB. Helminth-induced immune regulation: implications for immune responses to tuberculosis. PLoS Path. 2015;11(1):e1004582.
71. Chatterjee S, Kolappan C, Subramani R, Gopi PG, Chandrasekaran V, Fay MP, et al. Incidence of active pulmonary tuberculosis in patients with coincident filarial and/or intestinal helminth infections followed longitudinally in South India. PLoS One. 2014;9(4):e94603.

72. Brown M, Miiro G, Nkurunziza P, Watera C, Quigley MA, Dunne DW, et al. *Schistosoma mansoni*, nematode infections, and progression to active tuberculosis among HIV-1-infected Ugandans. Am J Trop Med Hyg. 2006;74(5):819–25.
73. Abate E, Elias D, Getachew A, Alemu S, Diro E, Britton S, et al. Effects of albendazole on the clinical outcome and immunological responses in helminth co-infected tuberculosis patients: a double blind randomised clinical trial. Int J Parasitol. 2015;45(2–3):133–40.
74. Potian JA, Rafi W, Bhatt K, McBride A, Gause WC, Salgame P. Preexisting helminth infection induces inhibition of innate pulmonary anti-tuberculosis defense by engaging the IL-4 receptor pathway. J Exp Med. 2011;208(9):1863–74.
75. Budischak SA, Sakamoto K, Megow LC, Cummings KR, Urban JF Jr, Ezenwa VO. Resource limitation alters the consequences of co-infection for both hosts and parasites. Int J Parasitol. 2015;45(7):455–63.
76. Ings TC, Montoya JM, Bascompte J, Bluthgen N, Brown L, Dormann CF, et al. Ecological networks--beyond food webs. J Anim Ecol. 2009;78(1):253–69.
77. O'Gorman EJ, Emmerson MC. Perturbations to trophic interactions and the stability of complex food webs. Proc Natl Acad Sci U S A. 2009;106(32):13393–8.
78. Scherber C, Eisenhauer N, Weisser WW, Schmid B, Voigt W, Fischer M, et al. Bottom-up effects of plant diversity on multitrophic interactions in a biodiversity experiment. Nature. 2010;468(7323):553–6.
79. DiMucci D, Kon M, Segre D. Machine learning reveals missing edges and putative interaction mechanisms in microbial ecosystem networks. mSystems. 2018;3(5):e00181-18.
80. Sangweme DT, Midzi N, Zinyowera-Mutapuri S, Mduluza T, Diener-West M, Kumar N. Impact of schistosome infection on *Plasmodium falciparum* malariometric indices and immune correlates in school age children in Burma Valley, Zimbabwe. PLoS Neg Trop Dis. 2010;4(11):e882.

# Chapter 15
# Climate Change Pathways and Potential Future Risks to Nutrition and Infection

Joacim Rocklöv, Clas Ahlm, Marilyn E. Scott, and Debbie L. Humphries

## Abbreviations

| | |
|---|---|
| $CO_2$ | Carbon dioxide |
| ENSO | El Niño-Southern Oscillation |
| GGCM | Global gridded crop models |
| GHG | Greenhouse gases |
| IPCC | Intergovernmental Panel on Climate Change |
| K | Potassium |
| LMIC | Lower- and middle-income countries |
| MUAC | Mid-upper arm circumference |
| N | Nitrogen |
| NHANES | National Health and Nutrition Examination Survey |
| P | Phosphorus |
| RCP | Representative Concentration Pathways |
| RVF | Rift Valley fever |
| SDG | Sustainable Development Goals |
| WHO | World Health Organization |

J. Rocklöv (✉)
Department of Public Health and Clinical Medicine, Section of Sustainable Health, Umeå University, Umeå, Sweden

Heidelberg Institute of Global Health, Heidelberg University, Heidelberg, Germany
e-mail: joacim.rocklov@umu.se

C. Ahlm
Department of Clinical Microbiology, Infection and Immunology, Umeå University, Umeå, Sweden

M. E. Scott
McGill University, Macdonald Campus, Sainte-Anne de Bellevue, QC, Canada
e-mail: marilyn.scott@mcgill.ca

D. L. Humphries
Department of Epidemiology of Microbial Disease, Yale School of Public Health, New Haven, CT, USA

© Springer Nature Switzerland AG 2021
D. L. Humphries et al. (eds.), *Nutrition and Infectious Diseases*, Nutrition and Health,
https://doi.org/10.1007/978-3-030-56913-6_15

**Key Points**
- Increasing $CO_2$ emission and climate change will have an impact on natural and social systems with consequences for global health.
- The amount of $CO_2$ emissions in the atmosphere and our adaptive responses will determine the degree of impact.
- Food systems are both a driver of climate change and heavily impacted by climate change. The food system is a large emitter of $CO_2$, and the impacts of climate change are expected to increase both macronutrient and micronutrient deficiencies.
- Critical food webs and food systems both on land and in the oceans are increasingly affected by climate change and concentrations of $CO_2$, thereby affecting nutritional status.
- Climate change is likely to influence infectious diseases through both its impact on survival and replication of pathogens, reservoirs, and vectors and the geographical range of transmission.
- As a consequence of observed and projected changes in climate, populations at risk of water- and vector-borne infectious diseases will likely increase, and current control efforts may be challenged in endemic areas.
- The synergistic impacts of undernutrition and infection with climate change are not yet well quantified, but current understanding of their interdependence suggests exacerbated negative impacts unless climate change is controlled.
- The 2030 Sustainable Development Goals intrinsically interrelate undernutrition, infection, and climate and lead to calls for action to urgently tackle these major global health challenges of the twenty-first century.

# Climate Change Pathways to Nutrition and Infection

The Intergovernmental Panel on Climate Change (IPCC) (see Box 15.1) has recently concluded that climate change has and will continue to affect terrestrial and ocean biodiversity and ecosystem stability and that climate change is altering the geographical distribution, abundance, and extinction probabilities of plant and animal species. IPCC highlights that these changes, in turn, will challenge food and water security and human health and that the most serious impacts can be avoided if $CO_2$

**Box 15.1 Climate Terminology**
**IPCC:** The Intergovernmental Panel on Climate Change is the United Nations body that is responsible for assessing the science related to climate change. It was initiated in 1988 and currently engages 195 member countries and thousands of voluntary scientists who contribute to assessments and special reports.

**Mitigation:** Refers to actions towards the reduction of carbon emissions that should reduce, stabilize, or reverse the trend of increasing atmospheric $CO_2$ levels.

**Adaptation:** Refers to planned or natural processes that lower exposure, vulnerability, and risk from climate change. Adaptation is mediated through policy, intervention programs, and local or regional capacity to resist, adapt, and manage the risks associated with climate change.

**Resilience**: Refers to the ability of a system (e.g., ecosystems, organizational systems, biological systems, other systems) to respond to change while retaining function and structure and options for future capacity [1].

emissions can be stabilized (see Box 15.2) [2, 3]. IPCC reports describe how melting of snow and ice and changes in precipitation are altering hydrologic systems, with effects on water quality and availability [3]. Many terrestrial and freshwater plant, animal, and insect species are shifting their seasonal activity windows, distribution range, and abundance, in response to climate and environmental change [2]. Coral bleaching and increasing ocean temperatures may be causing distributional range shifts among ocean species [2]. The altered seasonal activities, range shifts, and abundance patterns of marine species have spillover effects on the predator-prey dynamics, often with poleward shifts, for example, among fish and phytoplankton [2]. Based on a range of studies, negative impacts on crop

---

**Box 15.2 Climate Change Facts**

**Greenhouse gases:** *The concentration of greenhouse gases (GHGs) in the atmosphere has varied naturally throughout the history of the planet, but the speed of rise of concentrations since pre-industrial time has been alarmingly fast [5]. The current levels are around 400 ppm $CO_2$ today. The increased concentration of GHGs in the atmosphere traps solar energy and affects the energy balance of the climate system, which causes the warming trend. The changes observed over the past century are considered by the vast majority of climate scientists to be driven by human activities including the accelerated emissions of $CO_2$ associated with industrialization. This includes increased emissions from the food system (food production, food transport, and agricultural exploitation of land) [5]. The food system is estimated to cause between 19 and 29% of the annual global GHG emissions, the majority of which are attributed to agricultural production and associated changes in land-cover [6].*

*Observed climate changes: Since industrialization, the global mean surface temperature has increased by 0.87 °C, comparing 2006–2015 to 1850–1900. The number of cold days and nights has decreased, while the number of warm days and nights has increased globally. North America, Europe, and Australia have already observed a rise in the frequency of warm spells [3, 5]. There are observed increases in dryness and drought, especially in the Mediterranean region, but not at a global scale. More areas have an increased frequency and intensity of heavy precipitation [3]. The rate of the decrease of sea ice has been around 4%, 0.45 to 0.51 million $km^2$ per decade. The increasing $CO_2$ concentrations and the uptake of $CO_2$ in the oceans have contributed with high certainty to a 0.1 unit lowering of the ocean pH since the start of the industrialization, which has caused severe acidification of the oceans, especially in surface waters [3].*

*Future climate scenarios: The continuation and extent of future change in the twenty-first century and beyond depends on the concentration of carbon emissions in the atmosphere. This is highly dependent on human activities, and thus, climate model simulations project future changes according to scenarios of future emissions using Representative Concentration Pathways (RCPs). Table 15.1 describes the projected global and regional warming that would be associated with different RCPs of $CO_2$ according to a projected low (RCP2.6), low-medium (RCP4.5), high-medium (RCP6.0), and high (RCP8.5) carbon forcing of the climate system in 2081–2100 compared to 1980–2000. The model with lowest carbon forcing (RCP2.6) projects that a stabilization of $CO_2$ concentrations close to current levels of around 400 ppm at the end of this century would result in a 1.0 °C increase in global temperature, whereas the extreme scenario (RCP8.5) projects that $CO_2$ concentrations will reach 900 ppm and would result in a 3.7 °C increase in global temperature. Future temperature changes are highly dependent on future emissions and $CO_2$ concentrations. Estimates of changes in land temperature range from increases of 1.2 °C to 4.8 °C, but do not consider abrupt changes, so-called tipping points that might alter system dynamics, and lead to even larger changes [4].*

**Table 15.1** Scenarios of global warming under four different carbon emission trajectories presented globally, over land, over oceans, over the tropics, and over the polar Arctic and polar Antarctic areas [4]

| | Year 2081–2100 compared to 1980–2000 | | | |
| | RCP2.6 (ΔT in °C) | RCP4.5 (ΔT in °C) | RCP6.0 (ΔT in °C) | RCP8.5 (ΔT in °C) |
|---|---|---|---|---|
| Global | 1.0 | 1.8 | 2.2 | 3.7 |
| Land | 1.2 | 2.4 | 3.0 | 4.8 |
| Ocean | 0.8 | 1.5 | 1.9 | 3.1 |
| Tropics | 0.9 | 1.6 | 2.0 | 3.3 |
| Polar Arctic | 2.2 | 4.2 | 5.2 | 8.3 |
| Polar Antarctic | 0.8 | 1.5 | 1.7 | 3.1 |

yields (e.g., wheat and maize) are already more recurrent than positive impacts from currently observed climate change; this applies to many different crops in many regions, with the exception of high-altitude regions. While increasing $CO_2$ concentrations speed up growth and shorten the time to ripening for many crops, the increasing concentrations have negative effects on crop micronutrient content. Also, higher levels of tropospheric ozone damage plants. All these factors are amplified by human activities [2].

The extent of future change depends on the success of human efforts at mitigation of carbon emissions and pathways of stabilization. It also depends on natural biogeochemical feedback systems that lead to melting of ice and melting of permafrost with associated increases in methane emissions and reduce the capacity of oceans and forests to act as carbon sinks as temperatures rise. A stark contrast in the degree of change can even be seen in limiting the global average temperature increase to 1.5 °C compared to 2 °C, an aspiration of the ratified 2015 Paris Agreement. If emissions are not stabilized, the changes and impacts are predicted to increase exponentially beyond the twenty-first century, potentially limiting human life on Earth as we know it [4].

How will global health be affected? The Lancet Commission on Climate Change and Health has identified climate change as one of the largest challenges to global health over the twenty-first century [7]. Disease impacts from climate change are generally categorized by the degree to which climate change pathways *directly* or *indirectly* affect disease. Climate and climate hazards acting *directly* on health include, for example, injuries related to floods and heat stress where there is no, or little, mediation through biological systems and where vulnerability varies by social systems and demography. Disease impacts that are an *indirect* result of climate change are mediated through natural and social systems [8]. In the case of indirect effects, the climate hazard can be transformed into impacts on the biological and ecological system such as range shifts of vector and crop species and climate-induced changes on crop productivity or the vectorial capacity of disease vectors (see sections on "Impacts of Climate on Agriculture and Nutrition" and "Climate Change and Infectious Diseases"). Of note, mediation of impacts through biological systems and indirect pathways often gives rise to extended latent periods between the climate hazard and the health impacts, and such impacts are more challenging to study.

Vulnerabilities to climate and related biophysical hazards determine exposure and sensitivity of communities and individuals to health risks (see Box 15.3) and depend on a multitude of factors, including capacities of local public health and social protective systems [2]. The current trends of global urbanization and ongoing demographic transition in rural areas, and the concomitant economic and social change, are important contextual mediators of the impacts and vulnerabilities attributable to climate change. Pathways by which climate change intersects with water security, food security, and infectious diseases are introduced in the following overviews.

*Water insecurity* is a critical pathway by which climate change impacts food security, infectious diseases, and global health. Water is essential to health and food production, and scarcity impairs hygiene, reduces crop yields, and can increase waterborne infections [8]. Water scarcity is also associated with human conflict, with obvious and catastrophic health consequences [9]. Additional risks

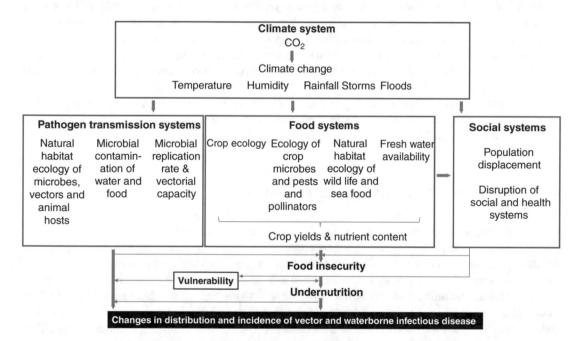

**Fig. 15.1** Pathways linking climate change to nutrition and infectious diseases

associated with water scarcity grow out of attempts to adapt to water scarcity. For example, collecting water in open containers has been reported to increase mosquito vector breeding, and using waste water for irrigation may also increase exposure to waterborne infections [10].

*Food insecurity* is another pathway by which climate change impacts global health and remains widespread despite dramatic progress over recent decades. The connection between food security and climate change is mediated through the impact of climate change on crop yields, fishery catches, animal production, and social systems, as well as the indirect impacts of reduced food on prevalence and severity of infectious diseases and decreased earning capacity. Social and economic systems play a fundamentally important role in food insecurity, regulating food prices, food availability, and the cash economy [8]. The impact of climate change on risks of malnutrition and micronutrient deficiencies and consequently for public health will be further discussed in section "Climate Change, Food Systems, and Nutrition."

*Infectious diseases* are another pathway by which climate change impacts global health, as pathogen success and transmission is often sensitive to climatic conditions. A graphical illustration of the pathways by which climate change can affect infectious diseases has been outlined in Fig. 15.1. The pathogens responsible for these diseases are a part of ecosystems where climate-related variables may affect their survival and replication outside the host, the distribution of their non-human vectors and hosts, and ecological associations of their non-human vectors and hosts with other competitors, predators, and prey within the ecosystem. Zoonotic infections often depend on multiple wild or domestic animals as reservoirs, making it difficult to explore the influences and impacts of social and environmental conditions on disease transmission. The emergence of infectious diseases in areas where they have previously not been observed can also depend on non-climatic drivers, such as bird migration routes (West Nile virus) and human mobility (dengue, chikungunya) [11]. Of 115 infectious disease threat events to Europe from 2008 to 2013, the top 5 drivers were travel and tourism, food and water quality, changes in the natural environment, global trade, and climate [11]. A combination of two or more drivers was responsible for most events, emphasizing the difficulty of isolating the effects of climate and environmental change as a single driver.

*Social and economic disruption* can be a potent result of climate change, leading to increasing vulnerability to various climate health risks, including extreme climatic events. The disruption of health-care services or health-care availability during severe storms and floods can lead to displacement and loss of income from disease or injuries, property damage, and disruption of hygiene. Such displacements and disruptions can cause vicious and indirect spirals with consequences for health and development [8].

While nutrition and infectious disease are not the only pathways by which climate change influences human health, they are interconnected and important. The remainder of this chapter will focus directly on these two pathways.

## Climate Change, Food Systems, and Nutrition

Climate change is impacted by nutrition, and food systems are in turn impacted by climate change. Agriculture and food production are important contributors to climate change, as between 19 and 29% of anthropogenic GHGs are related directly to the food system. Two big contributors are loss of forest carbon stores with deforestation and burning, when forests are cleared for agricultural land, and methane production. The indirect effects of deforestation to provide agricultural land include a reduction in carbon stores in trees and methane released from livestock and flooded rice paddies [6]. Reducing GHG emissions from the food system is thus essential to effectively mitigate climate change. This may involve changing dietary patterns, such as shifting western dietary practices to less red meat, which would reduce methane production and the amount of land required for livestock feed. In addition to dietary change, ranchers and farmers are experimenting with alternative animal production models, seeking approaches that reduce the carbon footprint of meat, particularly beef and pork [12–15]. Climate change may also be an important contributor to macronutrient and micronutrient undernutrition, as many lower-income tropical and sub-tropical countries are likely to face reduced agricultural yield and fish harvest potential in the future [16, 17]. Micronutrient undernutrition is likely to be exacerbated by the increasing $CO_2$ levels, as there is a growing awareness of the reductions in nutrient density associated with increasing levels of $CO_2$. For example, at global $CO_2$ concentrations of 690 ppm, reductions in micronutrient density of key grains and tubers such as rice, wheat, barley, and potatoes are estimated to be 5–10% [18]. Although this reduction in zinc and iron, as well as protein, may seem small, at a population level, such changes can have a significant impact, especially in regions where undernutrition is already prevalent. Estimates suggest an additional 200 million people will be at risk of falling below recommended daily protein intake [18].

   The IPCC Fifth Assessment report in 2014 identified climate impacts on nutrition as one of the most important health impacts [19]. This finding has been developed further in new research studies providing a better description of the complex inter-linkages between social systems and food systems and the potential role of adaptation and mitigation. Emerging research suggests the potential to avert more than 500,000 deaths per year by 2050 if diets shift toward less red meat consumption and more fruit and vegetables [20]. Impacts could be substantially lower if carbon emissions are reduced sufficiently. Here we will describe and develop the relationship between climate change, food systems, and undernutrition, after first reviewing the pathways of interdependence for climate, nutrition, and health using a systems perspective. Changes in climate are expected to lead to changes in temperature, humidity, rainfall, storms, and floods, which in turn will affect crop yields and nutrient content as shown in Fig. 15.1.

## Impacts of Nutrition and Agriculture on Climate Change

Agricultural production and food availability are fundamental requirements for improved nutritional status, although that production can come with environmental costs. Over the second half of the last century, agricultural and technological innovations accelerating food production and food availability played an important role in keeping food production abreast of population growth, and global rates of undernutrition have fallen [18]. Although progress has been made, an estimated two billion people still suffer from micronutrient deficiencies, an estimated 790 million people have insufficient daily macronutrient intake, and undernutrition is estimated to be an underlying cause of half of the deaths among children worldwide [21]. In the future, the need for food will continue to increase due to population growth, demographic transitions, and longevity, with an increasing global population along with greater demands for a western diet [22].

   Increasing agricultural production has historically been due to a combination of increasing the landmass under cultivation and new innovations that lead to greater yields. From 1992 to 2015, global agricultural lands increased by 7.1% primarily due to forest clearing and simultaneously decreased by 4.4% primarily due to encroachment of human settlements [23]. Future increases in agricultural food production are expected to occur at a slower rate than over the past two decades and may not keep pace with population needs [24, 25]. Key challenges are the decreasing availability of crop land due to urbanization and land degradation [25] and the environmental consequences of climate change and human activities [26].

   Livestock production represents another important source of GHGs from within the agricultural sector, responsible for an estimated 12% of anthropogenic GHGs [14]. Changing agriculture systems to adopt more sustainable intensification of livestock [14], managing grazing lands to increase carbon sequestration in soil [27], and adopting mitigation strategies to minimize GHG from livestock [28] are all important approaches to reduce the climate impact of agriculture.

   Within the agricultural sector, food choices play an important role in GHG emissions. Limiting the impacts of agriculture on GHGs would best be accomplished by reducing livestock consumption and by shifting livestock production systems to reduce emissions (see previous section). In an analysis of American diets drawn from the National Health and Nutrition Examination Survey (NHANES), researchers found that one or two items in a daily food record, were often responsible for a large proportion of GHGs associated with producing the food for the day [29]. Thus changing one or two food items, such as replacing steak with grilled chicken, could reduce GHGs associated with an individual's daily food consumption by over 50% [30]. Such changes can also help counteract the epidemic of macronutrient overnutrition, which can yield substantial health co-benefits and reductions of chronic diseases [19, 20].

## *Impacts of Climate on Agriculture and Nutrition*

A synthesis of the literature by Cline in 2007 estimated reductions of up to 50% of agricultural production potential by the year 2080, with considerable geographic variability [16]. Later estimates using a large range of climate change scenarios and around 30 different crop impact models confirmed this result in some regions as illustrated in Fig. 15.2 [31]. While northern countries (Canada, Northern Europe, Siberia) are predicted to see increases in yields of maize, wheat, rice, and soy, more tropical regions in Latin America, Africa, and Asia are predicted to see decreases in production of wheat and maize, with less changes in rice and soy (see Fig. 15.2).

Carbon emissions, and particularly atmospheric $CO_2$, are believed to affect food production systems, undernutrition, and the vulnerability to infectious disease globally. Figure 15.3 outlines key pathways of influence for these impacts.

### Factors Affecting Agricultural Yield

Agriculture is tightly connected to cultivation of land and achieving greater yields by practice and technology. Agricultural yields for both macronutrients and micronutrients depend on several biophysical conditions that are affected by or associated with climate change [18]. These are described below.

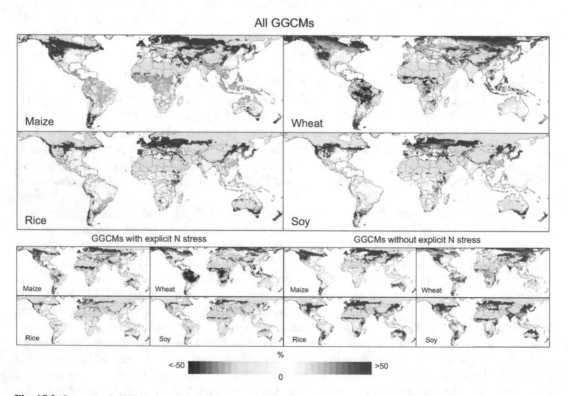

**Fig. 15.2** Impacts of climate change and $CO_2$ on major food crops from Rosenzweig et al. Median yield changes (%) for RCP8.5 (2070–2099 in comparison to 1980–2010 baseline) with $CO_2$ effects over five global circulation models estimated as ensemble means from many different crop impact models. Approach uses global gridded crop models (GGCMs), where the globe is divided by a grid into cells, for modelling purposes. (Reprinted from Rosenzweig et al. [31], with permission from PNAS)

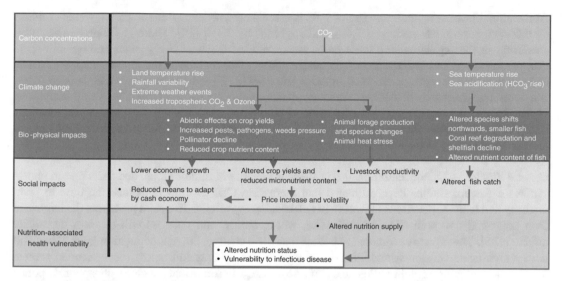

**Fig. 15.3** Pathways of carbon dioxide concentrations to altered nutrition status and vulnerability to infectious disease. (Amended from Myers et al. [18], published under a CC-BY SA license)

*Soil quality* There are at least 17 nutrients of relevance for crop development, although the most important micronutrients in the soil include nitrogen (N), phosphorus (P), and potassium (K) [32]. Nutrient cycles are complex since they incorporate a range of physical, chemical, and biological processes. In natural systems, nutrients in the soil are added through biomass decomposition, but in agriculture, nutrient-rich fertilizers are added due to loss of important soil nutrients from frequent harvesting. One of the consequences of use of fertilizers is that excess N and P are lost from the land in runoff which can pollute neighboring waters and bodies of water downstream. Different soils naturally hold different amounts of nutrients, with sandy soils holding less and clay soils holding more [32]. High amounts of soil organic matter create the dark and brown color of a nutrient-rich soil. The pH of soil is also important for determining bioavailability of the macro- and micronutrients in the soil to the crops. Soil erosion is a large problem with conventional agricultural practices, particularly when compared to organic and conservation agriculture, and is driven in part by higher rates of deforestation and desertification.

*Sunlight* Crops absorb sunlight through their leaves and use the sunlight as energy for photosynthesis that converts $CO_2$ and water into carbohydrates and oxygen. Carbohydrates contribute to vegetative and reproductive growth and increase crop biomass. Photosynthesis only occurs when the sun is above the horizon and is thus strongly seasonal closer to the north and south pole. The amount of sunlight reaching a crop is lower if the atmosphere holds more water vapor. While climate change is not expected to influence availability of solar energy, geoengineering solutions to reduce global warming could reflect sunlight back into space using light shields, and this would reduce sunlight available for plant growth and photosynthesis. Impacts on sunlight reduction would be greatest in the middle latitudes, both north and south of the equator [33]. In some locations, the resulting benefit of reduced global warming may offset reduced plant growth, but in others it could result in reduced agricultural production [33].

*Temperature and water* Crop yields are highly sensitive to temperature and water abundance, and overall ambient temperatures above 30 °C will generally lead to lower yields for rain-fed crops [18]. Without irrigation, water stress is partly related to temperature and dryness and evaporation of soil and crops, and partly to precipitation patterns in relation to the ability of the soil to absorb the water [18].

At the global level, a temperature rise of 1 °C is associated with reductions in global yields of wheat by 6.0%, rice by 3.2%, maize by 7.4%, and soybeans by 3.1% [34]. There is strong geographical clustering in the regions where these crops are grown, with wheat being much more common in Europe, the USA, and India, rice in Asia, maize across most regions of the globe except for Africa, and soybeans being more common in America and Asia [34]. High temperatures can damage plants and accelerate plant growth leading to reduced plant nutrient density, with negative overall impacts on yields. As global temperatures rise, adaptation of production practices will be necessary in locations where such conditions are becoming more frequent. This may involve, for example, introducing or increasing irrigation to maintain or increase yields [34].

*Carbon dioxide* $CO_2$ concentration also influences the growth rate of crops, due to its role in photosynthesis. Recent studies have estimated that increasing $CO_2$ levels will reduce the time to plant maturity and lead to reductions of 5–10% in nutrient density of zinc, iron, and protein of the harvested crop at around 550 ppm $CO_2$ [18, 35]. Rice, wheat, barley, and potatoes will be most negatively affected [35]. The effect is estimated to be less than 10% change, but at a population level, it can still have a significant impact. An additional 200 million people may fall below recommended protein intakes, and existing protein deficiencies could worsen. Micronutrients such as phosphorus, potassium, calcium, sulfur, magnesium, iron, zinc, copper, and manganese may be reduced in rice, wheat, maize, and potatoes by 5–10% from an increase from current $CO_2$ concentrations of 400–690 ppm [36], potentially placing an additional 100–200 million people at risk of zinc deficiency and exacerbating deficiency for more than one billion people. This change in $CO_2$ levels would correspond to a future RCP scenario between RCP6.5 and RCP8.5. The reduction of iron may be especially problematic as iron deficiency is the most common micronutrient deficiency [37], affecting approximately 30% of the global population [38], including a majority of children between 1 and 5 years of age [18].

*Combined effects* Projecting future impacts of temperature, $CO_2$ and precipitation on crop yields with climate change is complicated by adaptations in human management of yields that seek to prevent and compensate for production losses, so such mitigations would need to be considered in realistic models. The projected reduction of crop production could be up to 50% of wheat and maize in Africa and South America in low latitude areas and 25% at the end of the twenty-first century in the RCP8.5 emission trajectory, including the combined effects of $CO_2$ and its effects on the climate system [31]. There would also be estimated increases in crop productivity in temperate regions, such as North America and Europe, for example, for rice and soy (Fig. 15.2) [31]. However, individual model simulation results exhibit considerable variability in future impact estimates, and adaptations to overcome the falling yields have not been accounted for in these estimates. Adaptation (altered harvest of cultivation dates, change in crop varieties, and change in irrigation practices) improved yields by 7–15% in a meta-review study based on the data generated in the IPCC fourth assessment report [39]. These estimates did not consider more "radical" coping strategies such as switching crops, reallocating land from crops to grazing, or incorporating sustainable cropping strategies. The crop yield model estimates also do not incorporate effects from ozone, pollination, pests, or labor [18].

*Ozone* Ozone is also important to consider. High levels of ground-level ozone are formed by human activities and high temperatures, when sunlight reacts with volatile organic compounds from fossil fuel exhaust. Ozone formation is highly associated with vehicular traffic and climate change [40]. During warm and sunny days, ozone concentrations accumulate [40] and can have toxic effects on plants as ozone hinders photosynthesis, reduces crop growth, and reduces crop yields [18]. Ground-level ozone is formed locally, but can be transported long distances by air masses. It has been estimated that ozone concentrations of 54–75 ppb found in reasonably highly polluted areas can reduce yields of rice, soybeans, and wheat by 8–25% [18]. Climate change is anticipated to increase ground-level ozone, leading to direct mortality and morbidity from its toxic effects on humans, as well as indirect consequences through its negative impact on plant growth and yields [18, 40–42]. However, the impact on food production has not been well quantified.

*Insects* Insects play important roles in the food system, with both negative (e.g., pests and pathogens they carry) and positive (e.g., pollinators) impacts. Climate change projections show that reductions in insect biodiversity can be substantial for a large group of insects at a global warming of 1.5 °C, with even larger effects at higher future $CO_2$ concentration levels [43].

*Pests* The term "pest" refers to fungi, weeds, pathogens, and insects that reduce crop yields. Climate change may benefit insect pests and thus lower crop yields. Changes in temperature and rainfall have been shown to decouple the regulators of pest outbreaks. For example, the regional outbreak of cotton bollworm in North China was attributed to the combination of climate change and agricultural intensification [44]. Increasing temperatures have also been linked to increased abundance of olive fruit flies, with negative economic impacts on small olive farms, as well as on ecological services provided by these farms such as biodiversity, soil conservation, and fire prevention [45]. Pest distribution may expand towards the poles as the ability of pests to overwinter improves, leading to increased rates of herbivory and crop damage [18]. Crops often lack natural protection against invasive pests, requiring adaptation to handle these challenges. However, given the shorter generation time of insects, it is likely that they will rapidly evolve to the challenges of a changing climate.

Increased $CO_2$ can interact with both plants and pests and the effects can give rise to complex changes [18]. Atmospheric gas composition affects both plants and their insect pests. Elevated $CO_2$ and temperature alter plant biochemistry in ways that may reduce pest populations. As plants provide a food source to the pests, reduced protein or micronutrient content in agricultural crops may be insufficient as a food source for the pests, and this may have negative consequences not only for their reproduction but also for defense against their pathogens [46]. Ozone is a plant toxin that alters plant biosynthetic pathways needed to produce the volatile cues that pests use to find plants and to stimulate egg-laying [47]. In aphids, the direction of the impact of ozone depends on the duration of plant exposure and the age of the plant [47]. Similarly, the impact of increased $CO_2$ levels depends on insect physiology and behavior, traits that differ substantially among insect pests [47]. Furthermore, both plants and pests are embedded in a larger community that includes pathogens, competitors, and predators, each of which responds to atmospheric gas composition [47].

*Pollinators* Pollinators are affected by climate and environmental change, with observed shifts in distribution, loss of biodiversity, and extinction of insect species with critical stabilization functions within the ecosystem [18, 43]. Insect pollinators are also directly affected by pesticides used to limit crop damage. Given that insect pollinators contribute 75% of global crops [48], and one third of global food [49], the possibility that climate change may negatively influence insect pollinators is of considerable concern. Elevated temperatures have been shown to impair the ability of carrots to produce volatiles that are needed to attract pollinators to the crop and to lower nectar sugar concentrations, both of which would reduce pollination of carrots [49]. $CO_2$ concentrations affect the protein content of pollen that is a key nutrient source for pollinators, therefore indirectly affecting pollinator overwintering and survival [18]. However, a study on insect pollinators concluded that, whereas climate change was likely to decrease watermelon pollination by managed bee colonies, pollination by native, wild pollinators was projected to compensate [48]. Modeling estimates of hypothetical global pollinator declines suggest that this decline will lead to increasing child mortality and birth defects from lack of vitamin A and folate and also increase chronic diseases by reducing consumption of healthy foods [43].

## Oceans

The ocean provides human populations with foods rich in nutrients such as protein, iron, zinc, omega-3 fatty acids, and vitamins. Today, fish alone is estimated to be an essential source of at least 20% of the intake of food and micronutrients for over one billion people worldwide. Fish availability and consumption is also likely affected by climate change, with changes in fishing yields due to changes in ocean ecosystems, range shifts of species, and acidification of the ocean causing a severe decrease in coral reef habitats [17, 18]. The loss of coral reef habitat may be as large as 92% by 2100 [50], but the overall effects from acidification on fish food webs and their associated dynamics need to be better understood [17, 18]. The effects of ocean warming on plankton overall are thought to be very important due to the cumulative dependencies through marine food webs, despite spatial differences. Ocean warming is also expected to reduce overall fat content within some fish, secondary to its negative impacts on phytoplankton, with potential effects that ripple up through the marine food chain [17, 18]. The effect of $CO_2$ concentrations on fish catch is not well understood. Multi-model ensemble projections of fishery catches based on climate change scenarios suggest that, by year 2050, plankton reductions could already lead to a potential reduction of 2–13% in the global fish catch under the high $CO_2$ concentration RCP8.5 scenario [51]. Another modeling study suggested a reduction of around 20% of tropical fish biomass by 2050 in a high $CO_2$ concentration future, due to ocean warming and oxygen reductions [52].

Globally, the impact of climate change on marine food webs and fisheries is expected to be the greatest on poor and island populations that are heavily dependent on marine food sources [53]. The global decline in fish may lead to 1.4 billion people vulnerable to deficiencies from vitamin $B_{12}$ and omega-3 fatty acids with an additional 845 million at risk of deficiencies of iron, zinc, and vitamin A [17]. Considerable uncertainties exist in the impact and the reaction of the marine food web ecosystem to anthropogenic and climate changes, so estimates should be interpreted carefully. Over the last decade, overfishing has also started to decrease the global fish catch [54]. The concomitant impacts of overfishing and climate change may cause additional negative impacts on marine production that have not yet been well considered in climate change impact projections.

## Food Prices and Food Trade

Food prices will likely be affected by climate changes, with estimates suggesting increases from 31 to 106% for wheat, rice, and maize by 2050 depending on population growth and carbon concentrations. Although this would likely have a negative impact overall on the world population, it could benefit farmers. Growth of the gross domestic product can be anticipated in some areas, and this may outweigh the increased prices of crops, so overall impacts are still unclear. A recent study concluded that economic growth occurring in the shared socioeconomic scenario has the potential to improve global nutrition status [55], although other analyses raise concerns about assumptions of ongoing socioeconomic growth [56]. Under the scenarios of Nelson et al., the poorest countries will still suffer macronutrient deficits, and many countries will continue to have micronutrient deficits, suggesting that the greatest challenge ahead may be to supply sufficiently nutrient-rich diets [55]. A limitation of the socioeconomic scenarios embraced by the IPCC is that they do not consider impacts of climate change on socioeconomic development, but lean toward narratives of highly positive economic growth spanning different development trajectories [57].

Over the last 30 years, there has been an increase in the number of countries with sufficient energy availability (i.e., >2500 kcal or >10.5 MJ) per capita per day, thanks to global trade, but a decrease in the number of countries who are self-sufficient in dietary energy [58]. This increased reliance on food trade contributes directly to climate change because of increased reliance on transportation systems for moving agricultural products internationally.

## Malnutrition

Nutritional status refers broadly to the levels of both macronutrients (protein, energy, and fat) and micronutrients (vitamins and minerals) (see Chap. 2) [59]. A recent Lancet Commission highlights that climate change is intimately tied with global epidemics of undernutrition and obesity, a combination the Commission refers to as a "Global Syndemic" [60]. The term "syndemic" is used because 1) climate change, undernutrition, and obesity overlap in time and space; 2) they interact through common drivers such as food and agriculture, transportation, and land use; and 3) they are linked through feedback loops associated with governance, business, economics, ecology, and health. Together, they will be a major cause of ill-health not only of the environment but also of individuals and populations, and therefore, the Commission recommends a set of policy approaches that can synergistically address climate change, undernutrition, and obesity [60].

*Undernutrition* Among all the potential health impacts of climate change, undernutrition is considered to be the most important [61], in large part because reliance on domestic food production and undernutrition are already high in regions where food production is likely to be most negatively affected by climate change. For example, climate change is expected to most directly impact smallholder subsistence farming households [62], communities in resource-limited countries and marginal agricultural ecosystems, and regions that rely on a single cash crop whose yields are highly sensitive to climate change [61]. Unfortunately, opportunities for adaptation are more limited in these regions, thus further increasing the potential health impacts.

Although the number of studies is limited, there is evidence that more frequent and more prolonged floods and droughts, variability in rainfall, higher temperature, and crop failure negatively influence child growth and thus climate-related variables at least indirectly contribute to child malnutrition [63]. One pathway is that populations reliant on wheat, rice, or barley may experience increased deficiencies of protein, zinc, and iron as these crops are sensitive to higher atmospheric $CO_2$ that reduces protein, zinc, and iron concentrations in the plants [63]. Not only do these deficiencies impair child growth, but they also increase the risk of infection. Macronutrient deficiencies have been associated with 53% of the infectious disease deaths in LMIC countries [64, 65], and worldwide, 13% of respiratory tract infections, 10% of malaria cases, and 8% of diarrheal episodes have been attributed to zinc deficiency [66]. Overviews of the relationship between nutritional status and infection and specific nutrients and infections are provided in Chaps. 1 and 2 [59, 67].

*Overnutrition* In the past two decades, there has been increasing interest in pathways by which the obesity epidemic and climate change might be interrelated (see systematic review by An et al. [68]). It is hypothesized that behavioral responses to climate change alter thermogenesis in a way that leads to increased accumulation of brown and beige fat [69]. Thermoregulation by mammals is driven by average ambient temperature. The increasing pattern of avoiding cold and hot temperatures by staying indoors, often in air-conditioned rooms, decreases energy expenditure and allows for fat accumulation, especially when combined with less physical activity that is often associated with indoor lifestyles [69]. Food price shocks following crop failures due to floods or droughts have been shown to shift food choices toward less expensive high-fat, high-sugar diets that increase body fat [70]. Also, fetal and infant undernutrition predisposes children to obesity. Thus, as climate change increases undernutrition in young children, it may subsequently increase obesity [60].

On the other hand, increases in obesity and western dietary patterns associated with obesity are considered as an important driver of climate change [30]. Reasons proposed include increased $CO_2$ emissions associated with higher overall food intake, with a preference for foods known to contribute to climate change, and with the additional fuels needed to transport a heavier population [68]. Obesity may also increase with urbanization and population shifts secondary to climate change as populations transition to a western-like diet at lower incomes when in urban settings [71].

If dietary aspirations and patterns in richer countries and in limited resource settings were to move toward diets that are more reliant on plant products such as fruits and vegetables, the benefits would potentially reduce the epidemic of macronutrient overnutrition while also reducing $CO_2$ emissions from livestock production. A recent modeling study integrating impacts of climate models with current diets on health estimated that, without such intentional shifts, climate changes will likely decrease fruit and vegetable production and consumption globally. The impacts of such decreases in consumption are projected to lead to increases in cardiovascular disease deaths that are twice as high as the estimated increases in deaths from macronutrient undernutrition [20].

## Climate Change and Infectious Disease

Climate change is expected to facilitate more conducive conditions for many insect- and waterborne diseases. This is happening in a time characterized by reductions in major climate-sensitive diseases, such as malaria [72, 73]. The downward trends observed in prevalence of many infectious diseases can be attributed to general improvements in sanitation, health care, public health prevention programs, innovation, land use, and environmental change [74]. However, even if these downward trends continue, climate change can cause marginal (or more dramatic increases) in infectious diseases, associated with large additional disease burdens and costs. Many climate-sensitive diseases will increase their potential for transmission under projected climate scenarios, challenging the further success of disease control programs and eradication campaigns [75]. The risk of further emergence of climate-sensitive infections in new areas will continue, such as malaria in the highlands of Africa [76] and cholera and arboviruses in temperate areas [72, 77, 78]. Observational studies from control programs in sub-Saharan Africa indicate that climate change may decrease the effectiveness of anti-malaria interventions [79]. The reason is not well understood, but it is well known that climate change can increase vectorial capacity and, in turn, malaria's Basic Reproduction Number ($R_0$), thus requiring more effort to achieve the same control effect in a population. Theoretical studies also suggest that climate change has the potential to accelerate evolution of drug resistance [80].

In this section we explore various climate-sensitive pathogens which can be particularly detrimental for countries with limited resources. We focus on several major mosquito-borne arboviruses that cause disease in humans (e.g., dengue and chikungunya) or that are zoonotic, affecting animals and humans (e.g., Rift Valley fever). We also explore malaria, waterborne diseases, and helminth infections. As zoonotic pathogens constitute a large proportion of human infectious diseases and essentially include most of the emerging and re-emerging diseases [81], we address some of their developments over the last decades, describing their dependence and dynamics in relation to climate variability and change, within the context of other important drivers of infection emergence and incidence.

## *Arboviruses*

Arboviral diseases represent one of the important disease groups that is increasing globally. The total impact of arboviruses on global health is large, due to the high morbidity and mortality in endemic areas that substantially contributes to the overall disease burden with consequences for the public health and economy in affected countries (see Chap. 10) [82]. The frequent and large epidemics may cause constraints in the public health sector that may interfere with other important investments in health, for instance, prevention of undernutrition in children. The most important arbovirus, dengue, is widely spread and is estimated to infect up to 390 million with around 100 million clinical cases

**Box 15.4 El Niño and La Niña**

*What Are They? El Niño and La Niña are opposite phases of what is known as the El Niño-Southern Oscillation (ENSO) circulation cycle. During El Niño periods, there is a substantially higher than normal sea surface temperature in the equatorial Pacific Ocean for at least 5 months leading to complex subsequent changes in the weather patterns in Oceania, Asia, Africa, and the Americas related to its effects on the trade winds. The relationship between El Niño and local weather is highly sensitive to location. A general feature during El Niño events is higher than normal temperatures in Northern America and in the affected Asian and Oceanian regions with risk for droughts, whereas floods are more common in South America. During La Niña the pattern is opposite with higher risk of floods in Asia and Oceania and parts of the Americas.*

*Risk of infection: Infectious agents that are highly sensitive to El Niño episodes include malaria, cholera, dengue, chikungunya, Rift Valley fever, and leptospirosis, with increased outbreak risk and incidence [89–94]. The delay between El Niño or La Niña observations in the Pacific and their impacts on local weather patterns provide a window that can be used to prevent outbreaks. Scientists have suggested that these delays can be used proactively for preparing a response to control outbreaks and limit disease risks [93].*

each year [83]. According to WHO, it is estimated that each year around 500,000 cases with severe dengue require hospitalization with 2.5% case fatality rate [84]. Viruses transmitted by the invasive *Aedes aegypti* and *Aedes albopictus* mosquitoes include dengue and chikungunya, both of which have caused large epidemics within endemic areas with a history of transmission, as well as more frequent outbreaks in previously unaffected regions [77]. Specifically, dengue, chikungunya, and Zika are spreading and (re-)emerging in new areas [85–88]. In many areas, epidemics co-occur with the climatic anomalies of El Niño events (see Box 15.4) [72, 89, 90]. Unfortunately, transmission of these diseases is favored by development due to the increasing trends in human mobility and urbanization that provide ideal breeding grounds for the mosquito vectors.

Dengue, chikungunya, Zika, and yellow fever, diseases spread by the *Ae. aegypti* and *Ae. albopictus* mosquitoes, share dependencies associated with vector survival and behavior in response to climate conditions. Vector abilities, such as probability of becoming infected and viral replication enabling transmission of virus to humans during feeding, are highly climate dependent but also depend on virus-vector-specific interactions. Overall, many of the parameters of importance are factored into the vectorial capacity metric, which first emerged as a concept in malaria research [95] and which incorporates the vector parameters of importance for transmission and epidemics. The vectorial capacity is closely related to the Basic Reproduction Number, $R_0$, used for infectious diseases and which is defined as the average number of subsequent infections resulting from one infectious case in a totally immunologically naïve population assuming homogeneous mixing [96]. The vectorial capacity for *Aedes* vectors is highly related to climatic conditions, especially daily mean temperature and temperature diurnal variability [96]. Current trends show substantial global increases in vectorial capacity for both *Ae. aegypti* and *Ae. albopictus* (Fig. 15.4), even when excluding the vector to human abundance component (Fig. 15.4). Vectorial capacity is further projected to increase substantially into the future, with increases in most sub-tropical and tropical zones and decreases only in the dry and extremely hot areas of the Middle East and the Sahara and Sahel regions.

*Ae. aegypti* is the principal vector of dengue, chikungunya, Zika, and yellow fever and is thriving globally with urbanization and population crowding. It is, however, more a tropical and sub-tropical vector. In contrast, *Ae. albopictus* has developed the ability to arrest its development and thus survive winters in colder temperate climates. Thus, the global distribution of endemic dengue transmission is highly related to the areas where *Ae. aegypti* survives. Transmission through *Ae. albopictus* can co-occur in these areas and likely plays a role in the transmission, but in areas outside the *Ae. aegypti*

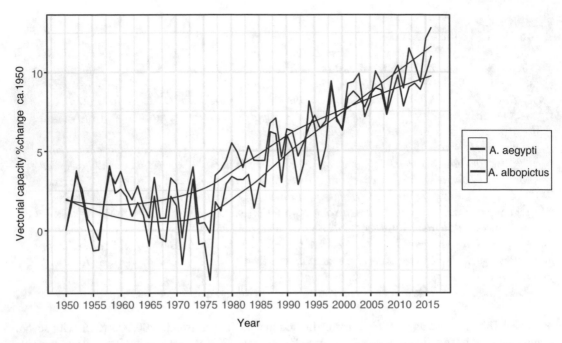

**Fig. 15.4** The aggregated global annual relative change in vectorial capacity of dengue for the vectors *Aedes aegypti* and *Ae. albopictus* 1950 to 2017. (Reprinted from Watts et al. [72], with permission from Elsevier)

zone, *Ae. albopictus* mostly contributes to smaller outbreaks of dengue and sporadic epidemics of chikungunya, such as in the temperate areas in the Mediterranean region of Europe. The life cycle of both vectors depends highly on temperature and rainfall patterns. This has been documented and included in both simulation models and empirical studies [97–101]. According to many studies, *Ae. aegypti* and *Ae. albopictus* will continue to disperse and increase in numbers from the tropical to subtropical to temperate areas across the globe [85, 101], catalyzed by the high population mobility [85]. The change in invasion and abundance is, however, highly dependent on the route of further carbon emissions, with the high RCP8.5 scenario contrasting fundamentally to the low RCP2.6 scenario (Fig. 15.5).

The deadly yellow fever virus is preventable by vaccination. However, still around 47 countries in Africa and South and Central America are endemic for, or at risk of, yellow fever outbreaks. There are an estimated 84,000–170,000 severe cases and 29,000–60,000 deaths annually. During larger outbreaks there is sometimes a worrying global shortage of vaccine.

While evidence on interactions between arboviral diseases such as dengue and chikungunya and nutritional status are limited (see Chap. 10) [82], the overlapping distributions of dengue in Asia and Africa with regions having the highest prevalence of undernutrition, and regions with greatest potential threat of climate change impacts (Fig. 15.5) highlight the importance of further attention to this nexus.

Rift Valley fever (RVF) is another example of a climate-sensitive arbovirus which causes hemorrhagic fever in both humans and animals, with serious consequences for rural populations in many African countries. Periodic epidemics occur especially in Eastern Africa (Kenya, Somalia, Tanzania) and other countries of the African continent and more recently on the Arabian Peninsula [102, 103]. Climate change with flooding that increases the abundance of competent mosquito vectors is understood to be a key driver for this lesser known emerging infection [104]. RVF causes a lethal infection in young ruminants, and outbreaks are characterized by mass abortions. Recently it was found that it may also induce abortions in humans [105]. No human vaccines or treatments are currently available.

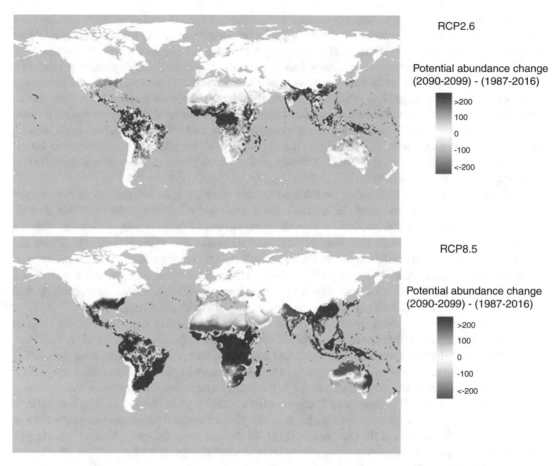

RCP2.6

Potential abundance change
(2090-2099) - (1987-2016)

>200
100
0
-100
<-200

RCP8.5

Potential abundance change
(2090-2099) - (1987-2016)

>200
100
0
-100
<-200

**Fig. 15.5** The simulated change in the potential of *Aedes aegypti* abundance in relation to climate change scenarios RCP2.6 compared with RCP8.5 at 2090–2099 compared to 1987–2016. (Reprinted from Liu-Helmersson et al. [101], published under a CC-BY license)

For decades RVF has caused transboundary outbreaks among humans and livestock in developing countries of eastern and southern Africa, leading to catastrophic economic impacts including export embargoes in large regions of Africa. Since RVF causes abortions and greater than 95% perinatal mortality in sheep, goats, cattle, and camel herds used for meat and dairy production, the epidemics can result in threats to food availability and nutritional status. There is a growing concern that RVF may spread to the American continent, Asia, and Europe through animal trade or spread of mosquito vectors [106, 107].

## Malaria

Malaria transmission is highly climate sensitive, and the main vectors are mosquitos of the genus *Anopheles* [108]. *Anopheles spp.* are sensitive to climate in terms of their breeding, survival, and behavior [95, 109]. The forces of development associated with malaria control and eradication programs are, however, a much more influential driver of malaria distribution and prevalence. Today, the less climate-sensitive and more widespread malaria parasite *Plasmodium vivax* is abundant only sporadically compared to its historical distribution, while the tropical malaria parasite *P. falciparum* is responsible for the majority of malaria disease and deaths on the African continent. Studies have attributed changes in climate to be the cause of the lower success of recent control and eradication products in countries such as Zambia [110]. Relatively higher disease burdens are predicted in a future characterized by accelerated climate change and less economic growth, although control programs and economic development more broadly are expected to be stronger drivers of future disease epidemiology than climate change [75]. A systematic review undertaken to investigate how socioeconomic, public health, and environmental factors interact with the epidemiology of malaria concluded that the influence of environmental factors on malaria epidemiology diminished when statistical analyses controlled for interventions [74]. This highlights the importance of considering interventions in future climate projections of malaria and potential opportunities for adaptation when malaria spreads into, for example, the African highlands [76].

Given the increasing areas suitable for malarial vectors in many endemic regions due to climate change, the resulting increase in malaria transmission may counteract the reductions due to anti-malaria interventions [79] and potentially also affect the spread of malaria drug resistance with the changes in prevalence of malaria [80]. Regarding the debate on the role of climate change driving the increasing risk of malaria in African highlands, there is clear support for such an effect, but as always, the situation of emergence is complicated. Multiple co-acting factors are likely to have contributed and are important to consider for understanding risk and vulnerabilities, including migration, land use, agricultural practice, demographics, and health and public health services [76].

Caminade et al. projected an overall change in the population at risk of malaria in the African highlands and southern Africa under five different climate models for malaria suitability. However, the simulations did not capture development and socioeconomic changes other than population growth, which may affect the model projections [111]. At the very high end of emissions and carbon concentrations (RCP8.5), the malaria situation was predicted to be substantially worse, with potential risks beyond the African highlands and southern Africa mentioned above [111]. The five models exhibited a fair amount of inter-model variability in the predictions and projections of population at risk, especially at the fringes of the distribution [111]. To date, none of the projections of malaria risk or incidence have considered co-occurring effects from climate change or undernutrition, which need to be properly investigated.

There has long been an understanding of the influence of nutritional status on malaria susceptibility and severity, with extensive efforts to understand the role of protein energy malnutrition (PEM) and iron as either risk factors for severe disease or protective factors against severe disease (see Chap. 11) [112]. While malaria control programs and efforts to improve nutrition and food security are leading to reductions in risk for both conditions in the Asian regions, East Africa remains of particular concern for both malaria and undernutrition, as all countries in the East Africa region except Ethiopia have seen increases in malaria cases from 2010 to 2017 [113], and the prevalence of malnutrition in East Africa remains the highest on the continent [114]. Impacts of iron deficiency are of particular importance given concerns about potential reduction of iron content in key grain crops with increases in atmospheric $CO_2$ [35].

## Waterborne Infections

Globally, there are about ten known pathogenic non-toxigenic cholera bacteria of the *Vibrio* species (spp.) including the common *Vibrio vulnificus*, *V. parahaemolyticus*, and *V. alginolyticus*. *Vibrio* species thrive in nutrient-rich waters with low or moderate salinity such as estuarine coastal waters and cause gastrointestinal infections when exposed sea food is consumed or severe necrotizing ulcers and septicemia when the bacteria colonize open wounds of swimmers or waders [78, 115]. Increases in water surface temperatures with climate change, medium salinity, high chlorophyll, and certain plankton concentrations lead to an increased growth rate of *Vibrio* spp. [78, 115]. *Vibrio* concentrations can be measured in filter-feeding mollusks, such as oysters, clams, and mussels. Overall, the suitability of the estuarine environment for *Vibrio* has increased in northern hemisphere, especially in the Baltic sea and along the northern US east coast (Fig. 15.6) [72].

The global disease burden of non-toxigenic cholera infections caused by *Vibrio spp.* is relatively unknown, but in the USA there are an estimated 80,000 infections and 100 deaths per year (https://www.cdc.gov/vibrio/index.html). A linear and increasing relationship between sea surface temperatures above 16°C and *Vibrio* incidence has been established by combining remotely sensed images of sea surface temperature and individual geo-tagged and time stamped case data from the Baltic (Fig. 15.7) [115]. The further risk projected in regions with warming seas from climate change depend directly on the generalizability of projected patterns of warming of the Baltic, in combination with salt concentration and chlorophyll [115].

In addition to the non-toxigenic cholera *Vibrio* infections, toxigenic cholera has also been shown to be climate sensitive throughout history and thrives in warmer surface waters. Toxigenic cholera strains are more dependent on co-existing infections in humans and are highly sensitive to good hygiene, sanitation, and treatment practices [116]. The feared toxigenic cholera is more abundant in resource-constrained settings and highly sensitive to disruption of social and health systems, which is common after natural disasters including those associated with El Niño events, i.e., floods [117].

Other waterborne pathogens, such as *Giardia, Cryptosporidium, Escherichia coli*, and norovirus, are also dependent on weather and climate for proliferation. Growth of the pathogens is regulated by water temperature and the release into water bodies used for distribution of household and drinking water, which is more common during floods and after rainfall [118]. Drought and water scarcity have also been linked to worsening water quality. Symptoms of gastrointestinal disease may be more widespread than disease surveillance data suggest. Sanitation, hygiene, and technological innovations contribute to reduce much illness. In Sweden, innovation in water treatment practice has been shown to reduce the overall reports of gastrointestinal symptoms [119].

## *Helminth Infections*

Other infections, including snail-transmitted schistosomiasis and vector-borne nematode infections [120, 121], as well as leptospirosis [94] are also highly climate sensitive due to their respective vector biology and exposure pathways to human infections and are likely to exhibit changes in distribution and spread in response to climate changes. A variety of helminth infections may be impacted by climate change (see review by Blum and Hotez [121]). The importance of temperature and rainfall on soil-transmitted helminths is described in Chap. 12 [122]. Impacts of climate change on important helminths transmitted by insect vectors and by aquatic snails are explored below.

***Nematodes and insect vectors***   Insects have evolved an optimum temperature range for development and survival of eggs, larvae, and pupae and for maturation, feeding, and reproduction of adults [123]. Shifts in temperature associated with climate change may reduce the abundance of vectors in regions where the vectors currently thrive, if temperatures drop below or increase above this optimum range. However, in regions where vectors cannot survive, the shift in temperature may allow the vector to expand its range, hence increasing transmission. The development of the parasite in the vector is also sensitive to temperature [123]. When temperatures are optimal for the adult mosquito and the larval parasites, female mosquitoes may be able to lay more batches of eggs, which would require more frequent blood meals, thus increasing transmission potential, so long as the interval between blood meals is sufficient to allow the parasite larvae to become infective.

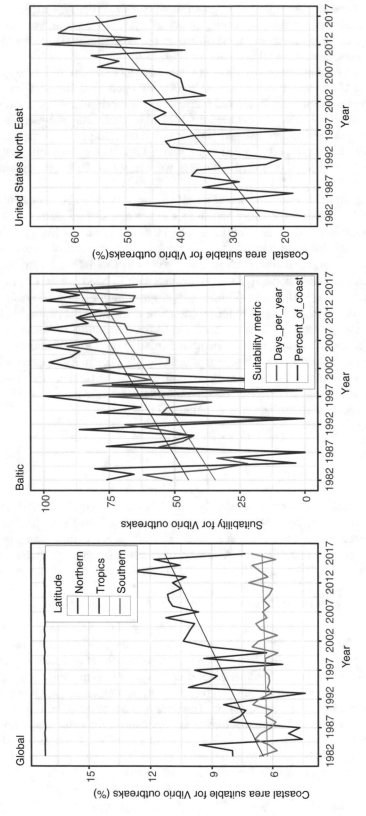

**Fig. 15.6** The suitability of *Vibrio* abundance in selected regions in response to ocean warming. (Reprinted from Watts et al. [72], with permission from Elsevier)

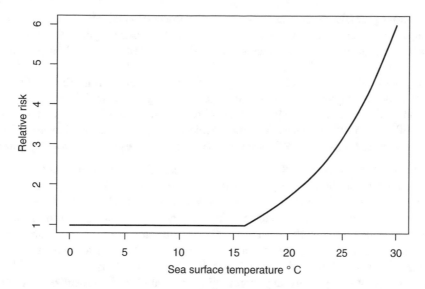

**Fig. 15.7** The relationship between sea surface temperature and individual risk of infection of *Vibrio* spp. along the Swedish coast. (Reprinted from Semenza et al. [115], an open-access journal published with support from the National Institute of Environmental Health Sciences, National Institutes of Health. All content is public domain unless otherwise noted)

Given the complex set of vector and parasite responses to temperature, and given that strains of vectors adapt to local conditions, it is challenging to make a generalized prediction about the impact of climate change on these diseases. However, an African study exploring potential impacts on lymphatic filariasis, a nematode infection caused by *Brugia malayi* and transmitted by mosquitoes, concluded that there is a high probability that disease will spread into West Africa and that the number of cases of disease may double when considering the impacts of climate change together with population growth [124]. With regard to onchocerciasis caused by *Onchocerca volvulus* and transmitted by blackflies, projections indicate that small increases in monthly average temperature will increase blackfly abundance and development of parasites to the infective larval stage, thus expanding the distribution of the disease [125]. However, the field data on blackfly abundance suggest that their numbers may decrease [125]. As with temperature, climate-induced changes in rainfall are also likely to influence the seasonal availability and suitability of insect breeding sites. Increased frequency and severity of droughts may limit or even eradicate insect vectors from some regions. Increased frequency and severity of floods may benefit blackflies that rely on fast-running water and mosquitoes that use temporary pools of water for breeding. However, severe floods may also wash away insect eggs and aquatic larvae. Nevertheless, there are strong biological reasons to anticipate that climate change will alter the geographical distribution of vector-borne nematode infections.

***Trematodes and aquatic snails*** Schistosomiasis is also likely to be strongly influenced by climate change. This trematode parasite requires freshwater snails for completion of its life cycle. As with insect vectors, there is a temperature optimum for growth, reproduction, and survival of aquatic snails and for development of the larval parasites within the snail. When applying a 1.5 °C increase in temperature, Yang and Bergquist [120] concluded that transmission of the three main species of *Schistosoma* would increase. It is important to note that the association with rates of transmission and disease is unlikely to be linear given the complex dynamics involved. Furthermore, the response of snail and parasite to multiple stresses can influence their biology. It is well known that infected snails have a dramatic increase in egg-laying during the period of parasite development, a response called "fecundity compensation." However, this response disappeared when snails were also exposed to drought conditions [126]. Even more surprising was the observation that drought conditions increased the output of infective cercariae from the snails. This study further exemplifies the difficulty in anticipating the net consequences of climate change on snail or insect vectors and their parasites.

***Implications for nutrition*** In an effort to increase food production within urban settings and simultaneously offset negative impacts of climate change, rooftop gardens are often promoted. There has been concern that these gardens may provide ideal breeding sites for *Culex* mosquitoes that transmit filariasis as well as the West Nile virus. An experimental study in Hong Kong, however, found that the number of mosquitoes trapped on roofs was not affected by the presence of a rooftop garden [127].

High-intensity *Onchocerca* infections have been associated with vitamin A deficiency [128], and blindness resulting from chronic infection with *Onchocerca* has historically led communities to relocate away from fertile river valleys to avoid transmission [129]. River blindness is less common now, but skin conditions have been shown to also negatively impact agricultural production. In Nigeria, farmers with severe onchocercal skin disease cultivated less of their farmland and were unable to compensate for lost income from other sources [130]. Filariasis can also be extremely debilitating causing severe lymphedema, and chronic schistosomiasis is associated with anemia and reduced work capacity [131]. Thus, any increase in, or expansion of, transmission associated with climate change is likely to have economic implications for their families and communities, including reduced access to food.

## Foodborne Infections

Foodborne infections result from ingestion of food (often raw fruits and vegetables) that is contaminated with bacterial pathogens and parasites. These outbreaks typically cause diarrheas but can be serious and in the case of immunosuppressed individuals can be life-threatening (see Chaps. 4 and 8) [132, 133]. Of the variety of ways in which climate change is likely to influence the risk of foodborne disease outbreaks, improved survival of the environmental stages in response to rising air and ocean temperatures, increased dispersal onto crops as a result of increased precipitation, and extreme weather events leading to major flooding are a few examples [134, 135].

Increased air temperatures are likely to increase the numbers and activity of flies that act as mechanical vectors of foodborne pathogens, transferring the bacteria onto foods. A recent modeling study found that transmission by insect vectors captured data on incidence of *Campylobacter* cases in Ontario, Canada [136]. Furthermore, their model showed that the incidence of *Campylobacter* cases was more sensitive to fly activity than fly population size. Using a medium-low climate scenario, a 25% increase in fly activity resulted in a 31.7% increase in incidence of *Campylobacter* cases in 2080 under a medium-low climate scenario.

*Vibrio* is considered as both a waterborne and a foodborne infection. As noted above, rising ocean temperatures have the potential to increase the risk of outbreaks of *Vibrio* bacteria on shellfish, particularly oysters, because the bacteria replicate at higher rates when water temperatures are higher. For example, the incidence of illnesses due to *Vibrio* contamination of oysters has been found to be higher during El Niño years when coastal water temperatures are higher than average [137].

Perhaps of most concern, however, is the impact of floods following extreme weather events, as floods can transport pathogens onto agricultural lands and thus increase the exposure to foodborne pathogens. For example, in September 2018, the North Carolina Department of Agriculture and Food Services released a warning during Hurricane Florence that crops exposed to floodwaters could not be used for human or animal food consumption because of potential contamination with foodborne pathogens and chemical toxins and toxins from mold growing on stored crops [138]. They specifically listed leafy greens, tomatoes, corn, peanuts, sweet potatoes, watermelon, winter squash, and products stored in bulk that might get wet and contaminated (e.g., grains, nuts, corn).

Much of the evidence on climate-related increases in foodborne outbreaks comes from developed countries. Yet, the same foodborne pathogens occur in developing countries where pre-existing malnutrition is likely to increase the risk of severe disease following exposure to foodborne pathogens and where mitigation against climate change may not be as effective as in developed countries. Furthermore, farmers in developing countries will be severely affected if their produce and grains cannot be used for human or animal consumption. In subsistence farming settings, families that attempt to prevent foodborne disease may also be reducing their already limited access to food. Thus, climate change is likely to increase the risk of foodborne pathogens and to reduce availability of fresh fruits and vegetables, with potential implications for nutritional status of vulnerable populations.

## The 2030 Sustainable Development Goals

The vision for the transformation of the global society presented in the UN global Sustainable Development Goals (SDGs) highlights the intersection of climate change, nutrition, and infection (see Table 15.2).

The climate action goal (SDG 13) relates to conversion of societies to clean energy and adaptation to protect vulnerable sectors and populations, as described in section "Climate Change Pathways to Nutrition and Infection." SDG 13 embraces the fact that emissions are a global issue which needs to be solved with global partnerships, such as the Paris Agreement. This goal is related to life on land and life on water and impacts directly on human nutrition and infection through social systems, hunger, health, and hygiene and sanitation as schematically illustrated in Fig. 15.8. In addition to the climate action goal, other SDGs of relevance include four social systems goals and two more natural systems goals. The four social systems goals most relevant to the climate/infection/nutrition nexus focus on ending poverty, reducing undernutrition, reducing disease, and increasing water quality and sanitation standards. The two additional natural systems SDGs of greatest relevance focus on life underwater and life on land. Table 15.2 highlights the focus and relevance of each of the identified SDGs for this chapter.

## Gaps and Future Directions

Taken together, the combined impact of climate change, undernutrition, obesity, and infectious disease on health is a very important area of emerging interest. If ignored, there will potentially be very serious consequences. Researchers will be challenged as they attempt to consider the complexity of direct and indirect pathways of impact, combined with potentially unanticipated latent effects.

Utilizing a One Health approach, where animal, human, plant, and environmental health are integrated, would strengthen assessment of the complex interplay between climate change, environment, infectious agents, their hosts, vectors, and the impact on human health [139]. As One Health effectively engages disciplines of medicine, public health, veterinary medicine, and environmental sciences and ecology [140], this approach will be useful for investigating outbreaks of vector-borne and zoonotic infections and for creating policies which need cross-sectoral collaboration such as for surveillance and control.

Models that consider the impacts of climate change on agriculture, nutrition, and/or infectious disease will be strengthened if pathways of effect, such as ozone, pollination, and pests, as well as

**Table 15.2** Global Sustainable Development Goals 2015–2030 (SDGs) in relation to climate change, mitigation of carbon emissions, and its relation to nutrition and infection (see https://sustainabledevelopment.un.org)

| SDG | Topic | Relevance |
|---|---|---|
| SDG1 Ending poverty | Aspires to reduce extreme poverty and vulnerability and a strive to universal social protection systems | Poor populations exhibit higher vulnerability to undernutrition and infection and to climate change<br>Highly related to risks of, and protection from, impacts of climate change |
| SDG 2 Zero hunger | Strives to reduce undernutrition and its consequences by preventing its causes | Ending hunger and achieving food security and improved nutrition are highly related<br>Links of poverty, climate action, and life on land and under water outlined in section "Climate Change, Food Systems, and Nutrition" |
| SDG 3 Good health and well-being | Advance global public health and well-being by reducing preventable diseases, infectious diseases affecting vulnerable populations, and neglected diseases affecting the poorest | Despite advancements in longevity and control of infectious diseases, major infectious diseases are still prevalent. Some diseases are climate sensitive and interrelated to the other goals (Fig. 15.1). Some are on the rise and may, or have already, spread to new areas or see increased potential for transmission, reducing effectiveness of control and increasing risks of drug resistance as described (section "Climate Change and Infectious Disease")<br>Achieving good health and well-being intrinsically depends on managing the combined impacts of climate change on infection and nutrition and finding ways to promote sustainable food systems and stabilize the $CO_2$ emission pathway (sections "Climate Change, Food Systems, and Nutrition" and "Climate Change and Infectious Disease") |
| SDG 6 Clean water and sanitation | Increase water quality and sanitation standards globally | Closely related to health (sections "Climate Change, Food Systems, and Nutrition" and "Climate Change and Infectious Disease"). Identifies water scarcity, floods, enhanced pathogen growth with global warming, and lack of wastewater management as key factors for successful achievement of the 2030 SDGs |
| SDG 13 Climate action | Increase use of clean energy, reduce carbon emissions, and catalyze adaption to reduce vulnerabilities and residual impacts | Relates to conversion of societies to clean energy and adaptation to protect vulnerable sectors and populations (section "Climate Change Pathways to Nutrition and Infection")<br>Embraces fact that emissions are global issue to be solved with global partnerships, such as the Paris Agreement<br>Related to life on land and life on water and impacts directly on human nutrition and infection through social systems, hunger, health, and hygiene and sanitation (Fig. 15.8) |
| SDG 14 Life under water | Protect oceans and sea life from reduction in biodiversity, overfishing, pollution, acidification, and ecosystem collapse and protect populations and wildlife depending on oceans | Focuses on health of ocean ecosystems and the terrestrial systems and populations that depend on the oceans |
| SDG 15 Life on land | Preserve forests for biodiversity and for as carbon sinks, reduces risks of desertification | Identifies forests as important for food security and for combating climate change by acting as carbon sinks<br>Goal is compromised by expansion of food systems and industrialized food production |

variation in assumptions about socioeconomic development trajectories are incorporated. This will be of particular importance when comparing mitigation/resilience approaches.

With increased transdisciplinary dialogue, less obvious pathways of effect are likely to emerge, and researchers are encouraged to be attentive to such possibilities.

Including this nexus in analysis of potential impacts of climate mitigation and resilience approaches will be essential for minimizing unintended negative consequences.

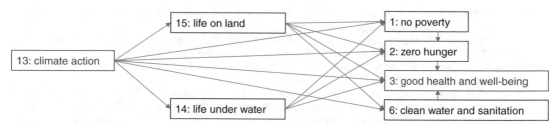

**Fig. 15.8** SDG interdependence on climate and environmental change and nutrition and infection. Of the 17 global goals of sustainable development (SDGs), this figure outlines the connections between the 7 SDGs most closely linked to climate change, infections, and nutrition. The three goals on the left and middle focus on preserving and protecting environmental systems, while the four goals on the right side are more broadly focused on human well-being. Each of the four SDGs on the right side of outline goals for improving human well-being that will be enhanced with the achievement of SDGs 13–15 and will be challenging to achieve for all without significant progress on SDGs 13–15

# References

1. Nelson DR, Adger WN, Brown K. Adaptation to environmental change: contributions of a resilience framework. Annu Rev Environ Resour. 2007;32:395–419.
2. Field CB, Barros VR, Dokken DJ, Mach KJ, Mastrandrea MD, Bilir TE, et al. Climate change 2014: impacts, adaptation, and vulnerability. Part A: global and sectoral aspects. Contribution of Working Group II to the Fifth Assessment report of the Intergovernmental Panel on Climate Change. IPCC. 2014.
3. Hoegh-Guldberg O, Jacob D, Taylor M, Bindi M, Brown S, Camilloni I, et al. Impacts of 1.5°C global warming on natural and human systems. In: Masson-Delmotte V, Zhai P, Pörtner O, Roberts D, Skea J, Shukla PR, et al., editors. Global warming of 1.5°C. An IPCC special report on the impacts of global warming of 1.5°C above pre-industrial levels and related global greenhouse gas emission pathways, in the context of strengthening the global response to the threat of climate change, sustainable development, and efforts to eradicate poverty: IPCC; 2018.
4. Collins M, Knutti R, Arblaster J, Dufresne J-L, Fichefet T, Friedlingstein P, et al. Long-term climate change: projections, commitments and irreversibility. In: Stocker TF, Qin D, Plattner G-K, Tignor M, Allen SK, Boschung J, et al., editors. Climate change 2013: the physical science basis. Contribution of Working Group I to the Fifth Assessment report of the Intergovernmental Panel on Climate Change: Cambridge University Press; 2013.
5. Stocker TF, Qin D, Plattner G-K, Tignor M, Allen SK, Boschung J, et al. Climate change 2013: the physical science basis. Contribution of Working Group I to the Fifth Assessment Report of the Intergovernmental Panel on Climate Change. IPCC; 2013.
6. Vermeulen SJ, Campbell BM, Ingram JS. Climate change and food systems. Annu Rev Environ Resour. 2012;37:195–222.
7. Costello A, Abbas M, Allen A, Ball S, Bell S, Bellamy R, et al. Managing the health effects of climate change: lancet and University College London Institute for Global Health Commission. Lancet. 2009;373(9676):1693–733.
8. McMichael AJ, Lindgren E. Climate change: present and future risks to health, and necessary responses. J Intern Med. 2011;270(5):401–13.
9. van Baalen S, Mobjork M. Climate change and violent conflict in East Africa: integrating qualitative and quantitative research to probe the mechanisms. Int Stud Rev. 2018;20(4):547–75.
10. Beebe NW, Cooper RD, Mottram P, Sweeney AW. Australia's dengue risk driven by human adaptation to climate change. PLoS Negl Trop Dis. 2009;3(5):e429.
11. Semenza JC, Lindgren E, Balkanyi L, Espinosa L, Almqvist MS, Penttinen P, et al. Determinants and drivers of infectious disease threat events in Europe. Emerg Infect Dis. 2016;22(4):581–9.
12. Foley JA, Ramankutty N, Brauman KA, Cassidy ES, Gerber JS, Johnston M, et al. Solutions for a cultivated planet. Nature. 2011;478(7369):337–42.
13. Gomiero T, Pimentel D, Paoletti MG. Environmental impact of different agricultural management practices: conventional vs. organic agriculture. Crit Rev Plant Sci. 2011;30(1–2):95–124.
14. Havlik P, Valin H, Herrero M, Obersteiner M, Schmid E, Rufino MC, et al. Climate change mitigation through livestock system transitions. Proc Natl Acad Sci U S A. 2014;111(10):3709–14.
15. Scherr SJ, Sthapit S, Mastny L. Mitigating climate change through food and land use, Worldwatch report 179. Washington, DC: Instituto Worldwatch; 2009.
16. Cline WR. Global warming and agriculture: impact estimates by country. Washington, DC: Center for Global Development: Peterson Institute for International Economics; 2007. p. xv, 186.

17. Golden CD, Allison EH, Cheung WW, Dey MM, Halpern BS, McCauley DJ, et al. Nutrition: fall in fish catch threatens human health. Nature. 2016;534(7607):317–20.
18. Myers SS, Smith MR, Guth S, Golden CD, Vaitla B, Mueller ND, et al. Climate change and global food systems: potential impacts on food security and undernutrition. Annu Rev Public Health. 2017;38:259–77.
19. Woodward A, Smith KR, Campbell-Lendrum D, Chadee DD, Honda Y, Liu Q, et al. Climate change and health: on the latest IPCC report. Lancet. 2014;383(9924):1185–9.
20. Springmann M, Mason-D'Croz D, Robinson S, Garnett T, Godfray HC, Gollin D, et al. Global and regional health effects of future food production under climate change: a modelling study. Lancet. 2016;387(10031):1937–46.
21. International Food Policy Research Institute. Global nutrition report 2015: actions and accountability to advance nutrition and sustainable development. Washington, DC: IFPRI; 2015.
22. Popkin BM, Adair LS, Ng SW. Global nutrition transition and the pandemic of obesity in developing countries. Nutr Rev. 2012;70(1):3–21.
23. Mousivand A, Arsanjani JJ. Insights on the historical and emerging global land cover changes: the case of ESA-CCI-LC datasets. Appl Geogr. 2019;106:82–92.
24. Godfray HC, Beddington JR, Crute IR, Haddad L, Lawrence D, Muir JF, et al. Food security: the challenge of feeding 9 billion people. Science. 2010;327(5967):812–8.
25. Roberts DP, Mattoo AK. Sustainable agriculture—enhancing environmental benefits, food nutritional quality and building crop resilience to abiotic and biotic stresses. Agriculture (Basel). 2018;8(1):8.
26. Food and Agriculture Organization of the United Nations. The state of food and agriculture: climate change, agriculture and food security. Rome: FAO; 2016.
27. Reeder JD, Schuman GE. Influence of livestock grazing on C sequestration in semi-arid mixed-grass and short-grass rangelands. Environ Pollut. 2002;116(3):457–63.
28. Hermansen JE, Kristensen T. Management options to reduce the carbon footprint of livestock products. Anim Front. 2011;1(1):33–9.
29. Rose D, Willits-Smith A, Heller M. Diet and planetary health: single-item substitutions significantly reduce the carbon footprint of self-selected diets reported in NHANES (OR20-08-19). Curr Dev Nutr. 2019;3(Suppl 1) https://doi.org/10.1093/cdn/nzz047.OR20-08-19.
30. Rose D, Willits-Smith A, Heller M. Diet and planetary health: single-item substitutions significantly reduce the carbon footprint of self-selected diets reported in NHANES (OR20-08-19). Curr Dev Nutr. 2019;3:1.
31. Rosenzweig C, Elliott J, Deryng D, Ruane AC, Muller C, Arneth A, et al. Assessing agricultural risks of climate change in the 21st century in a global gridded crop model intercomparison. Proc Natl Acad Sci U S A. 2014;111(9):3268–73.
32. Parikh SJ, James BR. Soil: the foundation of agriculture. Nat Educ Knowl. 2012;3(10):2.
33. Proctor J, Hsiang S, Burney J, Burke M, Schlenker W. Estimating global agricultural effects of geoengineering using volcanic eruptions. Nature. 2018;560(7719):480–3.
34. Zhao C, Liu B, Piao S, Wang X, Lobell DB, Huang Y, et al. Temperature increase reduces global yields of major crops in four independent estimates. Proc Natl Acad Sci U S A. 2017;114(35):9326–31.
35. Myers SS, Zanobetti A, Kloog I, Huybers P, Leakey AD, Bloom AJ, et al. Increasing CO2 threatens human nutrition. Nature. 2014;510(7503):139–42.
36. Loladze I. Hidden shift of the ionome of plants exposed to elevated CO(2)depletes minerals at the base of human nutrition. eLife. 2014;3:e02245.
37. Bailey RL, West KP Jr, Black RE. The epidemiology of global micronutrient deficiencies. Ann Nutr Metab. 2015;66(Suppl 2):22–33.
38. McLean E, Cogswell M, Egli I, Wojdyla D, de Benoist B. Worldwide prevalence of anaemia, WHO Vitamin and Mineral Nutrition Information System, 1993–2005. Public Health Nutr. 2009;12(4):444–54.
39. Challinor AJ, Watson J, Lobell DB, Howden SM, Smith DR, Chhetri N. A meta-analysis of crop yield under climate change and adaptation. Nat Clim Chang. 2014;4(4):287–91.
40. Ebi KL, McGregor G. Climate change, tropospheric ozone and particulate matter, and health impacts. Environ Health Perspect. 2008;116(11):1449–55.
41. Orru H, Andersson C, Ebi KL, Langner J, Astrom C, Forsberg B. Impact of climate change on ozone-related mortality and morbidity in Europe. Eur Respir J. 2013;41(2):285–94.
42. Sheffield PE, Knowlton K, Carr JL, Kinney PL. Modeling of regional climate change effects on ground-level ozone and childhood asthma. Am J Prev Med. 2011;41(3):251–7; quiz A3.
43. Warren R, Price J, Graham E, Forstenhaeusler N, VanDerWal J. The projected effect on insects, vertebrates, and plants of limiting global warming to 1.5 degrees C rather than 2 degrees C. Science. 2018;360(6390):791–5.
44. Ouyang F, Hui C, Ge S, Men XY, Zhao ZH, Shi PJ, et al. Weakening density dependence from climate change and agricultural intensification triggers pest outbreaks: a 37-year observation of cotton bollworms. Ecol Evol. 2014;4(17):3362–74.

45. Ponti L, Gutierrez AP, Ruti PM, Dell'Aquila A. Fine-scale ecological and economic assessment of climate change on olive in the Mediterranean Basin reveals winners and losers. Proc Natl Acad Sci U S A. 2014;111(15):5598–603.
46. Trebicki P, Dader B, Vassiliadis S, Fereres A. Insect-plant-pathogen interactions as shaped by future climate: effects on biology, distribution, and implications for agriculture. Insect Sci. 2017;24(6):975–89.
47. Boullis A, Francis F, Verheggen FJ. Climate change and tritrophic interactions: will modifications to greenhouse gas emissions increase the vulnerability of herbivorous insects to natural enemies? Environ Entomol. 2015;44(2):277–86.
48. Rader R, Reilly J, Bartomeus I, Winfree R. Native bees buffer the negative impact of climate warming on honey bee pollination of watermelon crops. Glob Chang Biol. 2013;19(10):3103–10.
49. Broussard MA, Mas F, Howlett B, Pattemore D, Tylianakis JM. Possible mechanisms of pollination failure in hybrid carrot seed and implications for industry in a changing climate. PLoS One. 2017;12(6):e0180215.
50. Speers AE, Besedin EY, Palardy JE, Moore C. Impacts of climate change and ocean acidification on coral reef fisheries: an integrated ecological-economic model. Ecol Econ. 2016;128:33–43.
51. Cheung WWL, Jones MC, Reygondeau G, Stock CA, Lam VWY, Frolicher TL. Structural uncertainty in projecting global fisheries catches under climate change. Ecol Model. 2016;325:57–66.
52. Cheung WWL, Watson R, Pauly D. Signature of ocean warming in global fisheries catch. Nature. 2013;497(7449):365–8.
53. Lotze HK, Tittensor DP, Bryndum-Buchholz A, Eddy TD, Cheung WWL, Galbraith ED, et al. Global ensemble projections reveal trophic amplification of ocean biomass declines with climate change. Proc Natl Acad Sci U S A. 2019;116(26):12907–12.
54. Pauly D, Zeller D. Catch reconstructions reveal that global marine fisheries catches are higher than reported and declining. Nat Comm. 2016;7:10244.
55. Nelson G, et al. Income growth and climate change effects on global nutrition security to mid-century. Nat Sustain. 2018;1(December 2018):773–81.
56. Butler CD. Infectious disease emergence and global change: thinking systemically in a shrinking world. Infect Dis Poverty. 2012;1(1):5.
57. Riahi K, van Vuuren DP, Kriegler E, Edmonds J, O'Neill BC, Fujimori S, et al. The Shared Socioeconomic Pathways and their energy, land use, and greenhouse gas emissions implications: an overview. Global Environ Chang. 2017;42:153–68.
58. Porkka M, Kummu M, Siebert S, Varis O. From food insufficiency towards trade dependency: a historical analysis of global food availability. PLoS One. 2013;8(12):e82714.
59. Barffour MA, Humphries DL. Core principles: infectious disease risk in relation to macro and micronutrient status. In: Humphries DL, Scott ME, Vermund SH, editors. Nutrition and infectious disease: shifting the clinical paradigm: Humana Press; 2020.
60. Swinburn BA, Kraak VI, Allender S, Atkins VJ, Baker PI, Bogard JR, et al. The global syndemic of obesity, undernutrition, and climate change: the lancet commission report. Lancet. 2019;393(10173):791–846.
61. Watts N, Amann M, Ayeb-Karlsson S, Belesova K, Bouley T, Boykoff M, et al. The Lancet countdown on health and climate change: from 25 years of inaction to a global transformation for public health. Lancet. 2018;391(10120):581–630.
62. Brown ME, Funk CC. Climate. Food security under climate change. Science. 2008;319(5863):580–1.
63. Phalkey RK, Aranda-Jan C, Marx S, Hofle B, Sauerborn R. Systematic review of current efforts to quantify the impacts of climate change on undernutrition. Proc Natl Acad Sci U S A. 2015;112(33):E4522–9.
64. Schaible UE, Kaufmann SH. Malnutrition and infection: complex mechanisms and global impacts. PLoS Med. 2007;4(5):e115.
65. Pelletier DL, Frongillo EA Jr, Schroeder DG, Habicht JP. The effects of malnutrition on child mortality in developing countries. Bull World Health Organ. 1995;73(4):443–8.
66. Bernstein AS, Myers SS. Climate change and children's health. Curr Opin Pediatr. 2011;23(2):221–6.
67. Humphries DL, Scott ME, Vermund SH. Pathways linking nutritional status and infectious disease. In: Humphries D, Scott ME, Vermund SH, editors. Nutrition and infectious disease: shifting the clinical paradigm: Humana Press; 2020.
68. An R, Ji M, Zhang S. Global warming and obesity: a systematic review. Obes Rev. 2018;19(2):150–63.
69. Turner JB, Kumar A, Koch CA. The effects of indoor and outdoor temperature on metabolic rate and adipose tissue – the Mississippi perspective on the obesity epidemic. Rev Endocr Metab Disord. 2016;17(1):61–71.
70. Husband A. Climate change and the role of food price in determining obesity risk. Am J Public Health. 2013;103(1):e2.
71. Popkin BM. The nutrition transition and obesity in the developing world. J Nutr. 2001;131(3):871S–3S.
72. Watts N, Amann M, Arnell N, Ayeb-Karlsson S, Belesova K, Berry H, et al. The 2018 report of the Lancet Countdown on health and climate change: shaping the health of nations for centuries to come. Lancet. 2018;392(10163):2479–514.

73. Gething PW, Smith DL, Patil AP, Tatem AJ, Snow RW, Hay SI. Climate change and the global malaria recession. Nature. 2010;465(7296):342–5.

74. Sadoine ML, Smargiassi A, Ridde V, Tusting LS, Zinszer K. The associations between malaria, interventions, and the environment: a systematic review and meta-analysis. Malar J. 2018;17(1):73.

75. Beguin A, Hales S, Rocklöv J, Åsröm C, Louis V, Sauerborn R. The opposing effects of climate change and socio-economic development on the global distribution of malaria. Glob Environ Change. 2011;21(4):6.

76. Chaves LF, Koenraadt CJ. Climate change and highland malaria: fresh air for a hot debate. Q Rev Biol. 2010;85(1):27–55.

77. Lillepold K, Rocklov J, Liu-Helmersson J, Sewe M, Semenza JC. More arboviral disease outbreaks in continental Europe due to the warming climate? J Travel Med. 2019;26(5):pii:taz017.

78. Vezzulli L, Grande C, Reid PC, Helaouet P, Edwards M, Hofle MG, et al. Climate influence on Vibrio and associated human diseases during the past half-century in the coastal North Atlantic. Proc Natl Acad Sci U S A. 2016;113(34):E5062–71.

79. Ssempiira J, Kissa J, Nambuusi B, Mukooyo E, Opigo J, Makumbi F, et al. Interactions between climatic changes and intervention effects on malaria spatio-temporal dynamics in Uganda. Parasite Epidemiol Control. 2018;3(3):e00070.

80. Artzy-Randrup Y, Alonso D, Pascual M. Transmission intensity and drug resistance in malaria population dynamics: implications for climate change. PLoS One. 2010;5(10):e13588.

81. Woolhouse ME, Gowtage-Sequeria S. Host range and emerging and reemerging pathogens. Emerg Infect Dis. 2005;11(12):1842–7.

82. Villamor E, Villar LA. Nutrition and arboviral infections. In: Humphries DL, Scott ME, Vermund SH, editors. Nutrition and infectious disease: shifting the clinical paradigm: Humana Press; 2020.

83. Bhatt S, Gething PW, Brady OJ, Messina JP, Farlow AW, Moyes CL, et al. The global distribution and burden of dengue. Nature. 2013;496(7446):504–7.

84. World Health Organization. Dengue and Severe Dengue Geneva. [updated 4 Nov 2019]. https://www.who.int/en/news-room/fact-sheets/detail/dengue-and-severe-dengue. Accessed 6 Dec 2019.

85. Kraemer MUG, Reiner RC Jr, Brady OJ, Messina JP, Gilbert M, Pigott DM, et al. Past and future spread of the arbovirus vectors Aedes aegypti and Aedes albopictus. Nat Microbiol. 2019;4(5):854–63.

86. Ramadona AL, Tozan Y, Lazuardi L, Rocklöv J. A combination of incidence data and mobility proxies from social media predicts the intra-urban spread of dengue in Yogyakarta, Indonesia. PLoS Negl Trop Dis. 2019;13(4):e0007298.

87. Rocklov J, Tozan Y, Ramadona A, Sewe MO, Sudre B, Garrido J, et al. Using big data to monitor the introduction and spread of chikungunya, Europe, 2017. Emerg Infect Dis. 2019;25(6):1041–9.

88. Struchiner CJ, Rocklov J, Wilder-Smith A, Massad E. Increasing dengue incidence in Singapore over the past 40 years: population growth, climate and mobility. PLoS One. 2015;10(8):e0136286.

89. Liyanage P, Tissera H, Sewe M, Quam M, Amarasinghe A, Palihawadana P, et al. A spatial hierarchical analysis of the temporal influences of the El Nino-Southern Oscillation and weather on dengue in Kalutara District, Sri Lanka. Int J Environ Res Public Health. 2016;13(11):pii:E1087.

90. Flahault A, de Castaneda RR, Bolon I. Climate change and infectious diseases. Public Health Rev. 2016;37:21.

91. Cazelles B, Chavez M, McMichael AJ, Hales S. Nonstationary influence of El Nino on the synchronous dengue epidemics in Thailand. PLoS Med. 2005;2(4):e106.

92. Fisman DN, Tuite AR, Brown KA. Impact of El Nino Southern Oscillation on infectious disease hospitalization risk in the United States. Proc Natl Acad Sci U S A. 2016;113(51):14589–94.

93. Yang XB, Scherm H. El Nino and infectious disease. Science. 1997;275(5301):739.

94. Weinberger D, Baroux N, Grangeon JP, Ko AI, Goarant C. El Nino Southern Oscillation and leptospirosis outbreaks in New Caledonia. PLoS Negl Trop Dis. 2014;8(4):e2798.

95. Smith DL, Battle KE, Hay SI, Barker CM, Scott TW, McKenzie FE. Ross, macdonald, and a theory for the dynamics and control of mosquito-transmitted pathogens. PLoS Pathog. 2012;8(4):e1002588.

96. Rocklöv JT, Tozan Y. Climate change and the rising infectiousness of dengue. Emerg Top Life Sci. 2019;3(2):133–42.

97. Kraemer MU, Sinka ME, Duda KA, Mylne A, Shearer FM, Brady OJ, et al. The global compendium of Aedes aegypti and Ae. albopictus occurrence. Sci Data. 2015;2:150035.

98. Liyanage P, Rocklöv J, Tissera H, et al. Evaluation of intensified dengue control measures with interrupted time series analysis in the Panadura Medical Officer of Health division in Sri Lanka: a case study and cost-effectiveness analysis. Lancet Planetary Health. 2019;3(5):211–8.

99. Metelmann S, Caminade C, Jones AE, Medlock JM, Baylis M, Morse AP. The UK's suitability for Aedes albopictus in current and future climates. J R Soc Interface. 2019;16(152):20180761.

100. Liu-Helmersson J, Rocklöv J, Sewe M, Brännström Å. Climate change may enable Aedes aegypti infestation in major European cities by 2100. Environ Res. 2019;172:7.

101. Liu-Helmersson J, Brännström Å, Sewe M, Semenza J, Rocklöv J. Estimating past, present and future trends in the global distribution and abundance of the arbovirus vector Aedes aegypti under climate change scenarios. Front Public Health. 2019;7:148.
102. Hassan OA, Ahlm C, Sang R, Evander M. The 2007 Rift Valley fever outbreak in Sudan. PLoS Negl Trop Dis. 2011;5(9):e1229.
103. Nanyingi MO, Munyua P, Kiama SG, Muchemi GM, Thumbi SM, Bitek AO, et al. A systematic review of Rift Valley Fever epidemiology 1931–2014. Infect Ecol Epidemiol. 2015;5:28024.
104. Anyamba A, Chretien JP, Small J, Tucker CJ, Formenty PB, Richardson JH, et al. Prediction of a Rift Valley fever outbreak. Proc Natl Acad Sci U S A. 2009;106(3):955–9.
105. Baudin M, Jumaa AM, Jomma HJE, Karsany MS, Bucht G, Naslund J, et al. Association of Rift Valley fever virus infection with miscarriage in Sudanese women: a cross-sectional study. Lancet Glob Health. 2016;4(11):e864–e71.
106. Mansfield KL, Banyard AC, McElhinney L, Johnson N, Horton DL, Hernandez-Triana LM, et al. Rift Valley fever virus: a review of diagnosis and vaccination, and implications for emergence in Europe. Vaccine. 2015;33(42):5520–31.
107. Scoglio CM, Bosca C, Riad MH, Sahneh FD, Britch SC, Cohnstaedt LW, et al. Biologically informed individual-based network model for Rift Valley fever in the US and evaluation of mitigation strategies. PLoS One. 2016;11(9):e0162759.
108. Sinka ME, Bangs MJ, Manguin S, Rubio-Palis Y, Chareonviriyaphap T, Coetzee M, et al. A global map of dominant malaria vectors. Parasit Vectors. 2012;5:69.
109. Brady OJ, Godfray HC, Tatem AJ, Gething PW, Cohen JM, McKenzie FE, et al. Vectorial capacity and vector control: reconsidering sensitivity to parameters for malaria elimination. Trans R Soc Trop Med Hyg. 2016;110(2):107–17.
110. Bennett A, Yukich J, Miller JM, Keating J, Moonga H, Hamainza B, et al. The relative contribution of climate variability and vector control coverage to changes in malaria parasite prevalence in Zambia 2006–2012. Parasit Vectors. 2016;9(1):431.
111. Caminade C, Kovats S, Rocklov J, Tompkins AM, Morse AP, Colon-Gonzalez FJ, et al. Impact of climate change on global malaria distribution. Proc Natl Acad Sci U S A. 2014;111(9):3286–91.
112. Kim HH, Bei AK. Nutritional frameworks in malaria. In: Humphries DL, Scott ME, Vermund SH, editors. Nutrition and infectious disease: shifting the clinical paradigm: Humana Press; 2020.
113. World Health Organization. World malaria report. Geneva: World Health Organization; 2018. Contract No.: Licence: CC BY-NC-SA 3.0 IGO.
114. UNICEF. The State of Food Security and Nutrition in the World 2018 2018 [updated 2018-09-11T10:53:32+00:00].
115. Semenza JC, Trinanes J, Lohr W, Sudre B, Lofdahl M, Martinez-Urtaza J, et al. Environmental suitability of vibrio infections in a warming climate: an early warning system. Environ Health Perspect. 2017;125(10):107004.
116. Koelle K, Rodo X, Pascual M, Yunus M, Mostafa G. Refractory periods and climate forcing in cholera dynamics. Nature. 2005;436(7051):696–700.
117. Hsueh BY, Waters CM. Combating cholera. F1000Res. 2019;8:589.
118. Tornevi A, Axelsson G, Forsberg B. Association between precipitation upstream of a drinking water utility and nurse advice calls relating to acute gastrointestinal illnesses. PLoS One. 2013;8(7):e69918.
119. Tornevi A, Simonsson M, Forsberg B, Save-Soderbergh M, Toljander J. Efficacy of water treatment processes and endemic gastrointestinal illness – a multi-city study in Sweden. Water Res. 2016;102:263–70.
120. Yang GJ, Bergquist R. Potential impact of climate change on schistosomiasis: a global assessment attempt. Trop Med Infect Dis. 2018;3:4.
121. Blum AJ, Hotez PJ. Global "worming": climate change and its projected general impact on human helminth infections. PLoS Negl Trop Dis. 2018;12(7):e0006370.
122. Scott ME, Koski K. Soil-transmitted helminths – does nutrition make a difference? In: Humphries DL, Scott ME, Vermund SH, editors. Nutrition and infectious disease: shifting the clinical paradigm: Humana Press; 2020.
123. Afrane YA, Githeko AK, Yan G. The ecology of Anopheles mosquitoes under climate change: case studies from the effects of deforestation in East African highlands. Ann N Y Acad Sci. 2012;1249:204–10.
124. Slater H, Michael E. Predicting the current and future potential distributions of lymphatic filariasis in Africa using maximum entropy ecological niche modelling. PLoS One. 2012;7(2):e32202.
125. Cheke RA, Basanez MG, Perry M, White MT, Garms R, Obuobie E, et al. Potential effects of warmer worms and vectors on onchocerciasis transmission in West Africa. Philos Trans R Soc Lond Ser B Biol Sci. 2015;370(1665) https://doi.org/10.1098/rstb.2013.0559.
126. Gleichsner AM, Cleveland JA, Minchella DJ. One stimulus-two responses: host and parasite life-history variation in response to environmental stress. Evolution. 2016;70(11):2640–6.
127. Wong GKL, Jim CY. Do vegetated rooftops attract more mosquitoes? Monitoring disease vector abundance on urban green roofs. Sci Total Environ. 2016;573:222–32.
128. Storey DM. Filariasis: nutritional interactions in human and animal hosts. Parasitology. 1993;107(Suppl):S147–58.

129. Nwoke BE. The socio-economic aspects of human onchocerciasis in Africa: present appraisal. J Hyg Epidemiol Microbiol Immunol. 1990;34(1):37–44.
130. Oladepo O, Brieger WR, Otusanya S, Kale OO, Offiong S, Titiloye M. Farm land size and onchocerciasis status of peasant farmers in south-western Nigeria. Tropical Med Int Health. 1997;2(4):334–40.
131. King CH, Dickman K, Tisch DJ. Reassessment of the cost of chronic helmintic infection: a meta-analysis of disability-related outcomes in endemic schistosomiasis. Lancet. 2005;365(9470):1561–9.
132. Berkley JA. Bacterial infections and nutrition – a primer. In: Humphries DL, Scott ME, Vermund SH, editors. Nutrition and infectious disease: shifting the clinical paradigm: Humana Press; 2020.
133. Siddiqui F, Belayneh G, Bhutta ZA. Nutrition and diarrheal disease and enteric pathogens. In: Humphries DL, Scott ME, Vermund SH, editors. Nutrition and infectious disease: shifting the clinical paradigm: Humana Press; 2020.
134. Hellberg RS, Chu E. Effects of climate change on the persistence and dispersal of foodborne bacterial pathogens in the outdoor environment: a review. Crit Rev Microbiol. 2016;42(4):548–72.
135. Pozio E. How globalization and climate change could affect foodborne parasites. Exp Parasitol. 2019:107807.
136. Cousins M, Sargeant JM, Fisman D, Greer AL. Modelling the transmission dynamics of Campylobacter in Ontario, Canada, assuming house flies, Musca domestica, are a mechanical vector of disease transmission. R Soc Open Sci. 2019;6(2):181394.
137. Taylor M, Cheng J, Sharma D, Bitzikos O, Gustafson R, Fyfe M, et al. Outbreak of Vibrio parahaemolyticus associated with consumption of raw oysters in Canada, 2015. Foodborne Pathog Dis. 2018;15(9):554–9.
138. North Carolina Department of Agriculture and Consumer Services. Flood crops cannot be used for human food. North Carolina, 18 Sept 2018.
139. Coker R, Rushton J, Mounier-Jack S, Karimuribo E, Lutumba P, Kambarage D, et al. Towards a conceptual framework to support one-health research for policy on emerging zoonoses. Lancet Infect Dis. 2011;11(4):326–31.
140. Gebreyes WA, Dupouy-Camet J, Newport MJ, Oliveira CJ, Schlesinger LS, Saif YM, et al. The global one health paradigm: challenges and opportunities for tackling infectious diseases at the human, animal, and environment interface in low-resource settings. PLoS Negl Trop Dis. 2014;8(11):e3257.

# Chapter 16
# Public Health and Clinical Implications of Nutrition-Infection Interactions

Sten H. Vermund, Marilyn E. Scott, and Debbie L. Humphries

## Abbreviations

| | |
|---|---|
| ACE2 | Angiotensin-converting enzyme 2 |
| COVID-19 | Coronavirus disease 2019 |
| DALYs | Disability-adjusted life years |
| DNA | Deoxyribonucleic acid |
| EED | Environmental enteric dysfunction |
| H1N1 | Influenza A virus subtype H1N1 |
| HAZ | Height-for-age Z score |
| HIV/AIDS | Human immunodeficiency virus/acquired immunodeficiency syndrome |
| ICU | Intensive care unit |
| MCN | Maternal child nutrition |
| MERS | Middle East respiratory syndrome |
| PEPaNIC | Early versus Late Parenteral Nutrition in the Pediatric Intensive Care Unit |
| PICU | Pediatric intensive care unit (PICU) |
| RNA | Ribonucleic acid |
| SARS | Severe acute respiratory syndrome |
| SARS-CoV-2 | Severe acute respiratory syndrome coronavirus 2 |
| STH | Soil-transmitted helminth |
| WHO | World Health Organization |

S. H. Vermund (✉) · D. L. Humphries
Epidemiology of Microbial Disease, Yale School of Public Health, Yale University, New Haven, CT, USA
e-mail: sten.vermund@yale.edu; debbie.humphries@yale.edu

M. E. Scott
Institute of Parasitology, McGill University, Ste-Anne de Bellevue, QC, Canada
e-mail: marilyn.scott@mcgill.ca

© Springer Nature Switzerland AG 2021
D. L. Humphries et al. (eds.), *Nutrition and Infectious Diseases*, Nutrition and Health,
https://doi.org/10.1007/978-3-030-56913-6_16

**Key Points**
- Infectious diseases are profoundly influenced by the nutritional status of their human hosts.
- Undernutrition may make it easier to acquire an infection and may compromise the host immune response, exacerbating the severity of the clinical course and making it harder to clear the organism.
- Overnutrition (overweight and obesity) is also associated with adverse reactions for human hosts with infections, including SARS-CoV-2, the virus that causes COVID-19.
- Causal relationships are complex, given that macro- and micronutrients are consumed together and teasing out a single element that is in deficit tends to be speculative.
- Improved nutrition, including adequate, but not excessive intake of needed macro- and micronutrients, can reduce infectious risks and augment vigorous immune responses.

# Introduction

Nutrition in clinical settings addresses the dietary nourishment of both healthy and ill individuals, as everyone depends upon nutrition, air, and water as fundamental necessities of life. In the face of infection, nutritional needs often differ from baseline needs, and optimized nutrition is a part of the recovery and healing process. Nutritional status may affect an individual's susceptibility when exposed to an infectious pathogen [1], and suboptimal nutrition can exacerbate the virulence of an organism and/or the pathogenic consequences of a given infectious disease [2–6].

As reviewed in Chap. 2 [7], deficiencies of macronutrients, such as protein-calorie malnutrition [8–10], predispose individuals to more frequent infections and more serious outcomes by compromising protective features such as cellular and humoral immunity, mucosal immunity, and the integrity of integumentary and mucosal surfaces, e.g., the skin, oropharyngeal cavity, and gut [11–20]. Furthermore, an excess of macronutrients as manifested in obesity may also predispose to infections [21]. For example, obesity is a predisposing factor for type 2 diabetes mellitus which, in turn, results in increased immunologic and physiologic risk for infections [22]. There has been long-standing speculation of an infectious etiology for at least some pancreatic changes that might lead to type 1 or 2 diabetes [23, 24]. Micronutrient deficiencies that can predispose to infection or exacerbate the severity of infections include a range of vitamins (e.g., A, B complex, C, D, and E) and minerals (e.g., iodine, iron, zinc, selenium, copper, fluoride, magnesium, and manganese) [7]. The impact of micronutrient deficiencies on infection are often most clinically severe in persons with underlying illnesses or in children under the age of 5 years [25].

Clinical management of specific nutritional deficiencies and excesses in the context of disease is covered in clinical nutrition texts [26–31], and public health approaches are regularly covered in public health nutrition textbooks [32, 33] and publications such as the 2013 *Lancet* series on Maternal and Child Nutrition (MCN). The 2013 *Lancet* series was focused on resource-limited settings and identified several nutrition-specific public health interventions that could decrease severe malnutrition as measured by stunting and severe wasting if effectively implemented. The recommended interventions included two for pregnant women (balanced energy protein supplementation and multiple micronutrient supplementation), several for infants and young children (breastfeeding promotion, complementary feeding education and supplementation, vitamin A supplementation), as well as interventions for populations (folic acid fortification), for children with diarrhea (zinc supplementation), and for malnourished children (management of severe and moderate acute malnutrition) [34]. While the 2013 *Lancet* MCN series focused on direct approaches to reducing malnutrition, it is important to note that the top five global infectious causes of death in children (pneumonia, diarrhea, malaria, measles, and human immunodeficiency virus/acquired immunodeficiency syndrome (HIV/

AIDS)) are all exacerbated by nutritional deficiencies [35]. Diarrhea-causing enteric infections are more severe in malnourished individuals [36], nutrition therapy can improve outcomes for individuals with HIV and tuberculosis (TB) [37], and malaria morbidity is complicated in the presence of host malnutrition [38].

Lower respiratory infections such as pneumonia are the fourth highest global cause of death across all ages [39], with increased risk in both children under 5 years of age and the elderly [40]. Given that the challenge of infectious diseases such as pneumonia and influenza is not restricted to resource-poor settings, and is increasingly evident in affluent societies, renewed attention to the intersection of nutrition and infection is timely. Another global population at increased risk of both malnutrition and infectious diseases is the elderly. In this chapter we will provide brief summaries of the key points from preceding chapters and then synthesize overarching and integrative themes relating to clinical and public health implications.

## Ancient Traditions

Prior to the era of modern medicine, nutritional considerations were paramount among ancient healthcare workers. Socrates, Hippocrates, and their contemporaries highlighted the differences, and the synergies, between foods and medicines [41–43]. Similarly, the Chinese had such adages as, "When you see a seriously ill patient, think first of his/her dietary needs; when these have been attended to, he/she may be given appropriate medication" (attributed to Hu Se-hui in the year 1330) and "Before prescribing medicine, explain to the patient what foods to avoid" (attributed to an old Chinese saying) [44]. In Africa, adaptations of food to accommodate genetic food intolerances and an emphasis on complementary food groups are documented [45]. In the Americas, nutrition was a highlighted element of medicine and health for indigenous populations in antiquity [46]. Enteral nutritional interventions were promulgated as far back as 3500 B.C. and have been documented in texts of ancient Egyptians, Indians, and Chinese [47].

In the modern era, nutritional researchers are studying the evolution of dietary patterns from prehistoric times through the agricultural transition to modern diets and are revising our understanding of health impacts of those transitions [48]. While historically the development of agriculture was thought to lead to improved human health, recent analyses of human remains around the globe have shown the opposite; a higher prevalence of skeletal pathological conditions paired with a decrease in mobility and a general decrease in skeletal strength are noted with the agricultural transition [49–51]. The more recent nutrition transition, with increases in salt, sugar, fat, processed grains, calories, and fried foods, continues the trend to worsening overall nutrition, particularly in urban settings [52, 53]. While attending to the recent dietary changes described in the nutrition transition literature, it is important not to romanticize the agricultural diet, given the prevalence of macro- and/or micronutrient deficiencies that have been associated with it [54–60]. A better understanding of human diets from prehistory to today may provide important insights for reducing the high rates of global diet-related diseases.

## Foundations of Nutrition/Infection Relationships

Given the variety of manifestations of infections and the ubiquitous influence of macro- and/or micronutrient status on responses to infection, an understanding of the intersection of nutrition and infection is vital for the fields of nutrition, nursing, public health, infectious diseases, and clinical medicine. The need for expertise in multiple disciplines has challenged this area of research.

While it has long been understood that infections can disrupt normal intake, digestion, and/or deployment of nutrients in ways that undermine the host's nutritional status, nutritional status can in turn influence exposure to the infectious organism, movement of the pathogen across host barriers, seeding of appropriate sites within the host, pathogen replication, and immunological responses [61]. Prior undernutrition can also alter the clinical course of an infectious disease, the effectiveness of vaccines that rely on a functional immune response, and the response to drugs that interact with specific nutritional parameters or with recent food intake. Relationships between a single infection and a single nutrient deficiency may not represent the clinically relevant question as such studies overlook important interactions that occur among pathogens and among nutritional deficiencies with critical clinical and public health implications.

## Conceptual Frameworks and Causality

Clinical decision-making, both at the individual and population levels, depends on an accurate understanding of causation within the context of complex interactions, an understanding which is derived from a critical assessment of available evidence. Chapters 1 and 14 present frameworks for conceptualizing host-pathogen relationships around nutrition and infection [61, 62]. Chapter 1 reviews criteria that have been suggested to better document causality with a focus on those that are relevant to nutrition-infection interactions [61]. From a design perspective, establishing causation in a context of multiple nutrient deficiencies and, perhaps, multiple infections is extremely challenging, especially given the difficulty of directly extrapolating mechanisms identified under controlled animal experiments to natural human populations. Observational studies provide insights, but the myriad of potential influencing factors make it difficult to draw conclusions [61]. Moreover, few epidemiological studies carefully consider the varied impact of nutrition on the different stages of infection, from transmission to disease to recovery. Therefore, in developing clear clinical frameworks for decisions regarding specific conditions, it is important to consider definitions of nutritional status in order to characterize macro- and/or micronutrient deficiencies, variability in study methods and conclusions, and the implications of covariates (see Chap. 11) [38]. We provide an example where explicit causal criteria have been used to better interpret available evidence on interactions between *Leishmania* and nutrition (Box 16.1).

As demonstrated in Box 16.1, application of clear causal criteria to existing evidence could help to clarify areas of consensus and gaps in knowledge. Progress in infectious disease control will be enhanced as we more rigorously consider how to evaluate evidence of causation, a process that is particularly important given increasing awareness that many, if not most, outcome measures of nutrition and of infection are influenced by their complex network of interactions. Hypotheses should

---

**Box 16.1 Leishmaniasis and Malnutrition**

Leishmaniasis is caused by a protozoan microorganism transmitted by the bite of an infected female phlebotomine sandfly. Over 1 billion people globally live in endemic areas with between 600,000 and 1,000,000 new cases estimated to occur per year worldwide [63]. Much of the evidence addressing the relationship between nutritional status and leishmaniasis is summarized in a recent review [64]. We focus here on one of the potential pathways identified in Chap. 1: impacts of macronutrient malnutrition on risk of infection. We then apply the causal criteria described in Chap. 1, strength, consistency, biological gradient, coherence, temporality, experimental design, plausibility, analogy, and specificity to the evidence supporting the two pathways. The evidence is summarized in Table 16.1.

**Table 16.1** Causal analysis[a] of nutritional risk and *Leishmania* infections [65–72]

| Hypothesis: Adults with high BMI are at increased risk of *Leishmania* infection | | |
|---|---|---|
| | | References and key findings |
| Epidemiological evidence | Strength | da Cunha [65], epidemiological study of an endemic community in Brazil found that adults infected with cutaneous *Leishmania* had significantly higher BMI and rates of overweight/obesity than adults who were not infected; Barbosa [66], in a retrospective study of human visceral leishmaniasis concluded that chronic diseases such as obesity are an important risk factor for visceral leishmaniasis |
| | Consistency | Insufficient studies to assess |
| | Biological gradient | Insufficient studies to assess |
| | Coherence | Results from da Cunha [65] and Barbosa [66] align with animal model data; in contrast, Ali [72] estimated a relative risk of visceral leishmaniasis of 5.9 for adults and children with low BMI vs. high BMI (BMI <18 vs. BMI ≥18), although obesity was not present in the study; no other studies identified |
| | Temporality | No relevant studies identified |
| Animal models, clinical trials, intervention studies | Experimental design | Tavares [67], volatile organic compounds (VOCs) from human volunteers can attract *Phlebotomine*; Sarnaglia [71], mice with diet-induced obesity had significantly increased parasite *Leishmania major* burdens in the liver and spleen than control mice; Martins [68], mice fed a hypercaloric diet had a higher parasite burden with *L. major* than well-nourished mice |
| | Plausibility | Kirstein [69], more female sandflies were attracted to a trap with a sugar/yeast mixture (SYM) than males, and sandflies were more attracted to the SYM than to lights; Tavares [67], VOCs from human volunteers can attract *Phlebotomine*; Pinto [70]. host size proportional to attractiveness to *Phlebotomine* |
| | Analogy | In mice infected with *L. major*, Sarnaglia [71] and Martins [68] show higher parasite burden when fed hypercaloric diets vs. normal diets |
| | Specificity | Underlying mechanisms driving this relationship are as yet unclear, so availability of alternate explanations cannot be ruled out |

[a]Definitions of causality terms:
  *Strength* – size of the relationship, effect size
  *Consistency* – similar findings observed in different regions and age groups
  *Biological gradient* – dose-response effects
  *Coherence* – results are coherent with current knowledge about nutrition and the specific infection
  *Temporality* – observed time sequence of hypothesized cause followed by effect
  *Experimental design* – clinical trials, randomized study designs, and animal models can provide this kind of evidence
  *Plausibility* – plausible biological pathways can be identified for the hypothesized relationship
  *Analogy* – findings from animal models or similar pathogens that address the hypothesized relationship in that system
  *Specificity* – no other likely explanation exists

be tested that are theory-based, explicitly naming and assessing causal criteria for given infection-nutrition interactions [73]. It is particularly important to be clear on what relationships are being examined in a given context, and the ability to isolate specific relationships may be very difficult in complex situations such as co-infections.

An ecological perspective (see Chap. 14) proposes the use of a trophic, or feeding, framework to better study the real-world situation of co-occurring infections [62]. Applying a trophic approach to studying co-infection and nutrition requires inclusion of co-occurring infections and nutritional deficiencies in conceptual models, decisions about variables to measure, and realistic analysis plans of adequate complexity to test the hypotheses. In a clinical setting, considering physiological demands of co-occurring infections could augment information from clinical assessments as clinicians weigh the challenges of simultaneously responding to multiple pathogens and nutritional deficiencies.

## Principles of Nutrition and Immunology

Chapters 2 and 3 provide foundations in nutrition and immunology that are important for untangling intersecting relationships [7, 106]. Adequate nutritional status is important for normal proliferation and differentiation of all immune cell types, as well as antibody and cytokine production. Several micronutrients such as iron, vitamin A, and zinc are involved in pro-inflammatory responses to infection, providing early resistance to invading pathogens. Nutrients such as vitamin A, vitamin K, and thiamin moderate the strength of inflammatory responses, limiting autoimmune reactions. Antioxidant vitamins, minerals, and amino acids protect the integrity of immune cell membranes from toxicities of free radicals.

A vigorous immune system depends on energy and nutrients supplied by diet; thus, the immune response of nutritionally marginal persons may be compromised. With severe, chronic, or repeated infections, the nutritional status of even a previously well-nourished host can be compromised through damage of host tissues, suboptimal food intake or food intolerance, malabsorption and nutrient loss, higher metabolic demands for nutrients, and perturbed nutrient transport or storage. That malnutrition compromises host immune defenses is a fundamental underpinning of the observed risk of increased virulence of organisms and pathogenicity of infections among malnourished populations [74]. Epithelial surfaces, particularly at mucosal sites, are important first-line defenses against pathogens, and multiple nutrients are involved in integrity of those surfaces. Specific macro- and micronutrients with essential roles in mucosal integrity include fatty acids, the amino acids proline and threonine, zinc, and vitamin A. The innate immune system responds rapidly to infection, differentiates among classes of pathogens, and can clear most microbial challenges. The adaptive immune system provides pathogen-specific immunity to protect against pathogens that evade the innate system. Both the innate and adaptive systems provide an integrated defense against specific types of pathogens, typically engaging IgM, IgG, and cellular mechanisms. Deficiencies in protein, energy, and specific nutrients can impair host defenses against infection, thus increasing the risk and severity of infections.

## Types of Infectious Diseases and Influence of Nutrition

In Chaps. 4, 5, 6, and 7, the authors provide primers on bacterial, viral, protozoan, and helminth pathogens and explain how each may be affected by, and in turn affect, host nutritional status.

### Bacterial Infections (See Chap. 4) [75]

Bacteria can be found throughout the body, and one of the current areas of research is the balance between commensal and pathogenic bacteria at different physiological sites. Much recent attention has been paid to the microbiome. The intestinal microbiome is influenced by diet, including probiotic dietary compounds such as oligosaccharides that favor bacterial growth, by antibacterial compounds such as antibodies and lysozymes (present in breastmilk and artificially added to commercial infant formulas), and by ingestion of probiotic bacterial components or potentially pathogenic bacteria. In turn, the gut microbiome has substantial influence on what and how food-derived nutrients are absorbed.

Environmental enteric dysfunction (EED) is characterized by chronic intestinal inflammation, increased permeability, and reduced nutrient absorptive surface. EED is also characterized by presence of bacterial pathogens. It is most prevalent in low-income individuals in lower-income countries and is associated with both wasting and stunting in children. Reduced mucosal integrity and mucosal immune abnormalities prevalent with severe EED lead to an increased translocation (i.e., gut-to-bloodstream) of bacterial products that cause chronic inflammation and local and systemic immune dysfunction. Vitamin A, vitamin C, zinc, and iron are all vital to aid mucosal and systemic immune protection from bacterial infections and from translocated bacterial products. Trials such as the Early versus Late Parenteral Nutrition in the Pediatric Intensive Care Unit (PEPaNIC) study provide important insights into the clinical implicationsutrition therapy decisions on infections. The PEPaNIC study compared initiation of parenteral feeding at 24 hours vs. 1 week in undernourished children entering a pediatric intensive care unit (PICU); the investigators found that amino acid supplementation was associated with new infections and increased intensive care unit (ICU) care, whereas supplementation with glucose alone was associated with fewer infections and earlier ICU release [76].

## Viral Infections (See Chap. 5) [77]

Both innate and adaptive immune responses are important for protection from viral infections, and adequate nutrition is essential for their function. Multiple kinds of malnutrition, including obesity/overnutrition and micronutrient deficiencies, have been shown to increase risk for viral infections such as influenza in adults and children. Micronutrients of interest for viral infections include vitamins B complex, C, D, and E and minerals such as magnesium, iron, selenium, and zinc. However, few studies have tested nutritional interventions as treatment for viral infections such as influenza. Several studies have shown that supplementing hospitalized influenza patients with vitamin C reduced complications and duration of ICU stay [78]. Given the importance of good nutrition for effective immune responses against influenza, the parallel global challenges of increasing overweight and obesity and the contrasting ongoing burden of undernutrition may exacerbate the risk for influenza epidemics and pandemics despite vaccination efforts. In turn, mitigation of global malnutrition may enhance influenza control by improving vaccine immunogenicity and blunting the clinical severity of infection.

## Protozoan Infections (See Chap. 6) [79]

Among the human diseases caused by pathogenic protozoa, those protozoans acquired via ingestion (e.g., *Giardia lamblia* and *Entamoeba histolytica*) are most notably affected by dietary factors through possible impacts on transmission, pathogenicity, and immunity. Undernutrition (particularly protein deficiency) can increase the virulence of protozoal diseases due to adverse effects on immunity. Prevention or treatment of malnutrition could improve a host's ability to immunologically respond to protozoans. Diarrheal diseases caused by a variety of intestinal protozoa lead to malabsorption and contribute, in turn, to undernutrition. While animal models have shown that deficiencies of vitamins A and $B_{12}$ are associated with increased parasitemia from the *Trypanosoma spp.* parasites but that vitamin E deficiency is associated with decreased *Trypanosoma spp.* parasitemia [80–82], few studies have directly addressed potential roles for nutritional supplementation in human protozoan infections.

## Helminth Infections (See Chap. 7) [83]

Helminth infections remain common in resource-limited regions, particularly in tropical areas, generally co-occurring with malnutrition. Helminth infections contribute to the cycle of poverty that restrains economic development. Helminth parasitism can limit appetite, growth, development, and physical and cognitive abilities, especially in children bearing heavy worm burdens. Helminths can interfere with absorption of macronutrients and some micronutrients. Although anthelmintic-based control programs have reduced the numbers of heavily infected individuals most likely to have complications and have decreased the morbidity associated with many parasitic helminths, between 1.5 and 2 billion people remain infected with helminths worldwide.

## Examples of Nutrition/Infection Interactions

Chapters 8, 9, 10, 11, and 12 build on the materials in Chaps. 1, 2, 3, 4, 5, 6, and 7 to investigate the broader implications of nutrition-infection interactions with respect to specific pathogens or diseases. Case studies cover five prevalent and burdensome conditions: diarrhea, HIV and TB, arboviruses, malaria, and soil-transmitted helminth (STH) infections.

### Diarrhea (See Chap. 8) [36]

In the context of diarrheal disease, clinicians need to be aware of the impact of nutritional status on both the infectious agents and the host. Malnutrition increases the pathogenicity of diarrhea-causing organisms, adversely affecting the components of the gut barrier, including the gut microbiome and gut mucosa. Malnutrition generally reduces the ability of the immune system to mount adequate responses against diarrhea-causing pathogens, although some components of the immune system remain unaffected or are enhanced in response to malnutrition. Diarrheal disease progresses faster, leads to more severe symptoms, takes longer to resolve, and has worse outcomes in malnourished individuals. Antibiotics, though lifesaving in some circumstances, can have detrimental effects on the gut microbiome, impairing a key defense mechanism against gut pathogens. Infection by some pathogens (e.g., *Entamoeba histolytica*) is paradoxically less likely in malnourished individuals.

### HIV/TB (See Chap. 9) [37]

HIV infection is transmitted when mucous membranes or damaged tissues of an uninfected individual contact bodily fluids (blood or blood products, semen, breast milk, and rectal or vaginal secretions) that contain the HIV virus. The most common routes of HIV infection are through sexual activity and contact with infected blood via medical procedures and use of injected drugs with shared, contaminated needles/syringes. Suboptimally treated HIV can be associated with serious and lethal malnutrition, as with the "wasting syndrome" reported in the 1980s, and with gastrointestinal infections like cryptosporidiosis that can cause debilitating malabsorption and diarrhea.

Tuberculosis (TB) can be more severe in immunocompromised persons. When less than optimally treated, it can cause a severe wasting syndrome related to its debilitating pulmonary, gastrointestinal, and systemic effects. The interaction of nutrition with both HIV and TB is bidirectional, as individuals who are undernourished have an increased risk of infection and those infected with HIV or TB are likely to develop nutritional abnormalities. Several micronutrient deficiencies are postulated to exacerbate risk both of HIV acquisition and disease progression. Less is known about micronutrients and TB. Many people living with HIV who have been on antiretroviral therapy for many years are now overweight or even obese, with metabolic abnormalities or metabolic syndrome. This may be related to lifestyle, diet, and/or side effects of some antiretroviral medications.

## Arboviruses (See Chap. 10) [84]

The role of the host's nutritional status is still uncertain vis-à-vis the risk of progression to severe forms of dengue disease, the most common mosquito-borne viral infection worldwide. While observational studies suggest that pediatric obesity may be related to adverse dengue disease outcomes, causality is uncertain. Investigators have reported inverse relations between severity of dengue disease and nutrient status biomarkers, including fatty acids, amino acids, vitamin D, and some minerals, but it is unclear whether these relations represent an effect of the nutritional status on the outcome of infection or an effect of the infection on the biomarkers. Small randomized trials of vitamin E and zinc supplements to patients with dengue fever have shown protective effects against intermediate outcomes leading to severe disease. Metabolomic studies of dengue and chikungunya infections have identified viral-induced alterations in fatty acid metabolism that may play a role in both viral replication and pathology [85]. The implications of such alterations are not yet fully understood.

## Malaria (See Chap. 11) [38]

Malaria and malnutrition both display nonspecific clinical symptoms, which make diagnosis and surveillance efforts difficult, especially in low-resource settings. The interactions between malaria and malnutrition are complex, as the *Plasmodium* pathogens need access to host nutrients such as iron for replication and reproduction. Clinical manifestations of malaria differ based on the specific species of *Plasmodium*, the type of host malnutrition (micronutrient deficiency, protein-energy malnutrition), and geosocial factors. An influential study in a refugee camp in Niger concluded that severely malnourished individuals who participated in a refeeding program experienced a rapid increase in malaria parasitemia and that refeeding needed to be done with care [86]. The ensuing controversy continued with the results of a study in Zanzibar reported in 2006 from an area with ongoing malaria transmission. In the absence of malaria control efforts, children who were not iron deficient but who received iron and folate supplementation were at increased risk of severe adverse events from malaria [87]. Was malaria less pathogenic in malnourished children? Childhood nutritional interventions in areas of high malaria risk should first consider malaria diagnosis and treatment before nutritional supplementation commences. To better delineate nutritional influences on malaria, it is important to carefully characterize macro- and/or micronutrient deficiencies, carefully plan study designs that align with the research questions, and thoroughly explore implications of covariates. Poor host nutritional status may increase susceptibility to malaria infection, although when specific categories of micro- and micronutrition malnutrition are considered, evidence is less clear. Public health interventions to combat malnutrition in areas endemic to malaria should consider the potential impacts on vulnerable populations of interactions with malaria.

## Soil-Transmitted Helminths (STH) (Chap. 12) [88]

STH infections are transmitted by contact with eggs and larvae that live in soil. As such, food- and agriculture-related risks for exposure to STHs can be minimized by agricultural interventions and health education. However, in many parts of the world, increasing water scarcity may increase use of wastewater for irrigation and therefore the risk of STH exposure. From the parasite perspective, STH larvae rely on host chemical cues to locate a host and migrate to their preferred site in the gastrointestinal tract. High-protein and high-carbohydrate diets improve feeding by adult worms because excess of these macronutrients reduces concentrations of a host protein that blocks worm feeding. In contrast, energy restriction and vitamin D deficiency may reduce STH egg production. Protein, energy, zinc, and selenium deficiencies prolong STH survival by impairing the anti-inflammatory Th2 response needed for STH expulsion, and protein, energy, and zinc deficiencies also blunt the pro-inflammatory Th1 response. From the host perspective, STH infections alter host nutritional status by modulating molecular signaling of appetite and taste receptors and by reducing absorption of macro-nutrients, β-carotene, and iron with consequences for growth. Low host iron increases pathology associated with hookworm infection. However, the anti-inflammatory response to STH infections reduces pathology associated with such chronic diseases/conditions as obesity, diabetes, and inflammatory bowel diseases. There is only limited overall evidence that deworming improves nutritional status, that supplementation reduces STH infection, and that combined interventions are more effective than single interventions.

## *The Bigger Picture*

The last section of the book – Chaps. 13, 14, and 15 – looks at nutrition-infection interactions from the wider lenses of the clinician concerned about drug-nutrient interactions, the community ecologist interested in interactions among co-occurring pathogens, and climate scientists charged with projecting how global climate change is likely to shift the nutrition-infectious disease dynamic.

### Nutritional Factors Affect Pharmaceuticals Used in Treatment of Infectious Diseases (Chap. 13) [89]

It is important for clinicians to be aware of the wide range of interactions between antimicrobial agents (antibacterial, antiviral, antifungal, antiparasitic) and nutrients (i.e., drug-nutrition interaction) [89]. A meal, a specific food, a food component (including a nutrient), and overall nutritional status may all influence the physiologic disposition of an antimicrobial agent. If a drug-nutrition interaction is not recognized and addressed, an altered drug concentration may adversely influence clinical progress and outcome including the risk for drug resistance. An antimicrobial regimen may influence whole body nutritional status, metabolic status, the microbiome, and the concentration of individual nutrients. Reduced efficacy or failure of antiviral, antibiotic, antifungal, and anthelmintic drugs may be a consequence of deficiencies of specific micro- or macronutrients and may increase the rate at which pathogens evolve resistance to these drugs. In turn, antibiotics, though lifesaving, have detrimental effects on the gut, skin, vaginal, and other microbiomes and key defense mechanisms against gut, skin, and genital tract pathogens (See Chap. 8).

Modern information management systems give us powerful tools to assess the interaction of nutrition, particularly current diet, and antiviral, antibacterial, antifungal, and antiparasitic drugs. Few clinicians can remember the myriad of drug-nutrition combinations that might increase or decrease drug levels to a suboptimal effect. Hence, drug-drug interaction databases are often helpfully enhanced with data on drug-food interactions as well [90, 91]. To summarize this complex issue, a short guide is provided by *Consumer Reports* for common interactions [92]. We have adapted this guide to show what consumer groups are doing to inform patients and clinicians alike (Table 16.2).

### The Community Ecologist Perspective (Chap. 14) [62]

Ezenwa suggests that analyzing two levels of competition between co-occurring infections, resource competition, and immune system competition, along with intensity of infections may help to explain heterogeneity in outcomes with particular co-infections [62]. Despite the frequency of multiple

**Table 16.2** Common food and drug interactions

| Type of food | Don't mix with | The reason |
|---|---|---|
| Bananas, green leafy vegetables, oranges, salt substitutes | ACE inhibitors, e.g., captopril, enalapril, and lisinopril, used to lower blood pressure (BP) and/or treat heart failure. Avoid mixing with some diuretics, e.g., triamterene, used to reduce fluid retention and treat high BP | These high-potassium foods help provide electrical signals to heart muscle and other cells. Increased potassium levels may lead to an irregular heartbeat or heart palpitations—which could be deadly |
| Broccoli, Brussels sprouts, cabbage, kale, spinach | Blood thinners, e.g., warfarin | These vitamin K-laden foods can reduce drugs' ability to thin the blood. In people with heart disease, that could trigger a heart attack or stroke. Once on warfarin, maintain a consistent diet, i.e., do not overload on leafy greens |
| Real black licorice (or supplements with licorice extract) | Digoxin, used to treat heart failure and abnormal heart rhythms. It's also best not to consume with most BP drugs, blood thinners, and birth control pills | Real black licorice and products with licorice extract (i.e., not licorice-flavored candy) contain glycyrrhizin, which can cause an irregular heartbeat or death with digoxin. Glycyrrhizin may reduce BP drug effectiveness, intensify side effects of blood thinners, and, with birth control pills, raise BP and lower potassium levels |
| Cheese, yogurt, milk, calcium supplements, antacids with calcium | Tetracycline | Calcium can interfere with the body's ability to absorb it. Best to take tetracycline 1 hour before or 2 hours after eating |
| Alcohol, avocados, bananas, chocolate, salami; aged, pickled, fermented, or smoked foods, e.g., processed cheeses, anchovies, dry sausage | Drugs used to treat bacterial infections, e.g., metronidazole and linezolid | These foods and beverages contain tyramine, an amino acid that can cause BP to spike if taken with linezolid. Alcohol and metronidazole together can cause nausea, stomach cramping, and vomiting |
| Soybean flour, walnuts | Thyroid drugs such as levothyroxine | These high-fiber foods can prevent absorbing thyroid medications. With a high-fiber diet, consider taking at bedtime for better absorption rather than a half-hour before breakfast (as usually recommended) |

Adapted from *Consumer Reports* [92]

infections and malnutrition, only a small fraction of studies address the issue of simultaneous additional infections. Applying a trophic framework can help advance our understanding of how co-infection affects nutrition using the example of helminths and malaria and, reciprocally, how nutrition affects co-infection using the example of tuberculosis and helminths [62].

## Climate Science (Chap. 15) [93]

The public health and clinical challenges resulting from nutrition-infection interactions are likely to increase due to climate change. The expanded geographical distribution of pathogens, combined with reduced food availability, and with social upheaval especially in coastal regions, is likely to expand the set of overlapping infections and nutrient deficiencies within a given population [93]. Food systems are both a driver of climate change and heavily affected by climate change. The food system, particularly animal grazing and husbandry, is a large emitter of $CO_2$, and the impacts of climate change are expected to increase both macronutrient and micronutrient deficiencies. Climate change is likely to influence infectious diseases both through its impact on nutritional status and through its impact on the geographical range of transmission, notably for vector-borne and water-borne agents. Increasing $CO_2$ emissions and climate change will alter natural and social systems with consequences for global health that are most severe in tropical and polar regions. The synergistic impacts of undernutrition and infection with climate change are not yet well quantified, but current understanding of their interdependence suggests exacerbated negative impacts unless climate change is controlled. The volume of greenhouse gas emissions in the atmosphere and our adaptive responses will determine the degree of impact on critical food webs and food systems both on land and in the oceans [93].

## Clinical and Public Health Relevance of the Bidirectional Nature of the Relationship between Nutrition and Infection

In the seminal 1968 WHO monograph by Scrimshaw, Taylor, and Gordon, the authors concluded with several synthesis statements (see Box 16.2). Their synthesis speaks to the challenge of extracting the key points from diverse and heterogeneous pathogens and contexts, with caveats such as "usually," "generally," and "can be" for all the relationships they describe (see Box 16.2). Today the burgeoning scientific evidence in this area is beyond the scope of any small group to synthesize. Instead, in this section, we have drawn out key points made by authors of different chapters in this book that highlight the clinical and public relevance of the relationship between nutrition and infectious diseases and also note that nutritional status impacts both diagnosis and treatment of infectious diseases.

We emphasize the bidirectional and synergistic nature of the interactions, which complicate our ability to interpret cross-sectional data whether in epidemiological studies or clinical settings given that the temporality and direction of influence cannot be clearly characterized. The bidirectional interactions raise questions about the optimum sequence of interventions. Should infections be cleared before nutrient interventions, as is suggested with childhood malaria? Should efforts to improve growth, especially linear growth, focus more directly on control of infections in addition to improvements in diets? Which interventions will most rapidly improve population health in the most effective and expeditious ways? All of these research questions require attention at the level of specific infections and nutrients but also at the level of general principles as demonstrated by Scrimshaw et al. (see Box 16.2).

---

**Box 16.2 Examples of effects of Malnutrition on Resistance to Infection** [94]
- Almost always synergistic (bacteria, helminths, protozoa)
- Antagonistic or synergistic (systemic viral, helminth, protozoa)
- Synergism most common with extracellular pathogens
- Antagonism common with intracellular pathogens; possible if organism depends on host enzymes or metabolites
- General malnutrition usually synergistic, can be antagonistic with viruses and protozoans
- Protein deficiencies generally synergistic, rare antagonism with specific amino acid deficiencies
- Vitamin A deficiency regularly synergistic
- Deficiencies of B vitamins both antagonistic and synergistic
- Vitamin C deficiency is synergistic but some antagonistic
- Mineral deficiencies may be synergistic or antagonistic

## Poor Nutritional Status May Increase Severity of Infections

Clinicians must consider malnutrition (over- and undernutrition) when assessing patients with infectious diseases. There are several overlapping pathways through which macro- and micronutrient deficiencies affect the immune system and in turn infectious diseases. Undernutrition, understood to be acting through effects on immunity, can increase the virulence of protozoal diseases such as malaria and some diarrheal pathogens and prolong survival of STH infections. Malnutrition directly affects the integrity of the gut barrier including the gut microbiome and gut mucosa. Diarrheal diseases, whether viral, protozoan, or bacterial, progress faster, lead to more severe symptoms, take longer to resolve, and generally have worse outcomes in malnourished individuals. Data on connections between obesity/overnutrition and increased risk of infectious disease are also growing. Immunosuppressive diseases increase risk of infectious diseases, especially fungal diseases and opportunistic agents that only rarely afflict persons with normal immune systems.

## Infectious Diseases May Contribute to Malnutrition

Patients with infectious diseases may be at risk of developing malnutrition, and appropriate precautions need to be taken. Infections can alter nutritional status by increasing nutritional needs, decreasing intake, or increasing nutrient loss. These pathways may occur individually or together, thus potentially increasing the impact on the host.

Infections can increase nutritional requirements through changes in metabolic rate or increases in specific needs. For example, resting energy expenditure is higher in asymptomatic HIV infection [95], and children with measles benefit from vitamin A supplementation [96]. Decreased appetite has been observed children infected with gastrointestinal nematodes, as seen in Egyptian children with strongyloidiasis who had higher concentrations of leptin, a protein that decreases appetite [97], and in Kenyan schoolchildren whose appetites improved 4 months after deworming for hookworm, trichuriasis, and ascariasis [98]. Decreased absorption happens with conditions such as diarrhea, when the intestinal transit time is decreased, and also when intestinal functioning is decreased such as with amebiasis and EED (see Chap. 4) [75]. Increased nutrient loss results from tissue damage or blood loss and can occur secondary to the acute physiological response to infection. Pathogen invasion, leading to bleeding and tissue breakdown, can result in catabolism of muscle tissues that provides a fuel source during infection and contributes to excretion of nitrogen from tissue breakdown [99–101]. The acute phase response to infections is also associated with changes in micronutrient metabolism such as when vitamin A excretion accelerates [102].

## Malnutrition May Protect Against Infections

While malnutrition generally increases infectious disease risk, some specific infections benefit if the host is malnourished, as with early evidence from some studies of malaria in children. Drawing conclusions about such antagonistic relationships is complicated by the inability to actively test such relationships in human beings and the risk of declaring such an antagonistic relationship prematurely. Thus, scientific evidence needs to include detailed analysis of biological plausibility of antagonism, animal models demonstrating such antagonism, and ideally, epidemiological evidence in humans.

## Combined Malnutrition and Infection May Affect Chronic Disease

With the global burden of disease from overweight and obesity accounting for 3.8% of disability-adjusted life years (DALYs) and affecting over 35% of men and women [103], clinicians need to be aware of the bidirectional impacts of malnutrition and infection in the context of obesity and overweight. There are two primary routes of influence, one through infections that alter systemic inflammation and the other through associations of obesity and overweight with micronutrient deficiencies. Helminth infections that lower systemic inflammation are associated with decreased risk of chronic diseases such as diabetes and metabolic syndrome [104]. Obesity and overweight are inversely associated with serum levels of both fat-soluble (A and D) and water-soluble (thiamin, folate, $B_6$, and $B_{12}$) vitamins [105] that are key elements of effective immune responses (Chaps. 2 and 3) [7, 106]. Diabetes increases risk of some bacterial infections including a two- to four-fold increase in risk of tuberculosis leading to a growing co-epidemic of diabetes and tuberculosis [107].

## Nutritional Status and Practices May Affect Infectious Disease Prevention

Public health activities aimed at infectious disease prevention are primarily focused on reducing exposure and susceptibility and improving early detection and treatment. Of these, reducing susceptibility by enhancing the immune response through vaccination may be affected by nutritional practices and status. Exposure to food-borne illnesses may be affected by compliance with dietary recommendations, particularly around infant and young child feeding and recommendations for increasing fruit and vegetable consumption [108–113].

Extensive research has explored relationships between malnutrition and vaccine efficacy, with inconsistent findings. Vaccines currently in widespread use include whole live attenuated and killed vaccines, as well as protein conjugates, virus-like particles, and epitope constructs [114]. Oral vaccines such as the cholera vaccine generally require an effective mucosal immune response, whereas injected vaccines stimulate a systemic response, with or without notable mucosal immunity, depending on the vaccine and its target organism. A study comparing children in Nicaragua and Sweden following the same oral cholera vaccine regimen found significantly lower vibriocidal antibodies in the children in Nicaragua [115], and studies in animal models demonstrate reduced mucosal immunity to oral vaccines such as cholera and *Salmonella* in mice on a low-protein diet [116]. A cohort study of Senegalese children following vaccination with the *Bordetella pertussis* toxin identified nutritional status as measured by height-for-age Z score (HAZ) and season as significant modulators of the antibody response [117]. The underperformance of oral poliovirus vaccine in children with high rates of enteric pathogens, such as in Gaza, has been overcome by use of combined killed and live attenuated vaccines [118–122]. While the differences in human immune responses to selected vaccines cannot be definitively attributed to nutritional status, malnutrition and dysbiosis of the enteric microbiome have both led to decreased efficacy of several oral vaccines. The heterogeneity of nutritional status in human populations and variations in microbiological exposures and immune responses prior to vaccination all increase the complexity of this topic.

## Nutritional Factors May Affect Disease Diagnosis

Diagnostic tests for infectious diseases typically focus either on the host response to an infection or on direct detection of the pathogen or its genetic material. Antibody tests assess host responses, as do a range of emerging methods such as enzymatic responses, biomarkers, gene expression, and activity-based diagnostics [123]. Diagnostic tests that rely on antibody detection may lose sensitivity due to malnutrition, whether protein deficiency or deficiencies of vitamin A, some B vitamins, and selenium that may be associated with decreased antibody production [106].

Pathogen detection includes antigen and nucleic acid detection (RNA or DNA depending on the organism), often with amplification methods, and microbial culture-based methods [124, 125]. Direct observation of parasite eggs in stool or organisms in the bloodstream is still used commonly, as with STH and malaria. Diagnostic tests relying on pathogen detection may be affected if pathogen development or proliferation is altered due to impaired nutrition status, as noted in polyparasitism and immunodiagnostics [126].

## Need for Integrated Action

Protein-energy malnutrition, including both overnutrition and undernutrition, together with micronutrient deficiencies, is a leading challenge for global health. Population-level impacts of malnutrition-infection interactions cannot be addressed without the successful collaboration of the public health, medical and nutrition professions with veterinarians, entomologists, ecologists, environmental scientists, and social scientists. A collaborative "OneHealth" perspective that emphasizes the mutual influences of animal and environmental health on humans is critical for conceptualizing new approaches to prevention, control, and treatment [127]. From a global population of less than 2.6 billion in 1950 to a population of 7.8 billion in mid-2020, human pressures on natural environments have grown. HIV/AIDS emerged from primates in forests of central Africa and was likely transferred to hunters who would bloody their hands when capturing or skinning the animals for bushmeat [128]. The emergence of the novel coronavirus, SARS-CoV-2, causing a devastating pulmonary disease, COVID-19, is another such example, discussed below.

An improvement in nutritional status of individuals and of populations would have additional benefits in reducing severity of co-existing infectious diseases. While current research often focuses on single infections and nutrients in the name of clarity, a trophic framework such as that proposed by Ezenwa [62] may form a foundation for more rigorous assessment of nutritional infections with multiple co-infections. Combining ecological approaches with epidemiological data in the context of co-infection and nutrition can shed light on complex co-infection-nutrition interactions.

## A Post-Script on Modern Medicine and Clinical Care

This book is focused on the global challenges of nutrition-infection interactions inherent in community health, with an emphasis on resource limited settings. There is also a vast array of nutrition-infection interactions that are related directly to modern medicine and clinical care that are beyond the scope of this book. Persons now can live longer lives, even with immunosuppressive diseases or conditions, including the proportion of persons aging beyond what was typical over the previous millennia.

Vulnerable populations for nutrition-infection interactions are many. Some are defined by age, given the relatively less robust immune responses of infants and children, particularly those born preterm, and of the elderly, particularly if frail or infirm. Others are vulnerable due to preexisting conditions, as with pregnant women and immunosuppressed hosts who have not been treated to optimize immune system reconstitution, e.g., cancer, HIV, and severe rheumatologic conditions, and other debilitating conditions. Some persons have comorbidities that, in themselves, increase nutrition and/or infection risk, as with substance use disorders, e.g., alcoholism and opioid use disorder.

## Opportunistic Infections

Nosocomial and opportunistic infections have become of major concern in hospitals, and both are associated with both nutritional antecedents and consequences. For example, fungal infections and nosocomial bacteria (often multidrug-resistant) are serious impediments to more successful cancer and transplant outcomes. The US Centers for Disease Control and Prevention highlights *Staphylococcus aureus, Pseudomonas aeruginosa,* and *Escherichia coli* as the most common nosocomial infections in such sites as the urinary tract, lungs, surgical sites, gastrointestinal tract, skin, and bloodstream (bacteremia or septicemia). Other texts focus on nosocomial/hospital-acquired infections and those that are characterized as opportunistic infections of immunosuppressed hosts [129–143]. Nutritionally impaired individuals are at especially high risk of death from multiple-drug-resistant organisms such as *Candida auris* or *Enterococcus spp.* Infections that occur in immunosuppressed hosts that impair lung or gut function like esophageal candidiasis, *Pneumocystis spp.* pneumonia, or cryptosporidiosis can be associated with devastating nutritional consequences. Methicillin-resistant *Staphylococcus aureus* (MRSA) is a scourge with both nutritional antecedents and consequences. Textbooks of clinical nutrition are the best source for these themes.

## Severe Acute Respiratory Syndrome Coronavirus 2 (SARS-CoV-2) and COVID-19 Disease

In late December 2019, initial reports of a novel coronavirus emerged in Wuhan, China. COVID-19 spread rapidly, and by November 2020, over 61 million individuals had tested positive, infections were present in every country, and over 1.4 million deaths globally were attributed to the infection. COVID-19 is an enveloped, positive-sense single-stranded RNA that binds to angiotensin-converting enzyme 2 (ACE2), similar to two previously identified coronaviruses, the causal agents for severe acute respiratory syndrome (SARS), Middle East respiratory syndrome (MERS), and four coronaviruses recognized first that just cause cold symptoms. It is believed that SARS-CoV-2 leapt into humans in 2019 from bats, plausibly through an intermediate wild host sold in Chinese markets for food [144]. Even COVID-19 is nutritionally linked, as mortality rates have been far higher in obese infected persons [145–153].

Given the slow global response to the pandemic, when countries eventually recognized the importance of taking action, community spread of the virus was already substantial in many countries. At that point the primary options for prevention were non-pharmaceutical interventions such as closing schools and public spaces to reduce exposure, use of masks and personal hand/face hygiene, and physical distancing (>2 m advised). The dramatic global drop in economic activity, including increases in global unemployment reported by the International Labour Organization [154], was associated with increased rates of hunger and food insecurity due to lost wages and employment opportunities [155–160]. In addition, the global food system suffered large-scale losses, with farmers unable to sell their products and consumers unable to connect with the producers [161, 162]. Stay-in-residence advisories spawned sedentary lifestyles in many persons used to more exercise [163]. Consequences of these dimensions of the COVID-19 pandemic are unknown to say nothing of impacts of medical care deferred by persons not accessing health services.

To date, there are only a few studies addressing nutritional influences on previous coronavirus infections, although several studies have identified selenium, vitamin D, and vitamin C as critical nutrients. An ecological analysis of population-level variation in selenium status in China noted a correlation between regions with higher selenium levels and higher cure rates for COVID-19 [164]. An ecological analysis of population-level variation in vitamin D status also noted higher rates of COVID-19 infection in countries with lower vitamin D status, supporting the need for additional research investigating whether the relationship might be causal [165, 166].

Obesity has been identified as a risk factor for severe disease from COVID-19, in part due to extra chest pressure when ventilator use is indicated. Recent studies have seen similar patterns of increased risk for individuals with obesity and overweight for both seasonal influenza and the pandemic H1N1 circulating in 2008 and 2009 [167]. Karlsson and colleagues recently reviewed potential pathways between influenza infection and obesity, noting that animal models and laboratory research suggest obesity-related hormone changes, chronic inflammation observed with obesity, and changes in the microbiome associated with obesity may all contribute to the inability to control inflammation associated with worse outcomes from influenza [167]. The same pattern of inability to control inflammation associated with worse outcomes from COVID-19 appears to be a critical driver of high mortality rates [150, 168–173].

# Conclusion

The importance of interactions between nutrition and infection was formally recognized as early as 1959 [174]. At that time the scientific community had only begun to comprehend the magnitude of complexities that we now know to exist. Today, rather than being at the point where public health and clinical decisions are obvious, many seem to be less tractable and fraught with risk. How can we move forward effectively and efficiently when not only malnutrition and infectious diseases from the past are still present but also when new pandemics are likely to emerge and when climate change is likely to expand the distribution and magnitude of both infectious diseases and malnutrition?

Infectious disease experts bemoan the fact that clinical and public health providers may not have adequate backgrounds to optimize infectious disease prevention, diagnosis, and treatment. Nutritional scientists are frequently dismayed that clinical and public health providers are often ignorant of the details of the role of nutrition in prevention. All can agree to the vital importance of nutrition-infection education for health and public health providers, yet more needs to be done.

We come back to the one of the statements at the end of the Scrimshaw, Taylor, and Gordon 1968 WHO monograph: "[w]here both malnutrition and exposure to infection are serious, as they are in most tropical and developing countries, successful control of these conditions depends upon efforts directed equally against both" [94]. While the emphasis at that time was on tropical and developing countries, today we see emerging infections threatening populations around the world, independent of socioeconomic status and geography. We need a new effort to raise the consciousness of today's generation of global health workers, clinicians, researchers, and policymakers as to the importance of nutrition in affecting infectious disease virulence and pathogenicity [94] and the pathways by which nutrition alters risk of pathogen acquisition or transmission. We hope that by compiling current knowledge, together with a conceptual framework for clarifying the research evidence and enhancing the research agenda for nutrition and infection interactions, future scientists, clinicians, and public health practitioners will have a strong foundation that guides scientific discoveries integrating nutrition and prevention and control of infectious diseases in the future.

# References

1. Rota PA, Moss WJ, Takeda M, de Swart RL, Thompson KM, Goodson JL. Measles. Nat Rev Dis Primers. 2016;2:16049.
2. Weger-Lucarelli J, Auerswald H, Vignuzzi M, Dussart P, Karlsson EA. Taking a bite out of nutrition and arbovirus infection. PLoS Negl Trop Dis. 2018;12(3):e0006247.
3. Gerwien F, Skrahina V, Kasper L, Hube B, Brunke S. Metals in fungal virulence. FEMS Microbiol Rev. 2018;42(1):fux050.
4. Palmer LD, Skaar EP. Transition metals and virulence in bacteria. Annu Rev Genet. 2016;50:67–91.
5. Sheldon JR, Laakso HA, Heinrichs DE. Iron acquisition strategies of bacterial pathogens. Microbiol Spectr. 2016;4:2.
6. Neyrolles O, Wolschendorf F, Mitra A, Niederweis M. Mycobacteria, metals, and the macrophage. Immunol Rev. 2015;264(1):249–63.
7. Barffour MA, Humphries DL. Core principles: infectious disease risk in relation to macro and micronutrient status. In: Humphries DL, Scott ME, Vermund SH, editors. Nutrition and infectious disease: shifting the clinical paradigm. New York: Humana Press, an imprint of Springer Science+Business Media; 2020.
8. Koethe JR, von Reyn CF. Protein-calorie malnutrition, macronutrient supplements, and tuberculosis. Int J Tuberc Lung Dis. 2016;20(7):857–63.
9. Sirisinha S. The pleiotropic role of vitamin A in regulating mucosal immunity. Asian Pac J Allergy Immunol. 2015;33(2):71–89.
10. Rodriguez L, Cervantes E, Ortiz R. Malnutrition and gastrointestinal and respiratory infections in children: a public health problem. Int J Environ Res Public Health. 2011;8(4):1174–205.
11. Yoshii K, Hosomi K, Sawane K, Kunisawa J. Metabolism of dietary and microbial vitamin B family in the regulation of host immunity. Front Nutr. 2019;6:48.
12. Lazar V, Ditu LM, Pircalabioru GG, Gheorghe I, Curutiu C, Holban AM, et al. Aspects of gut microbiota and immune system interactions in infectious diseases, immunopathology, and cancer. Front Immunol. 2018;9:1830.
13. Okumura R, Takeda K. Maintenance of intestinal homeostasis by mucosal barriers. Inflamm Regen. 2018;38:5.
14. Ma N, Guo P, Zhang J, He T, Kim SW, Zhang G, et al. Nutrients mediate intestinal bacteria-mucosal immune crosstalk. Front Immunol. 2018;9:5.
15. Gil A, Plaza-Diaz J, Mesa MD. Vitamin D: classic and novel actions. Ann Nutr Metab. 2018;72(2):87–95.
16. Indrio F, Martini S, Francavilla R, Corvaglia L, Cristofori F, Mastrolia SA, et al. Epigenetic matters: the link between early Nutrition, microbiome, and long-term health development. Front Pediatr. 2017;5:178.
17. Torow N, Marsland BJ, Hornef MW, Gollwitzer ES. Neonatal mucosal immunology. Mucosal Immunol. 2017;10(1):5–17.
18. Blanton LV, Barratt MJ, Charbonneau MR, Ahmed T, Gordon JI. Childhood undernutrition, the gut microbiota, and microbiota-directed therapeutics. Science. 2016;352(6293):1533.
19. Rosselot AE, Hong CI, Moore SR. Rhythm and bugs: circadian clocks, gut microbiota, and enteric infections. Curr Opin Gastroenterol. 2016;32(1):7–11.
20. Bostick JW, Zhou L. Innate lymphoid cells in intestinal immunity and inflammation. Cell Mol Life Sci. 2016;73(2):237–52.
21. Green WD, Beck MA. Obesity altered T cell metabolism and the response to infection. Curr Opin Immunol. 2017;46:1–7.
22. Frydrych LM, Bian G, O'Lone DE, Ward PA, Delano MJ. Obesity and type 2 diabetes mellitus drive immune dysfunction, infection development, and sepsis mortality. J Leukoc Biol. 2018;104(3):525–34.
23. Hainer V, Zamrazilova H, Kunesova M, Bendlova B, Aldhoon-Hainerova I. Obesity and infection: reciprocal causality. Physiol Res. 2015;64(Suppl 2):S105–19.
24. Xiao L, Van't Land B, van de Worp W, Stahl B, Folkerts G, Garssen J. Early-life nutritional factors and mucosal immunity in the development of autoimmune diabetes. Front Immunol. 2017;8:1219.
25. Farhadi S, Ovchinnikov RS. The relationship between nutrition and infectious diseases: a review. Biomed Biotechnol Res J. 2018;2(3):168.
26. Heimburger DC, Ard JD. Handbook of clinical nutrition. 4th ed. London: Mosby; 2006.
27. Katz DL. Nutrition in clinical practice. Philadelphia: Lippincott Williams & Wilkins; 2014.
28. Thompson JJ, Manore M. Nutrition: an applied approach United States of America. New York: Pearson Education, Inc; 2017.
29. Insel P, Ross D, McMahon K, Bernstein M. Nutrition. 6th ed. Burlington: Jones & Bartlett Learning; 2016.
30. Width M, Reinhard T. The essential pocket guide for clinical nutrition. Philadelphia: Wolters Kluwer Health; 2018.
31. Kleinman RE, Greer FR. Pediatric nutrition. Elk Grove Village: American Academy of Pediatrics; 2020.
32. Gibney M, Margetts B, Kearney J, Arab L. Public health nutrition: the nutrition society textbook series. Hoboken: Wiley-Blackwell; 2004. p. 302–16.

33. Stein N. Public health nutrition. Sudbury: Jones & Bartlett Publishers; 2014.
34. Bhutta ZA, Das JK, Rizvi A, Gaffey MF, Walker N, Horton S, et al. Evidence-based interventions for improvement of maternal and child nutrition: what can be done and at what cost? Lancet. 2013;382(9890):452–77.
35. Katona P, Katona-Apte J. The interaction between nutrition and infection. Clin Infect Dis. 2008;46(10):1582–8.
36. Siddiqui F, Belayneh G, Bhutta ZA. Nutrition and diarrheal disease and enteric pathogens. In: Humphries DL, Scott ME, Vermund SH, editors. Nutrition and infectious disease: shifting the clinical paradigm. New York: Humana Press, an imprint of Springer Science+Business Media; 2020.
37. Baum M, Tamargo JA, Wanke C. Nutrition in HIV and tuberculosis. In: Humphries DL, Scott ME, Vermund SH, editors. Nutrition and infectious disease: shifting the clinical paradigm. New York: Humana Press, an imprint of Springer Science+Business Media; 2020.
38. Kim HH, Bei AK. Nutritional frameworks in malaria. In: Humphries DL, Scott ME, Vermund SH, editors. Nutrition and infectious disease: shifting the clinical paradigm. New York: Humana Press, an imprint of Springer Science+Business Media; 2020.
39. World Health Organization. Global Health Observatory (GHO) data: top 10 causes of death Geneva, Switzerland. Geneva: World Health Organization; 2020; updated 2020. Available from: https://www.who.int/gho/mortality_burden_disease/causes_death/top_10/en/.
40. G. B. D. Lower Respiratory Infections Collaborators. Estimates of the global, regional, and national morbidity, mortality, and aetiologies of lower respiratory infections in 195 countries, 1990–2016: a systematic analysis for the Global Burden of Disease Study 2016. Lancet Infect Dis. 2018;18(11):1191–210.
41. Totelin L. When foods become remedies in ancient Greece: the curious case of garlic and other substances. J Ethnopharmacol. 2015;167:30–7.
42. Wilkins J. Good food and bad: nutritional and pleasurable eating in ancient Greece. J Ethnopharmacol. 2015;167:7–10.
43. Touwaide A, Appetiti E. Food and medicines in the Mediterranean tradition. A systematic analysis of the earliest extant body of textual evidence. J Ethnopharmacol. 2015;167:11–29.
44. Hume EH. Doctors east, doctors west. Originally published as: Hume EH. *Doctors East, Doctors West: an American Physician's Life in China* (New York: WW Norton & Company, Inc., 1946) ed. Changsha: Yuelu Publishing House; 1994.
45. Curtin PD. Nutrition in African history. J Interdiscip Hist. 1983;14(2):371–82.
46. Borchers AT, Keen CL, Stern JS, Gershwin ME. Inflammation and native American medicine: the role of botanicals. Am J Clin Nutr. 2000;72(2):339–47.
47. Vassilyadi F, Panteliadou AK, Panteliadis C. Hallmarks in the history of enteral and parenteral nutrition: from antiquity to the 20th century. Nutr Clin Pract. 2013;28(2):209–17.
48. Larsen CS. Biological changes in human-populations with agriculture. Annu Rev Anthropol. 1995;24:185–213.
49. Cordain L, Eaton SB, Miller JB, Mann N, Hill K. The paradoxical nature of hunter-gatherer diets: meat-based, yet non-atherogenic. Eur J Clin Nutr. 2002;56(Suppl 1):S42–52.
50. Cordain L, Eaton SB, Sebastian A, Mann N, Lindeberg S, Watkins BA, et al. Origins and evolution of the Western diet: health implications for the 21st century. Am J Clin Nutr. 2005;81(2):341–54.
51. Eaton SB, Cordain L. Evolutionary aspects of diet: old genes, new fuels. Nutritional changes since agriculture. World Rev Nutr Diet. 1997;81:26–37.
52. Popkin BM. The nutrition transition and obesity in the developing world. J Nutr. 2001;131(3):871S–3S.
53. Popkin BM, Adair LS, Ng SW. Global nutrition transition and the pandemic of obesity in developing countries. Nutr Rev. 2012;70(1):3–21.
54. Chen JD, Xu H. Historical development of Chinese dietary patterns and nutrition from the ancient to the modern society. World Rev Nutr Diet. 1996;79:133–53.
55. Wahlqvist ML. Diversification in indigenous and ethnic food culture. Forum Nutr. 2005;57(57):52–61.
56. Berry EM, Arnoni Y, Aviram M. The Middle Eastern and biblical origins of the Mediterranean diet. Public Health Nutr. 2011;14(12A):2288–95.
57. Kulkarni AD, Sundaresan A, Rashid MJ, Yamamoto S, Karkow F. Application of diet-derived taste active components for clinical nutrition: perspectives from ancient Ayurvedic medical science, space medicine, and modern clinical nutrition. Curr Pharm Des. 2014;20(16):2791–6.
58. James WPT, Johnson RJ, Speakman JR, Wallace DC, Fruhbeck G, Iversen PO, et al. Nutrition and its role in human evolution. J Intern Med. 2019;285(5):533–49.
59. Radd-Vagenas S, Kouris-Blazos A, Singh MF, Flood VM. Evolution of Mediterranean diets and cuisine: concepts and definitions. Asia Pac J Clin Nutr. 2017;26(5):749–63.
60. Greiner AK, Papineni RV, Umar S. Chemoprevention in gastrointestinal physiology and disease. Natural products and microbiome. Am J Physiol Gastrointest Liver Physiol. 2014;307(1):G1–15.
61. Humphries DL, Scott ME, Vermund SH. Pathways linking nutritional status and infectious disease. In: Humphries D, Scott ME, Vermund SH, editors. Nutrition and infectious disease: shifting the clinical paradigm. New York: Humana Press, an imprint of Springer Science+Business Media; 2020.

62. Ezenwa VO. Co-infection and nutrition: integrating ecological and epidemiological perspectives. In: Humphries DL, Scott ME, Vermund SH, editors. Nutrition and infectious disease: shifting the clinical paradigm. New York: Humana Press, an imprint of Springer Science+Business Media; 2020.

63. World Health Organization. Leishmaniasis Geneva, Switzerland. Geneva: World Health Organization; 2020. https://www.who.int/leishmaniasis/en/. Accessed 2 July 2020.

64. Nweze JA, Nweze EI, Onoja US. Nutrition, malnutrition, and leishmaniasis. Nutrition. 2020;73:110712.

65. da Cunha DF, de Carvalho da Cunha SF, Nunes AG, Silva-Vergara ML. Is an increased body mass index associated with a risk of cutaneous leishmaniasis? Rev Soc Bras Med Trop. 2009;42(5):494–5.

66. Barbosa JF, de Figueiredo SM, Lyon S, Caligiorne RB. An 8-year retrospective study of human visceral leishmaniasis. Curr Clin Pharmacol. 2016;11(4):265–9.

67. Tavares DDS, Salgado VR, Miranda JC, Mesquita PRR, Rodrigues FM, Barral-Netto M, et al. Attraction of phlebotomine sandflies to volatiles from skin odors of individuals residing in an endemic area of tegumentary leishmaniasis. PLoS One. 2018;13(9):e0203989.

68. Martins VD, Silva FC, Caixeta F, Carneiro MB, Goes GR, Torres L, et al. Obesity impairs resistance to Leishmania major infection in C57BL/6 mice. PLoS Negl Trop Dis. 2020;14(1):e0006596.

69. Kirstein OD, Faiman R, Gebreselassie A, Hailu A, Gebre-Michael T, Warburg A. Attraction of Ethiopian phlebotomine sand flies (Diptera: Psychodidae) to light and sugar-yeast mixtures (CO 2). Parasit Vectors. 2013;6(1):341.

70. Pinto M, Campbell-Lendrum DH, Lozovei A, Teodoro U, Davies C. Phlebotomine sandfly responses to carbon dioxide and human odour in the field. Med Vet Entomol. 2001;15(2):132–9.

71. Sarnaglia GD, Covre LP, Pereira FE, HL DEMG, Faria AM, Dietze R, et al. Diet-induced obesity promotes systemic inflammation and increased susceptibility to murine visceral leishmaniasis. Parasitology. 2016;143(12):1647–55.

72. Ali A. Visceral leishmaniasis in Southern Ethiopia II. Nutritional risk factors. Ethiop J Health Dev. 1997;11:2.

73. Albers R, Bourdet-Sicard R, Braun D, Calder PC, Herz U, Lambert C, et al. Monitoring immune modulation by nutrition in the general population: identifying and substantiating effects on human health. Br J Nutr. 2013;110(Suppl 2):S1–30.

74. National Institute of Allergy and Infectious Diseases. Overview of the immune system. Bethesda: National Institute of Health; updated 30 Dec 2013. https://www.niaid.nih.gov/research/immune-system-overview. Accessed 2 July 2020.

75. Berkley JA. Bacterial infections and nutrition – a primer. In: Humphries DL, Scott ME, Vermund SH, editors. Nutrition and infectious disease: shifting the clinical paradigm. New York: Humana Press, an imprint of Springer Science+Business Media; 2020.

76. van Puffelen E, Hulst JM, Vanhorebeek I, Dulfer K, Van den Berghe G, Verbruggen S, et al. Outcomes of delaying parenteral nutrition for 1 week vs initiation within 24 hours among undernourished children in Pediatric intensive care: a subanalysis of the PEPaNIC randomized clinical trial. JAMA Netw Open. 2018;1(5):e182668.

77. Green WD, Karlsson EA, Beck MA. Viral infections and nutrition: influenza virus as a case study. In: Humphries DL, Scott ME, Vermund SH, editors. Nutrition and infectious disease: shifting the clinical paradigm. New York: Humana Press, an imprint of Springer Science+Business Media; 2020.

78. Hemila H. Vitamin C and infections. Nutrients. 2017;9(4):339.

79. Wiser MF. Nutrition and protozoan pathogens of humans -- a primer. In: Humphries DL, Scott ME, Vermund SH, editors. Nutrition and infectious diseases: shifting the clinical paradigm. New York: Humana Press, an imprint of Springer Science+Business Media; 2020.

80. Lee CM, Aboko-Cole F, Fletcher J. Effect of malnutrition on susceptibility of mice to Trypanosoma musculi: vitamin A-deficiency. Z Parasitenkd. 1976;49(1):1–10.

81. Thomaskutty KG, Lee CM. Interaction of nutrition and infection: macrophage activity in vitamin B12-deficient rats infected with Trypanosoma lewisi. J Natl Med Assoc. 1987;79(4):441–6.

82. Thomaskutty KG, Lee CM. Interaction of nutrition and infection: effect of vitamin B12 deficiency on resistance to Trypanosoma lewisi. J Natl Med Assoc. 1985;77(4):289–99.

83. Geary TG, Haque M. Human helminth infections. In: Humphries DL, Scott ME, Vermund SH, editors. Nutrition and infectious disease: shifting the clinical paradigm. New York: Humana Press, an imprint of Springer Science+Business Media; 2020.

84. Villamor E, Villar LA. Nutrition and arboviral infections. In: Humphries DL, Scott ME, Vermund SH, editors. Nutrition and infectious disease: shifting the clinical paradigm. New York: Humana Press, an imprint of Springer Science+Business Media; 2020.

85. Byers NM, Fleshman AC, Perera R, Molins CR. Metabolomic insights into human arboviral infections: dengue, chikungunya, and zika viruses. Viruses. 2019;11(3):225.

86. Murray MJ, Murray NJ, Murray AB, Murray MB. Refeeding-malaria and hyperferraemia. Lancet. 1975;1(7908):653–4.

87. Sazawal S, Black RE, Ramsan M, Chwaya HM, Stoltzfus RJ, Dutta A, et al. Effects of routine prophylactic supplementation with iron and folic acid on admission to hospital and mortality in preschool children in a high malaria transmission setting: community-based, randomised, placebo-controlled trial. Lancet. 2006;367(9505):133–43.

88. Scott ME, Koski K. Soil-transmitted helminths – does nutrition make a difference? In: Humphries DL, Scott ME, Vermund SH, editors. Nutrition and infectious disease: shifting the clinical paradigm. New York: Humana Press, an imprint of Springer Science+Business Media; 2020.

89. Boullata JI. Drug-nutrition interactions in infectious diseases. In: Humphries DL, Scott ME, Vermund SH, editors. Nutrition and infectious disease: shifting the clinical paradigm. New York: Humana Press, an imprint of Springer Science+Business Media; 2020.

90. Drugs.com. Drugs interaction checker: drugs.com; updated 2 Dec 2019. https://www.drugs.com/drug_interactions.html. Accessed 2 July 2020.

91. American Heart Association. Medication interactions: food, supplements and other drugs; updated 30 Oct 2014.

92. Consumer Reports. Food and drug interactions you need to know about: what you eat and drink can interfere with the effectiveness of your meds. Consumer Reports on Health. 2017.

93. Rocklov J, Ahlm C, Scott ME, Humphries DL. Climate change pathways and potential future risks to nutrition and infection. In: Humphries DL, Scott ME, Vermund SH, editors. Nutrition and infectious disease: shifting the clinical paradigm. New York: Humana Press, an imprint of Springer Science+Business Media; 2020.

94. Scrimshaw NS, Taylor CE, Gordon JE. Interactions of nutrition and infection. Monogr Ser World Health Organ. 1968;57:3–329.

95. Batterham MJ. Investigating heterogeneity in studies of resting energy expenditure in persons with HIV/AIDS: a meta-analysis. Am J Clin Nutr. 2005;81(3):702–13.

96. Fawzi WW, Chalmers TC, Herrera MG, Mosteller F. Vitamin A supplementation and child mortality. A meta-analysis. JAMA. 1993;269(7):898–903.

97. Yahya RS, Awad SI, Kizilbash N, El-Baz HA, Atia G. Enteric parasites can disturb leptin and adiponectin levels in children. Arch Med Sci. 2018;14(1):101–6.

98. Stephenson LS, Latham MC, Adams EJ, Kinoti SN, Pertet A. Physical fitness, growth and appetite of Kenyan school boys with hookworm, Trichuris trichiura and Ascaris lumbricoides infections are improved four months after a single dose of albendazole. J Nutr. 1993;123(6):1036–46.

99. Radrizzani D, Iapichino G, Cambisano M, Bonetti G, Ronzoni G, Colombo A. Peripheral, visceral and body nitrogen balance of catabolic patients, without and with parenteral nutrition. Intensive Care Med. 1988;14(3):212–6.

100. Cashman MD, Wightkin WT, Madden JE, Phillips RS. Massive azoturia and failure to achieve positive nitrogen balance in a botulism patient. JPEN J Parenter Enteral Nutr. 1986;10(3):316–8.

101. Leverve X, Guignier M, Carpentier F, Serre JC, Caravel JP. Effect of parenteral nutrition on muscle amino acid output and 3-methylhistidine excretion in septic patients. Metabolism. 1984;33(5):471–7.

102. Stephensen CB, Alvarez JO, Kohatsu J, Hardmeier R, Kennedy JIJ, Gammon RBJ. Vitamin A is excreted in the urine during acute infection. Am J Clin Nutr. 1994;60(3):388–92.

103. Ng M, Fleming T, Robinson M, Thomson B, Graetz N, Margono C, et al. Global, regional, and national prevalence of overweight and obesity in children and adults during 1980–2013: a systematic analysis for the Global Burden of Disease Study 2013. Lancet. 2014;384(9945):766–81.

104. Wiria AE, Sartono E, Supali T, Yazdanbakhsh M. Helminth infections, type-2 immune response, and metabolic syndrome. PLoS Pathog. 2014;10(7):e1004140.

105. Thomas-Valdes S, Tostes M, Anunciacao PC, da Silva BP, Sant'Ana HMP. Association between vitamin deficiency and metabolic disorders related to obesity. Crit Rev Food Sci Nutr. 2017;57(15):3332–43.

106. Stephensen CB. Primer on immune response and interface with malnutrition. In: Humphries DL, Scott ME, Vermund SH, editors. Nutrition and infectious disease: shifting the clinical paradigm. New York: Humana Press, an imprint of Springer Science+Business Media; 2020.

107. Segura-Cerda CA, Lopez-Romero W, Flores-Valdez MA. Changes in host response to Mycobacterium tuberculosis infection associated with type 2 diabetes: beyond hyperglycemia. Front Cell Infect Microbiol. 2019;9:342.

108. Porter JDH, Gaffney C, Heymann D, Parkin W. Food-borne outbreak of Giardia-Lamblia. Am J Public Health. 1990;80(10):1259–60.

109. Scavia G, Alfonsi V, Taffon S, Escher M, Bruni R, De Medici D, et al. A large prolonged outbreak of hepatitis A associated with consumption of frozen berries, Italy, 2013–14. J Med Microbiol. 2017;66(3):342–9.

110. Berhe B, Bugssa G, Bayisa S, Alemu M. Foodborne intestinal protozoan infection and associated factors among patients with watery diarrhea in Northern Ethiopia; a cross-sectional study. J Health Popul Nutr. 2018;37(1):5.

111. Kaindi DW, Schelling E, Wangoh JM, Imungi JK, Farah Z, Meile L. Risk factors for symptoms of gastrointestinal illness in rural town Isiolo, Kenya. Zoonoses Public Health. 2012;59(2):118–25.

112. Nimri LF. Cyclospora cayetanensis and other intestinal parasites associated with diarrhea in a rural area of Jordan. Int Microbiol. 2003;6(2):131–5.

113. Koumans EH, Katz DJ, Malecki JM, Kumar S, Wahlquist SP, Arrowood MJ, et al. An outbreak of cyclosporiasis in Florida in 1995: a harbinger of multistate outbreaks in 1996 and 1997. Am J Trop Med Hyg. 1998;59(2):235–42.

114. Stern PL. Key steps in vaccine development. Ann Allergy Asthma Immunol. 2020;125:17.

115. Hallander HO, Paniagua M, Espinoza F, Askelof P, Corrales E, Ringman M, et al. Calibrated serological techniques demonstrate significant different serum response rates to an oral killed cholera vaccine between Swedish and Nicaraguan children. Vaccine. 2002;21(1–2):138–45.

116. Rho S, Kim H, Shim SH, Lee SY, Kim MJ, Yang BG, et al. Protein energy malnutrition alters mucosal IgA responses and reduces mucosal vaccine efficacy in mice. Immunol Lett. 2017;190:247–56.

117. Gaayeb L, Pincon C, Cames C, Sarr JB, Seck M, Schacht AM, et al. Immune response to Bordetella pertussis is associated with season and undernutrition in Senegalese children. Vaccine. 2014;32(27):3431–7.

118. Lasch EE, Abed Y, Abdulla K, El Tibbi AG, Marcus O, El Massri M, et al. Successful results of a program combining live and inactivated poliovirus vaccines to control poliomyelitis in Gaza. Rev Infect Dis. 1984;6(Suppl 2):S467–70.

119. Lasch EE, Abed Y, Gerichter CB, Massri ME, Marcus O, Hensher R, et al. Results of a program successfully combining live and killed polio vaccines. Isr J Med Sci. 1983;19(11):1021–3.

120. Goldblum N, Gerichter CB, Tulchinsky TH, Melnick JL. Poliomyelitis control in Israel, the West Bank and Gaza Strip: changing strategies with the goal of eradication in an endemic area. Bull World Health Organ. 1994;72(5):783–96.

121. Tulchinsky T, Abed Y, Handsher R, Toubassi N, Acker C, Melnick J. Successful control of poliomyelitis by a combined OPV/IPV polio vaccine program in the West Bank and Gaza, 1978–93. Isr J Med Sci. 1994;30(5–6):489–94.

122. Tulchinsky T, Abed Y, Shaheen S, Toubassi N, Sever Y, Schoenbaum M, et al. A ten-year experience in control of poliomyelitis through a combination of live and killed vaccines in two developing areas. Am J Public Health. 1989;79(12):1648–52.

123. Soleimany AP, Bhatia SN. Activity-based diagnostics: an emerging paradigm for disease detection and monitoring. Trends Mol Med. 2020;26(5):450–68.

124. Relman D. Pathogen discovery, detection, and diagnostics. Microbial threats to health: emergence, detection, and response Appendix C, Washington. Washington D.C.: The National Academies; 2003. p. 313–30.

125. Schenz J, Weigand MA, Uhle F. Molecular and biomarker-based diagnostics in early sepsis: current challenges and future perspectives. Expert Rev Mol Diagn. 2019;19(12):1069–78.

126. Buck AA, Anderson RI, MacRae AA. Epidemiology of poly-parasitism. III. Effects on the diagnostic capacity of immunological tests. Tropenmed Parasitol. 1978;29(2):145–55.

127. Zinsstag J, Mackenzie JS, Jeggo M, Heymann DL, Patz JA, Daszak P. Mainstreaming one health. EcoHealth. 2012;9(2):107–10.

128. Peeters M, Courgnaud V, Abela B, Auzel P, Pourrut X, Bibollet-Ruche F, et al. Risk to human health from a plethora of simian immunodeficiency viruses in primate bushmeat. Emerg Infect Dis. 2002;8(5):451–7.

129. Wenzel RP, editor. Prevention and control of nosocomial infections. 4th ed. Philadelphia: Lippincott Williams & Wilkin; 2002.

130. Hawkey P. Nocosomial pneumonia. Lung biology in health and disease, Vol. 150: WR Jarvis, Ed., C. Lenfant, Executive Ed. Marcel Dekker, Inc., New York, NY, USA, 2000. ISBN 0-8247-0384-7. J Antimicrob Chemother. 2001;47(6):907–8.

131. Rello J. Nosocomial pneumonia: Wiley Online Library; 2007.

132. Morrow L, Baughman R. Contemporary diagnosis and management of nosocomial pneumonias. Newtown: Handbooks in Health Care Co; 2009.

133. Center for Disease Control. National nosocomial infections study report. 1974

134. Donelli G. Biofilm-based nosocomial infections. Basel: MDPI AG – Multidisciplinary Digital Publishing Institute; 2015. ISBN 978-3-03842-135-1.

135. Dunn AS. Essentials of hospital medicine: a practical guide for clinicians. Hackensack: World Scientific; 2012.

136. Mathur P. Hospital acquired infections: prevention & control. New Delhi: Wolters Kluwer Health; 2010.

137. Charney W. Epidemic of medical errors and hospital-acquired infections: systemic and social causes. Boca Raton: CRC Press; 2012.

138. Calfee DP. Crisis in hospital-acquired, healthcare-associated infections. Annu Rev Med. 2012;63:359–71.

139. Muralidhar V, Muralidhar S. Hospital acquired infections power strategies for clinical practice. Tunbridge Wells: Anshan; 2007; ISBN 978-1-905740-55-0.

140. Bartlett JG, Pham PA, Shah M. The Bartlett pocket guide to HIV/AIDS treatment. Frederick: PPham and JBriggs LLC; 2019. ISBN 978-0-9967333-7-32019.

141. Georgiev VS. Opportunistic infections: treatment and prophylaxis. Totowa: Humana Press; 2003; ISBN 978-1-58829-009-0 %L RC112.G45 2003.

142. Gupta RK. Pathology of opportunistic infections: an illustrative atlas. New York/Berlin Heidelberg: Springer. ISBN 978-981-10-1668-4; 2016.

143. Galanda CD. AIDS-related opportunistic infections. New York: Nova Biomedical Books; 2009.

144. Zhou P, Yang XL, Wang XG, Hu B, Zhang L, Zhang W, et al. A pneumonia outbreak associated with a new coronavirus of probable bat origin. Nature. 2020;579(7798):270–3.

145. Dietz W, Santos-Burgoa C. Obesity and its implications for COVID-19 mortality. Obesity (Silver Spring). 2020;28(6):1005.

146. Zhang F, Xiong Y, Wei Y, Hu Y, Wang F, Li G, et al. Obesity predisposes to the risk of higher mortality in young COVID-19 patients. J Med Virol. 2020. https://doi.org/10.1002/jmv.26039.
147. Luzi L, Radaelli MG. Influenza and obesity: its odd relationship and the lessons for COVID-19 pandemic. Acta Diabetol. 2020;57(6):759–64.
148. Zhao L. Obesity accompanying COVID-19: the role of epicardial fat. Obesity (Silver Spring). 2020;28:1837.
149. Muniyappa R, Gubbi S. COVID-19 pandemic, coronaviruses, and diabetes mellitus. Am J Physiol Endocrinol Metab. 2020;318(5):E736–E41.
150. Chiappetta S, Sharma AM, Bottino V, Stier C. COVID-19 and the role of chronic inflammation in patients with obesity. Int J Obes. 2020;44:1790.
151. Palaiodimos L, Kokkinidis DG, Li W, Karamanis D, Ognibene J, Arora S, et al. Severe obesity, increasing age and male sex are independently associated with worse in-hospital outcomes, and higher in-hospital mortality, in a cohort of patients with COVID-19 in the Bronx, New York. Metabolism. 2020;108:154262.
152. Butler MJ, Barrientos RM. The impact of nutrition on COVID-19 susceptibility and long-term consequences. Brain Behav Immun. 2020;87:53.
153. Klang E, Kassim G, Soffer S, Freeman R, Levin MA, Reich DL. Morbid obesity as an independent risk factor for COVID-19 mortality in hospitalized patients younger than 50. Obesity (Silver Spring). 2020;28(9):1595–9.
154. International Labor Organization. As job losses escalate, nearly half of global workforce at risk of losing livelihoods [Press release]: ILO; 2020. [updated 29 Apr 2020].
155. The Lancet Global H. Food insecurity will be the sting in the tail of COVID-19. Lancet Glob Health. 2020;8(6):e737.
156. Perez-Escamilla R, Cunningham K, Moran VH. COVID-19, food and nutrition insecurity and the wellbeing of children, pregnant and lactating women: a complex syndemic. Matern Child Nutr. 2020;16:e13036.
157. McLinden T, Stover S, Hogg RS. HIV and food insecurity: a syndemic amid the COVID-19 pandemic. AIDS Behav. 2020;24(10):2766–69.
158. Kalu B. COVID-19 in Nigeria: a disease of hunger. Lancet Respir Med. 2020;8:556.
159. Shammi M, Bodrud-Doza M, Towfiqul Islam ARM, Rahman MM. COVID-19 pandemic, socioeconomic crisis and human stress in resource-limited settings: a case from Bangladesh. Heliyon. 2020;6(5):e04063.
160. Rashid SF, Theobald S, Ozano K. Towards a socially just model: balancing hunger and response to the COVID-19 pandemic in Bangladesh. BMJ Glob Health. 2020;5(6):e002715.
161. Dickinson M. Food frights: COVID-19 and the specter of hunger. Agric Human Values. 2020;37:589–90.
162. Moran D, Cossar F, Merkle M, Alexander P. UK food system resilience tested by COVID-19. Nat Food. 2020;1:242.
163. Pecanha T, Goessler KF, Roschel H, Gualano B. Social isolation during the COVID-19 pandemic can increase physical inactivity and the global burden of cardiovascular disease. Am J Physiol Heart Circ Physiol. 2020;318(6):H1441–H6.
164. Zhang J, Taylor EW, Bennett K, Saad R, Rayman MP. Association between regional selenium status and reported outcome of COVID-19 cases in China. Am J Clin Nutr. 2020;111:1297.
165. Ilie PC, Stefanescu S, Smith L. The role of vitamin D in the prevention of coronavirus disease 2019 infection and mortality. Aging Clin Exp Res. 2020;32(7):1195–98.
166. Rhodes JM, Subramanian S, Laird E, Kenny RA. Editorial: low population mortality from COVID-19 in countries south of latitude 35 degrees North supports vitamin D as a factor determining severity. Aliment Pharmacol Ther. 2020;51(12):1434–7.
167. Karlsson EA, Milner JJ, Green WD, Rebeles J, Schultz-Cherry S, Beck MA. Influence of obesity on the response to influenza infection and vaccination. In: Mechanisms and manifestations of obesity in lung disease. London: Elsevier; 2019. p. 227–59.
168. Zabetakis I, Lordan R, Norton C, Tsoupras A. COVID-19: the inflammation link and the role of nutrition in potential mitigation. Nutrients. 2020;12(5):1466.
169. Kim J, Nam JH. Insight into the relationship between obesity-induced low-level chronic inflammation and COVID-19 infection. Int J Obes. 2020;44:1541.
170. Korakas E, Ikonomidis I, Kousathana F, Balampanis K, Kountouri A, Raptis A, et al. Obesity and COVID-19: immune and metabolic derangement as a possible link to adverse clinical outcomes. Am J Physiol Endocrinol Metab. 2020;319:E105.
171. Michalakis K, Ilias I. SARS-CoV-2 infection and obesity: common inflammatory and metabolic aspects. Diabetes Metab Syndr. 2020;14(4):469–71.
172. Hamer M, Kivimaki M, Gale CR, David Batty G. Lifestyle risk factors, inflammatory mechanisms, and COVID-19 hospitalization: a community-based cohort study of 387,109 adults in UK. Brain Behav Immun. 2020;87:184.
173. Urra JM, Cabrera CM, Porras L, Rodenas I. Selective CD8 cell reduction by SARS-CoV-2 is associated with a worse prognosis and systemic inflammation in COVID-19 patients. Clin Immunol. 2020;217:108486.
174. Scrimshaw NS, Taylor CE, Gordon JE. Interactions of nutrition and infection. Am J Med Sci. 1959;237(3):367–403.

# Index

© Springer Nature Switzerland AG 2021

D. L. Humphries et al. (eds.), *Nutrition and Infectious Diseases*, Nutrition and Health, https://doi.org/10.1007/978-3-030-56913-6